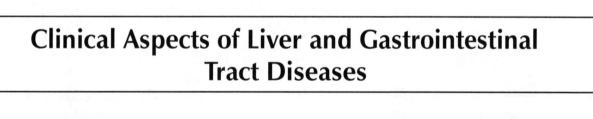

Clinical Aspects of Liver and Gastrointestinal Tract Diseases

Clinical Aspects of Liver and Gastrointestinal Tract Diseases

Editor: Adan Bowler

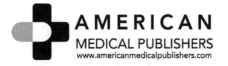

AMERICAN
MEDICAL PUBLISHERS
www.americanmedicalpublishers.com

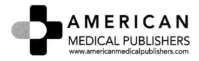

Cataloging-in-Publication Data

Clinical aspects of liver and gastrointestinal tract diseases / edited by Adan Bowler.
    p. cm.
Includes bibliographical references and index.
ISBN 978-1-63927-986-9
1. Liver--Diseases. 2. Gastrointestinal system--Diseases. 3. Liver--Diseases--Treatment.
4. Gastrointestinal system--Diseases--Treatment. 5. Liver--Diseases--Diagnosis.
6. Gastrointestinal system--Diseases--Diagnosis. I. Bowler, Adan.
RC845 .C55 2023
616.362--dc23

American Medical Publishers,
41 Flatbush Avenue,
1st Floor, New York,
NY 11217, USA

ISBN 978-1-63927-986-9 (Hardback)

Contents

Permissions

List of Contributors

Index

Preface

Liver disease is a condition that can affect and damage liver function. There are various diseases that can affect the liver, which include hepatitis, fascioliasis, alcoholic liver disease, cirrhosis, fatty liver disease and liver cancer. Their symptoms depend on the cause and may include jaundice, altered consciousness and confusion, coagulopathy, and thrombocytopenia. Liver diseases also have bleeding symptoms that take place in gastrointestinal tract, which is a passageway from the mouth to the anus. There are various diseases affecting the gastrointestinal system, which include cancer, infections and inflammation. The diagnosis of liver diseases can be done by liver function tests, while diagnosis of gastrointestinal tract diseases can be done by various imaging methods. Treatment of liver diseases includes medications such as ursodeoxycholic acid and steroid-based drugs, which strive to slow down the progression of the disease. Gastrointestinal tract diseases can be treated with medications and surgery in severe cases. This book contains some recent studies on liver and gastrointestinal tract diseases. Its aim is to present researches that have advanced the frontiers in the clinical management of these diseases.

This book is a comprehensive compilation of works of different researchers from varied parts of the world. It includes valuable experiences of the researchers with the sole objective of providing the readers (learners) with a proper knowledge of the concerned field. This book will be beneficial in evoking inspiration and enhancing the knowledge of the interested readers.

In the end, I would like to extend my heartiest thanks to the authors who worked with great determination on their chapters. I also appreciate the publisher's support in the course of the book. I would also like to deeply acknowledge my family who stood by me as a source of inspiration during the project.

Editor

Brucella abortus Infection Elicited Hepatic Stellate Cell-Mediated Fibrosis Through Inflammasome-Dependent IL-1β Production

Paula Constanza Arriola Benitez[1], Ayelén Ivana Pesce Viglietti[1], Marco Tulio R. Gomes[2], Sergio Costa Oliveira[2], Jorge Fabián Quarleri[3], Guillermo Hernán Giambartolomei[1] and María Victoria Delpino[1*]

[1] Instituto de Inmunología, Genética y Metabolismo (INIGEM), Universidad de Buenos Aires, CONICET, Buenos Aires, Argentina, [2] Department of Biochemistry and Immunology, Institute of Biological Sciences, Federal University of Minas Gerais, Belo Horizonte, Brazil, [3] Instituto de Investigaciones Biomédicas en Retrovirus y Sida (INBIRS), Universidad de Buenos Aires, CONICET, Buenos Aires, Argentina

*Correspondence:
María Victoria Delpino
mdelpino@ffyb.uba.ar

In human brucellosis, the liver is frequently affected. *Brucella abortus* triggers a profibrotic response on hepatic stellate cells (HSCs) characterized by inhibition of MMP-9 with concomitant collagen deposition and TGF-β1 secretion through type 4 secretion system (T4SS). Taking into account that it has been reported that the inflammasome is necessary to induce a fibrotic phenotype in HSC, we hypothesized that *Brucella* infection might create a microenvironment that would promote inflammasome activation with concomitant profibrogenic phenotype in HSCs. *B. abortus* infection induces IL-1β secretion in HSCs in a T4SS-dependent manner. The expression of caspase-1 (Casp-1), absent in melanoma 2 (AIM2), Nod-like receptor (NLR) containing a pyrin domain 3 (NLRP3), and apoptosis-associated speck-like protein containing a CARD (ASC) was increased in *B. abortus*-infected HSC. When infection experiments were performed in the presence of glyburide, a compound that inhibits NLRP3 inflammasome, or A151, a specific AIM2 inhibitor, the secretion of IL-1β was significantly inhibited with respect to uninfected controls. The role of inflammasome activation in the induction of a fibrogenic phenotype in HSCs was determined by performing *B. abortus* infection experiments in the presence of the inhibitors Ac-YVAD-cmk and glyburide. Both inhibitors were able to reverse the effect of *B. abortus* infection on the fibrotic phenotype in HSCs. Finally, the role of inflammasome in fibrosis was corroborated *in vivo* by the reduction of fibrotic patches in liver from *B. abortus*-infected ASC, NLRP, AIM2, and cCasp-1/11 knock-out (KO) mice with respect to infected wild-type mice.

Keywords: *Brucella*, inflammasome, fibrosis, hepatic stellate cells, IL-1β

INTRODUCTION

Human brucellosis is a zoonosis that induces a chronic and debilitating disease caused by *Brucella* species that manifests itself with a broad clinical spectrum (1, 2). Liver involvement in human brucellosis is usually documented, given the well-characterized tropism of *Brucella* for the reticuloendothelial system (1, 2). The incidence of liver involvement in active brucellosis has ranged from 5 to 53% or more (2).

Inflammasome activation has been documented in several liver diseases. Accordingly, it has been postulated that the upregulation of IL-1β and IL-18 secretion leads to myofibroblast differentiation with concomitant increase of collagen and TGF-β expression (3). In addition, it was established that inflammasome components are present in hepatic stellate cells (HSCs) and could regulate their function (3). The consequences of activation of inflammasome pathway were also confirmed *in vivo*, demonstrating its key role in liver fibrosis (4).

The activation and release of IL-1β and IL-18 requires two distinct signals. TLR engagement by pathogen or endogenous signal induces the expression of the precursor forms of these cytokines (pro–IL-1β and pro–IL-18), after which NLR-dependent activation of caspase-1 regulates their proteolytic processing and release (5). Activation of inflammasome by *Brucella abortus* infection has been previously demonstrated in bone marrow-derived macrophages and dendritic cells (6, 7). In these cells, *B. abortus* induces the secretion of IL-1β, in a process in which NLRP3 is necessary for activation of ASC inflammasome and the concomitant activation of caspase-1 and maturation and secretion of IL-1β (6, 7). In addition, ASC inflammasomes are also essential for IL-1β secretion induced by *B. abortus* infection in astrocytes and microglia (8). The first signal can be triggered by various pathogen-associated molecular patterns (PAMPs) via TLR activation. In the case of *B. abortus* infection inflammasome activation, the second signal involved the presence of a functional type 4 secretion system (T4SS) and DNA-sensing inflammasome receptor AIM2, in bone marrow-derived macrophages, and Mal/TIRAP and TLR-2 are the main signaling involved in astrocytes and microglia (8).

Previously, we have demonstrated that upon infection of HSCs, *B. abortus* triggers a profibrotic response characterized by inhibition of MMP-9 secretion inducing concomitant collagen deposition and transforming growth factor (TGF)-β1 secretion in a way that involves a functional T4SS and its effectors protein BPE005 (9). Taking into account that inflammasome has been documented to be necessary to induce activation to a fibrotic phenotype of HSCs, we hypothesized that *Brucella* infection might create a microenvironment that would promote inflammasome activation and concomitant profibrogenic phenotype in HSCs. The results of the study are presented here.

MATERIALS AND METHODS

Bacterial Culture

Brucella abortus S2308 DsRed-expressing *B. abortus* S2308 or the isogenic *B. abortus virB10* polar mutants were grown overnight in 10 ml of tryptic soy broth (Merck, Buenos Aires, Argentina) with constant agitation at 37°C. Bacteria were harvested and the inocula were prepared as described previously (10).

To obtain heat-killed *B. abortus* (HKBA), bacteria were washed five times for 10 min each in sterile PBS, heat killed at 70°C for 20 min, aliquoted, and stored at −70°C until they were used. The total absence of *B. abortus* viability after heat killing was verified by the absence of bacterial growth on tryptose soy agar.

All live *Brucella* manipulations were performed in biosafety level 3 facilities located at the Instituto de Investigaciones Biomédicas en Retrovirus y SIDA (INBIRS).

Cell Culture

LX-2 cell line, a spontaneously immortalized human HSC line, was kindly provided by Dr. Scott L. Friedman (Mount Sinai School of Medicine, New York, NY). LX-2 cells were maintained in DMEM (Life Technologies–Invitrogen, Carlsbad, CA, USA) and supplemented with 2 mM L-glutamine, 100 U/ml penicillin, 100 μg/ml streptomycin, and 2% (v/v) fetal bovine serum (FBS; Gibco–Invitrogen, Carlsbad, CA, USA). All cultures were grown at 37°C and 5% CO_2.

Cellular Infection

LX-2 cells were seeded in 24-well-plates and infected with *B. abortus* S2308, DsRed-expressing *B. abortus* S2308, or its isogenic mutants at multiplicities of infection (MOI) of 100 and 1000. After the bacterial suspension was dispensed, the plates were centrifuged for 10 min at 2,000 rpm and then incubated for 2 h at 37°C under a 5% CO_2 atmosphere. Cells were extensively washed with DMEM to remove extracellular bacteria and incubated in medium supplemented with 100 μg/ml gentamicin and 50 μg/ml streptomycin to kill extracellular bacteria. LX-2 cells were harvested at different times to determine cytokine production, MMP secretion, and collagen deposition.

Neutralization Experiments

Neutralization experiments were performed with 5 μM of Bay 11-7082, an inhibitory compound of the nuclear factor-κB (NF-κB), 50 μM of glybenclamide (glyburide), an inhibitor of the NLRP3 inflammasome, 50 μM of general caspase inhibitor Z-VAD-FMK, or 50 μM of caspase 1 inhibitor Y-VAD-FMK (all inhibitors were from Sigma-Aldrich). The cells were treated for 1 h with each inhibitor before infection.

AIM2 inflammasome complex formation was prevented using 3 μM of A151, a DNA sequence that inhibits in a competitive manner the immunostimulatory DNA. A151 (5-TTAGGGTTAG GGTTAGGGTTAGGG-3) and the control C151 (5-TTCAA ATTCAAATTCAAATTCAAA-3) constructs were synthesized with a phosphorothioate backbone. To determine the implication of IL-1β, neutralization experiments were performed by adding 50 ng/ml of ANAKINRA, the inhibitor of IL-1 receptor, and the natural antagonist IL-1Ra (R&D Systems). Recombinant human IL-1β (rIL-1β, R&D Systems) at a concentration of 50 ng/ml was used as a positive control.

mRNA Preparation and Quantitative PCR

RNA from LX-2 cells was isolated using the Quick-RNA MiniPrepKit (Zymo Research) and 1 μg of RNA was subjected to reverse transcription using Improm-II Reverse Transcriptase (Promega). PCR analysis was performed with StepOne real-time PCR detection system (Life Technology) using SYBR Green as fluorescent DNA binding dye. The primer sets used for amplification were as follows: β-actin sense: 5′-AACAGTCCGC CTAGAAGCAC-3′, β-actin antisense: 5′-CGTTGACATCCG TAAAGACC-3′; NLRP3 sense: 5′-CCACAAGATCGTGAGAA AACCC-3′; NLRP3 antisense: 5′-CGGTCCTATGTGCTC GTCA-3′; IL-1β sense: 5′-AGCTACGAATCTCCGACCAC-3′; IL-1β antisense: 5′-CGTTATCCCATGTGTCGAAGAA-3′; ASC sense: 5′-TGGATGCTCTGTACGGGAAG-3′; ASC antisense: 5′-CCAGGCTGGTGTGAAACTGAA-3′; Capase-1 sense: 5′-TTT CCGCAAGGTTCGATTTTCA-3′ Caspase-1 antisense: 5′-GGCATCTGCGCTCTACCATC-3′; AIM2 sense: 5′-TGGCAA AACGTCTTCAGGAGG-3′; AIM2 antisense: 5′-AGCTT GACTTAGTGGCTTTGG-3′.

The amplification cycle for Caspase-1, ASC, and β-actin was 95°C for 15 s, 58°C for 30 s, and 72°C for 60 s; the amplification cycle for IL-1β, NLRP3, and AIM2 was 95°C for 15 s, 61°C for 30 s, and 72°C for 60 s. All primer sets yielded a single product of the correct size. Relative expression levels were normalized against β-actin.

Immunofluorescence

LX-2 cells were infected with *B. abortus*, and after 24 h, cells were fixed in 4% paraformaldehyde for 10 min at room temperature, permeabilized with 0.3% Triton X-100 (Roche Diagnostics GmbH, Mannheim, Germany) for 10 min, and blocked with PBS containing 1% BSA for 1 h. Infected cells were stained with mouse anti-ASC (Santa Cruz Biotechnology) diluted in 0.1% PBS–Tween 20 overnight at 4°C. Cells then were incubated with rabbit anti-mouse Alexa Fluor 488 (Molecular Probes, Life Technologies) diluted in 0.1% PBS–Tween for 4 h at room temperature. 4,6-Diamidine-2-phenylindole (DAPI) was used for nuclear staining, and cells were stained for 30 min at room temperature. After washing in PBS, cells were mounted and then analyzed by fluorescence microscopy. Confocal images were analyzed using FV-1000 confocal microscope with an oil immersion Plan Apochromatic 60× NA1.42 objective (Olympus).

Zymography

Gelatinase activity was assayed by the method of Hibbs et al. with modifications, as described (11–13). Briefly, a total of 20 μl of cell culture supernatants from infected LX-2 cells cultured in the presence or not of the inhibitors Bay 11-7082, glyburide, Y-VAD-FMK, A151, control C151, and ANAKINRA at the concentrations mentioned above was mixed with 5 μl of 5× loading buffer [0.25 M Tris (pH 6.8), 50% glycerol, 5% SDS, and bromophenol blue crystals] and loaded onto 10% SDS-PAGE gels containing 1 mg/ml gelatin (Sigma-Aldrich, Buenos Aires, Argentina). After electrophoresis, gels were washed with a solution containing 50 mM Tris–HCl (pH 7.5) and 2.5% Triton X-100 (buffer A) for 30 min and with buffer A added with 5 mM

CaCl₂ and 1 μM ZnCl₂ for 30 min and were later incubated with buffer A with an additional 10 mM CaCl₂ and 200 mM NaCl for 48 h at 37°C. This denaturation/renaturation step promotes MMP activity without the proteolytic cleavage of pro-MMP. Gelatin activity was visualized by the staining of the gels with 0.5% Coomassie blue. Unstained bands indicated the presence of gelatinase activity, and their positions in the gel indicate the molecular weights of the enzymes involved.

Measurement of Cytokine Concentrations

Secretion of TGF-β1 and IL-1β in the supernatants was quantified by ELISA (BD Biosciences).

Assessment of Collagen Deposition—Sirius Red Staining

Collagen deposition was quantified using Sirius red (Sigma-Aldrich, Argentina SA), a strong anionic dye that binds strongly to collagen molecules (14). Sirius red staining was performed as was described (15). Briefly, Sirius red was dissolved in saturated aqueous picric acid at a concentration of 0.1%. Bouin's fluid (for cell fixation) was prepared by mixing 15 ml saturated aqueous picric acid with 5 ml of 35% formaldehyde and 1 ml of glacial acetic acid. Cell layers were fixed with 1 ml of Bouin's fluid for 1 h. Afterwards, culture plates were washed three times with deionized water. Culture dishes were air dried before adding 1 ml of Sirius red dye reagent. Cells were stained for 18 h with mild shaking. The stained cell layers were extensively washed with 0.01 N hydrochloric acid to remove all unbound dye. The stained material was dissolved in 0.2 ml of 0.1 N sodium hydroxide by shaking for 30 min. The dye solution was transferred to microtiter plates, and OD was measured using a microplate reader (Thermo Scientific) at 550 nm against 0.1 N sodium hydroxide as a blank.

Lipoproteins and LPS

Brucella abortus lipidated outer membrane protein 19 (LOmp19) and unlipidated Omp19 (U-Omp19) were obtained as described (16). Both contained <0.25 endotoxin U/μg of protein as assessed by Limulus Amebocyte Lysates (Associates of Cape Cod). *B. abortus* S2308 LPS and *Escherichia coli* O111k58H2 LPS were provided by I. Moriyon. The synthetic lipohexapeptide (tripalmitoyl S-glyceryl-Cys-Ser- Lys4-OH [Pam3Cys]) was purchased from Boehringer Mannheim (Mannheim, Germany).

DNA From *B. abortus*

Brucella abortus DNA was purified using the kit Wizard® Genomic DNA (Promega) following the instructions of the manufacturer. *Brucella* DNA was measured spectrophotometrically. Transient transfections of LX-2 cells with 2 μg/ml of *B. abortus* DNA were carried out using Lipofectamine 2000 (Invitrogen), following the manufacturer's instructions. After the purification step, an aliquot of 100 μg of DNA was treated with DNase I (1 U/mg) DNA (Zymo Research) according to the instructions of the manufacturer.

Hepatic Fibrosis in a Mouse Model

Mouse strains used in this study included apoptosis-associated speck-like protein containing a CARD (ASC), Nod-like receptor (NLR) containing a pyrin domain 3 (NLRP3), absent in melanoma 2 (AIM2), and caspase-1 (Casp-1)/11 knock-out (KO) mice, as described previously (8), and C57BL/6 wild-type (WT) mice (provided by Federal University of Minas Gerais, Belo Horizonte, Brazil). Six- to eight-week-old mice were infected through the intraperitoneal route with 5×10^5 CFU of *B. abortus* S2308. Mice were born from breeding pairs that were housed under controlled temperature (22 ± 2°C) and artificial light under a 12-h cycle period. Mice were kept under specific pathogen-free conditions in positive-pressure cabinets and provided with sterile food and water *ad libitum*.

All animal procedures were performed according to the rules and standards for the use of laboratory animals of the National Institutes of Health. Animal experiments were approved by the Institutional Committee for the Care and Use of Laboratory Animals (CICUAL, permit number: 287/2015). Histological examination of liver was carried out at week 4 post-infection after routine fixation and paraffin embedding. Five-micrometer-thick sections were cut and stained with Masson's trichrome stain. Masson's trichrome staining was conducted according to the manufacturer's instructions (Sigma-Aldrich). Collagen-positive areas were visualized by light microscopy and quantified using Image Pro-Plus 6.0 software (Media Cybernetics, Inc.).

Statistical Analysis

Statistical analysis was performed with one-way ANOVA, followed by *post-hoc* Tukey test (a single-step multiple comparison statistical test that finds means that are significantly different from each other) using GraphPad Prism 4.0 software. Data were presented as mean ± SEM.

RESULTS

B. abortus Infection Induces IL-1β Secretion by LX-2 Cells via T4SS

It has been established that inflammasome components are present in HSCs and could regulate their function (3). To determine if *B. abortus* infection induces inflammasome activation, LX-2 cells were infected with *B. abortus* and the secretion of IL-1β was evaluated in culture supernatants by ELISA 24 h post-infection. *B. abortus* infection induces the secretion of IL-1β by LX-2 cells (**Figure 1A**). The T4SS encoded by *virB* genes was first involved in the capacity of *Brucella* to establish an intracellular replication niche in several cell types (17). In addition, this system has been involved in the induction of inflammatory response during *B. abortus* infection (18) and also in the inflammasome signaling activation (7). Therefore, experiments were conducted to determine if the T4SS could be involved in the secretion of IL-1β induced by *B. abortus* in LX-2 cells. To this end, LX-2 cells were infected with *B. abortus* and its

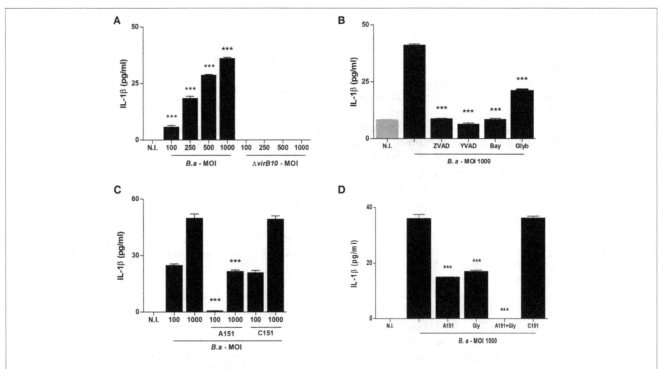

FIGURE 1 | *B. abortus* infection induces IL-1β in a VirB-dependent manner. LX-2 cells were infected with *B. abortus* (*B.a*) and its *vir*B10 isogenic mutant (Δ*vir*B10) at an MOI of 100–1000 and 24 h post-infection; IL-1β secretion was determined by ELISA in culture supernatants **(A)**. Effect of Z-VAD-FMK (ZVAD), Y-VAD-FMK (YVAD), Bay 11-7082 (Bay) and glybenclamide (Glyb) during *B. abortus* infection (MOI 1000) on IL-1β secretion **(B)**. Effect of A151 and the control 151 (C151) during *B. abortus* infection on IL-1β secretion **(C)**. Effect of Glyb plus A151 on IL-1βsecretion during *B. abortus* infection (MOI 1000). Data are given as the means ± SD from at least three individual experiments. ***P < 0.001 vs. cells infected with Δ*vir*B10 **(A)** or vs. infected and untreated cells **(B–D)**.

isogenic *B. abortus virB10* mutant, and IL-1β secretion induced by *B. abortus* was dependent on the expression of a functional T4SS, since the levels or IL-1β did not differ significantly between LX-2 cells infected with *B. abortus virB10* mutant and uninfected controls (**Figure 1A**). Taken together, our results indicated that *B. abortus* infection induces IL-1β secretion in a mechanism that is dependent on the presence of a functional T4SS.

IL-1β Secretion Induced by *B. abortus* Infection Is Dependent on Caspase-1 and NLRP3

Caspase-1 plays a fundamental role in innate immunity as the protease that activates the pro-inflammatory cytokines pro-IL-1β and pro-IL-18. Caspase-1 itself is activated in different inflammasome complexes; however, activation of the NLRP3 inflammasome has been frequently implicated in the development of fibrosis (19). To determine the role of caspase-1 and NLRP3 in IL-1β secretion by *B. abortus*-infected LX-2 cells, we performed the infection of LX-2 cells in the presence

of specific pharmacological inhibitors. Inhibition of caspase-1 using the general caspase inhibitor Z-VAD-FMK or the specific caspase-1 inhibitor Ac-YVAD-cmk completely abrogated the secretion of IL-1β secretion induced by *B. abortus* infection of LX-2 cells (**Figure 1B**). When infection experiments were performed in the presence of Bay compound that inhibits NFκB, the secretion of IL-1β was significantly inhibited. However, glyburide, a compound that inhibits NLRP3, partially inhibits IL-1β secretion with respect to untreated cells (**Figure 1B**). Taken together, these results indicated that caspase-1 and NLRP3 are involved in the secretion of IL-1β by *B. abortus*-infected LX-2 cells.

IL-1β Secretion Induced by *B. abortus* Infection Is Also Dependent on AIM2

AIM2 inflammasome has been previously involved in the induction of IL-1β secretion in a T4SS-dependent manner during *B. abortus* infection of bone marrow derived macrophages and dendritic cells (6, 7). Since the inhibition of NLRP3 did not

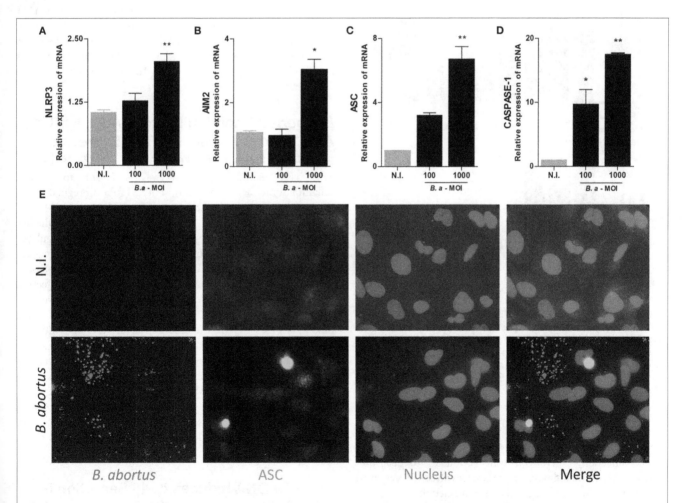

FIGURE 2 | *B. abortus* induces inflammasome in LX-2 cells. LX-2 cells were infected with *B. abortus* at MOI of 100 and 1000; at 24 h, post-infection levels of NLRP3 **(A)**, AIM2 **(B)**, ASC **(C)**, Caspase 1 **(D)**, and IL-1β **(E)** were determined by RT-qPCR. LX-2 cells were infected with Ds-Red *B. abortus* and ASC speck were revealed by immunofluorescence with a specific antibody labeled with Alexa 488. Nuclei were stained with DAPI. Data are given as the means ± SD from at least three individual experiments. *P < 0.05; **P < 0.01 vs. non-infected cells (N.I.).

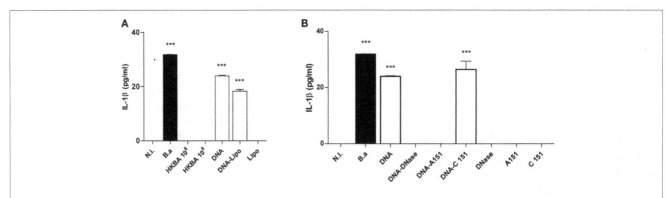

FIGURE 3 | DNA from *B. abortus* induces IL-1β. **(A)** LX-2 cells were infected with *B. abortus* (*B.a*) at MOI 1000 or treated with heat-killed *B. abortus* (HKBA) (1 × 10^6 and 1 × 10^8 bacteria/ml), 2 μg/ml of DNA, DNA and lipofectamine (DNA + Lipo), and lipofectamine alone as control (Lipo); IL-1β secretion was measured in culture supernatant after 24 h by ELISA. Determination of IL-1β in culture supernatants from LX-2 cells treated with DNA, DNA and A151, DNA and C151 as control, DNA treated with DNAse I, and DNAse I alone as control **(B)**. Data are given as the means ± SD from at least three individual experiments. ***P < 0.001 vs. non-infected cells (N.I.).

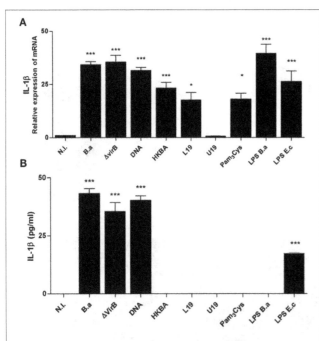

FIGURE 4 | L-Omp19 induces mRNA of IL-1β. **(A)** LX-2 cells were infected with *B. abortus* (*B.a*) and its *virB10* isogenic mutant (Δ*vir*B10) at MOI 1000, or incubated with DNA (2 μg/ml), heat-killed *B. abortus* (HKBA) (1 × 10^6 and 1 × 10^8 bacteria/ml), L-Omp19 (1,000 ng/ml), U-Omp19 (1,000 ng/ml), *B. abortus* LPS (1,000 ng/ml), Pam$_3$Cys (50 ng/ml), or *E. coli* LPS (100 ng/ml). Determination of IL-1β mRNA by RT-qPCR **(A)** and IL-1β secretion by ELISA **(B)**. Data are given as the means ± SD from at least three individual experiments. *P < 0.05; ***P < 0.001 vs. non-infected cells (N.I.).

completely abrogate the secretion of IL-1β in response to *B. abortus* infection, experiments were conducted to determine whether AIM2 inflammasome is also involved in caspase-1 activation. To this end, LX-2 cells were infected in the presence of A151, the oligodeoxinucleotide sequence that inhibits AIM2 or the sequence control C151. Our results indicated that AIM2 inflammasome contributes to IL-1β production by *B. abortus*-infected LX-2 cells, since the secretion of IL-1β was significantly

inhibited when cells were treated with A151 with respect to untreated cells or cells treated with C151 (**Figure 1C**). When infection experiments were performed in the presence of A151 and glyburide administered in conjunction, the production of IL-1β was completely abrogated (**Figure 1D**). Taken together, these results indicated that NLRP3 and AIM2 inflammasomes are involved in the secretion of IL-1β by *B. abortus*-infected LX-2 cells.

B. abortus Infection Induces ASC, NLRP3, AIM2, and Caspase-1 mRNA Expression and ASC Speck Formation in LX-2 Cells

The basal AIM2 expression was sufficient to initiate inflammasome activation (20), but NLRP3 upregulation is necessary to initiate the activation of inflammasome (21, 22). Then, experiments were conducted to determine whether expression of inflammasome components could be upregulated during *B. abortus* infection. To this end, we determine the mRNA transcription of ASC, NLRP3, AIM2, and caspase-1 by RT-qPCR. Our results indicated that *B. abortus* infection induces an increase in ASC, NLRP3, AIM2, and caspase-1 mRNA transcription in LX-2 cells (**Figures 2A–D**). Most inflammasomes require oligomerization of ASC and thus the presence of ASC specks is a direct evidence of inflammasome activation. After infection with *B. abortus*, the formation of ASC specks was detected using specific antibodies by a fluorescence microscope. ASC specks were formed in *B. abortus*-infected LX-2 cells, but these structures were not detectable in non-infected cells. This indicates that *B. abortus* infection induces inflammasome assembly and consequently ASC speck formation (**Figure 2E**).

Brucella DNA Induces IL-1β Secretion in LX-2 Cells

IL-1β secretion was dependent on bacteria viability since stimulation of LX-2 cells with heat-killed *B. abortus* (HKBA) was unable to induce IL-1β (**Figure 3A**).

It has been recently demonstrated that *Brucella* DNA is involved in IL-1β secretion via activation of caspase-1 through the AIM2 inflammasome in macrophages and dendritic cells (6, 7). Therefore, we decided to test whether *Brucella* genomic DNA could be the putative ligand for AIM2 in the context of the inflammasome activation in LX-2 cells. To this end, *Brucella* DNA was transfected into LX-2 cells using lipofectamine or added to the culture medium to determine IL-1β secretion. *Brucella* DNA induced IL-1β secretion by LX-2 cells when it was added to the culture medium and also in transfected cells (**Figure 3A**). To determine if AIM2 inflammasome is involved in the secretion of IL-1β induced by *Brucella* DNA, experiments were performed in the presence of A151, the oligodeoxinucleotide that inhibits AIM2 or its oligodeoxinucleotide control C151. AIM2 is involved in the secretion of IL-1β induced by *Brucella* DNA, since A151 abrogated its secretion (**Figure 3B**). Additionally, DNase I treatment significantly reduced or abrogated *Brucella* DNA-induced IL-1β secretion (**Figure 3B**), demonstrating that

bacterial DNA participates or is a major agonist that activates the inflammasome.

PAMPs Associated to Inflammasome Activation

For the production of IL-1β, PAMPs via TLRs and NLRs function in concert. PAMPs induce the expression of the precursor form of this cytokine (pro-IL-1β), and NLR-dependent CASP-1 activation induces its proteolytic processing and release (5). Hence, to assess the role of *Brucella* PAMPs, LX-2 cells were stimulated with HKBA and mRNA expression of IL-1β was determined by RT-qPCR. Our results indicated that HKBA was able to induce IL-1β expression at the mRNA level (**Figure 4A**) without IL-1β release, which demonstrated that viability is crucial for IL-1β protein production.

Previous observations indicated that LPS and lipoproteins from *B. abortus* are crucial for inflammatory responses induced by *B. abortus* in different models *in vivo* and *in vitro* (16, 23–26). Cells were then incubated with LPS from *B. abortus* and

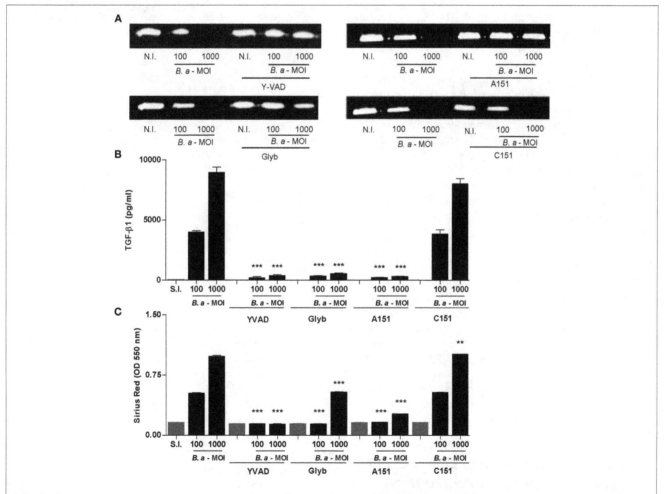

FIGURE 5 | Inflammasome is involved in profibrogienic response of LX-2 cells. LX-2 cells were infected with *B. abortus* at MOI of 100 and 1000 in the presence or not of Z-VAD-FMK (ZVAD), Y-VAD-FMK (YVAD), Bay 11-7082 (Bay), and glybenclamide (Glyb). At 24 h after infection, supernatants were harvested to analyze MMP-9 production by zymography **(A)** and TGF-β1 secretion by ELISA **(B)**. Quantification of collagen deposition was revealed by Sirius red staining by OD readings at 550 nm at 10 days post-infection **(C)**. Data are given as the means ± SD of duplicates. **P < 0.01; ***P < 0.001 vs. non-infected cells (N.I.).

lipidated Omp19 (L-Omp19) as a *Brucella* lipoprotein model, and the expression of IL-1β mRNA was determined by RT-qPCR. Our results indicated that L-Omp19 and LPS induce an increase in IL-1β mRNA expression in LX-2 cells. IL-1β mRNA expression induced by Omp19 was dependent on the lipid moiety of the molecule because unlipidated Omp19 (U-Omp19) did not induce IL-1β mRNA expression. The requirement for lipidation was further supported by the fact that Pam3Cys, a lipohexapeptide with an irrelevant peptide sequence, also induced the production of mRNA of IL-1β (**Figure 4A**). As expected, the presence of IL-1β at the protein level was not detected in supernatants of cultures of LX-2 cells treated with LPS or L-Omp19 (**Figure 4B**). Taken together, these results indicated that *B. abortus* lipoproteins and LPS induce mRNA of IL-1β in LX-2 cells.

The Inflammasome Pathway Is Involved in the Profibrogenic Response of LX-2 Cells Upon *B. abortus* Infection

It has been demonstrated that inflammasome activation has a variety of functional consequences for HSCs, including enhanced collagen 1 and TGF-β expression (4). Previously, we have demonstrated that upon infection of LX-2 cells, *B. abortus* inhibits MMP-9 secretion and induces concomitant collagen and TGF-β1 secretion (15). Therefore, experiments were conducted to determine the role of the inflammasome in the induction of a fibrogenic phenotype in LX-2 cells during *B. abortus* infection. To this end, the levels of secretion of MMP-9, TGF-β, and collagen deposition were determined in LX-2 cells infected with *B. abortus* in the presence of different inflammasome inhibitors. When infection experiments were performed in the presence of YVAD, glyburide, or A151, the effect of *B. abortus* infection on MMP-9 expression, collagen deposition, and TGF-β secretion on LX-2 cells was partially reversed with respect to untreated infected cells (**Figure 5**). These results indicated that NLRP3 and AIM2 inflammasome are involved in the induction of profibrogenic phenotype in LX-2 cells.

IL-1β Is Involved in the Induction of a Profibrogenic Phenotype

Caspase-1 is required not only for IL-1β secretion but also for IL-18 secretion. To determine the role of IL-1β in the induction of a fibrotic phenotype, infection experiments were performed in the presence of the inhibitor of IL-1 receptor, the natural antagonist IL-1Ra (ANAKINRA). As shown in **Figure 6**, ANAKINRA abrogated the ability of *B. abortus* to inhibit MMP-9 and to induce collagen deposition. These results indicate that IL-1β could be a key cytokine during inflammasome activation involved in the fibrogenic phenotype triggered by *B. abortus* infection.

NLRP3 and AIM2 Influence Liver Fibrosis in Livers From *B. abortus*-Infected Mice

Finally, to verify the *in vivo* significance of our hypothesis, Casp-1, ASC, NLRP3, and AIM2 KO mice and WT mice, as control, were infected with *B. abortus*, and 4 weeks later, animals were sacrificed to determine the role of inflammasome in the liver fibrosis. Accordingly with our previous results, Masson's

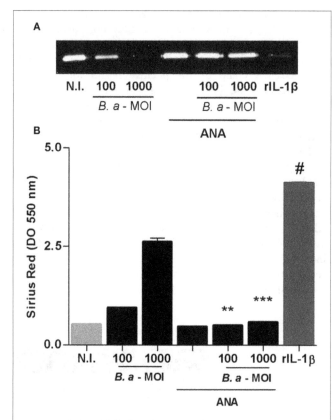

FIGURE 6 | IL-1β is involved in the induction of a profibrogenic phenotype. LX-2 cells were infected with *B. abortus* at MOI of 100 and 1000 in the presence or not of ANAKINRA (ANA). Determination of MMP-9 at 24 h post-infection in culture supernatants by zymography **(A)**. Recombinant human IL-1-β, (rIL-1β) (50 ng/ml) was used as a positive control. Quantification of collagen deposition was revealed by Sirius red staining by OD readings at 550 nm at 10 days post-infection **(B)**. Data are given as the means ± SD of duplicates. **$P < 0.01$; ***$P < 0.001$ vs. untreated cells. #$P < 0.001$ vs. non-infected cells (N.I.).

trichrome staining revealed the presence of fibrotic patch in livers from *B. abortus*-infected mice with respect to uninfected control (9, 15). In contrast, Casp-1, ASC, NLRP3, and AIM2 KO animals presented a significant reduction in the fibrotic patch (**Figure 7**). No fibrotic patch was observed in mice inoculated with saline (data not shown). These results indicated that inflammasomes NLRP2 and AIM2 play a key role in the modulation of fibrosis during *B. abortus* infection.

DISCUSSION

The liver is frequently affected in patients with active brucellosis, as revealed by the presence of histopathology lesions, such as granulomas, inflammatory infiltrates, and necrosis of liver parenchyma (27, 28).

Fibrosis is an intrinsic response to chronic persistent liver injury that results in a wound-healing process to mitigate the damage, but can also lead to scar formation. Inflammasome activation may play an important role in this process (19).

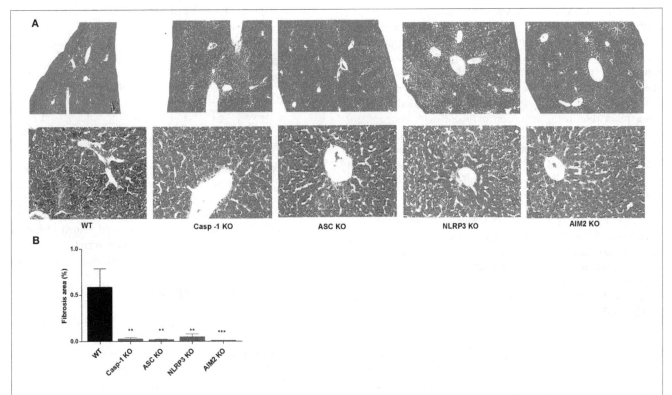

FIGURE 7 | NLRP3 and AIM2 influence liver fibrosis in livers from *B. abortus*-infected mice. Representative photomicrographs of liver sections from control mice, *B. abortus*-infected mice WT, Casp-1, ASC, NLRP3, and AM2 KO mice (n5) stained with Masson's trichrome staining. The top panels show images taken at the original magnification (×100), and the bottom panels show a detail of collagen patches (magnification, ×400) **(A)**. Collagen-positive areas were quantified using Image Pro-Plus 6.0 software **(B)**. Data are given as the means ± SD from at least three individual experiments. ***P* < 0.01; ****P* < 0.001 vs. wild type (WT).

In the present study, we demonstrated that *B. abortus* infection activates the inflammasome with concomitant secretion of IL-1β in HSC leading to upregulation of a profibrogenic phenotype.

Inflammasomes have emerged as critical signaling molecules of innate immune system involved in liver fibrosis. Inflammasomes are intracellular multiprotein complexes that act as regulators of inflammation and cell destiny. They respond to several danger signals by activating caspase-1 by the release of proinflammatory cytokines IL-1β and IL-18 (29). In particular, the NLRP3 inflammasome has been frequently implicated in the pathogenesis of chronic inflammatory liver diseases that causes liver fibrosis (30).

HSCs are the main cells involved in extracellular matrix deposition during liver fibrosis (31). In this process, the NLRP3 inflammasome has been involved in the functional changes in HSCs, including upregulation of the expression of collagen and TGF-β (4, 32), in findings that were confirmed by performing the knocking in NLRP3 (33).

Previous studies performed in dendritic cells, macrophages, and glial cells indicate that *Brucella* is sensed by ASC-dependent inflammasomes, mainly NLRP3 and AIM2, that induce caspase-1 activation with pro-inflammatory response (6, 8, 34, 35). Accordingly, in *Brucella*-infected HSCs, the secretion of IL-1β depends on NLRP3 and AIM2 inflammasomes. In this context, the participation of PAMPs in the activation of the inflammasome

and the secretion of IL-1β must be discussed. The activation and release of IL-1β requires two distinct signals. The first signal can be triggered by various pathogen-associated molecular patterns via TLR activation, which induces the synthesis of pro–IL-1β. The second signal is provided by the activation of the inflammasome and caspase-1 leading to IL-1β processing. During *B. abortus* infection, the induction of IL-1β at mRNA level was independent of bacterial viability and induced at least by two structural bacterial components, including lipoproteins and LPS. However, the second signal requires bacterial viability and the presence of a functional T4SS and *B. abortus* DNA. The T4SS is encoded by *vir*B genes that play a main role in *Brucella* intracellular replication (17), and it has also been involved in the immune response to *Brucella* infection (7, 18). Bacteria utilize the T4SS to deliver effectors to eukaryotic cells. In LX-2 cells, *B. abortus* *vir*B10 mutant was unable to induce IL-1β secretion, and it could suggest that *Brucella* T4SS is involved in the transport of effector molecules that act via NLRP3 and/or AIM2 to activate inflammasomes. This is in agreement with our other finding in which we demonstrate that HKBA does not induce the secretion of IL-1β by LX-2 cells.

In vitro studies have shown that IL-1β promotes the proliferation and myofibroblast transdifferentiation of HSCs with substantial increased levels of their fibrogenic markers (36–38). Activated caspase-1 could also cleave pro-IL-18 into its active form IL-18, and this cytokine has also been involved in fibrosis induction (38, 39). In a murine model of non-alcoholic steatohepatitis, fibrosis was not reversed by IL-1Ra treatment, indicating that other regulators of NLRP3 inflammasome are involved in fibrogenesis promotion (33). However, our experiments performed in *B. abortus*-infected HSCs in the presence of ANAKINRA, a version of the human interleukin-1 receptor antagonist, indicated that IL-1β secreted by HSCs has a main role in the induction of TGF-β with concomitant collagen deposition and inhibition of MMP-9 secretion. This role of IL-1β in the myofibroblast transdifferentiation with concomitant fibrosis is not exclusive for HSCs; accordingly, it has been previously described in endothelial and epithelial cell transdifferentiation and fibrosis (40–42).

These results and previous findings suggest that the interaction of *Brucella* with innate immunity *in vivo* may result in an increase of inflammatory response that results in liver fibrosis. Inflammasomes would dictate this fibrotic phenotype. Consequently, *B. abortus* infection induces fibrosis in mice that was reduced in mice lacking AIM2 or NLRP3.

Together, these results indicated that upon infection of HSCs, *B. abortus* triggers AIM2 and NLRP3 inflammasome activation with concomitant IL-1β secretion in a mechanism that is dependent on a functional T4SS and DNA. This

IL-1β is implicated in the induction of fibrotic phenotype in HSC.

ETHICS STATEMENT

This animal study was reviewed and approved by CICUAL-Facultad de Medicina, Universidad de Buenos Aires.

AUTHOR CONTRIBUTIONS

MD conceived and designed the experiments, supervised experiments, interpreted the data, and wrote the manuscript. PA, MG, and AP performed the experiments. PA analyzed the data and wrote sections of the manuscript. SO, JQ, and GG supported the work with key suggestions and helped with data interpretation. All authors reviewed the manuscript.

ACKNOWLEDGMENTS

We thank Horacio Salomón and the staff of the Instituto de Investigaciones Biomédicas en Retrovirus y Sida (INBIRS) for their assistance with biosafety level 3 laboratory uses. PA and AP are recipients of a fellowship from CONICET. JQ, GG, and MD are members of the Research Career of CONICET.

REFERENCES

Pappas G, Akritidis N, Bosilkovski M, Tsianos E. Brucellosis. *N Engl J Med.* (2005) 352:2325–36. doi: 10.1056/NEJMra050570

Madkour MM. Osteoarticular brucellosis. In: Madkour MM, editor. *Madkour's Brucellosis.* 2nd ed. Berlin: Springer-Verlag. (2001). p. 74– 84. doi: 10.1007/978-3-642-59533-2_8

Alegre F, Pelegrin P, Feldstein AE. Inflammasomes in liver fibrosis. *Semin Liver Dis.* (2017) 37:119–27. doi: 10.1055/s-0037-1601350

Watanabe A, Sohail MA, Gomes DA, Hashmi A, Nagata J, Sutterwala FS, et al. Inflammasome-mediated regulation of hepatic stellate cells. *Am J Physiol Gastrointest Liver Physiol.* (2009) 296:G1248–57. doi: 10.1152/ajpgi.90223.2008

Miao EA, Andersen-Nissen E, Warren SE, Aderem A. TLR5 and Ipaf: dual sensors of bacterial flagellin in the innate immune system. *Semin Immunopathol.* (2007) 29:275–88. doi: 10.1007/s00281-007-0078-z

Costa Franco MMS, Marim FM, Alves-Silva J, Cerqueira D, Rungue M, Tavares IP, et al. AIM2 senses *Brucella abortus* DNA in dendritic cells to induce IL-1beta secretion, pyroptosis and resistance to bacterial infection in mice. *Microbes Infect.* (2018) 21:85–93. doi: 10.1016/j.micinf.2018.09.001

Gomes MT, Campos PC, Oliveira FS, Corsetti PP, Bortoluci KR, Cunha LD, et al. Critical role of ASC inflammasomes and bacterial type IV secretion system in caspase-1 activation and host innate resistance to *Brucella abortus* infection. *J Immunol.* (2013) 190:3629–38. doi: 10.4049/jimmunol.1202817

Miraglia MC, Costa Franco MM, Rodriguez AM, Bellozi PM, Ferrari CC, Farias MI, et al. Glial cell-elicited activation of brain microvasculature in response to *Brucella abortus* infection requires ASC inflammasome-dependent IL-1beta production. *J Immunol.* (2016) 196:3794–805. doi: 10.4049/jimmunol.1500908

Arriola Benitez PC, Rey Serantes D, Herrmann CK, Pesce Viglietti AI, Vanzulli S, Giambartolomei GH, et al. The effector protein BPE005 from *Brucella abortus* induces collagen deposition and matrix metalloproteinase 9 downmodulation via transforming growth factor beta1 in hepatic stellate cells. *Infect Immun.* (2016) 84:598–606. doi: 10.1128/IAI. 01227-15

Scian R, Barrionuevo P, Rodriguez AM, Arriola Benitez PC, Garcia Samartino C,

Fossati CA, et al. *Brucella abortus* invasion of synoviocytes inhibits apoptosis and induces bone resorption through RANKL expression. *Infect Immun.* (2013) 81:1940–51. doi: 10.1128/IAI.01366-12

Hibbs MS, Hasty KA, Seyer JM, Kang AH, Mainardi CL. Biochemical and immunological characterization of the secreted forms of human neutrophil gelatinase. *J Biol Chem.* (1985) 260:2493–500.

Scian R, Barrionuevo P, Giambartolomei GH, De Simone EA, Vanzulli SI, Fossati CA, et al. Potential role of fibroblast-like synoviocytes in joint damage induced by *Brucella abortus* infection through production and induction of matrix metalloproteinases. *Infect Immun.* (2011) 79:3619– 32. doi: 10.1128/IAI.05408-11

Scian R, Barrionuevo P, Giambartolomei GH, Fossati CA, Baldi PC, Delpino MV. Granulocyte-macrophage colony-stimulating factor- and tumor necrosis factor alpha-mediated matrix metalloproteinase production by human osteoblasts and monocytes after infection with *Brucella abortus. Infect Immun.* (2011) 79:192–202. doi: 10.1128/IAI.00934-10

Tullberg-Reinert H, Jundt G. *In situ* measurement of collagen synthesis by human bone cells with a sirius red-based colorimetric microassay: effects of transforming growth factor beta2 and ascorbic acid 2- phosphate. *Histochem Cell Biol.* (1999) 112:271–6. doi: 10.1007/s004180 050447

Arriola Benitez PC, Scian R, Comerci DJ, Serantes DR, Vanzulli S, Fossati CA, et al. *Brucella abortus* induces collagen deposition and MMP-9 downmodulation in hepatic stellate cells via TGF-beta1 production. *Am J Pathol.* (2013) 183:1918–27. doi: 10.1016/j.ajpath.2013. 08.006

Giambartolomei GH, Zwerdling A, Cassataro J, Bruno L, Fossati CA, Philipp MT. Lipoproteins, not lipopolysaccharide, are the key mediators of the proinflammatory response elicited by heat-killed *Brucella abortus. J Immunol.* (2004) 173:4635–42. doi: 10.4049/jimmunol.173.7.4635

Comerci DJ, Martinez-Lorenzo MJ, Sieira R, Gorvel JP, Ugalde RA. Essential role of the VirB machinery in the maturation of the *Brucella abortus*-containing vacuole. *Cell Microbiol.* (2001) 3:159–68. doi: 10.1046/j.1462-5822.2001.00102.x

Roux CM, Rolan HG, Santos RL, Beremand PD, Thomas TL, Adams LG, et al. *Brucella* requires a functional Type IV secretion system to elicit innate immune responses in mice. *Cell Microbiol.* (2007) 9:1851– 69. doi: 10.1111/j.1462-5822.2007.00922.x

Szabo G, Csak T. Inflammasomes in liver diseases. *J Hepatol.* (2012) 57:642– 54. doi: 10.1016/j.jhep.2012.03.035

Rathinam VA, Jiang Z, Waggoner SN, Sharma S, Cole LE, Waggoner L, et al. The AIM2 inflammasome is essential for host defense against cytosolic bacteria and DNA viruses. *Nat Immunol.* (2010) 11:395– 402. doi: 10.1038/ni.1864

Franchi L, Eigenbrod T, Nunez G. Cutting edge: TNF-alpha mediates sensitization to ATP and silica via the NLRP3 inflammasome in the absence of microbial stimulation. *J Immunol.* (2009) 183:792–6. doi: 10.4049/jimmunol.0900173

Bauernfeind FG, Horvath G, Stutz A, Alnemri ES, MacDonald K, Speert D, et al. Cutting edge: NF-kappaB activating pattern recognition and cytokine receptors license NLRP3 inflammasome activation by regulating NLRP3 expression. *J Immunol.* (2009) 183:787–91. doi: 10.4049/jimmunol.0901363

Zwerdling A, Delpino MV, Barrionuevo P, Cassataro J, Pasquevich KA, Garcia Samartino C, et al. Brucella lipoproteins mimic dendritic cell maturation induced by *Brucella abortus. Microbes Infect.* (2008) 10:1346– 54. doi: 10.1016/j.micinf.2008.07.035

Zwerdling A, Delpino MV, Pasquevich KA, Barrionuevo P, Cassataro J, Garcia Samartino C, et al. *Brucella abortus* activates human neutrophils. *Microbes Infect.* (2009) 11:689–97. doi: 10.1016/j.micinf.2009.04.010

Garcia Samartino C, Delpino MV, Pott Godoy C, Di Genaro MS, Pasquevich KA, Zwerdling A, et al. *Brucella abortus* induces the secretion of proinflammatory mediators from glial cells leading to astrocyte apoptosis. *Am J Pathol.* (2010) 176:1323–38. doi: 10.2353/ajpath.2010.090503

Oliveira SC, de Oliveira FS, Macedo GC, de Almeida LA, Carvalho NB. The role of innate immune receptors in the control of *Brucella abortus* infection: toll-like receptors and beyond. *Microbes Infect.* (2008) 10:1005– 9. doi: 10.1016/j.micinf.2008.07.005

Akritidis N, Tzivras M, Delladetsima I, Stefanaki S, Moutsopoulos HM, Pappas G. The liver in brucellosis. *Clin Gastroenterol Hepatol.* (2007) 5:1109– 12. doi: 10.1016/j.cgh.2006.08.010

Madkour MM. Gastrointestinal brucellosis. Madkour MM, editor. *Madkour's Brucellosis.* 2nd ed. Berlin: Springer-Verlag (2001). p. 150–8. doi: 10.1007/978-3-642-59533-2_13

Latz E, Xiao TS, Stutz A. Activation and regulation of the inflammasomes. *Nat Rev Immunol.* (2013) 13:397–411. doi: 10.1038/nri3452

Henao-Mejia J, Elinav E, Jin C, Hao L, Mehal WZ, Strowig T, et al. Inflammasome-mediated dysbiosis regulates progression of NAFLD and obesity. *Nature.* (2012) 482:179–85. doi: 10.1038/nature10809

Bataller R, Brenner DA. Liver fibrosis. *J Clin Invest.* (2005) 115:209– 18. doi: 10.1172/JCI24282

Mederacke I, Hsu CC, Troeger JS, Huebener P, Mu X, Dapito DH, et al. Fate tracing reveals hepatic stellate cells as dominant contributors to liver fibrosis independent of its aetiology. *Nat Commun.* (2013) 4:2823. doi: 10.1038/ncomms3823

Wree A, McGeough MD, Pena CA, Schlattjan M, Li H, Inzaugarat ME, et al. NLRP3 inflammasome activation is required for fibrosis development in NAFLD. *J Mol Med.* (2014) 92:1069–82. doi: 10.1007/s00109-014-1170-1

Campos PC, Gomes MTR, Marinho FAV, Guimaraes ES, de Moura Lodi Cruz MGF, Oliveira SC. *Brucella abortus* nitric oxide metabolite regulates inflammasome activation and IL-1beta secretion in murine macrophages. *Eur J Immunol.* (2019) 49:1023–37. doi: 10.1002/eji.201848016

Costa Franco MM, Marim F, Guimaraes ES, Assis NRG, Cerqueira DM, Alves-Silva J, et al. *Brucella abortus* triggers a cGAS-independent STING pathway to induce host protection that involves guanylate- binding proteins and inflammasome activation. *J Immunol.* (2018) 200:607– 22. doi: 10.4049/jimmunol.1700725

Yaping Z, Ying W, Luqin D, Ning T, Xuemei A, Xixian Y. Mechanism of interleukin-1beta-induced proliferation in rat hepatic stellate cells from different levels of signal transduction. *Apmis.* (2014) 122:392– 8. doi: 10.1111/apm.12155

Reiter FP, Wimmer R, Wottke L, Artmann R, Nagel JM, Carranza MO, et al. Role of interleukin-1 and its antagonism of hepatic stellate cell proliferation and liver fibrosis in the Abcb4(-/-) mouse model. *World J Hepatol.* (2016) 8:401–10. doi: 10.4254/wjh.v8.i8.401

Artlett CM. Inflammasomes in wound healing and fibrosis. *J Pathol.* (2013) 229:157-67. doi: 10.1002/path.4116

Tanino A, Okura T, Nagao T, Kukida M, Pei Z, Enomoto D, et al. Interleukin- 18 deficiency protects against renal interstitial fibrosis in aldosterone/salt- treated mice. *Clin Sci.* (2016) 130:1727–39. doi: 10.1042/CS20160183

Leaf IA, Nakagawa S, Johnson BG, Cha JJ, Mittelsteadt K, Guckian KM, et al. Pericyte MyD88 and IRAK4 control inflammatory and fibrotic responses to tissue injury. *J Clin Invest.* (2017) 127:321–34. doi: 10.1172/JCI87532

Fan JM, Huang XR, Ng YY, Nikolic-Paterson DJ, Mu W, Atkins RC, et al. Interleukin-1 induces tubular epithelial-myofibroblast transdifferentiation through a transforming growth factor-beta1-dependent mechanism in vitro. *Am J Kidney Dis.* (2001) 37:820–31. doi: 10.1016/S0272-6386(01)80132-3

Rieder F, Kessler SP, West GA, Bhilocha S, de la Motte C, Sadler TM, et al. Inflammation-induced endothelial-to-mesenchymal transition: a novel mechanism of intestinal fibrosis. *Am J Pathol.* (2011) 179:2660– 73. doi: 10.1016/j.ajpath.2011.07.042

2

Dapagliflozin Alleviates Hepatic Steatosis by Restoring Autophagy via the AMPK-mTOR Pathway

Liuran Li[1†], Qinghua Li[1†], Wenbin Huang[2], Yibing Han[1], Huiting Tan[1], Min An[1], Qianru Xiang[1], Rui Zhou[3]*, Li Yang[1,4]* and Yanzhen Cheng[1]*

[1]Department of Endocrinology, Zhujiang Hospital, Southern Medical University, Guangzhou, China, [2]Department of Hepatobiliary Surgery II, Zhujiang Hospital, Southern Medical University, Guangzhou, China, [3]Department of Pathology, School of Basic Medical Sciences, Southern Medical University, Guangzhou, China, [4]Department of Nutrition, Zhujiang Hospital, Southern Medical University, Guangzhou, China

*Correspondence:
Yanzhen Cheng
chengyzx@163.com
Li Yang
yangli19762009@163.com
Rui Zhou
yaruisunny@sina.com

[†]These authors have contributed equally to this work

As a newly approved oral hypoglycaemic agent, the sodium-glucose cotransporter 2 (SGLT2) inhibitor dapagliflozin, which is derived from the natural product phlorizin can effectively reduce blood glucose. Recent clinical studies have found that dapagliflozin alleviates non-alcoholic fatty liver disease (NAFLD), but the specific mechanism remains to be explored. This study aimed to investigate the underlying mechanism of dapagliflozin in alleviating hepatocyte steatosis *in vitro* and *in vivo*. We fed the spontaneous type 2 diabetes mellitus rats with high-fat diets and cultured human normal liver LO2 cells and human hepatocellular carcinoma HepG2 cells with palmitic acid (PA) to induce hepatocellular steatosis. Dapagliflozin attenuated hepatic lipid accumulation both *in vitro* and *in vivo*. In Zucker diabetic fatty (ZDF) rats, dapagliflozin reduced hepatic lipid accumulation via promoting phosphorylation of acetyl-CoA carboxylase 1 (ACC1), and upregulating lipid β-oxidation enzyme acyl-CoA oxidase 1 (ACOX1). Furthermore, dapagliflozin increased the expression of the autophagy-related markers LC3B and Beclin1, in parallel with a drop in p62 level. Similar effects were observed in PA-stimulated LO2 cells and HepG2 cells. Dapagliflozin treatment could also significantly activated AMPK and reduced the phosphorylation of mTOR in ZDF rats and PA-stimulated LO2 cells and HepG2 cells. We demonstrated that dapagliflozin ameliorates hepatic steatosis by decreasing lipogenic enzyme, while inducing fatty acid oxidation enzyme and autophagy, which could be associated with AMPK activation. Moreover, our results indicate that dapagliflozin induces autophagy via the AMPK-mTOR pathway. These findings reveal a novel clinical application and functional mechanism of dapagliflozin in the treatment of NAFLD.

Keywords: NAFLD, AMPK, mTOR, autophagy, dapagliflozin

INTRODUCTION

Non-alcoholic fatty liver disease (NAFLD), the most common liver disease worldwide, is characterized by the hepatic fat accumulation in patients without alcohol abuse (Angulo, 2002). Metabolic syndromes, such as obesity and hyperglycaemia, predispose patients to developing severe NAFLDs, including nonalcoholic steatohepatitis (NASH), liver cirrhosis, and hepatocellular carcinoma (Lu et al., 2018). In patients with type 2 diabetes mellitus (T2DM), the prevalence rate of NAFLD is approximately 70%, among which 20% develops advanced fibrosis, revealing the high correlation between diabetes and NAFLD (Bril et al., 2016). In fact, NAFLD is only one outcome of multisystem diseases, in which the most frequent causes of high morbidity and mortality are cardiovascular diseases, extrahepatic malignant tumors and liver-related complications (Adams et al., 2017). At present, the common measures for NAFLD treatment are restricted to diet adjustment, exercise and bariatric surgery, due to lacking of effective and safe medications. Therefore, a pharmacological treatment for NAFLD is urgently required.

Dapagliflozin, a sodium-glucose cotransporter 2 (SGLT2) inhibitor, is a novel antidiabetic agent that is approved for the treatment of T2DM by based on its ability to inhibit SGLT2-mediated renal glucose reabsorption. In addition to providing effective glycaemic control, dapagliflozin help decrease body weight, reduce rate of cardiovascular death, and possibly slow the progression of diabetic kidney diseases (Dhillon, 2019). Dapagliflozin has been reported to alleviate hepatic steatosis in patients with type 2 diabetes and NAFLD; however, whether the improvement in liver steatosis is related to the reduction in body weight by dapagliflozin cannot be ruled out (Kurinami et al., 2018; Shimizu et al., 2019). A recent study suggested that dapagliflozin attenuated SGLT2 expression, which could prevent excessive glucose absorption and increase AMPK phosphorylation in HFD-induced obese mice or OA-stimulated HuS-E/2 cells (Chiang et al., 2020), but the explicit mechanism has not yet been fully clarified. Thus, whether dapagliflozin can moderate hepatic steatosis independent of hypoglycaemic control and body weight loss requires further investigation.

Acetyl-CoA carboxylase 1 (ACC1), a rate-controlling enzyme in *de novo* lipogenesis, plays a crucial role in fatty acid metabolism. Inhibition of ACC1 can significantly reduce hepatic steatosis and hepatic insulin resistance (Brownsey et al., 1997; Goedeke et al., 2018). Acyl-CoA oxidase 1 (ACOX1), a rate-limiting enzyme in the peroxisomal β-oxidation pathway, promotes catabolism of very long–chain fatty acids. ACOX1-deficient mice exhibit spontaneous hepatic steatosis and steatohepatitis (Sheridan et al., 2011; Moreno-Fernandez et al., 2018). Hepatic lipid accumulation is caused by an imbalance between lipid synthesis and lipid degradation, which are mediated through several pathways, such as increased *de novo* lipogenesis and reduced fatty acid oxidation. AMPK is a vital energy sensor that regulates hepatic lipid metabolism (Madiraju et al., 2016). mTOR, a crucial downstream target of AMPK, negatively regulates autophagy (Kim and Guan, 2015). It was reported that the hepatic autophagy was suppressed by inhibiting AMPK, which caused the development of hepatic steatosis (You et al., 2004). Although the pathogenesis of NAFLD is elusive, increasing evidence suggests that impaired autophagy plays a vital role in the development of NAFLD. In the present study, we investigated the protective effect of the SGLT2 inhibitor dapagliflozin in alleviating NAFLD both *in vivo* and *in vitro*, and further clarified the role of AMPK activation in ameliorating hepatic lipid accumulation and the involvement of the AMPK-mTOR signaling pathway in autophagy induction.

MATERIALS AND METHODS

Antibodies and Reagents

Protein expression was assessed by immunoblot analysis of cell lysates (20–60 μg) in RIPA buffer in the presence of the following antibodies: including anti-p-AMPK (Affinity, AF3423), anti-AMPK (Affinity, AF6423), anti-p-ACC1 (Cell Signaling Technology, 11818s), anti-ACC1(Cell Signaling Technology, 4190s), anti-ACOX1 (Santa Cruz Biotechnology, sc-517306), anti-p-mTOR (Affinity, AF3308), anti-mTOR (Affinity, AF6308), anti-SGLT2 (Abcam, ab37296), anti-LC3B (Cell Signaling Technology, 12741S), anti-Beclin1 (Cell Signaling Technology, 4122s), anti-p62/SQSTM1 (Proteintech, 18420-1-AP), and anti-GAPDH (Abcam, ab8245).

Unless otherwise specified, all chemicals were purchased from Sigma-Aldrich (St. Louis, MO, United States). Dulbecco's modified Eagle's medium (DMEM), fetal bovine serum (FBS, Gibco) were obtained from Gibco; palmitate (PA) was obtained from Sigma-Aldrich (P9767); compound C (Comp C) was purchased from AbMole (M2238), chloroquine (CQ, S4157) and dapagliflozin (S1548) were bought from Selleck; and Oil Red O and triglyceride detection kit (G1262; BC0625) were obtained from Solarbio.

Animal Model

Eight-week-old male Zucker Diabetic Fatty (ZDF, fa/fa) rats and Zucker lean (ZL, fa/+) rats were purchased from the Laboratory Animal Center of Vital River [Beijing, China; license number, SYXK (Yue) 2011–0,074]. Five ZL rats and 10 male ZDF rats, at 8 weeks of age, were fed with a high-fat diet Purina #5008 for 4 weeks to induce diabetes. At the age of 12 weeks, the ZDF rats were randomly separated into two groups ($n = 5$ in each group) including: the diabetic control group (ZDF) and the diabetic group treated with dapagliflozin (ZDF + Dapa). In addition, the rats in ZL group were used as the non-diabetic controls. High-fat diet Purina #5008 was provided from 8 weeks of age to the end of the experiment. The rats in the ZDF + Dapa group were administered with dapagliflozin at a dosage of 1.0 mg/kg/day using intragastric gavage, while the ZL group and the ZDF group were treated with a vehicle via gavage as control. The interventions had been maintained for 9 weeks. Glucose levels of all the rats in different groups were measured every week. At the age of 21 weeks, all rats were anesthetized and sacrificed, blood was collected via the tail vein, and liver tissues were weighed at once after sampling and then stored at −80°C for subsequent measurements. All animal experimental procedures were performed with the approval of the Southern Medical University Animal Care and Use Committee in accordance with established ethical guidelines for animal studies (Resolution No. L2015039).

Oral Glucose Tolerance Tests

Oral glucose tolerance tests (2 g/kg of body weight) were performed on overnight fasted rats using a glucometer, and the blood samples were obtained from the tail vein at 0, 30, 60, and 120 min to measure blood glucose levels. Ultimately, the area under the curve (AUC) of blood glucose was calculated by the trapezoidal method (AUC = 1/4*fasting glucose +1/2*30-min glucose +3/4*60-min glucose +1/2*120-min glucose).

Cell Viability Assay

Cell viability assays of HepG2 cells and LO2 cells were carried out using Cell Counting Kit 8 (CCK8) (Dojindo; Kumamoto, Japan). Cells were plated into 96-well plates at a density of 1×10^4 cells per well and cultured overnight. Then, the culture medium was replaced by DMEM supplemented with PA (0.3 mM) and dapagliflozin (0, 10, 20, 40, 80, and 100 µg/ml). After incubation for 24 h, 10 µL CCK-8 reagent and 90 µL DMEM were added to each well for an additional 2 h of cultivation and the absorbance value was analyzed with a microplate reader at the wavelength of 450 nm.

Cell Culture and Treatments

Immortalized normal human hepatocyte-derived liver cells (LO2) and human hepatocellular carcinoma cells (HepG2) were obtained from Shanghai Institute of Cellular Biology of Chinese Academy of Sciences. When cultured in DMEM supplemented with 10% FBS at 37°C in a humidified incubator containing 5% CO_2, the cells were treated with 0.3 mM PA for 24 h to create the hepatocyte steatosis model *in vitro*. Then, hepatocytes were exposed to dapagliflozin at a concentration of 20 µM with or without chloroquine for 24 h. To study the effect of AMPK inhibition on autophagy, cells were treated with 10 µM compound C (Comp C) for 24 h.

Western Blot Analysis

HepG2 cells, LO2 cells and rat liver tissues were extracted in RIPA lysis buffer with protease inhibitor (Beyotime, Biotechnology). Phosphatase inhibitor was added to detect phosphorylated proteins. The protein concentrations of the lysates were quantified using the BCA Protein Assay Kit (Beyotime). Equal amounts of proteins were size-separated on a 10% SDS-polyacrylamide gel and then electroblotted onto PVDF membranes. Membranes were blocked by using a blocking reagent (0.1% Tween 20 and 5% Bovine Serum Albumin in TBS) for 1 h and subsequently incubated with specific primary antibodies (1:1,000) against LC3B, AMPK, p-AMPK, p62, Beclin1, ACC1, p-ACC1, ACOX1, p-mTOR, mTOR, SGLT2, and GAPDH overnight at 4 °C. After incubation with the secondary antibodies (1:10,000) for 1 h at room temperature, the signals were developed with an ECL luminescent kit and detected using enhanced chemiluminescence detection system (Pierce, Rockford, IL). The protein bands were analyzed densitometrically by ImageJ, and GAPDH protein was used as an internal control.

RNA Isolation and Quantitative Real-Time PCR Analysis

Total RNA was extracted from liver tissues and cells using TRIzol reagent and reverse-transcribed into cDNA according to the manufacturer's protocols. A quantitative PCR (qPCR) analysis was performed using SYBR Green PCR master mix (Applied Biosystems; Foster City, CA) on a 7,500 Fast Real-Time PCR system to examine the expression of related genes. The sequences of the primers used in this study are listed in (**Supplementary Table S1**). The expression levels of the target genes were normalized to that of GAPDH, and the ΔΔcycle threshold method was used for the quantitative analysis. All reagents in this study including those for RNA preparation, reverse transcription and quantitative real-time PCR analysis were purchased from Takara (Japan).

Immunofluorescence Staining

Immunofluorescence staining was performed according to standard protocols. Cells were fixed with 4% paraformaldehyde for 10 min, permeabilized in 0.25% Triton X-100 for 15 min and blocked with 5% normal goat serum for 1 h. Samples were incubated with primary antibodies against SGLT2 (1:100) and LC3B (1:100) at 4°C overnight followed by the incubation with secondary antibodies (1:100; Jackson Laboratories) for 1 h at room temperature, and the staining of 4′,6-diamidino-2-phenylindole (DAPI; 1:100; Invitrogen) for 4min. All cells were observed and captured under an Olympus FluoView FV1000 confocal microscope (Olympus, Hamburg, Germany). For the quantitative analysis, the average score of selected areas was calculated using Image Pro Plus 6.0 software (Media Cybernetics, Inc., Rockville, MD, United States).

Intracellular Lipid Droplets Staining

The accumulation of intracellular lipid droplets was detected by BODIPY 493/503 staining. Hepatocytes were treated with the indicated concentrations of PA and dapagliflozin for 24 h. Subsequently, the cells were fixed with 4% paraformaldehyde and stained with 1 µg/ml BODIPY 493/503 for 30 min at 37°C. Cell images and fluorescence intensity were visualized and quantified using an Olympus FluoView FV1000 confocal microscope.

Oil Red O Staining and Cellular Triglyceride Assays

Lipid droplets were visualized and quantified by Oil Red O (ORO) staining. According to the instructions, the cells were fixed with ORO fixative for 20min, and stained with newly prepared ORO staining solution for 20 min. After washing with 60% isopropanol, they were restained by Mayer hematoxylin for 2 min. Then, red-stained lipid droplets were subsequently observed and imaged using a light microscope (Olympus, Japan) at 400 × magnification. To quantify the intracellular lipid accumulation, the TG content in HepG2 cells and LO2 cells was measured using a Triglyceride Content Detection Kit according to the manufacturer's recommended protocols.

Liver Histopathological Examination

For Oil Red O staining, 8-µm-thick frozen sections were prepared and stained with freshly diluted Oil Red O staining solution for 20 min. After washed with 60% isopropanol, the sections were re-stained by Mayer hematoxylin for 2 min. The histological features of the samples were observed and imaged using a light microscopy. For hematoxylin and eosin (H&E) staining, the liver tissue was fixed in 4% formalin for 24 h, and then maintained in 70% alcohol for subsequent processing in paraffin for the histological studies. Paraffin sections were cut at 3 µm before paraffin removal. Then slices were obtained and stained with hematoxylin-eosin reagents.

Immunohistochemistry Staining (IHC)

IHC was used to detect the expression of proteins in 3 µm sections from formalin-fixed and paraffin-embedded tissue specimens as previously described (Tang et al., 2019). The tissues were

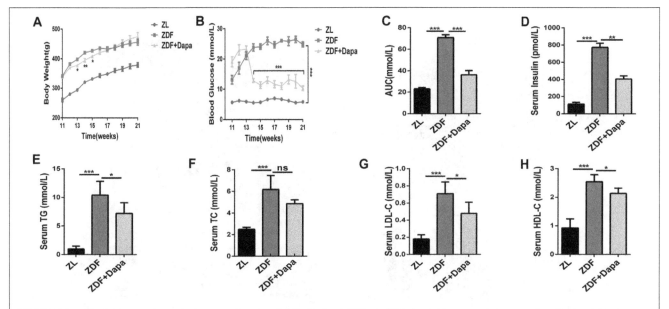

FIGURE 1 | Dapagliflozin improves glucose intolerance and regulates lipid metabolism in ZDF rats. **(A)** Body weight was recorded every week and body weight gain was measured at the end of the 21st week. **(B)** Blood glucose levels were monitored throughout the entire experiment. **(C)** The area under the curve (AUC) of blood glucose was calculated by the trapezoidal method. **(D)** Serum insulin levels were evaluated in groups. **(E–H)** Serum levels of TG, TC, LDL-C, and HDL-C were evaluated in groups. ZL: ZL rats as a normal control, ZDF: ZDF rats fed with a high-fat diet, ZDF + Dapa: dapagliflozin-treated ZDF rats. Data are expressed as the means ± SEM of five animals per group. *$p < 0.05$, **$p < 0.01$, and ***$p < 0.001$ compared with the ZDF rat group.

incubated with primary antibodies (1:200) against LC3B, Beclin1, p62, and SGLT-2 at 4°C overnight, followed by incubation with the secondary antibody. Then the sections were stained with a 3,3′-diaminobenzidine solution for 3 min and counterstained with Mayer's hematoxylin. Photomicrographs were captured under an optical microscope at 400 × magnification. Image-Pro Plus 6.0 software was used to select the same brown-yellow color as the unified standard for judging the positiveness of all photos, and analyze each photo to get the cumulative optical density value (IOD) of each photo and the pixel area of to be tested (AREA). The area density value (IOD/AREA) was obtained, and a larger value corresponded to a higher positive expression level.

Statistical Analysis

The results are expressed as the mean ± SEM. Comparisons between two groups were assessed using a *t*-test. Statistical analyses were performed using SPSS 20.0 statistical software and GraphPad Prism 6.02. Statistical significance was defined as a *p* value of <0.05.

RESULTS

Dapagliflozin Improves Glucose Intolerance and Regulates Lipid Metabolism in ZDF Rats

The ZDF rat is a recognized T2DM animal model characterized with overweight, impaired glucose tolerance and hyperlipidemia due to the leptin receptor mutation (Al-awar et al., 2016). To confirm the influence of dapagliflozin on the metabolic phenotypes

of ZDF rats *in vivo*, body weight and blood glucose were weekly assessed in different groups. As shown in **Figure 1A**, the body weight of ZDF rats was significantly higher than that of ZL rats from 11 to 21 weeks. In the first three weeks after the administration of dapagliflozin, the body weight of ZDF rats began to decrease significantly compared to that of the ZDF rats without treatments. At the end of the experiment, the body weights of the ZDF + Dapa and ZDF groups showed no significant difference. In addition, the blood glucose level in the treatment group was dramatically reduced throughout the entire experiment (**Figure 1B**). To investigate the effect of dapagliflozin on glucose tolerance, OGTTs were performed on all animals without anesthesia after an overnight fast. As demonstrated in **Figure 1C**, the AUC revealed that the ZL group was tolerant of glucose, while the rats in ZDF group had an impaired tolerance to glucose. However, the impaired glucose tolerance was significantly improved after dapagliflozin administration. In addition, dapagliflozin treatment also improved whole body insulin sensitivity in this ZDF rat model as reflected by a significant reduction in plasma insulin concentrations (**Figure 1D**).

To evaluate the effect of dapagliflozin on lipid metabolism, serum lipid profiles including total cholesterol (TC), triglyceride (TG), low-density lipoprotein cholesterol (LDL-C) and high-density lipoprotein cholesterol (HDL-C) levels were tested in groups. Compared with the ZL rats, the ZDF rats exhibited markedly increased serum levels of TC, TG and LDL-C, indicating an impaired lipid metabolism. Compared with the ZDF rats, the ZDF rats with the dapagliflozin treatments showed significant decrease in the abnormally elevated serum TG and LDL-C levels, although the TC levels were not statistically impacted by the dapagliflozin intervention (**Figures 1E–H**).

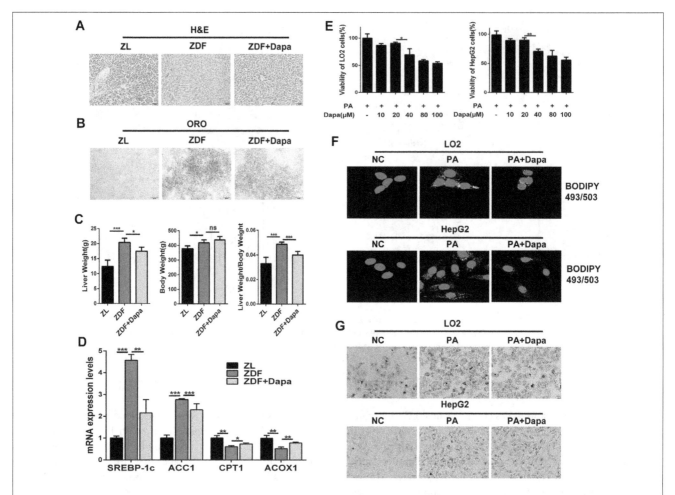

FIGURE 2 | Dapagliflozin alleviates hepatic lipid accumulation in ZDF rats and PA-stimulated LO2 and HepG2 cells. **(A, B)** Liver sections were stained with H&E (Scale bars: 50 μm)and Oil Red O (Scale bars: 20 μm). **(C)** Liver/body weight ratio was calculated by liver weight (g)/body weight (g). **(D)** The mRNA expression levels of hepatic lipogenic genes ACC1, SREBP-1c, and fatty acid oxidation genes CPT1 and ACOX1 were examined by real-time q-PCR **(E)** CCK-8 assays indicate the effect of dapagliflozin (10, 20, 40, 80, and 100 μmol/L) on the viability of HepG2 cells and LO2 cells. **(F)** HepG2 cells and LO2 cells were stained with 1 μg/ml BODIPY 493/503 and fluorescence images were captured by a confocal microscope. **(G)** LO2 and HepG2 cells were stained with Oil Red O. Scale bars: 20 μm. Data are expressed as the means ± SEM from three independent experiments. *$p < 0.05$, **$p < 0.01$, and ***$p < 0.001$.

Dapagliflozin Alleviates Hepatic Lipid Accumulation in ZDF Rats and PA-Stimulated LO2 and HepG2 Cells

To determine whether dapagliflozin alleviated hepatic lipid accumulation *in vivo*, the liver/body weight ratio and hepatic lipid accumulation in hepatic histology were evaluated in groups. The histological observation of H&E and Oil Red O staining indicated that dapagliflozin administration apparently alleviated hepatic steatosis through reducing the fatty degeneration of hepatocytes and intracellular lipid droplet formation (**Figures 2A,B**). As shown in **Figure 2C**, significant differences in body weight were not observed between the ZDF rats with or without dapagliflozin treatment, but the liver weight and the liver/body weight ratio were dramatically reduced in comparison with those of the ZDF group. Moreover, dapagliflozin treatment downregulated the expression of several hepatic lipogenic genes including ACC1 and SREBP-1c, and

upregulated genes related to fatty acid oxidation, such as CPT1 and ACOX1 (**Figure 2D**).

Next, we examined the effect of dapagliflozin on lipid accumulation in LO2 and HepG2 cells. Prior to testing the effect of dapagliflozin in cells *in vitro*, a CCK-8 assay was performed to evaluate the cytotoxic effects of dapagliflozin on hepatic cells, and the results showed that dapagliflozin had a limited effect on the viability of LO2 cells and HepG2 cells, even at a concentration up to 20 μmol/L (**Figure 2E**). As shown in **Figure 2F**, the fluorescence intensity of BODIPY 493/503-stained lipid droplets was decreased after dapagliflozin administration in cells. To further confirm the lipid clearance effects of dapagliflozin in hepatic cells, we stained lipid droplets with Oil Red O (ORO). Exposure to 0.3 mM PA for 24 h dramatically increased the intracellular lipid accumulation in LO2 cells and HepG2 cells, whereas cotreatment with dapagliflozin could obviously attenuate the PA-induced lipid accumulation in both of hepatic cell lines (**Figure 2G**). Taken together, these findings indicated that dapagliflozin prevented

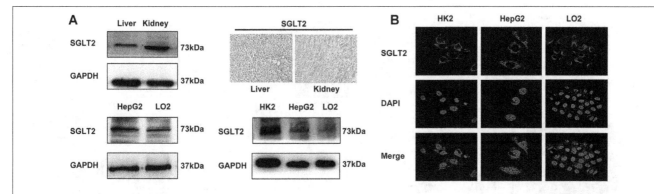

FIGURE 3 | Expression of SGLT2 in rat liver and LO2 and HepG2 cells. **(A)** Western blot analysis and IHC staining demonstrate the protein expression level of SGLT2 in rat liver and kidney tissues. **(B)** Western blot analysis and immunofluorescence staining show the expression of SGLT2 in human hepatic cell lines.

against hepatic lipid deposition in ZDF rats and PA-stimulated hepatic cells.

Expression of SGLT2 in Rat Liver, LO2 Cells and HepG2 Cells

To determine whether dapagliflozin exerted its effects by targeting on SGLT2, we investigated the expression of SGLT2 in LO2, HepG2, HK2 cells, and animal tissues by Western blot, immunofluorescence and immunohistochemistry analyses. As shown in **Figure 3A**, the Western blot analysis showed a band in the liver with the same molecular weight as that in the kidney, which indicates the expression of SGLT2 in rat liver. Immunohistochemical staining also confirmed the expression of SGLT2 predominantly on the cell membrane in both kidney and liver tissues. In addition, immunofluorescence staining and Western blot analysis indicated the expression of SGLT2 in LO2 cells and HepG2 cells (**Figure 3B**).

Dapagliflozin Induces Autophagy and Regulates Fatty Acid Metabolism in ZDF Rats and PA-Stimulated LO2 and HepG2 Cells

We examined the autophagic alterations in the rat liver and compared the effects with PA-stimulated LO2 and HepG2 cells. Detection of autophagy and the expression of autophagy-related genes were evaluated by Western blot analysis and immunohistochemistry (IHC) in the liver tissue of each group. Immunohistochemical staining showed that dapagliflozin administration significantly increased the expression of LC3B and Beclin1, but decreased that of p62 in the liver of ZDF rats (**Figure 4A**). As shown in **Figure 4B**, dapagliflozin significantly upregulated the levels of LC3B-II and Beclin1 and decreased the levels of p62 compared with the ZDF group. In addition, the administration of dapagliflozin increased ACC1 phosphorylation and significantly upregulated fatty acid oxidation gene ACOX1 (**Figure 4C**). These data suggested that dapagliflozin induced autophagy and improved cellular lipid metabolism in ZDF rats.

Moreover, the effects of dapagliflozin on the LC3B expression in PA-induced hepatocytes were detected by immunofluorescence staining and Western blot assays. Administration of dapagliflozin

dramatically increased the expression of LC3B, as indicated by the enhanced fluorescence intensity (**Figures 4D,E**). Consistently, the Western blot assays demonstrated that dapagliflozin increased the expression of LC3B-II and Beclin1, and inhibited the expression of p62, which strongly indicated the enhancement of autophagy (**Figures 4F,G**). Similar outcomes on ACC1 phosphorylation and ACOX1 protein expression were also observed after dapagliflozin administration in PA-stimulated LO2 cells and HepG2 cells (**Figures 4H,I**). To assess the influence of dapagliflozin on autophagy, we pharmacologically blocked autophagosome-lysosome fusion using chloroquine diphosphate (CQ, 20 μmol/L), a lysosomal inhibitor. As shown in (**Figures 4J,K**), cotreatment with CQ abolished the effect of dapagliflozin on reducing lipid accumulation, indicating that involvement of autophagy in dapagliflozin alleviated hepatic lipid accumulation.

Dapagliflozin Induces Autophagy via the AMPK-mTOR Pathway *in vitro* and *in vivo*

To test whether autophagy is activated via the AMPK-mTOR pathway, the protein expression of AMPK and mTOR was examined *in vitro* and *in vivo*. As shown in **Figures 5A–C**, the p-AMPK/AMPK ratio was elevated in dapagliflozin-treated ZDF rats or hepatocytes, while the p-mTOR/mTOR ratio was significantly reduced. Then, to determine the association of AMPK activation with dapagliflozin-induced autophagy, AMPK inhibitor compound C (Comp C) was used to block AMPK phosphorylation in hepatic cells. Treatment with Comp C reversed the effect of dapagliflozin on cellular lipid deposition, indicating the involvement of the AMPK pathway in dapagliflozin-mediated protection against hepatic steatosis (**Figures 5D,E**).

DISCUSSION

NAFLD is a burgeoning health problem worldwide and has become a significant risk factor for both hepatic and cardiometabolic mortality (Al-awar et al., 2016). However, effective drugs approved for the treatment of NAFLD are still lacking. SGLT2 inhibitors are listed as a new class of oral anti-hyperglycaemic medications for the pharmacological management of T2DM (Chaudhury et al., 2017).

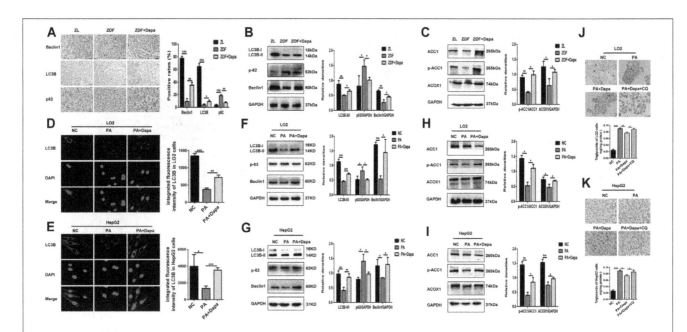

FIGURE 4 | Dapagliflozin induces autophagy and regulates fatty acid metabolism in ZDF rats and PA-stimulated LO2 and HepG2 cells. **(A)** IHC staining detected the expression of LC3B, Beclin-1 and p62 in hepatic tissue. Scale bars: 20 μm. Data are expressed as the means ± SEM of five animals per group. *$p <$ 0.05, **$p <$ 0.01, and ***$p <$ 0.001 compared with the ZDF rat group. **(B)** Western blot analysis evaluated the protein expression levels of LC3B, Beclin-1, and p62 in rats. **(C)** Western blot analysis detected the expression of ACC1, p-ACC1, and ACOX1 in the livers of rats. **(D, E)** LC3B immunofluorescence staining showed the endogenous LC3B level of LO2 and HepG2 cells. **(F, G)** Western blot analysis demonstrated the expression of LC3B, Beclin-1, and p62 in LO2 and HepG2 cells. **(H, I)** Western blot analysis detected the protein expression of ACC1, p-ACC1 and ACOX1 in cells. **(J, K)** LO2 and HepG2 cells were treated with 0.3 mM PA, 20 μM dapagliflozin and 20 μM chloroquine (CQ) for 24 h. The cells were stained with Oil Red O and intracellular TG was quantitatively analyzed. Scale bars: 20 μm. Data are expressed as the means ± SEM from three independent experiments. *$p <$ 0.05, **$p <$ 0.01, and ***$p <$ 0.001.

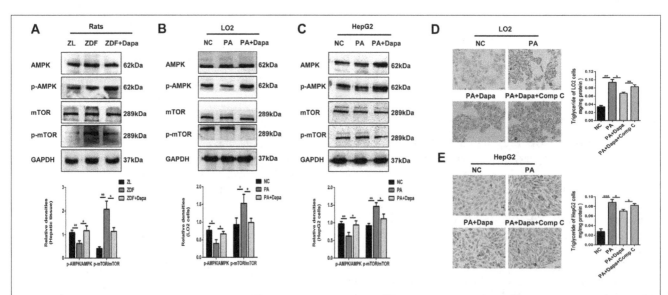

FIGURE 5 | Dapagliflozin induces autophagy via the AMPK-mTOR pathway *in vitro* and *in vivo*. **(A–C)** Western blot analysis evaluated the protein expression levels of p-AMPK, AMPK, p-mTOR, and mTOR in rats and cells. **(D, E)** LO2 and HepG2 cells were treated with 0.3 mM PA, 20 μM dapagliflozin and 10 μM compound C (Comp C) for 24 h. The cells were stained with Oil Red O and intracellular TG was quantitatively analyzed. Scale bars: 20 μm. Data are expressed as the means ± SEM from three independent experiments. *$p <$ 0.05, **$p <$ 0.01, and ***$p <$ 0.001.

A single-center retrospective observational study indicated that dapagliflozin and empagliflozin could improve the metabolic and hepatic disorders (Lee et al., 2018). Thus, it is of great significance to explore the underlying specific mechanisms of SGLT2 inhibitors in alleviating the diet-induced metabolic dysfunction and NAFLD. In the present study, we report a beneficial effect of dapagliflozin in

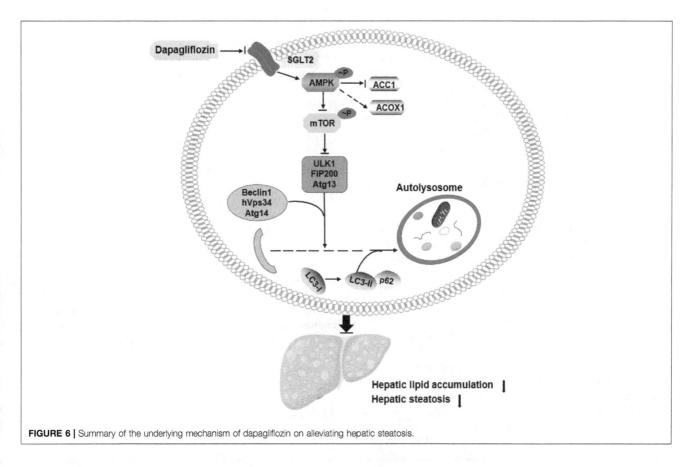

FIGURE 6 | Summary of the underlying mechanism of dapagliflozin on alleviating hepatic steatosis.

ameliorating hepatic steatosis by modulating AMPK-mediated autophagic activation. We observed for the first time that the dapagliflozin alleviated lipid accumulation and lipotoxicity, accompanied by induced autophagy in ZDF rats and PA-induced human hepatic cells, indicating that the antihepatosteatotic effects of dapagliflozin might be independent of its hypoglycaemic activities.

Previous studies have demonstrated that the excessive lipid accumulation can lead to cellular injury and death (Czaja, 2016; Li et al., 2020). In this study, we focused on the effects of dapagliflozin on hepatic steatosis and explored the relevant mechanism using hepatic cells and ZDF rats with obesity, NAFLD and metabolic dysfunction. Both LO2 cells and HepG2 cells were used to study the effects of dapagliflozin with the presence of PA. Our data showed that continuous intervention with dapagliflozin attenuated liver weight, lipotoxicity, dyslipidaemia, impaired glucose tolerance and hepatic lipid deposition in ZDF rats. Meanwhile, BODIPY 493/503 and ORO staining indicated that dapagliflozin prevented against intracellular lipid accumulation in PA-stimulated LO2 cells and HepG2 cells.

SGLT2 is a sodium-glucose transporter that is mainly expressed in the proximal convoluted tubules of the kidney, and its ubiquitous expression has also been detected in other human tissues (Uthman et al., 2018). Some studies have demonstrated that the protein expression of SGLT2 could be detected in the immortalized human primary hepatocytes HuS-E/2 cells, human hepatocellular carcinoma HepG2 cells and mouse hepatic tissue (Hawley et al., 2016; Kaji et al., 2018; Chiang et al., 2020). However, the SGLTs

family consists of 12 members, and the expression of these proteins in extrarenal tissues is controversial due to the lack of specific antibodies (Wright et al., 2011). In this study, we demonstrated the expression of SGLT2 in hepatic cell lines and rat liver tissues.

Autophagy is a pathway of lysosome degradation that can ameliorate the state of insulin resistance by regulating cellular lipid metabolism (Amir and Czaja., 2011). Currently, emerging evidence suggests that autophagy may be associated with the pathological and physiological changes of NAFLD (Park and Lee., 2014). Autophagy has been reported to delay the progression of NAFLD and protects against liver injury by decreasing hepatocyte lipid accumulation (Czaja, 2016). However, previous studies have not reported on the role of SGLT2 inhibitors in inducing autophagy and reducing hepatic lipid accumulation by directly targeting hepatocytes. Our data strongly suggest that dapagliflozin administration reduces the intracellular lipid accumulation and activates the autophagy machinery because increased autophagy markers (LC3B and Beclin1 protein levels), and decreased p62 levels were found *in vitro* and *in vivo*. Most importantly, this improvement effect was abolished by incubation with CQ, a lysosomal function inhibitor, suggesting the involvement of autophagy activation in dapagliflozin-mediated hypolipidaemic effects. Hepatic lipid accumulation is caused in part by increased intracellular *de novo* lipogenesis, in which the ACC1 enzyme catalyzes the first rate-controlling step (Goedeke et al., 2018; Ipsen et al., 2018). Specific knockout of ACC1 reduced *de novo* lipogenesis in hepatocytes and lipid accumulation in the liver of mice (Mao et al., 2006). ACOX1 is the rate-limiting enzyme in peroxisomal fatty acid oxidation (Xiao et al., 2020), and the deficiency of ACOX1 leads to hepatic lipid accumulation, inflammation and fibrosis (Ipsen et al., 2018). Thus, reducing *de novo* lipogenesis or increasing fatty acid oxidation will improve hepatic lipid accumulation. In this study, we demonstrated that dapagliflozin phosphorylated and inactivated ACC1 and increased the expression of ACOX1, which helped to alleviate cellular lipid accumulation *in vitro* and *in vivo*.

AMPK is a crucial metabolic regulator that not only inhibits energy-consuming pathways but also activates the energy-compensating process (Ha et al., 2015). Evidence shows that AMPK plays a critical role in autophagy induction in response to various cellular stresses, such as glucose starvation (Vingtdeux et al., 2010). In the liver, AMPK activation regulates metabolism by increasing catabolic pathways, such as autophagy (Alers et al., 2012) and fatty acid oxidation (Fernandez-Galilea et al., 2014), and decreasing anabolic pathways such as lipid synthesis (Zhou et al., 2001). In addition, mTOR, a downstream target of AMPK, negatively regulates autophagy activity (Kim et al., 2011). Our study demonstrated that dapagliflozin could increase the phosphorylation of AMPK, while suppressing the phosphorylation of mTOR in dapagliflozin-treated ZDF rats and cultured hepatic cells. Meanwhile this phenomenon was reversed by the AMPK specific inhibitor compound C, which strongly suggests that the effects of dapagliflozin on the amelioration in hepatic steatosis are directly mediated through AMPK activation. In addition, these results also illustrate that the AMPK-mTOR pathway plays an important role in the activation of autophagy in steatotic hepatic cells.

In summary, we demonstrated that dapagliflozin ameliorates hepatic steatosis by decreasing the *de novo* lipogenesis enzyme ACC1, increasing the fatty acid oxidation enzyme ACOX1 and inducing autophagy. These beneficial effects seem to be in part mediated through AMPK activation (**Figure 6**). In addition, our data indicate that dapagliflozin induces autophagy via the AMPK-mTOR pathway. Importantly, our findings suggest an important mechanism for the positive effects of dapagliflozin on alleviating hepatic steatosis and provide evidence for the novel clinical usage of dapagliflozin in NAFLD by targeting intracellular autophagy in hepatic cells.

ETHICS STATEMENT

The animal study was reviewed and approved by the Institutional Animal Care and Use Committee of Southern Medical University (Guangzhou, China).

AUTHOR CONTRIBUTIONS

YC, LY, and RZ led the study design and prepared the manuscript. LL and QL carried out the experiments. WH, YH and MA assisted in tissue sample collection. HT and QX performed data analysis and interpretation. All authors read and approved the final manuscript.

FUNDING

This work was supported by the National Natural Science Foundation of China (Grant No. 81500679), Science and Technology Plan of Guangdong Province (Grant No. 2017A020215045), the Science and Technology Plan Project of Guangzhou (Grant No. 202102020165) and Clinical Research Startup Program of Southern Medical University by High-level University Construction Funding of Guangdong Provincial Department of Education (Grant No. LC2016YM007).

REFERENCES

Adams, L. A., Anstee, Q. M., Tilg, H., and Targher, G. (2017). Non-alcoholic Fatty Liver Disease and its Relationship with Cardiovascular Disease and Other Extrahepatic Diseases. *Gut* 66, 1138–1153. doi:10.1136/gutjnl-2017-313884

Al-awar, A., Kupai, K., Veszelka, M., Szűcs, G., Attieh, Z., Murlasits, Z., et al. (2016). Experimental Diabetes Mellitus in Different Animal Models. *J. Diabetes Res.* 2016, 1–12. doi:10.1155/2016/9051426

Alers, S., Loffler, A. S., Wesselborg, S., and Stork, B. (2012). Role of AMPK-mTOR-Ulk1/2 in the Regulation of Autophagy: Cross Talk, Shortcuts, and Feedbacks. *Mol. Cell Biol.* 32, 2–11. doi:10.1128/MCB.06159-11

Amir, M., and Czaja, M. J. (2011). Autophagy in Nonalcoholic Steatohepatitis. *Expert Rev. Gastroenterol. Hepatol.* 5, 159–166. doi:10.1586/egh.11.4

Angulo, P. (2002). Nonalcoholic Fatty Liver Disease. *N. Engl. J. Med.* 346, 1221–1231. doi:10.1056/NEJMra011775

Bril, F., and Cusi, K. (2016). Nonalcoholic Fatty Liver Disease. *Endocrinol. Metab. Clin. North America* 45, 765–781. doi:10.1016/j.ecl.2016.06.005

Brownsey, R. W., Zhande, R., and Boone, A. N. (1997). Isoforms of Acetyl-CoA Carboxylase: Structures, Regulatory Properties and Metabolic Functions. *Biochem. Soc. Trans.* 25, 1232–1238. doi:10.1042/bst0251232

Chaudhury, A., Duvoor, C., Reddy Dendi, V. S., Kraleti, S., Chada, A., Ravilla, R., et al. (2017). Clinical Review of Antidiabetic Drugs: Implications for Type 2 Diabetes Mellitus Management. *Front. Endocrinol.* 8, 6. doi:10.3389/fendo.2017.00006

Chiang, H., Lee, J. C., Huang, H. C., Huang, H., Liu, H. K., and Huang, C. (2020). Delayed Intervention with a Novel SGLT2 Inhibitor NGI001 Suppresses Diet-induced Metabolic Dysfunction and Non-alcoholic Fatty Liver Disease in Mice. *Br. J. Pharmacol.* 177, 239–253. doi:10.1111/bph.14859

Czaja, M. J. (2016). Function of Autophagy in Nonalcoholic Fatty Liver Disease. *Dig. Dis. Sci.* 61, 1304–1313. doi:10.1007/s10620-015-4025-x

Dhillon, S. (2019). Dapagliflozin: A Review in Type 2 Diabetes. *Drugs* 79, 1135–1146. doi:10.1007/s40265-019-01148-3

Fernández-Galilea, M., Pérez-Matute, P., Prieto-Hontoria, P. L., Sáinz, N., López-Yoldi, M., Houssier, M., et al. (2014). α-Lipoic Acid Reduces Fatty Acid Esterification and Lipogenesis in Adipocytes from Overweight/obese Subjects. *Obesity* 22, 2210–2215. doi:10.1002/oby.20846

Goedeke, L., Bates, J., Vatner, D. F., Perry, R. J., Wang, T., Ramirez, R., et al. (2018). Acetyl-CoA Carboxylase Inhibition Reverses NAFLD and Hepatic Insulin Resistance but Promotes Hypertriglyceridemia in Rodents. *Hepatology* 68, 2197–2211. doi:10.1002/hep.30097

Ha, J., Guan, K.-L., and Kim, J. (2015). AMPK and Autophagy in Glucose/glycogen Metabolism. *Mol. Aspects Med.* 46, 46–62. doi:10.1016/j.mam.2015.08.002

Hawley, S. A., Ford, R. J., Smith, B. K., Gowans, G. J., Mancini, S. J., Pitt, R. D., et al. (2016). The Na+/Glucose Cotransporter Inhibitor Canagliflozin Activates AMPK by Inhibiting Mitochondrial Function and Increasing Cellular AMP Levels. *Diabetes* 65, 2784–2794. doi:10.2337/db16-0058

Ipsen, D. H., Lykkesfeldt, J., and Tveden-Nyborg, P. (2018). Molecular Mechanisms of Hepatic Lipid Accumulation in Non-alcoholic Fatty Liver Disease. *Cell. Mol. Life Sci.* 75, 3313–3327. doi:10.1007/s00018-018-2860-6

Kaji, K., Nishimura, N., Seki, K., Sato, S., Saikawa, S., Nakanishi, K., et al. (2018). Sodium Glucose Cotransporter 2 Inhibitor Canagliflozin Attenuates Liver Cancer Cell Growth and Angiogenic Activity by Inhibiting Glucose Uptake. *Int. J. Cancer* 142, 1712–1722. doi:10.1002/ijc.31193

Kim, J., Kundu, M., Viollet, B., and Guan, K.-L. (2011). AMPK and mTOR Regulate Autophagy through Direct Phosphorylation of Ulk1. *Nat. Cel Biol.* 13, 132–141. doi:10.1038/ncb2152

Kim, Y. C., and Guan, K.-L. (2015). mTOR: a Pharmacologic Target for Autophagy Regulation. *J. Clin. Invest.* 125, 25–32. doi:10.1172/JCI73939

Kurinami, N., Sugiyama, S., Yoshida, A., Hieshima, K., Miyamoto, F., Kajiwara, K., et al. (2018). Dapagliflozin Significantly Reduced Liver Fat Accumulation Associated with a Decrease in Abdominal Subcutaneous Fat in Patients with Inadequately Controlled Type 2 Diabetes Mellitus. *Diabetes Res. Clin. Pract.* 142, 254–263. doi:10.1016/j.diabres.2018.05.017

Lee, P. C. H., Gu, Y., Yeung, M. Y., Fong, C. H. Y., Woo, Y. C., Chow, W. S., et al. (2018). Dapagliflozin and Empagliflozin Ameliorate Hepatic Dysfunction Among Chinese Subjects with Diabetes in Part through Glycemic Improvement: A Single-Center, Retrospective, Observational Study. *Diabetes Ther.* 9, 285–295. doi:10.1007/s13300-017-0355-3

Li, Y., Zhang, Y., Ji, G., Shen, Y., Zhao, N., Liang, Y., et al. (2020). Autophagy Triggered by Oxidative Stress Appears to Be Mediated by the AKT/mTOR Signaling Pathway in the Liver of Sleep-Deprived Rats. *Oxidative Med. Cell Longevity* 2020, 1–11. doi:10.1155/2020/6181630

Lu, Y., Jiang, Z., Dai, H., Miao, R., Shu, J., Gu, H., et al. (2018). Hepatic Leukocyte Immunoglobulin-like Receptor B4 (LILRB4) Attenuates Nonalcoholic Fatty Liver Disease via SHP1-TRAF6 Pathway. *Hepatology* 67, 1303–1319. doi:10.1002/hep.29633

Madiraju, A. K., Alves, T., Zhao, X., Cline, G. W., Zhang, D., Bhanot, S., et al. (2016). Argininosuccinate Synthetase Regulates Hepatic AMPK Linking Protein Catabolism and Ureagenesis to Hepatic Lipid Metabolism. *Proc. Natl. Acad. Sci. USA* 113, E3423–E3430. doi:10.1073/pnas.1606022113

Mao, J., DeMayo, F. J., Li, H., Abu-Elheiga, L., Gu, Z., Shaikenov, T. E., et al. (2006). Liver-specific Deletion of Acetyl-CoA Carboxylase 1 Reduces Hepatic Triglyceride Accumulation without Affecting Glucose Homeostasis. *Proc. Natl. Acad. Sci.* 103, 8552–8557. doi:10.1073/pnas.0603115103

Moreno-Fernandez, M. E., Giles, D. A., Stankiewicz, T. E., Sheridan, R., Karns, R., Cappelletti, M., et al. (2018). Peroxisomal β-oxidation Regulates Whole Body Metabolism, Inflammatory Vigor, and Pathogenesis of Nonalcoholic Fatty Liver Disease. *JCI Insight* 3. doi:10.1172/jci.insight.93626

Park, H.-W., and Lee, J. H. (2014). Calcium Channel Blockers as Potential Therapeutics for Obesity-Associated Autophagy Defects and Fatty Liver Pathologies. *Autophagy* 10, 2385–2386. doi:10.4161/15548627.2014.984268

Sheridan, R., Lampe, K., Shanmukhappa, S. K., Putnam, P., Keddache, M., Divanovic, S., et al. (2011). Lampe1: an ENU-Germline Mutation Causing Spontaneous Hepatosteatosis Identified through Targeted Exon-Enrichment and Next-Generation Sequencing. *Plos One* 6, e21979. doi:10.1371/journal.pone.0021979

Shimizu, M., Suzuki, K., Kato, K., Jojima, T., Iijima, T., Murohisa, T., et al. (2019). Evaluation of the Effects of Dapagliflozin, a Sodium-Glucose Co-transporter-2 Inhibitor, on Hepatic Steatosis and Fibrosis Using Transient Elastography in Patients with Type 2 Diabetes and Non-alcoholic Fatty Liver Disease. *Diabetes Obes. Metab.* 21, 285–292. doi:10.1111/dom.13520

Tang, Y., Lu, Y., Chen, Y., Luo, L., Cai, L., Peng, B., et al. (2019). Pre-metastatic Niche Triggers SDF-1/CXCR4 axis and Promotes Organ Colonisation by Hepatocellular Circulating Tumour Cells via Downregulation of Prrx1. *J. Exp. Clin. Cancer Res.* 38, 473. doi:10.1186/s13046-019-1475-6

Uthman, L., Baartscheer, A., Schumacher, C. A., Fiolet, J. W. T., Kuschma, M. C.,

Hollmann, M. W., et al. (2018). Direct Cardiac Actions of Sodium Glucose Cotransporter 2 Inhibitors Target Pathogenic Mechanisms Underlying Heart Failure in Diabetic Patients. *Front. Physiol.* 9. doi:10.3389/fphys.2018.01575

Vingtdeux, V., Giliberto, L., Zhao, H., Chandakkar, P., Wu, Q., Simon, J. E., et al. (2010). AMP-activated Protein Kinase Signaling Activation by Resveratrol Modulates Amyloid-β Peptide Metabolism*. *J. Biol. Chem.* 285, 9100–9113. doi:10.1074/jbc.M109.060061

Wright, E. M., Loo, D. D. F., and Hirayama, B. A. (2011). Biology of Human Sodium Glucose Transporters. *Physiol. Rev.* 91, 733–794. doi:10.1152/physrev.00055.2009

Xiao, Z., Chu, Y., and Qin, W. (2020). IGFBP5 Modulates Lipid Metabolism and Insulin Sensitivity through Activating AMPK Pathway in Non-alcoholic Fatty Liver Disease. *Life Sci.* 256, 117997. doi:10.1016/j.lfs.2020.117997

You, M., Matsumoto, M., Pacold, C. M., Cho, W. K., and Crabb, D. W. (2004). The Role of AMP-Activated Protein Kinase in the Action of Ethanol in the Liver. *Gastroenterology* 127, 1798–1808. doi:10.1053/j.gastro.2004.09.049

Zhou, G., Myers, R., Li, Y., Chen, Y., Shen, X., Fenyk-Melody, J., et al. (2001). Role of AMP-Activated Protein Kinase in Mechanism of Metformin Action. *J. Clin. Invest.* 108, 1167–1174. doi:10.1172/JCI13505

3

T Lymphocyte-Mediated Liver Immunopathology of Schistosomiasis

Bing Zheng[1,2], Jianqiang Zhang[1], Hui Chen[1], Hao Nie[1,2], Heather Miller[3], Quan Gong[1,2*] and Chaohong Liu[4*]

[1] Department of Immunology, School of Medicine, Yangtze University, Jingzhou, China, [2] Clinical Molecular Immunology Center, School of Medicine, Yangtze University, Jingzhou, China, [3] Department of Intracellular Pathogens, National Institute of Allergy and Infectious Diseases, Bethesda, MD, United States, [4] Department of Pathogen Biology, School of Basic Medicine, Tongji Medical College, Huazhong University of Science & Technology, Wuhan, China

*Correspondence:
Quan Gong
gongquan1998@163.com
Chaohong Liu
chaohongliu80@126.com

The parasitic worms, *Schistosoma mansoni* and *Schistosoma japonicum*, reside in the mesenteric veins, where they release eggs that induce a dramatic granulomatous response in the liver and intestines. Subsequently, infection may further develop into significant fibrosis and portal hypertension. Over the past several years, uncovering the mechanism of immunopathology in schistosomiasis has become a major research objective. It is known that T lymphocytes, especially $CD4^+$ T cells, are essential for immune responses against *Schistosoma* species. However, obtaining a clear understanding of how T lymphocytes regulate the pathological process is proving to be a daunting challenge. To date, $CD4^+$ T cell subsets have been classified into several distinct T helper (Th) phenotypes including Th1, Th2, Th17, T follicular helper cells (Tfh), Th9, and regulatory T cells (Tregs). In the case of schistosomiasis, the granulomatous inflammation and the chronic liver pathology are critically regulated by the Th1/Th2 responses. Animal studies suggest that there is a moderate Th1 response to parasite antigens during the acute stage, but then, egg-derived antigens induce a sustained and dominant Th2 response that mediates granuloma formation and liver fibrosis. In addition, the newly discovered Th17 cells also play a critical role in the hepatic immunopathology of schistosomiasis. Within the liver, Tregs are recruited to hepatic granulomas and exert an immunosuppressive role to limit the granulomatous inflammation and fibrosis. Moreover, recent studies have shown that Tfh and Th9 cells might also promote liver granulomas and fibrogenesis in the murine schistosomiasis. Thus, during infection, T-cell subsets undergo complicated cross-talk with antigen presenting cells that then defines their various roles in the local microenvironment for regulating the pathological progression of schistosomiasis. This current review summarizes a vast body of literature to elucidate the contribution of T lymphocytes and their associated cytokines in the immunopathology of schistosomiasis.

Keywords: T lymphocyte, schistosomiasis, immunopathology, liver fibrosis, soluble egg antigen

INTRODUCTION

Human schistosomiasis is a zoonotic parasitic disease caused by schistosomes, which are digenetic trematodes. In nature, many species of *Schistosoma* exist, but the main human pathogens are *Schistosoma japonicum*, *Schistosoma mansoni*, and *Schistosoma haematobium*. There is an estimate of more than 230 million people in tropical countries around the world infected with *Schistosoma* species (1). Infection occurs when cercariae, the free-living larval form of schistosomes, are released from freshwater snails and penetrate a human host's skin, where they may remain in the host epidermis for ~72 h (2). Then, cercariae transform into schistosomula, the parasitic larvae form that enter the vasculature and travel via the pulmonary artery to the lungs, which they are then referred to as lung schistosomula (3). After exiting the lungs, schistosomula re-enter the venous circulation and finally migrate to the perivesicular venules (*S. haematobium*) or mesenteric venules (*S. japonicum*, *S. mansoni*), where they mature into worms and form copulating pairs. Paired adult worms migrate to the intestinal venous vasculature to release their eggs. Of the fertilized eggs released by the female, a portion is discharged via emunctory routes and hatch in freshwater, releasing free-living ciliated miracidia that invade snails and continue on the life cycle. However, a large portion of *S. haematobium* eggs may become trapped in the bladder and urogenital system, while the eggs of *S. japonicum* and *S. mansoni* become lodged in the intestinal wall and liver (4). The eggs then induce a local granulomas inflammatory response. The granulomas mainly consist of lymphocytes, macrophages, and eosinophils, which contain egg proteolytic enzymes to prevent tissue damage; however, the egg-induced granuloma also leads to chronic schistosomiasis. In this review, we will focus on *S. japonicum* and *S. mansoni*, both of which have been extensively studied and have also been used in mouse models to study liver immunopathology.

The basic pathological process of schistosomiasis includes acute and chronic phases of the disease. Acute schistosomiasis (sometimes referred to as Katayama fever) occurs most often in schistosome-endemic regions to naive individuals and to those who experience heavy reinfection. The major clinical manifestation of acute schistosomiasis includes a sudden onset of fever, fatigue, urticaria, eosinophilia, and abdominal tenderness. These symptoms occur weeks to months after schistosome infection because of worm maturation, egg production, and egg antigen-induced inflammatory granulomatous response (4, 5). Chronic schistosomiasis involves immune responses to the eggs within the liver and intestine, which causes formation of granuloma (6–9). Over time, the granulomatous response is gradually downregulated, leading to the progression of relatively tolerable chronic intestinal schistosomiasis. However, some patients will develop life-threatening hepatosplenic schistosomiasis accompanied by extensive hepatic and periportal fibrosis, portal hypertension, ascites, and gastrointestinal hemorrhage.

T lymphocytes are generally classified into CD4$^+$ T helper (Th) cells and CD8$^+$ cytotoxic T lymphocytes (CTLs). Th cells are important for host humoral and cellular immune responses against parasitic infections (6). The Th cells are further classified into several distinct Th phenotypes [Th1, Th2, Th17, follicular helper T cell (Tfh), Th9, and regulatory T cells (Tregs)] according to cytokine production and specialized functions. This review focuses on the role of various Th subsets and their associated cytokines in the immunopathogenesis of schistosomiasis.

THE ROLE OF Th1/Th2 RESPONSES IN THE IMMUNOPATHOLOGY OF SCHISTOSOMIASIS

An accumulation of evidence suggests that Th cells are involved in the immunopathogenesis of schistosomiasis. In athymic nude mice or mice without Th cells resulted in decreased granuloma size after infection by schistosomes (10, 11). The role of Th1/Th2 responses in schistosomiasis has been intensely investigated and reviewed (6, 9, 12). In the acute illness, parasite antigens elicit a moderate Th1 response, which is characterized by increased levels of proinflammatory cytokines, including tumor necrosis factor alpha (TNF-α), interferon gamma (IFN-γ), interleukin-1 (IL-1), and IL-6 (13). About 5–6 weeks post-infection, the schistosomula develop into mature worms. Female worms release fertilized eggs that stimulate the immune response via their soluble egg antigens (SEAs). SEA induces resident macrophages to secrete inflammatory cytokines and chemokines that stimulate the influx of lymphocytes, neutrophils, and monocytes, which initiates circumoval granulomatous inflammation (14). A clinical study comparing acutely and chronically infected patients showed that the level of TNF-α was elevated in the plasma of acutely infected patients and their peripheral blood mononuclear cells spontaneously secreted high levels of IL-1 and IL-6 and detectable levels of IFN-γ, while chronically infected patients produced little TNF-α or IFN-γ. Thus, higher levels of IFN-γ and proinflammatory cytokines in patients with acute illness show a dominant Th1 response (15). During the acute phase, the SEA-specifically activated CD4$^+$ Th cells release the Th1-type cytokines, IL-2 and IFN-γ, which mediate the establishment of early granulomas. Immunocytochemical examination *in situ* have confirmed the presence of Th1-type cytokine-producing cells within local microenvironments of the lesion in early granuloma formation (16). Although the granulomatous response is detrimental to the liver because of subsequent progression of hepatic fibrosis, the egg-induced granuloma is beneficial to the host. If the eggs are not sequestered effectively, continuously secreted egg antigens act as a stimulus and lead to uncontrolled inflammatory responses and permanent tissue damage. For instance, IL-4-deficient mice that cannot mount a normal Th2 response develop an unchecked Th1 response and die earlier than immunity intact mice when infected by *S. mansoni* (6). Similarly, in a Tamoxifen-induced IL-4 receptor α (IL-4Rα)-deficient mouse model, interrupting IL-4Rα-mediated signaling during the acute stage decreased protective Th2 responses, leading to severe disease and premature death (17). Therefore, moderate Th1 responses are involved in the acute schistosomiasis and early granuloma formation, whereas excessive polarization toward the Th1 response is detrimental to the host. The Th1 response during the early stage of schistosomiasis is downregulated by IL-4 and IL-10. IL-10-/IL-4-deficient mice develop extremely polarized Th1-type cytokine IFN-γ responses that lead to 100% mortality during the acute illness (18).

The immune response and immunopathology of schistosomiasis are a consequence of CD4$^+$ T-cell sensitization to egg antigens. Some of the major components of egg are implicated in the Th response in schistosomiasis, including glycoprotein IPSE/α1, ω1 (19, 20), lacto-N-fucopentaose III (21), and $S.$ $mansoni$-p40 (Sm-p40) (22), of which Sm-p40 is the most abundant egg component that can induce a strong Th1-polarized response (23). IPSE/α1 induces a mixed Th1/Th2 response and promote the development of hepatic granuloma (19), while lacto-N-fucopentaose III and ω1 directly act on dendritic cells (DCs) to enhance the Th2 response (21, 24). In addition, Th1-type responses could also be induced by the schistosome vaccine candidates MAP4 (25), egg-derived r38 (22, 26), rSmLy6B, rSmTSP6, and rSmTSP7 (27), and rSjCRT (28).

Compared to the Th1 response, the Th2 response exerts anti-inflammatory effects and regulates Th1-mediated immunopathology. SEA is considered to be the key factor in driving the dramatic transition from a Th1- to a Th2-dominated response. During the Th response transition, the interaction of CD40–CD40L, CD80/86–CD28, and B7-related protein 1-inducible costimulator (ICOS) are required for egg antigen-induced Th2 responses (29–31). In correlation with the Th2 transition, the cytokine profile is changed in that IFN-γ production is decreased, whereas Th2-type cytokines IL-4, IL-5, and IL-13 are increased (32). This has been shown in lymphocytes isolated from liver granulomas at 8 weeks, which secrete IL-4 and IL-5, but not IFN-γ. The mechanism underlying this switch to Th2 response has been deeply investigated. Lymphocytes from $S.$ $mansoni$ ova-infected signal transducer and activator of transcription (STAT6)-deficient mice produce minimal levels of Th2-type cytokines and enhanced IFN-γ production, which greatly reduces the size of pulmonary and hepatic granulomas (33). IL-4 signal is critical for the development of the Th2 response and animals treated with anti-IL-4 showed decreased Th2-type IL-4, IL-5, and IL-10 and increased Th1-type IL-2 and IFN-γ (34). IL-4 is recognized as the dominant cytokine for granuloma development and injection with neutralizing antibodies against IL-4 significantly suppresses splenic cell proliferation and hepatic granulomatous inflammation (35). Nevertheless, other studies showed that infected IL-4 knockout (KO) mice still have the ability to generate egg granulomas. Surprisingly, infected IL-4Rα-deficient mice exhibit only minimal hepatic granulomas and fibrosis, even though Th2-type cytokine production is similar to infected IL-4 KO mice, which demonstrates that the IL-4R signaling pathway, rather than IL-4, may be essential for egg granulomas (36). However, another Th2-type cytokine, IL-13, is known to be involved in granulomatous inflammation and fibrosis through the IL-4Rα signaling. Blocking IL-13 has been shown to be highly effective in treating an established and ongoing $S.$ $mansoni$ infection-induced fibrosis (37, 38). These results were further confirmed by studies using schistosome-infected IL-13 and IL-4-/IL-13-deficient mice (39). Furthermore, IL-13-deficient mice exhibit increased survival time, demonstrating the important role of IL-13 in the pathogenesis of schistosomiasis. In $vitro$ studies revealed that IL-13 stimulates collagen production in fibroblasts and has a direct role in collagen homeostasis of normal human skin and keloid fibroblasts (40, 41). Overall, it is known that IL-4 and IL-13 play redundant roles in the schistosomiasis granulomatous response, but IL-13 is not dependent on profibrotic cytokines or affected by Th1/Th2 cytokines.

The source of Th2-type cytokines are not only produced by Th2 cells but also secreted by other innate lymphocytes, such as type 2 innate lymphoid cells (ILC2s). The three epithelial cell-derived cytokines, IL-33, IL-25, and thymic stromal lymphopoietin (TSLP), act as crucial initiators of Th2 responses to induce ILC2s to produce IL-13, therefore promoting Th2-type immunity (42–44). It has been reported that IL-33 treatment promotes a Th2 response together with increased liver immunopathology, and these effects are prevented by anti-IL-33 monoclonal antibodies. Furthermore, IL-33 is a requisite for IL-13-, but not IL-4, driven Th2 responses during the pathology (45). Subsequent studies have further confirmed that IL-33 is involved in initiating Th2 pathology after schistosome infection via regulating IL-13 expression in hepatic stellate cells (46) and inducing polarization of M2 macrophages (47). However, another study demonstrated an overlapping role of IL-33, IL-25, and TSLP in a schistosome-induced lung granuloma and liver fibrosis model. They showed that simultaneous disruption of IL-33, IL-25, and TSLP signaling inhibited the progression of Th2 cytokine-driven liver fibrosis but that individual disruption of each had no effect (48).

In addition to SEA-induced specific Th2 responses, parasite-derived cysteine peptidases are also responsible for Th2 responses. For instance, during acute schistosomiasis, injection of outbred mice with $S.$ $mansoni$ cathepsin B1 (SmCB1) or $S.$ $mansoni$ cathepsin L3 (SmCL3) develops a polarized Th2-type immune environment that is harmful for the development of $S.$ $mansoni$ larvae and leads to significant reduction in worm burden and liver egg counts (49). A similar study also showed the effectiveness of a cysteine-peptidase-based vaccine that protects hamsters from schistosomiasis $haematobium$ by inducing Th2 immune responses (50). Therefore, the cysteine-peptidase-based vaccine has shown great potential to be further used in non-human primates, and even in humans, through inducing protective Th2 immune responses.

Although a strong Th2 response seems detrimental to the host, a Th2 response is indispensable for the survival of the host. Th2-deficient IL-4$^{-/-}$ mice are highly susceptible to infection and develop severe acute cachexia followed by death (51). Depletion of the Th2 response against the eggs results in tissue damage and increased host mortality and liver pathology due to proinflammatory Th1-type responses (52, 53). Clinical cases also demonstrate that more severe forms of hepatosplenic schistosomiasis is linked to low levels of Th2-type IL-5 and increased Th1-type IFN-γ and TNF-α (54). Therefore, Th2 immunity acts as a double-edged sword: on the one side, it protects the host to decrease the overall pathology and prevent excessive granulomatous inflammation, but on the other side, it causes liver immunopathological damage. Thus, the Th2-response-mediated egg granuloma is a necessary evil for host survival. Therefore, maintaining the proper balance of Th1/Th2 responses is important to control the excessive pathology of schistosomiasis. Previous studies demonstrated that excessively polarized Th1- or Th2-type cytokine responses induce different but equally detrimental pathologies after infection (18). IL-4/IL-10 double-deficient mice develop highly polarized Th1-type cytokine responses, exhibited by rapid weight loss during egg production and 100% acute mortality by week 9 post-infection. In contrast, IL-12/IL-10 double-deficient mice with highly polarized Th2-type cytokine responses develop increased hepatic fibrosis and mortality during the chronic stages of infection (18). Both Th1 and Th2 phases are downregulated by endogenous IL-10, which is produced by macrophages and T cells (55). Thus, IL-10 acts as an important regulator to prevent excessive Th1 and Th2 responses during the development of schistosomiasis.

Th17/IL-17 EXACERBATE THE EGG-INDUCED LIVER IMMUNOPATHOLOGY

The first notion of Th17 cells playing a role in schistosomiasis egg-induced granuloma formation came from experiments using knockout mice unable to produce IL-23, which drives the production of IL-17 by Th17 cells. In these experiments, IL-12p40$^{-/-}$ mice, incapable of producing IL-12 or IL-23, were highly resistant to liver pathology, whereas IL-12p35$^{-/-}$ mice, able to produce IL-23 but not IL-12, developed severe granuloma lesions (56). Granuloma formation is associated with high levels of IL-17 and treatment with anti-IL-17 neutralizing antibodies significantly inhibited hepatic granulomatous inflammation (56). Therefore, the IL-17-producing CD4$^+$ T-cell population driven by IL-23 was recognized as a separate lineage and designated as Th17 cells that contribute to severe immunopathology in schistosomiasis (56, 57).

The IL-23–IL-1–IL-17 axis plays an essential role in the development of severe forms of schistosomiasis (58). A study conducted on mice lacking the IL-23-specific subunit p19 revealed an impaired liver immunopathology together with a marked decrease in IL-17 in the granulomas, but not in the draining mesenteric lymph nodes (59). Subsequent studies conducted on high pathology-prone CBA mice and low pathology-prone C57BL/6 mice identified IL-23 and IL-1, derived from DCs stimulated by live schistosome eggs, as the critical host factors that drive IL-17 production (60, 61). S. mansoni-infected CBA mice possess more IL-17-producing cells in the spleen and granulomas when compared with C57BL/6 mice (62). It was later determined that egg antigens, but not adult worm antigens, preferentially induce the generation of Th17 cells. Lowering IL-17 levels by neutralizing anti-IL-17 antibodies can increase the parasite-specific antibody levels and supply partial protection against S. japonicum infection in mice (63). In addition, anti-IL-17 antibody markedly inhibited hepatic granulomatous

inflammation and hepatocyte necrosis partly through reducing the proinflammatory cytokines/chemokines and infiltrating neutrophils (64). Similar results were obtained with S. japonicum-infected IL-17RA-deficient mice that displayed decreased granulomatous inflammation, hepatic fibrosis, improved liver function, and high survival (65). Rutitzky et al. investigated the role of IL-17 and IFN-γ in schistosomiasis immunopathology using mice lacking either one or both cytokines. They found that IL-17-deficient mice show significantly reduced immunopathology associated with the increased levels of IFN-γ, whereas IFN-γ-deficient mice displayed exacerbated immunopathology as well as increased levels of IL-17. Hence, IL-17 plays a powerful pathogenic role in severe immunopathology in murine schistosomiasis that normally is restrained by IFN-γ (66). It has also been reported that T-bet$^{-/-}$ mice have significantly increased egg-induced hepatic immunopathology, with the absence of IFN-γ and increased IL-23p19, IL-17, and TNF-α in granulomas. Thus, T-bet-dependent signaling negatively regulates Th17-mediated schistosomiasis immunopathology (67).

Recent reports found that ICOS is essential for pathogenic-induced Th17 cell development. This was discovered by Wang et al., who found that ICOSL KO mice had lower levels of Th17-associated cytokines (IL-17/IL-21), IL-13, and TGF-β1, which is correlated with improved survival rate, alleviated liver granulomatous inflammation, and hepatic fibrosis development (68). In addition, CD209a (C-type lectin receptor), expressed on DCs, also proved to be essential for the development of Th17 cell responses in murine schistosomiasis (61, 69). CD209a-deficient CBA mice had decreased Th17 responses and developed reduced egg-induced liver immunopathology (69, 70). Clinical studies also demonstrated the positive correlation between the percentage of Th17 cells and bladder pathology in S. haematobium-infected children (62).

The above findings demonstrate that Th17/IL-17 exacerbate the egg-induced liver immunopathology in schistosomiasis. However, it should be noted that a recent study found that acute schistosome infection induced a transient Th17 response to cathepsin B1 cysteine proteases secreted by the worms and that, this early, Th17 response may determine the pathogenic progression of the infection (71).

Although the role of Th17/IL-17 in schistosomiasis liver immunopathology has been defined, the source of IL-17 is not completely clear. Generally, IL-17-producing cells include Th17 cells, CTL cells, γδT cells, and natural killer T cells. Some researchers ignore the source of IL-17, and others found that Th17 cells are the major IL-17-producing cell population that contributes to pulmonary granuloma induced by S. japonicum (72). However, some studies showed that innate γδ T cells are the major IL-17-producing cells that contribute to the formation of granuloma in murine schistosomiasis (73, 74). The above discrepant findings may result from the different granuloma models. In addition, aforementioned ILC2s mediate Th2-type immunity through secreting IL-13. The ILC3s, as counterparts to Th17 cells, engage in Th17 immunity-mediated mucosal homeostasis and defense (75). However, the exact role of ILC3s has not been clarified yet in the pathology of schistosomiasis.

Thus far, numerous studies have promoted our understanding of the basic immunopathogenesis of schistosomiasis; however, it should be noted that schistosome-induced liver immunopathologies are associated with *Schistosoma* species and host. Examples of this include that the cellular composition of the *S. japonicum* egg-induced granulomas are mainly neutrophils, whereas *S. mansoni*-induced granulomas consist of a higher ratio of mononuclear cells and eosinophils, with lower numbers of neutrophils (76, 77). The differences between *S. japonicum*- and *S. mansoni*-induced hepatic granuloma could be attributed to the secreted specific leukocyte-associated chemokines at the site of inflammation (77). A host's genetic background also affects infection intensity and pathology of schistosomiasis (78, 79). Nevertheless, most researchers perform their studies using BALB/c and C57BL/6 strain mice. Actually, schistosome-infected BALB/c and C57BL/6 mice only develop mild hepatic granulomatous inflammation; however, CBA and C3H mice develop a severe pathology with larger size and poorly confined granulomas (80). As previously discussed, mouse strain-dependent schistosomiasis pathology may arise from the difference of Ag-specific Th responses (62), such as *S. mansoni*-infected CBA mice displaying exacerbated granulomatous lesions when compared to C57BL/6 mice because of high ratios of IL-17-producing cells in the granulomas (62).

Tfh PROMOTES LIVER PATHOLOGY OF SCHISTOSOMIASIS

Tfh cells are a specialized Th subset equipped to provide B cell help (81). Gene microarrays revealed that the transcriptional profile of Tfh cells is different from Th1, Th2, and Th17 cells (82). Tfh cells are mainly located in the periphery of B-cell follicles in secondary lymphoid organs and are identified by expression of various molecules, such as surface receptors CXCR5, programmed death 1 (PD-1), ICOS, the transcription factor B-cell lymphoma 6 (Bcl-6), and the cytokine IL-21 (83–85). Tfh cells were found to differentiate from Th2 cells in germinal centers responding to SEA (86). *S. japonicum* recombinant protein, SjGST-32, also has the ability to induce the formation of Tfh cells in BALB/c mice, which promotes humoral immune responses and long-lived memory B cells (87). Functional studies on Tfh cells showed that downregulation of their cellular development leads to immune deficiencies and that Tfh cells are closely associated with autoimmune and chronic inflammatory disease (85, 88). *S. mansoni* eggs induce differentiation of Tfh, which is highly dependent on Notch expression on T cells. Notch-deficient mice show impaired germinal center formation and decreased secretion of high-affinity antibodies (89). Tfh expansion and antibody production in response to schistosome infection are negatively regulated by B7-H1 (programmed death ligand 1) that is expressed on B cells (90). Immunization of B7-H1$^{-/-}$ mice with SEA leads to increased numbers of Tfh cells compared to wild-type mice (90). Recent studies have demonstrated that Tfh cells promote liver granulomas and fibrogenesis in mice infected with *S. japonicum* (91, 92). Wang et al. found that, in murine schistosomiasis, Tfh cells accumulate in the splenic germinal center and that the Tfh phenotypic molecule, Bcl-6, and the Tfh-type cytokine, IL-21, correlate with progression of liver fibrosis (92). In addition, clinical studies have shown that Tfh cells are involved in immune responses for both acute and chronic human schistosomiasis (93, 94). The frequency of circulating PD-1$^+$CXCR5$^+$CD4$^+$ Tfh cells in the peripheral blood is increased in both acute and chronic schistosomiasis patients relative to healthy controls. However, the difference between acute and chronic schistosomiasis is that there is no correlation between percentages of PD-1$^+$CXCR5$^+$CD4$^+$ Tfh cells, memory B cells, or the level of immunoglobulin G (IgG) specific to *S. japonicum* antigen in acute schistosomiasis patients; however, frequency of PD-1$^+$CXCR5$^+$CD4$^+$ Tfh cells is positively correlated to the levels of IL-21 in sera and the levels of SEA-specific antibody in chronic schistosomiasis patients (93, 94). These findings demonstrate that Tfh cells might exhibit distinct mechanisms to regulate the immune response between acute and chronic schistosomiasis. In addition, IL-4-producing Tfh cells are presumed to be important for naturally acquired resistance to schistosome reinfection (95).

Th9 CELLS AND EGG-INDUCED HEPATIC GRANULOMATOUS AND FIBROSIS

Th9 cells are another unique subset of CD4$^+$ T cells recently characterized by their production of cytokine IL-9 after activation. The specific transcription factors for Th9 cells include PU.1 and IRF-4 (96, 97). Before discovery of the Th9 cell, IL-9 was thought to be a Th2-specific cytokine. Until 2008, it was reported that IL-9 could be secreted exclusively by distinct IL-9$^+$IL-10$^+$ Th cells lacking suppressive function (98). Th9 cells have been implicated in many diseases, such as allergic inflammation, autoimmune disorders, as well as helminth infections (96, 99, 100). Zhan et al. investigated the dynamics of splenic Th9 cells and IL-9 expression in liver and serum and found that the proportion of splenic Th9 cells and levels of IL-9 were significantly higher in *S. japonicum*-infected mice compared to uninfected controls. Moreover, dynamic changes of Th9, IL-9, and PU.1 levels were consistent with hepatic egg granulomatous inflammation (101). In agreement with these studies, Li et al. additionally showed that anti-IL-9 monoclonal antibody treatment significantly inhibits *S. japonicum*-induced hepatic granulomatous and fibrosing inflammation (102). The above findings indicate that Th9 cells may be involved in immunopathogenesis in murine schistosomiasis. However, a clinical investigation showed that the level of IL-9 in serum had no significant difference between acute and chronic schistosomiasis patients (103). Therefore, further studies are needed to clarify the defining roles of Th9 cells and IL-9 in the pathology of human schistosomiasis.

Tregs REGULATE THE GRANULOMATOUS INFLAMMATION AND FIBROSIS

In 1995, Sakaguchi et al. introduced regulatory T cells to the field of immunology (104). Tregs are a separate lineage of T cells that are responsible for maintaining immunological homeostasis, suppressing potentially deleterious activities of Th cells, as well as mediating the magnitude of immunity against invading pathogens (105). It has been conceded that two main types of Tregs exist: one is termed "inducible" Tregs (iTregs), which responds to infectious challenge, and the other is termed "natural" Treg (nTregs), which is an endogenous Tregs (106). The forkhead box protein 3 (Foxp3) is a unique transcription factor that can be used to separate nTregs from iTregs that have similar regulatory properties (107). The nTregs develop from a normal process of maturation in the thymus and serve as an essential subset of T cells in the periphery. The specific markers for nTregs include CD25, the T-cell inhibitory co-receptor CTLA-4, and the glucocorticoid-inducible TNF receptor (108, 109). The iTregs originate from conventional CD4$^+$ T cells that are exposed to specific stimulatory factors, such as a cocktail of cytokines or drugs (110). Currently, the iTregs identified include IL-10-producing Tr1 cells, TGF-β-producing T helper type 3 (Th3) cells, and regulatory CD4$^+$CD25$^+$Foxp3$^-$ cells (111, 112). Both iTregs and nTregs exert suppressive/regulatory effects to restrict immune-mediated pathology.

So far, numerous studies have demonstrated that both nTregs and iTregs represent key players in the regulation of schistosomiasis pathology. During schistosome infection, Tregs suppress DC activation, mediate Th2 responses, and inhibit granuloma development and fibrosis. After infection with *S. mansoni*, the percentage of granuloma nTregs (CD4$^+$ CD25$^+$ Foxp3$^+$) has a significant increase at 8 and 16 weeks of the infection (113). Similarly, schistosome eggs show the ability to induce a significant Foxp3$^+$ Treg cell response, which suggests that SEA may be the most potent inducer for the generation of nTregs during infection (114). Except for SEA, schistosome-derived molecules, such as lysophosphatidylserine (lyso-PS), identified as the TLR2-activating molecule, can also actively induce the development of IL-10-producing Tregs (115). Although the percentage of Tregs are elevated either following infection or egg immunization, the natural ratio between nTregs and effector T cells is remarkably stable during the progress of the egg-induced inflammation, suggesting that the expansion of effector T cells maybe closely regulated by the nTregs response.

With the progression into the chronic stage of egg-induced inflammation, the phenotype of nTregs is changed so that the frequency of CD103-expressing nTregs is strongly increased. CD103 binds integrin β7 to form the complete integrin molecule αEβ7, which is an activation marker for nTregs. Thus, increasing the CD103-expressing nTregs is required for immunosuppression during chronic schistosomiasis (116). Although numerous studies have characterized nTregs during schistosome infection, the exact mechanism of how nTregs regulate immunopathology is not yet clear. To address the functional role of Tregs in schistosomiasis, many studies used the CD4 and CD25 sorting of Tregs; however, this makes it difficult to distinguish the function of either Tregs because CD4$^+$CD25$^+$ compartment includes both nTregs and iTregs. Nevertheless, Baumgart et al. established nTregs depleted mice to evaluate the role of nTregs in egg-induced inflammation. They found that

both IFN-γ and IL-4 responses were increased following immunization, demonstrating that nTregs suppress both Th1 and Th2 responses (116), which is likely not associated with IL-10 (114).

In addition to nTregs, schistosomiasis infection also induces the production of iTregs (117, 118). It has been reported that IL-10, secreted from iTregs and Th2 cells, inhibits IL-12 production by CD40 agonist-stimulated DC and iTregs, thus suppressing development of egg-specific Th1 responses during schistosomiasis (118). Furthermore, IL-10-secreting iTregs isolated from the granuloma of chronically infected mice can inhibit CD4$^+$ T-cell proliferation (118), which is different from nTregs that do not appear to control the proliferation of T cells *in vivo* (116). Therefore, it is possible that both nTregs and iTregs have the ability to suppress both Th1 and Th2 responses. To investigate the importance of Tregs for controlling schistosomiasis liver pathology, adoptive transfer purified populations of CD25-depleted CD4$^+$ T cells into RAG-deficient mice (lack of mature T or B lymphocytes) lead to increased weight loss, liver damage, and mortality following infection, suggesting a strong capacity for Tregs to suppress liver pathology (117).

WHAT ABOUT THE ROLE OF CD8$^+$ T CELLS?

The role and mechanism of CD8$^+$ T cells in the process of schistosomiasis has been a somewhat neglected area of study. Early studies conducted in the pulmonary granuloma model demonstrated that CD8$^+$ T-cell deficiency increased granuloma formation by 70%, which was attributed to CD8$^+$ T-cell inhibition of Th2 maturation (119). However, a subsequent study found that granuloma formation and hepatic granulomatous reaction were unchanged in CD8$^+$ T-cell-deficient mice (120). Another study, using major histocompatibility complex (MHC) class II or I mutant mice to examine the role of CD4$^+$ and CD8$^+$ T cells in the pathology of schistosomiasis, found that schistosome-infected MHC I mutant mice developed normal granulomatous lesions, while in contrast, MHC II mutant mice failed to form egg granuloma (121). Therefore, CD8$^+$ T cells are not likely essential for regulating the immunopathology of schistosomiasis.

INNATE $\gamma\delta$ T CELLS IN SCHISTOSOMIASIS

The previously discussed T lymphocyte, the $\alpha\beta$ T cell, has TCR composed of two glycoprotein chains, α and β, while $\gamma\delta$ T cells, another subset of lymphocytes, are CD4$^-$CD8$^-$CD3$^+$ T cells with TCR encoded by the γ and δ genes (122). Generally, $\gamma\delta$ T cells consist of $\sim$5% of the circulating peripheral blood T cells, but in some infectious diseases, the enumeration of $\gamma\delta$ T cells exceeds 30% of the peripheral blood T cells (123). During schistosomiasis, the response to schistosome antigen is primarily mediated by activated CD4$^+$ $\alpha\beta$ T cells (33). However, it has also been reported that $\gamma\delta$ T cells are recruited to egg-induced granuloma in the murine schistosomiasis (124) and that the levels of γδ T cells are increased in schitosome-infected mice and patients (125, 126). However, an earlier study investigating the relative roles of αβ and γδ T cells in the immunopathology of schistosomiasis found that mutant mice lacking γδ T cells display vigorous formation of egg granulomas similar to normal mice, which demonstrates that granuloma formation is not dependent on γδT cells (127). In contrast with this study, another study identified two different γδ T cell subsets, including the Vγ1 γδ T cells that secrete IFN-γ only and the Vγ2 γδ T cells that secrete both IL-17A and IFN-γ (74). During *S. japonicum* infection, Vγ2 γδ T cells prevent hepatic fibrosis by recruiting neutrophils and secreting IL-17A (74). Thus, the role of innate γδ T cells in the pathology of schistosomiasis requires further investigation.

THE IMPACT OF OTHER IMMUNE CELLS ON CD4⁺ T CELLS AND REGULATION ON IMMUNOPATHOLOGY OF SCHISTOSOMIASIS

Over the past four decades, immunoregulation has been deeply studied in the context of schistosomiasis. T-cell subsets are influenced by macrophages, B cells, DCs, and eosinophils, of which macrophages represent nearly 30% of the total granuloma cells. Macrophages, similar to Th1 and Th2 cells, can be classified into two major types, classically activated macrophages (CAM/M1) and alternatively activated macrophages (AAM/M2). CAM polarization, stimulated by inflammatory cytokines, such as IFN-γ, IL-12, and IL-18, serve a vital role in the response to intracellular pathogens like *Mycobacterium tuberculosis* (128), whereas AAM polarization is dependent on Th2-type cytokines, such as IL-4 and IL-13, that induce the expression of arginase-1 (Arg-1), Ym-1, and Fizzl, which is mainly involved in allergic, cellular, and humoral responses to parasites (129). Egg-induced inflammation and liver fibrosis promotes the Th2 response, which in turn increases AAM polarization in granulomas (130). In several models of Th1-polarized mice, such as IL-4/IL-10 deficient, IL-4/IL-13 deficient, and egg/IL-12-immunized or macrophage-specific IL-4 deficient (131, 132), schistosome infection failed to induce the expression of Arg-1, demonstrating that Th2 cytokines are necessary for the development of Arg-1-expressing AAM. Moreover, Th1-polarized mice showed an increased inducible nitric oxide synthase response together with smaller granulomas and elevated mortality (131, 132). Thus, CAM polarization is associated with Th1 responses and Arg-1-expressing AAM is associated with Th2 responses and liver fibrosis progression.

The function of B cells has also been intensely investigated in schistosomiasis. Several studies have demonstrated that the B-cell number in the lymph nodes and spleen significantly increase during the schistosome infection, suggesting that B cells are important for host responses against schistosome infection (133, 134). Mice immunized with radiation-attenuated cercariae of *S. mansoni* showed reduced protection against challenge

infection in B-cell knockout mice compared to wild-type mice (135). IgE antibody against the worms, but not the eggs, has been closely associated with resistance to reinfection, and eosinophil-mediated antibody-dependent cellular cytotoxicity is the main immune mechanism to kill early schistosome larvae (136). Evidence shows that SEA-specific IgG1 is the main isotype released from the early granulomas and that, during the chronic infection stage, granulomas secrete a mixture of IgG1, IgG2, IgG3, and IgA (137). The antibodies produced within intragranulomas mainly function to downregulate the granuloma formation, and it has been found that immune complexes from chronic schistosomiasis patients can inhibit granuloma formation *in vitro* (138). In addition, research has been done on the regulatory role of B cells in schistosomiasis immunopathology and T-cell effector functions. A previous study has proven that B cells are important in promoting a strong Th2-type response to helminths (139). After SEA stimulation, mesenteric lymph cells from B-cell-deficient mice produce more Th1-type cytokines and less Th2-type cytokines compared to wild-type mice (140, 141). A recent study has shown that the absence of IL-4α signaling in B cells leads to increased mortality and pathology in *S. mansoni*-infected mice, which is attributed to decreased Th2 responses (142). These findings demonstrate that B cells are critical in directing and mediating Th cells toward Th2 responses. In addition, in a study about *S. mansoni*-mediated protection against experimental ovalbumin-induced allergic airway inflammation, the investigators found that splenic marginal zone CD1d⁺ B cells from schistosome-infected mice had the ability to secret IL-10 and induce generation of FoxP3⁺ Treg cells. Although B cells are essential for Th2 responses and Treg cell generation, B cells are not responsible for granuloma formation (140). However, a contrasting study showed that B-cell deficiency had no effect on Th2 responses but augmented tissue pathology (143). Therefore, further study is needed to clarify the role of B cells in immunopathology of schistosomiasis.

DCs are important antigen-presenting cells that have superior activity to stimulate naive T-cell activation and mediate the polarization of CD4⁺ T cells in response to invading pathogens. DCs determine Th differentiation through secreted polarizing cytokines. For example, *M. tuberculosis* infection induces DCs to produce IL-12 to elicit a strong IFN-γ-producing Th1 response, which leads to macrophage activation and killing of intracellular bacteria (144). Depletion of DCs in CD11c-diphtheria toxin receptor mice demonstrated that DCs are required to initiate Th2 responses in the *S. mansoni* infection (145). However, DC subsets, such as conventional CD11c⁺ DCs and some specialized DCs do not produce IL-4, which is important for Th2 polarization. Ma et al. uncovered a novel subset of CD11c⁺CD49b⁺FcεRI⁺ DCs that can produce IL-4 and subsequently promote Th2 differentiation in an IL-4-dependent manner (146). However, contradictory findings revealed that conventional DCs are critical subsets for Th2 effector cell development during acute *S. mansoni* infection (147). In fact, more researchers support the notion that DCs do not need to produce IL-4 to promote Th2 development (148–150) because IL-4-deficient DCs still show the ability to induce excellent Th2 responses (148). In addition, a recent study revealed an unrecognized role of type I IFN in the Th2 response, whereby IFN-I signaling is implicated in not only activating DCs but also enhancing DCs effective migration and antigen presentation during the *S. mansoni*-induced Th2 response (151). Thus, the exact mechanism by which DCs induce Th2 responses needs to be further clarified.

SUMMARY AND CONCLUDING COMMENTS

Schistosomiasis is a disease with profound impact on human health. At least 230 million people worldwide are affected by the parasitic disease (1). In the near future, we may face a situation where there is no available drug to treat schistosomiasis, as praziquantel is still the only effective drug being used to treat the disease and praziquantel resistance has been reported in endemic areas and in the laboratory (152, 153). Therefore, it is urgent to develop some alternative drugs to control schistosomiasis, including the use of vaccines (154–156). Schistosome infection can lead to acute febrile illness and chronic life-threatening hepatosplenic disease. As summarized in **Figure 1**, during the progression of the disease, Th cells

are activated and differentiated into distinct effector subsets, including Th1, Th2, Th17, Tfh, Th9, and Treg cells. Acute schistosomiasis is recognized as a Th1-dominated disease. Recent studies showed that Th17 and Tfh are also involved in the immune response of acute cases (71, 94). Chronic disease of hepatic granuloma formation and fibrosis are upregulated by Th2 and Th17 cells, mainly secreting IL-4 and IL-17, respectively (33, 63), and downregulated by Th1 and Treg cells (80, 113). The plasticity of Th cells are affected by the local microenvironment (e.g., cytokines and antigens of schistosomes) and regulated by various immune cells (e.g., macrophages, B cells, and DCs) through a complicated interacting network. Although we have acquired sufficient knowledge about the immunopathology of schistosomiasis, the effective strategies to restrain the development of granulomas and subsequent fibrosis are still lacking. A vaccine designed to skew the immune response toward the Th1 phenotype would be useful to prevent the development of fibrosis (80). However, murine studies have shown that extreme immune deviation toward either Th1 or Th2 results in increased pathology and premature death (18, 157). Most importantly, maintaining the balance of various effector T cells would be critical to prevent excessive pathology. While many researchers are focused on the Tregs-associated suppression and the powerful force of IL-10, successful immunotherapies will only be developed for schistosomiasis if we have a broader view

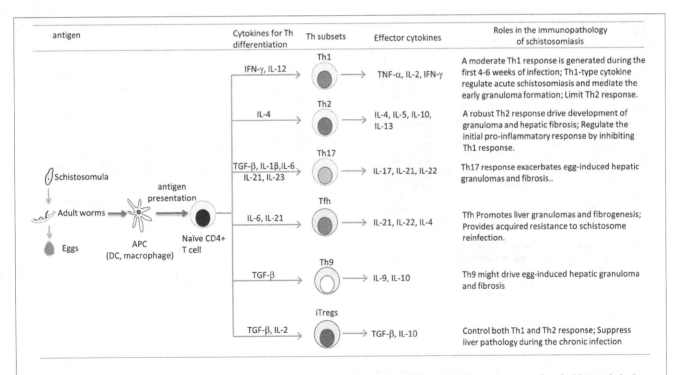

FIGURE 1 | T helper (Th) subsets differentiation and their roles in immunopathology of the murine schistosomiasis. During the progression of schistosomiasis, the schistosome antigen from schistosomula, adult worms, or eggs are captured and processed by antigen-presenting cells, such as dendritic cells (DCs) and macrophages; this leads to the production of various cytokines, and processed antigens are presented to naive CD4+ T cell in the form of major histocompatibility complex (MHC) class II-peptide complexes, then activated CD4+ T cells differentiate into Th1, Th2, Th17, Tfh, Th9, and Tregs, which are strictly regulated by the local microenvironment (e.g., cytokines and antigens of schistosomes) and cross-talk with various immune cells (e.g., macrophages, B cells, and DCs) through a complicated interacting network. It is generally thought that Th2, Th17 responses and Tfh, Th9 cells positively drive the development of pathology of chronic schistosomiasis, whereas the Th1 response counteracts Th2-mediated chronic pathology, and Tregs exert a suppressive effect on the immunopathology of schistosomiasis by inhibiting both Th1 and Th2 responses.

and deeper understanding of the mechanism of T-cell-mediated liver immunopathology.

AUTHOR CONTRIBUTIONS

CL organized the article. BZ wrote the draft. JZ, HC, HN and HM participated in the conception, discussion and revision of the draft. QG edited the language and figure.

REFERENCES

Vos T, Flaxman AD, Naghavi M, Lozano R, Michaud C, Ezzati M, et al. Years lived with disability (YLDs) for 1160 sequelae of 289 diseases and injuries 1990–2010: a systematic analysis for the Global Burden of Disease Study 2010. *Lancet.* (2012) 380:2163–96. doi: 10.1016/S0140-6736(12) 61729-2

He Y-X, Chen L, Ramaswamy K. *Schistosoma mansoni, S. haematobium,* and *S. japonicum*: early events associated with penetration and migration of schistosomula through human skin. *Exp Parasitol.* (2002) 102:99– 108. doi: 10.1016/S0014-4894(03)00024-9

Gobert GN, Chai M, McManus DP. Biology of the schistosome lung-stage schistosomulum. *Parasitology.* (2007) 134:453– 60. doi: 10.1017/ S0031182006001648

Colley DG, Bustinduy AL, Secor WE, King CH. Human schistosomiasis. *Lancet.* (2014) 383:2253–64. doi: 10.1016/S0140-6736(13)61949-2

Ross AG, Vickers D, Olds GR, Shah SM, McManus DP. Katayama syndrome. *Lancet Infect Dis.* (2007) 7:218–24. doi: 10.1016/S1473-3099(07)70053-1

Pearce EJ, MacDonald AS. The immunobiology of schistosomiasis. *Nat Rev Immunol.* (2002) 2:499–511. doi: 10.1038/nri843

Wilson MS, Mentink-Kane MM, Pesce JT, Ramalingam TR, Thompson R, Wynn TA. Immunopathology of schistosomiasis. *Immunol Cell Biol.* (2007) 85:148–54. doi: 10.1038/sj.icb.7100014

Burke ML, Jones MK, Gobert GN, Li YS, Ellis MK, McManus DP. Immunopathogenesis of human schistosomiasis. *Parasite Immunol.* (2009) 31:163–76. doi: 10.1111/j.1365-3024.2009.01098.x

Lundy SK, Lukacs NW. Chronic schistosome infection leads to modulation of granuloma formation and systemic immune suppression. *Front Immunol.* (2013) 4:39. doi: 10.3389/fimmu.2013.00039

Amsden AF, Boros DL, Hood AT. Etiology of the liver granulomatous response in *Schistosoma mansoni*-infected athymic nude mice. *Infect Immun.* (1980) 27:75–80. doi: 10.1128/IAI.27.1.75- 80.1980

Mathew RC, Boros DL. Anti-L3T4 antibody treatment suppresses hepatic granuloma formation and abrogates antigen-induced interleukin-2 production in *Schistosoma mansoni* infection. *Infect Immun.* (1986) 54:820–6. doi: 10.1128/ IAI.54.3.820-826.1986

Boros DL. T helper cell populations, cytokine dynamics, and pathology of the schistosome egg granuloma. *Microbes Infect.* (1999) 1:511– 6. doi: 10.1016/ S1286-4579(99)80090-2

Hiatt RA, Sotomayor ZR, Sanchez G, Zambrana M, Knight WB. Factors in the pathogenesis of acute schistosomiasis mansoni. *J Infect Dis.* (1979) 139:659–66. doi: 10.1093/infdis/139.6.659

Burke ML, McManus DP, Ramm GA, Duke M, Li Y, Jones MK, et al. Temporal expression of chemokines dictates the hepatic inflammatory infiltrate in a murine model of schistosomiasis. *PLoS Negl Trop Dis.* (2010) 4:e598. doi: 10.1371/journal.pntd.0000598

de Jesus AR, Silva A, Santana LB, Magalhaes A, de Jesus AA, de Almeida RP, et al. Clinical and immunologic evaluation of 31 patients with acute schistosomiasis mansoni. *J Infect Dis.* (2002) 185:98– 105. doi: 10.1086/324668

Bogen SA, Flores Villanueva PO, McCusker ME, Fogelman I, Garifallou M, el-Attar ES, et al. *In situ* analysis of cytokine responses in experimental murine schistosomiasis. *Lab Invest.* (1995) 73:252–8.

Nono JK, Ndlovu H, Aziz NA, Mpotje T, Hlaka L, Brombacher F. Host regulation of liver fibroproliferative pathology during experimental schistosomiasis via interleukin-4 receptor alpha. *PLoS Negl Trop Dis.* (2017) 11:e0005861. doi: 10.1371/journal.pntd.0005861

Hoffmann KF, Cheever AW, Wynn TA. IL-10 and the dangers of immune polarization: excessive type 1 and type 2 cytokine responses induce distinct forms of lethal immunopathology in murine schistosomiasis. *J Immunol.* (2000) 164:6406–16. doi: 10.4049/jimmunol.164.12.6406

Fahel JS, Macedo GC, Pinheiro CS, Caliari MV, Oliveira SC. IPSE/alpha- 1 of *Schistosoma mansoni* egg induces enlargement of granuloma but does not alter Th2 balance after infection. *Parasite Immunol.* (2010) 32:345– 53. doi: 10.1111/j.1365-3024.2009.01192.x

Dunne DW, Jones FM, Doenhoff MJ. The purification, characterization, serological activity and hepatotoxic properties of two cationic glycoproteins (alpha 1 and omega 1) from *Schistosoma mansoni* eggs. *Parasitology.* (1991) 103:225–36. doi: 10.1017/S0031182000059503

Wang Y, Da'Dara AA, Thomas PG, Harn DA. Dendritic cells activated by an anti-inflammatory agent induce CD4[+] T helper type 2 responses without impairing CD8[+] memory and effector cytotoxic T-lymphocyte responses. *Immunology.* (2010) 129:406–17. doi: 10.1111/j.1365-2567.2009. 03193.x

Cai Y, Langley JG, Smith DI, Boros DL. A cloned major *Schistosoma mansoni* egg antigen with homologies to small heat shock proteins elicits Th1 responsiveness. *Infect Immun.* (1996) 64:1750–5. doi: 10.1128/ IAI.64.5.1750-1755.1996

Hernandez HJ, Edson CM, Harn DA, Ianelli CJ, Stadecker MJ. Schistosoma mansoni: genetic restriction and cytokine profile of the CD4[+] T helper cell response to dominant epitope peptide of major egg antigen Sm-p40. *Exp Parasitol.* (1998) 90:122–30. doi: 10.1006/expr.1998.4309

Everts B, Perona-Wright G, Smits HH, Hokke CH, van der Ham AJ, Fitzsimmons CM, et al. Omega-1, a glycoprotein secreted by Schistosoma mansoni eggs, drives Th2 responses. *J Exp Med.* (2009) 206:1673– 80. doi: 10.1084/jem.20082460

Reis EAG, Mauadi Carmo TA, Athanazio R, Reis MG, Harn DA Jr. *Schistosoma mansoni* triose phosphate isomerase peptide MAP4 is able to trigger naive donor immune response towards a type-1 cytokine profile. *Scand J Immunol.* (2008) 68:169–76. doi: 10.1111/j.1365-3083.2008. 02131.x

Chen Y, Boros DL. The *Schistosoma mansoni* egg-derived r38 peptide- induced Th1 response affects the synchronous pulmonary but not the asynchronous hepatic granuloma growth. *Parasite Immunol.* (2001) 23:43– 50. doi: 10.1046/j.1365-3024.2001.00354.x

Egesa M, Lubyayi L, Tukahebwa EM, Bagaya BS, Chalmers IW, Wilson S, et al. *Schistosoma mansoni* schistosomula antigens induce Th1/Pro-inflammatory cytokine responses. *Parasite Immunol.* (2018) 40:e12592. doi: 10.1111/pim.12592

Ma LZ, Li DD, Yuan CX, Zhang XQ, Ta N, Zhao XC, et al. SjCRT, a recombinant *Schistosoma japonicum* calreticulin, induces maturation of dendritic cells and a Th1-polarized immune response in mice. *Parasites Vectors.* (2017) 10:570. doi: 10.1186/s13071-017-2516-7

MacDonald AS, Patton EA, La Flamme AC, Araujo MI, Huxtable CR, Bauman B, et al. Impaired Th2 development and increased mortality during *Schistosoma mansoni* infection in the absence of CD40/CD154 interaction. *J Immunol.* (2002) 168:4643–9. doi: 10.4049/jimmunol.168.9.4643

Hernandez HJ, Sharpe AH, Stadecker MJ. Experimental murine schistosomiasis in the absence of B7 costimulatory molecules: reversal of elicited T cell cytokine profile and partial inhibition of egg granuloma formation. *J Immunol.* (1999) 162:2884–9.

Rutitzky LI, Ozkaynak E, Rottman JB, Stadecker MJ. Disruption of the ICOS-B7RP-1 costimulatory pathway leads to enhanced hepatic immunopathology and increased gamma interferon production by CD4 T cells in murine schistosomiasis. *Infect Immun.* (2003) 71:4040–4. doi: 10.1128/IAI.71.7.4040-4044.2003

Pearce EJ, Caspar P, Grzych JM, Lewis FA, Sher A. Downregulation of Th1 cytokine production accompanies induction of Th2 responses by a parasitic helminth, Schistosoma mansoni. J Exp Med. (1991) 173:159– 66. doi: 10.1084/jem.173.1.159

Kaplan MH, Whitfield JR, Boros DL, Grusby MJ. Th2 cells are required for the Schistosoma mansoni egg-induced granulomatous response. J Immunol. (1998) 160:1850–6.

Cheever AW, Williams ME, Wynn TA, Finkelman FD, Seder RA, Cox TM, et al. Anti-IL-4 treatment of Schistosoma mansoni-infected mice inhibits development of T cells and non-B, non-T cells expressing Th2 cytokines while decreasing egg-induced hepatic fibrosis. J Immunol. (1994) 153:753–9.

Yamashita T, Boros DL. IL-4 influences IL-2 production and granulomatous inflammation in murine schistosomiasis mansoni. J Immunol. (1992) 149:3659–64.

Jankovic D, Kullberg MC, Noben-Trauth N, Caspar P, Ward JM, Cheever AW, et al. Schistosome-infected IL-4 receptor knockout (KO) mice, in contrast to IL-4 KO mice, fail to develop granulomatous pathology while maintaining the same lymphokine expression profile. J Immunol. (1999) 163:337–42.

Wynn TA. IL-13 effector functions. Annu Rev Immunol. (2003) 21:425– 56. doi: 10.1146/annurev.immunol.21.120601.141142

Chiaramonte MG, Cheever AW, Malley JD, Donaldson DD, Wynn TA. Studies of murine schistosomiasis reveal interleukin-13 blockade as a treatment for established and progressive liver fibrosis. Hepatology. (2001) 34:273–82. doi: 10.1053/jhep.2001.26376

Fallon PG, Richardson EJ, McKenzie GJ, McKenzie AN. Schistosome infection of transgenic mice defines distinct and contrasting pathogenic roles for IL-4 and IL-13: IL-13 is a profibrotic agent. J Immunol. (2000) 164:2585–91. doi: 10.4049/jimmunol.164.5.2585

Chiaramonte MG, Donaldson DD, Cheever AW, Wynn TA. An IL-13 inhibitor blocks the development of hepatic fibrosis during a T-helper type 2-dominated inflammatory response. J Clin Invest. (1999) 104:777– 85. doi:10.1172/JCI7325

Oriente A, Fedarko NS, Pacocha SE, Huang SK, Lichtenstein LM, Essayan DM. Interleukin-13 modulates collagen homeostasis in human skin and keloid fibroblasts. J Pharmacol Exp Ther. (2000) 292:988–94.

Fort MM, Cheung J, Yen D, Li J, Zurawski SM, Lo S, et al. IL-25 induces IL- 4, IL-5, and IL-13 and Th2-associated pathologies in vivo. Immunity. (2001) 15:985–95. doi: 10.1016/S1074-7613(01)00243-6

Soumelis V, Reche PA, Kanzler H, Yuan W, Edward G, Homey B, et al. Human epithelial cells trigger dendritic cell mediated allergic inflammation by producing TSLP. Nat Immunol. (2002) 3:673–80. doi: 10.1038/ni805

Schmitz J, Owyang A, Oldham E, Song Y, Murphy E, McClanahan TK, et al. IL-33, an interleukin-1-like cytokine that signals via the IL-1 receptor-related protein ST2 and induces T helper type 2-associated cytokines. Immunity. (2005) 23:479–90. doi: 10.1016/j.immuni.2005.09.015

Yu Y, Deng W, Lei J. Interleukin-33 promotes Th2 immune responses in infected mice with Schistosoma japonicum. Parasitol Res. (2015) 114:2911– 8. doi: 10.1007/s00436-015-4492-1

He X, Xie J, Wang Y, Fan X, Su Q, Sun Y, et al. Down-regulation of microRNA-203-3p initiates type 2 pathology during schistosome infection via elevation of interleukin-33. PLoS Pathog. (2018) 14:e1006957.doi:10.1371/journal.ppat.1006957

Peng H, Zhang Q, Li X, Liu Z, Shen J, Sun R, et al. IL-33 contributes to Schistosoma japonicum-induced hepatic pathology through induction of M2 macrophages. Sci Rep. (2016) 6:29844. doi: 10.1038/srep29844

Vannella KM, Ramalingam TR, Borthwick LA, Barron L, Hart KM, Thompson RW, et al. Combinatorial targeting of TSLP, IL-25, and IL-33 in type 2 cytokine-driven inflammation and fibrosis. Sci Transl Med. (2016) 8:337ra65. doi: 10.1126/scitranslmed.aaf1938

Tallima H, Dvorak J, Kareem S, Abou El Dahab M, Abdel Aziz N, Dalton JP, et al. Protective immune responses against Schistosoma mansoni infection by immunization with functionally active gut-derived cysteine peptidases alone and in combination with glyceraldehyde 3-phosphate dehydrogenase. PLoS Negl Trop Dis. (2017) 11:e0005443. doi: 10.1371/journal.pntd.0005443

Tallima H, Dalton JP, El Ridi R. Induction of protective immune responses against Schistosomiasis haematobium in hamsters and mice using cysteine peptidase-based vaccine. Front Immunol. (2015) 6:130. doi: 10.3389/fimmu.2015.00130

Brunet LR, Finkelman FD, Cheever AW, Kopf MA, Pearce EJ. IL-4 protects against TNF-alpha-mediated cachexia and death during acute schistosomiasis. J Immunol. (1997) 159:777–85.

Fallon PG, Smith P, Dunne DW. Type 1 and type 2 cytokine- producing mouse CD4+ and CD8+ T cells in acute Schistosoma mansoni infection. Eur J Immunol. (1998) 28:1408–16. doi: 10.1002/(SICI)1521- 4141(199804)28:04<1408::AID-IMMU1408>3.0.CO;2-H

La Flamme AC, Patton EA, Bauman B, Pearce EJ. IL-4 plays a crucial role in regulating oxidative damage in the liver during schistosomiasis. J Immunol. (2001) 166:1903–11. doi: 10.4049/jimmunol.166.3.1903

Mwatha JK, Kimani G, Kamau T, Mbugua GG, Ouma JH, Mumo J, et al. High levels of TNF, soluble TNF receptors, soluble ICAM-1, and IFN-gamma, but low levels of IL-5, are associated with hepatosplenic disease in human schistosomiasis mansoni. J Immunol. (1998) 160:1992–9.

Boros DL, Whitfield JR. Endogenous IL-10 regulates IFN-gamma and IL-5 cytokine production and the granulomatous response in Schistosomiasis mansoni-infected mice. Immunology. (1998) 94:481–7. doi: 10.1046/j.1365-2567.1998.00544.x

Rutitzky LI, Lopes da Rosa JR, Stadecker MJ. Severe CD4 T cell-mediated immunopathology in murine schistosomiasis is dependent on IL-12p40 and correlates with high levels of IL-17. J Immunol. (2005) 175:3920– 6. doi: 10.4049/jimmunol.175.6.3920

Harrington LE, Hatton RD, Mangan PR, Turner H, Murphy TL, Murphy KM, et al. Interleukin 17-producing CD4+ effector T cells develop via a lineage distinct from the T helper type 1 and 2 lineages. Nat Immunol. (2005) 6:1123–32. doi: 10.1038/ni1254

Shainheit MG, Lasocki KW, Finger E, Larkin BM, Smith PM, Sharpe AH, et al. The pathogenic Th17 cell response to major schistosome egg antigen is sequentially dependent on IL-23 and IL-1 beta. J Immunol. (2011) 187:5328– 35. doi: 10.4049/jimmunol.1101445

Rutitzky LI, Bazzone L, Shainheit MG, Joyce-Shaikh B, Cua DJ, Stadecker MJ. IL-23 is required for the development of severe egg- induced immunopathology in schistosomiasis and for lesional expression of IL-17. J Immunol. (2008) 180:2486–95. doi: 10.4049/jimmunol.18 0.4.2486

Shainheit MG, Smith PM, Bazzone LE, Wang AC, Rutitzky LI, Stadecker MJ. Dendritic cell IL-23 and IL-1 production in response to schistosome eggs induces Th17 cells in a mouse strain prone to severe immunopathology. J Immunol. (2008) 181:8559–67. doi: 10.4049/jimmunol.181.12.8559

Ponichtera HE, Shainheit MG, Liu BYC, Raychowdhury R, Larkin BM, Russo JM, et al. CD209a expression on dendritic cells is critical for the development of pathogenic Th17 cell responses in murine schistosomiasis. J Immunol. (2014) 192:4655–65. doi: 10.4049/jimmunol.1400121

Mbow M, Larkin BM, Meurs L, Wammes LJ, de Jong SE, Labuda LA, et al. T-helper 17 cells are associated with pathology in human schistosomiasis. J Infect Dis. (2013) 207:186–95. doi: 10.1093/infdis/jis654

Wen X, He L, Chi Y, Zhou S, Hoellwarth J, Zhang C, et al. Dynamics of Th17 cells and their role in Schistosoma japonicum infection in C57BL/6 mice. PLoS Negl Trop Dis. (2011) 5:e1399. doi: 10.1371/journal.pntd.0001399

Zhang Y, Chen L, Gao W, Hou X, Gu Y, Gui L, et al. IL-17 neutralization significantly ameliorates hepatic granulomatous inflammation and liver damage in Schistosoma japonicum infected mice. Eur J Immunol. (2012) 42:1523–35. doi: 10.1002/eji.201141933

Zhang YX, Huang DK, Gao WD, Yan J, Zhou WL, Hou X, et al. Lack of IL- 17 signaling decreases liver fibrosis in murine schistosomiasis japonica. Int Immunol. (2015) 27:317–25. doi: 10.1093/intimm/dxv017

Rutitzky LI, Stadecker MJ. Exacerbated egg-induced immunopathology in murine Schistosoma mansoni infection is primarily mediated by IL- 17 and restrained by IFN-gamma. Eur J Immunol. (2011) 41:2677– 87. doi: 10.1002/eji.201041327

Rutitzky LI, Smith PM, Stadecker MJ. T-bet protects against exacerbation of schistosome egg-induced immunopathology by regulating Th17-mediated inflammation. Eur J Immunol. (2009) 39:2470–81. doi: 10.1002/eji.200939325

Wang B, Liang S, Wang Y, Zhu X-Q, Gong W, Zhang H-Q, et al. Th17 down-regulation is involved in reduced progression of schistosomiasis fibrosis in ICOSL KO mice. PLoS Negl Trop Dis. (2015) 9:e3434.doi:10.1371/journal.pntd.0003434

Kalantari P, Morales Y, Miller EA, Jaramillo LD, Ponichtera HE, Wuethrich MA, et al. CD209a synergizes with dectin-2 and mincle to drive severe Th17 cell-mediated schistosome egg-induced immunopathology. Cell Rep. (2018) 22:1288–300. doi: 10.1016/j.celrep.2018.01.001

Kalantari P, Bunnell SC, Stadecker MJ. The C-type lectin receptor-driven, Th17 cell-mediated severe pathology in schistosomiasis: not all immune responses to helminth parasites are Th2 dominated. *Front Immunol.* (2019) 10:26. doi: 10.3389/fimmu.2019.00026

Soloviova K, Fox EC, Dalton JP, Caffrey CR, Davies SJ. A secreted schistosome cathepsin B1 cysteine protease and acute schistosome infection induce a transient T helper 17 response. *PLoS Negl Trop Dis.* (2019) 13:e7070. doi: 10.1371/journal.pntd.0007070

Chen D, Xie H, Luo X, Yu X, Fu X, Gu H, et al. Roles of Th17 cells in pulmonary granulomas induced by *Schistosoma japonicum* in C57BL/6 mice. *Cell Immunol.* (2013) 285:149–57. doi: 10.1016/j.cellimm.2013.09.008

Chen D, Luo X, Xie H, Gao Z, Fang H, Huang J. Characteristics of IL-17 induction by *Schistosoma japonicum* infection in C57BL/6 mouse liver. *Immunology.* (2013) 139:523–32. doi: 10.1111/imm.12105

Zheng L, Hu Y, Wang Y, Huang X, Xu Y, Shen Y, et al. Recruitment of neutrophils mediated by Vgamma2 gammadelta T cells deteriorates liver fibrosis induced by *Schistosoma japonicum* infection in C57BL/6 mice. *Infect Immun.* (2017) 85:e01020-16. doi: 10.1128/IAI.01020-16

Eberl G, Di Santo JP, Vivier E. The brave new world of innate lymphoid cells. *Nat Immunol.* (2015) 16:1–5. doi: 10.1038/ni.3059

Von Lichtenberg F, Erickson DG, Sadun EH. Comparative histopathology of schistosome granulomas in the hamster. *Am J Pathol.* (1973) 72:149–78.

Chuah C, Jones MK, Burke ML, McManus DP, Gobert GN. Cellular and chemokine-mediated regulation in schistosome-induced hepatic pathology. *Trends Parasitol.* (2014) 30:141–50. doi: 10.1016/j.pt.2013.12.009

Cheever AW, Duvall RH, Hallack TA Jr, Minker RG, Malley JD, Malley KG. Variation of hepatic fibrosis and granuloma size among mouse strains infected with *Schistosoma mansoni*. *Am J Trop Med Hyg.* (1987) 37:85– 97. doi: 10.4269/ajtmh.1987.37.85

Larkin BM, Smith PM, Ponichtera HE, Shainheit MG, Rutitzky LI, Stadecker MJ. Induction and regulation of pathogenic Th17 cell responses in schistosomiasis. *Semin Immunopathol.* (2012) 34:873–88. doi: 10.1007/s00281-012-0341-9

Stadecker MJ, Asahi H, Finger E, Hernandez HJ, Rutitzky LI, Sun J. The immunobiology of Th1 polarization in high-pathology schistosomiasis. *Immunol Rev.* (2004) 201:168–79. doi: 10.1111/j.0105-2896.2004.00197.x

King C. New insights into the differentiation and function of T follicular helper cells. *Nat Rev Immunol.* (2009) 9:757–66. doi: 10.1038/nri2644

Chtanova T, Tangye SG, Newton R, Frank N, Hodge MR, Rolph MS, et al. T follicular helper cells express a distinctive transcriptional profile, reflecting their role as non-Th1/Th2 effector cells that provide help for B cells. *J Immunol.* (2004) 173:68–78. doi: 10.4049/jimmunol.173.1.68

Breitfeld D, Ohl L, Kremmer E, Ellwart J, Sallusto F, Lipp M, et al. Follicular B helper T cells express CXC chemokine receptor 5, localize to B cell follicles, and support immunoglobulin production. *J Exp Med.* (2000) 192:1545– 52. doi: 10.1084/jem.192.11.1545

Crotty S. Follicular helper CD4 T cells (TFH). *Annu Rev Immunol.* (2011) 29:621–63. doi: 10.1146/annurev-immunol-031210-101400

King C, Tangye SG, Mackay CR. T follicular helper (TFH) cells in normal and dysregulated immune responses. *Annu Rev Immunol.* (2008) 26:741– 66. doi: 10.1146/annurev.immunol.26.021607.090344

Zaretsky AG, Taylor JJ, King IL, Marshall FA, Mohrs M, Pearce EJ. T follicular helper cells differentiate from Th2 cells in response to helminth antigens. *J Exp Med.* (2009) 206:991–99. doi: 10.1084/jem.20090303

Zhang JY, Gao WJ, Guo QR, Huang BB, Wang B, Xia GL, et al. Helminth protein vaccine induced follicular T helper cell for enhancement of humoral immunity against *Schistosoma japonicum*. *Biomed Res Int.* (2013) 2013:798164. doi: 10.1155/2013/798164

Tripodo C, Petta S, Guarnotta C, Pipitone R, Cabibi D, Colombo MP, et al. Liver follicular helper T-cells predict the achievement of virological response following interferon-based treatment in HCV-infected patients. *Antiviral Ther.* (2012) 17:111–18. doi: 10.3851/IMP1957

Auderset F, Schuster S, Fasnacht N, Coutaz M, Charmoy M, Koch U, et al. Notch signaling regulates follicular helper T cell differentiation. *J Immunol.* (2013) 191:2344–50. doi: 10.4049/jimmunol.1300643

Hams E, McCarron MJ, Amu S, Yagita H, Azuma M, Chen LP, et al. Blockade of B7-H1 (programmed death ligand 1) enhances humoral immunity by positively regulating the generation of T follicular helper cells. *J Immunol.* (2011) 186:5648–55. doi: 10.4049/jimmunol.1003161

Chen X, Yang X, Li Y, Zhu J, Zhou S, Xu Z, et al. Follicular helper T cells promote liver pathology in mice during *Schistosoma japonicum* infection. *PLoS Pathog.* (2014) 10:e1004097. doi: 10.1371/journal.ppat.1004097

Wang YY, Lin C, Cao Y, Duan ZL, Guan ZX, Xu J, et al. Up-regulation of interleukin-21 contributes to liver pathology of schistosomiasis by driving GC immune responses and activating HSCs in mice. *Sci Rep.* (2017) 7:16682. doi: 10.1038/s41598-017-16783-7

Zhang YM, Jiang YY, Wang YJ, Liu H, Shen YJ, Yuan ZY, et al. Higher frequency of circulating PD-1(high) CXCR5+CD4+ Tfh cells in patients with chronic schistosomiasis. *Int J Biol Sci.* (2015) 11:1049– 55. doi: 10.7150/ijbs.12023

Zhang YM, Wang YJ, Jiang YY, Pan W, Liu H, Yin JH, et al. T follicular helper cells in patients with acute schistosomiasis. *Parasites Vectors.* (2016) 9:321. doi: 10.1186/s13071-016-1602-6

Fairfax K, Nascimento M, Huang SCC, Everts B, Pearce EJ. Th2 responses in schistosomiasis. *Semin Immunopathol.* (2012) 34:863–71. doi: 10.1007/s00281-012-0354-4

Kaplan MH. Th9 cells: differentiation and disease. *Immunol Rev.* (2013) 252:104–15. doi: 10.1111/imr.12028

Zhao P, Xiao X, Ghobrial RM, Li XC. IL-9 and T(h)9 cells: progress and challenges. *Int Immunol.* (2013) 25:547–51. doi: 10.1093/intimm/dxt039

Dardalhon V, Awasthi A, Kwon H, Galileos G, Gao W, Sobel RA, et al. IL-4 inhibits TGF-beta-induced Foxp3+ T cells and, together with TGF- beta, generates IL-9+ IL-10+ Foxp3− effector T cells. *Nat Immunol.* (2008) 9:1347–55. doi: 10.1038/ni.1677

Anuradha R, George PJ, Hanna LE, Chandrasekaran V, Kumaran P, Nutman TB, et al. IL-4-, TGF-beta-, and IL-1-dependent expansion of parasite antigen-specific Th9 cells is associated with clinical pathology in human lymphatic filariasis. *J Immunol.* (2013) 191:2466–73. doi: 10.4049/jimmunol.1300911

Li H, Nourbakhsh B, Cullimore M, Zhang G-X, Rostami A. IL-9 is important for T-cell activation and differentiation in autoimmune inflammation of the central nervous system. *Eur J Immunol.* (2011) 41:2197– 206. doi: 10.1002/eji.201041125

Zhan TZ, Zhang TT, Wang YY, Wang XL, Lin C, Ma HH, et al. Dynamics of Th9 cells and their potential role in immunopathogenesis of murine schistosomiasis. *Parasites Vectors.* (2017) 10:305. doi: 10.1186/s13071-017-2242-1

Li L, Xie HY, Wang M, Qu JL, Cha HF, Yang Q, et al. Characteristics of IL- 9 induced by *Schistosoma japonicum* infection in C57BL/6 mouse liver. *Sci Rep.* (2017) 7:2343. doi: 10.1038/s41598-017-02422-8

Matos Sa Barreto AV, Nunes de lacerda GA, de Castro Figueiredo AL, Nunes Diniz GT, Souza Gomes EC, Coutinho Domingues AL, et al. Evaluation of serum levels of IL-9 and IL-17 in human *Schistosoma mansoni* infection and their relationship with periportal fibrosis. *Immunobiology.* (2016) 221:1351– 54. doi: 10.1016/j.imbio.2016.07.014

Sakaguchi S, Wing K, Miyara M. Regulatory T cells–a brief history and perspective. *Eur J Immunol.* (2007) 37:S116–23. doi: 10.1002/eji.2007 37593

Belkaid Y, Rouse BT. Natural regulatory T cells in infectious disease. *Nat Immunol.* (2005) 6:353–60. doi: 10.1038/ni1181

Jonuleit H, Schmitt E. The regulatory T cell family: distinct subsets and their interrelations. *J Immunol.* (2003) 171:6323– 7. doi: 10.4049/jimmunol.171.12.6323

Fontenot JD, Rasmussen JP, Williams LM, Dooley JL, Farr AG, Rudensky AY. Regulatory T cell lineage specification by the forkhead transcription factor foxp3. *Immunity.* (2005) 22:329–41. doi: 10.1016/j.immuni.2005.01.016

Piccirillo CA, Shevach EM. Naturally-occurring CD4+CD25+ immunoregulatory T cells: central players in the arena of peripheral tolerance. *Semin Immunol.* (2004) 16:81–8. doi: 10.1016/j.smim.2003. 12.003

Fontenot JD, Rudensky AY. A well adapted regulatory contrivance: regulatory T cell development and the forkhead family transcription factor Foxp3. *Nat Immunol.* (2005) 6:331–7. doi: 10.1038/ni1179

Barrat FJ, Cua DJ, Boonstra A, Richards DF, Crain C, Savelkoul HF, et al. *In vitro* generation of interleukin 10-producing regulatory CD4+ T cells is induced by immunosuppressive drugs and inhibited by T helper type 1 (Th1)- and Th2-inducing cytokines. *J Exp Med.* (2002) 195:603– 16. doi: 10.1084/jem.20011629

Bluestone JA, Abbas AK. Natural versus adaptive regulatory T cells. *Nat Rev Immunol.* (2003) 3:253–7. doi: 10.1038/nri1032

O'Garra A, Vieira PL, Vieira P, Goldfeld AE. IL-10-producing and naturally occurring CD4+ Tregs: limiting collateral damage. *J Clin Invest.* (2004) 114:1372–8. doi: 10.1172/JCI23215

Singh KP, Gerard HC, Hudson AP, Reddy TR, Boros DL. Retroviral Foxp3 gene transfer ameliorates liver granuloma pathology in *Schistosoma mansoni* infected mice. *Immunology*. (2005) 114:410–7. doi:10.1111/j.1365-2567.2004.02083.x

Taylor JJ, Mohrs M, Pearce EJ. Regulatory T cell responses develop in parallel to Th responses and control the magnitude and phenotype of the Th effector population. *J Immunol*. (2006) 176:5839–47. doi: 10.4049/jimmunol.176.10.5839

van der Kleij D, Latz E, Brouwers JFHM, Kruize YCM, Schmitz M, Kurt-Jones EA, et al. A novel host-parasite lipid cross-talk. Schistosomal lyso-phosphatidylserine activates toll-like receptor 2 and affects immune polarization. *J Biol Chem*. (2002) 277:48122–9. doi: 10.1074/jbc.M2069 41200

Baumgart M, Tompkins F, Leng J, Hesse M. Naturally occurring CD4$^+$ Foxp3$^+$ regulatory T cells are an essential, IL-10-independent part of the immunoregulatory network in *Schistosoma mansoni* egg-induced inflammation. *J Immunol*. (2006) 176:5374–87. doi:10.4049/jimmunol.176.9.5374

Hesse M, Piccirillo CA, Belkaid Y, Prufer J, Mentink-Kane M, Leusink M, et al. The pathogenesis of schistosomiasis is controlled by cooperating IL-10-producing innate effector and regulatory T cells. *J Immunol*. (2004) 172:3157–66. doi:10.4049/jimmunol.172.5.3157

McKee AS, Pearce EJ. CD25$^+$ CD4$^+$ cells contribute to Th2 polarization during helminth infection by suppressing Th1 response development. *J Immunol*. (2004) 173:1224–31. doi: 10.4049/jimmunol.173.2.1224

Chensue SW, Warmington KS, Hershey SD, Terebuh PD, Othman M, Kunkel SL. Evolving T cell responses in murine schistosomiasis. Th2 cells mediate secondary granulomatous hypersensitivity and are regulated by CD8$^+$ T cells *in vivo*. *J Immunol*. (1993) 151:1391–40.

Yap G, Cheever A, Caspar P, Jankovic D, Sher A. Unimpaired down-modulation of the hepatic granulomatous response in CD8 T-cell- and gamma interferon-deficient mice chronically infected with *Schistosoma mansoni*. *Infect Immun*. (1997) 65:2583–6. doi:10.1128/IAI.65.7.2583-2586.1997

Hernandez HJ, Wang Y, Tzellas N, Stadecker MJ. Expression of class II, but not class I, major histocompatibility complex molecules is required for granuloma formation in infection with *Schistosoma mansoni*. *Eur J Immunol*. (1997) 27:1170–6. doi: 10.1002/eji.1830270518

Hayday AC. [gamma][delta] cells: a right time and a right place for a conserved third way of protection. *Annu Rev Immunol*. (2000) 18:975–1026. doi: 10.1146/annurev.immunol.18.1.975

Bank I, Marcu-Malina V. Quantitative peripheral blood perturbations of gammadelta T cells in human disease and their clinical implications. *Clin Rev Allergy Immunol*. (2014) 47:311–33. doi:10.1007/s12016-013-8391-x

Sandor M, Sperling AI, Cook GA, Weinstock JV, Lynch RG, Bluestone JA. Two waves of gamma delta T cells expressing different V delta genes are recruited into schistosome-induced liver granulomas. *J Immunol*. (1995) 155:275–84.

Schwartz E, Rosenthal E, Bank I. Gamma delta T cells in non-immune patients during primary schistosomal infection. *Immun Inflamm Dis*. (2014) 2:56–61. doi: 10.1002/iid3.18

Yu X, Luo X, Xie H, Chen D, Li L, Wu F, et al. Characteristics of gammadelta T cells in *Schistosoma japonicum*-infected mouse mesenteric lymph nodes. *Parasitol Res*. (2014) 113:3393–401. doi: 10.1007/s00436-014- 4004-8

Iacomini J, Ricklan DE, Stadecker MJ. T cells expressing the γδ T cell receptor are not required for egg granuloma formation in schistosomiasis. *Eur J Immunol*. (1995) 25:884–88. doi: 10.1002/eji.1830250404

Holscher C, Atkinson RA, Arendse B, Brown N, Myburgh E, Alber G, et al. A protective and agonistic function of IL-12p40 in mycobacterial infection. *J Immunol*. (2001) 167:6957–66. doi: 10.4049/jimmunol.167.12.6957

Gordon S. Alternative activation of macrophages. *Nat Rev Immunol*. (2003) 3:23–35. doi:10.1038/nri978

Hesse M, Cheever AW, Jankovic D, Wynn TA. NOS-2 mediates the protective anti-inflammatory and antifibrotic effects of the Th1-inducing adjuvant, IL-12, in a Th2 model of granulomatous disease. *Am J Pathol*. (2000) 157:945–55. doi:10.1016/S0002-9440(10)64607-X

Hesse M, Modolell M, La Flamme AC, Schito M, Fuentes JM, Cheever AW, et al. Differential regulation of nitric oxide synthase-2 and arginase- 1 by type 1/type 2 cytokines *in vivo*: granulomatous pathology is shaped by the pattern of L-arginine metabolism. *J Immunol*. (2001) 167:6533–44. doi:10.4049/jimmunol.167.11.6533

Herbert DBR, Holscher C, Mohrs M, Arendse B, Schwegmann A, Radwanska M, et al. Alternative macrophage activation is essential for survival during schistosomiasis and downmodulates T helper 1 responses and immunopathology. *Immunity*. (2004) 20:623–35. doi: 10.1016/ S1074-7613(04)00107-4

Chensue SW, Boros DL. Modulation of granulomatous hypersensitivity. I. Characterization of T lymphocytes involved in the adoptive suppression of granuloma formation in *Schistosoma mansoni*-infected mice. *J Immunol*. (1979) 123:1409–14.

el-Cheikh MC, Bonomo AC, Rossi MI, Pinho Mde F, Borojevic R. Experimental murine schistosomiasis mansoni: modulation of the B-1 lymphocyte distribution and phenotype expression. *Immunobiology*. (1998) 199:51–62. doi: 10.1016/S0171-2985(98)80063-6

Jankovic D, Wynn TA, Kullberg MC, Hieny S, Caspar P, James S, et al. Optimal vaccination against Schistosoma mansoni requires the induction of both B cell- and IFN-gamma-dependent effector mechanisms. *J Immunol*. (1999) 162:345–51.

Dunne DW, Butterworth AE, Fulford AJ, Kariuki HC, Langley JG, Ouma JH, et al. Immunity after treatment of human schistosomiasis: association between IgE antibodies to adult worm antigens and resistance to reinfection. *Eur J Immunol*. (1992) 22:1483–94. doi: 10.1002/eji.183022 0622

Boros DL, Amsden AF, Hood AT. Modulation of granulomatous hypersensitivity. IV. Immunoglobulin and antibody production by vigorous and immunomodulated liver granulomas of *Schistosoma mansoni*-infected mice. *J Immunol*. (1982) 128:1050–3.

Goes AM, Gazzinelli G, Rocha R, Katz N, Doughty BL. Granulomatous hypersensitivity to *Schistosoma mansoni* egg antigens in human schistosomiasis. III. *In vitro* granuloma modulation induced by immune complexes. *Am J Trop Med Hyg*. (1991) 44:434–43. doi: 10.4269/ajtmh.1991.44.434

Harris N, Gause WC. To B or not to B: B cells and the Th2- type immune response to helminths. *Trends Immunol*. (2011) 32:80– 8. doi: 10.1016/j. it.2010.11.005

Hernandez HJ, Wang Y, Stadecker MJ. In infection with *Schistosoma mansoni*, B cells are required for T helper type 2 cell responses but not for granuloma formation. *J Immunol*. (1997) 158:4832–7.

Ferru I, Roye O, Delacre M, Auriault C, Wolowczuk I. Infection of B-cell- deficient mice by the parasite *Schistosoma mansoni*: demonstration of the participation of B cells in granuloma modulation. *Scand J Immunol*. (1998) 48:233–40. doi: 10.1046/j.1365-3083.1998.00376.x

Hurdayal R, Ndlovu HH, Revaz-Breton M, Parihar SP, Nono JK, Govender M, et al. IL-4-producing B cells regulate T helper cell dichotomy in type 1- and type 2-controlled diseases. *Proc Natl Acad Sci USA*. (2017) 114:E8430– 9. doi: 10.1073/pnas.1708125114

Jankovic D, Cheever AW, Kullberg MC, Wynn TA, Yap G, Caspar P, et al. CD4$^+$ T cell-mediated granulomatous pathology in schistosomiasis is downregulated by a B cell-dependent mechanism requiring Fc receptor signaling. *J Exp Med*. (1998) 187:619–29. doi: 10.1084/jem.187.4.619

Yamane H, Paul WE. Early signaling events that underlie fate decisions of naive CD4$^+$ T cells toward distinct T-helper cell subsets. *Immunol Rev*. (2013) 252:12–23. doi:10.1111/imr.12032

Phythian-Adams AT, Cook PC, Lundie RJ, Jones LH, Smith KA, Barr TA, et al. CD11c depletion severely disrupts Th2 induction and development *in vivo*. *J Exp Med*. (2010) 207:2089–96. doi: 10.1084/jem.201 00734

Ma YL, Huang FJ, Cong L, Gong WC, Bai HM, Li J, et al. IL-4- producing dendritic cells induced during *Schistosoma japonica* infection promote Th2 cells via IL-4-dependent pathway. *J Immunol*. (2015) 195:3769– 80. doi: 10.4049/jimmunol.1403240

Lundie RJ, Webb LM, Marley AK, Phythian-Adams AT, Cook PC, Jackson- Jones LH, et al. A central role for hepatic conventional dendritic cells in supporting Th2 responses during helminth infection. *Immunol Cell Biol*. (2016) 94:400–10. doi: 10.1038/icb.2015.114

MacDonald AS, Pearce EJ. Cutting edge: polarized Th cell response induction by transferred antigen-pulsed dendritic cells is dependent on IL-4 or IL-12 production by recipient cells. *J Immunol*. (2002) 168:3127– 30. doi: 10.4049/jimmunol.168.7.3127

Whelan M, Harnett MM, Houston KM, Patel V, Harnett W, Rigley KP. A filarial nematode-secreted product signals dendritic cells to acquire a phenotype that drives development of Th2 cells. *J Immunol*. (2000) 164:6453–60. doi: 10.4049/jimmunol.164.12.6453

MacDonald AS, Straw AD, Bauman B, Pearce EJ. CD8- dendritic cell activation status plays an integral role in influencing Th2 response development. *J Immunol*. (2001) 167:1982– 8. doi: 10.4049/jimmunol.167.4.1982

Webb LM, Lundie RJ, Borger JG, Brown SL, Connor LM, Cartwright AN, et al. Type I interferon is required for T helper (Th) 2 induction by dendritic cells. *EMBO J.* (2017) 36:2404–18. doi: 10.15252/embj.2016 95345

Ismail M, Metwally A, Farghaly A, Bruce J, Tao LF, Bennett JL. Characterization of isolates of *Schistosoma mansoni* from Egyptian villagers that tolerate high doses of praziquantel. *Am J Trop Med Hyg.* (1996) 55:214– 8. doi: 10.4269/ajtmh.1996.55.214

Couto FF, Coelho PM, Araujo N, Kusel JR, Katz N, Jannotti-Passos LK, et al. *Schistosoma mansoni*: a method for inducing resistance to praziquantel using infected *Biomphalaria glabrata* snails. *Mem Inst Oswaldo Cruz.* (2011) 106:153–7. doi: 10.1590/S0074-02762011000200006

Doenhoff MJ, Cioli D, Utzinger J. Praziquantel: mechanisms of action, resistance and new derivatives for schistosomiasis. *Curr Opin Infect Dis.* (2008) 21:659–67. doi: 10.1097/QCO.0b013e328318978f

Thomas CM, Timson D. The mechanism of action of praziquantel: can new drugs exploit similar mechanisms? *Curr Med Chem.* (2018). doi: 10.2174/0929867325666180926145537. [Epub ahead of print].

Bergquist R, Utzinger J, McManus DP. Trick or treat: the role of vaccines in integrated schistosomiasis control. *PLoS Negl Trop Dis.* (2008) 2:e244. doi: 10.1371/journal.pntd.0000244

Rutitzky LI, Hernandez HJ, Stadecker MJ. Th1-polarizing immunization with egg antigens correlates with severe exacerbation of immunopathology and death in schistosome infection. *Proc Natl Acad Sci USA.* (2001) 98:13243–8. doi: 10.1073/pnas.231258498

4

Rutaecarpine Ameliorates Ethanol-Induced Gastric Mucosal Injury in Mice by Modulating Genes Related to Inflammation, Oxidative Stress and Apoptosis

Sichen Ren[1,2], Ying Wei[1,2], Ruilin Wang[3], Shizhang Wei[1,2], Jianxia Wen[1,2], Tao Yang[2,4], Xing Chen[1,2], Shihua Wu[1,2], Manyi Jing[2], Haotian Li[2], Min Wang[2] and Yanling Zhao[2]*

[1]School of Pharmacy, Chengdu University of Traditional Chinese Medicine, Chengdu, China, [2]Department of Pharmacy, The Fifth Medical Center of Chinese PLA General Hospital, Beijing, China, [3]Integrative Medical Center, The Fifth Medical Center of Chinese PLA General Hospital, Beijing, China, [4]School of Clinical Medicine, Chengdu University of Traditional Chinese Medicine, Chengdu, China

*Correspondence:
Yanling Zhao
zhaoyl2855@126.com

Background: Rutaecarpine (RUT), a major quinazolino carboline alkaloid compound from the dry unripe fruit *Tetradium ruticarpum* (A. Juss.) T. G. Hartley, has various pharmacological effects. The aim of this present study was to investigate the potential gastroprotective effect of rutaecarpine on ethanol-induced acute gastric mucosal injury in mice and associated molecular mechanisms, such as activating Nrf2 and Bcl-2 via PI3K/AKT signaling pathway and inhibiting NF-κB.

Methods: Gastric ulcer index and histopathology was carried out to determine the efficacy of RUT in gastric ulceration, and the content of SOD, GSH in serum and CAT, MDA, MPO, TNF-α, IL-6, IL-1β in tissue were measured by kits. Besides, in order to illustrate the potential inflammatory, oxidative, and apoptotic perturbations, the mRNA levels of NF-κB p65, PI3K, AKT, Nrf2, Nqo1, HO-1, Bcl-2 and Bax were analyzed. In addition, the protein expression of NF-κB p65 and Nrf2 in cytoplasm and nucleus, AKT, p-AKT, Bcl-2 Bax and Caspase 3 were analyzed for further verification. Finally, immunofluorescence analysis was performed to further verify nuclear translocation of NF-κB p65.

Results: Current data strongly demonstrated that RUT alleviated the gross gastric damage, ulcer index and the histopathology damage caused by ethanol. RUT inhibited the expression and nuclear translocation of NF-κB p65 and the expression of its downstream signals, such as TNF-α, IL-6, IL-1β and MPO. Immunofluorescence analysis also verifies the result. In the context of oxidative stress, RUT improved the antioxidant milieu by remarkably upregulating the expression Nqo1 and HO-1 with activating Nrf2, and could remarkably upregulate antioxidant SOD, GSH, CAT and downregulate levels of MDA. Additionally, RUT activate the expression of Bcl-2 and inhibited the expression of downstream signals Bax and Caspase 3 to promote gastric cellular survival. These were confirmed by RUT activation of the PI3K/AKT pathway manifested by enhanced expression of PI3K and promotion of AKT phosphorylation.

Conclusion: Taken together, these results strongly demonstrated that RUT exerted a gastroprotective effect against gastric mucosal injury induced by ethanol. The underlying mechanism might be associated with the improvement of anti-inflammatory, anti-oxidation and anti-apoptosis system.

Keywords: rutaecarpine, ethanol, gastric mucosal injury, anti-inflammation, anti-oxidation, anti-apoptosis

INTRODUCTION

Gastric ulcer (GU) is a common multifactorial gastrointestinal disease worldwide, affecting the quality of life of millions of patients. According to the survey, 20–60 people out of every 100,000 population suffer from GUs, accounting for 5–10% of the world's mortality (Sung et al., 2010). Under normal physiological conditions, the mucosa maintains its integrity through defense, thus maintaining the gastric epithelial barrier and blood flow, as well as the presence of protective factors such as mucus, prostaglandins, bicarbonate, heat shock protein (HSP) and growth factors. Mucosal damage may occur when the toxic factors such as gastric acid, pepsin, bile acid, ethanol, *Helicobacter pylori* and nonsteroidal anti-inflammatory drugs (NSAIDs) invade and exceed the defense function load of gastric mucosa (Guth et al., 1979; Lee et al., 2017; Khan et al., 2018). Some other factors, such as inadequate dietary habits, excessive ethanol consumption, cigarette smoking, stress and hereditary predisposition, also may lead to the development of GU (Søreide et al., 2015; Jeon et al., 2020). Yet, the clinical treatment for the disease focuses on the use of antisecretory drugs such as H2 receptor antagonist (cimetidine) or proton pump inhibitors (omeprazole), antibiotics (clarithromycin), antacids (aluminum hydroxide), prostaglandin analogues and mucosal protective agents (bismuth) currently (Wallace, 2008). Although the use of these drug is associated with the problem of reoccurrence of GU and several undesirable side effects, the usage is still on the rise, which brings more risks (Piao et al., 2018). Therefore, the search for alternative drugs or natural resources has attracted many scholars.

With the deepening of the research on natural drugs, the characteristics of some natural drugs with rich sources and less side effects have been recognized. Rutaecarpine (RUT, **Figure 1**), a major quinazolino carboline alkaloid compound from the dry unripe fruit (named "Wu-Chu-Yu" in China) of *Tetradium ruticarpum* (A. Juss.) T. G. Hartley. It is a longstanding and multipurpose Chinese medicine traditionally used for the treatment of abdominal pain, vomiting and pyresis (Zhao et al., 2015). As one of the main active components of "Wu-Chu-Yu", RUT has a wide range of biological and pharmacological effects, such as diuresis, perspiration, uterotonic action, cardiovascular protection, improving brain function, protecting gastric mucosa, anti-inflammatory and anti-oxidation, and its pharmacological mechanism involves a variety of biological targets (Jia et al., 2010; Tian et al., 2019). Several *in vitro* studies acknowledged positive effect of RUT in peritoneal resident macrophages (Li et al., 2019), monocytes (Liu et al., 2016), osteoclast (Fukuma et al., 2018), HepG2 cells (Jin et al., 2017; Surbala et al., 2020) and Hepa-1c1c7 cells (Lee et al., 2012). Meanwhile, RUT has shown versatile beneficial effects on

several experimental models, such as colitis (Zhang et al., 2020), atherosclerosis (Luo et al., 2020), cerebral ischemia-reperfusion (Han et al., 2019), hypertension (Ma et al., 2019), Acute kidney injury (Liu et al., 2020a; Liu et al., 2020b), type 2 diabetic (Surbala et al., 2020), Alzheimer's disease (Ahmad et al., 2020; Huang et al., 2020) and so on. Notably, RUT exerted definite anti-inflammatory, anti-oxidation and anti-apoptosis effects in several experimental pathology with the signaling of NF-κB, Nrf2/HO-1, Bcl-2/Bax pathways (Jin et al., 2017; Li et al., 2019a; Li et al., 2019b; Han et al., 2019). Yet, few reports focused on the effect of RUT on the ethanol-induced gastric ulcer based on above pathways. Hence, the aim of the current study was to investigate the ameliorative activity of RUT on ethanol-induced gastric ulcer and explore its underlying mechanisms.

MATERIALS AND METHODS

Reagents

In this study, RUT (pure: ≥98%) were purchased from Chengdu Chroma-Biotechnology Company (Chengdu, China). As the positive control, omeprazole (OME) was supplied by AstraZeneca Research-based Biopharmaceutical Company (Sweden). Biochemical indicator kits for SOD (Cat.No.: A001-3-2), GSH (Cat.No.: A006-2-1), CAT (Cat.No.: A007-1-1), MDA (Cat.No.: A003-1-1) and MPO (Cat.No.: A044-1-1) were provided by the Nanjing Jiancheng Bioengineering Institute (Nanjing, China) and enzyme-linked immune sorbent assay (ELISA) kits for TNF-α (Cat.No.: ml002293), IL-6 (Cat.No.: ml002293) and IL-1β (Cat.No.: ml063132) were provided by Shanghai enzyme linked biology Co., Ltd. (Shanghai, China). All antibodies were provided by Cell Signaling Technology, Inc. (Danvers, MA, United States), Abcam plc. (Cambridge, United Kingdom) or Proteintech Group, Inc. (Rosemont, IL, USA), and the specific information is shown in **Table 1**. All other experimental supplies were purchased from commercial sources.

Animals and Treatments

A total of 50 male specific pathogen-free (SPF) KM mice weighting 20 ± 2 g were obtained from SPF (Beijing) Biotechnology Co., Ltd. (Permission No. SCXK-(A) 2012-0004). All the animals were maintained in the same temperature (25 ± 2°C) and lighting (12:12 h light:dark cycle) conditions for 1 w and provided with water and standard chow ad libitum. All experimental procedures were approved by the Animal Experiment Committee of Fifth Medical Centre, General Hospital of Chinese People's Liberation Army, and carried out in accordance with the guidelines of the Council on Animal Care of Academia Sinica.

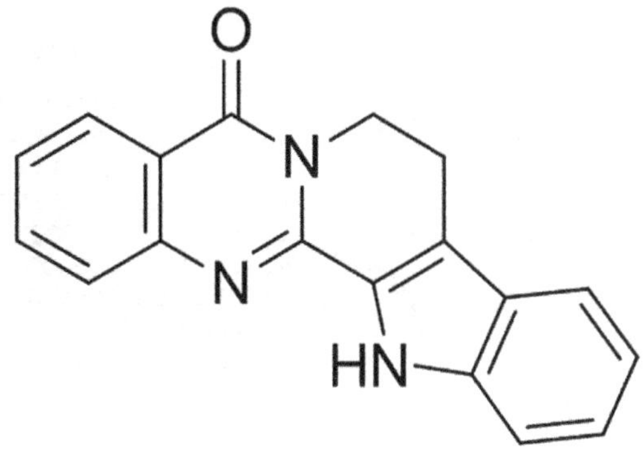

FIGURE 1 | The chemical structure of rutaecarpine.

TABLE 1 | Antibodies information.

Antibodies	Dilution	Manufacturers	Cat. No.
For western blot analysis			
Rabbit anti-NF-κB p65	1:1,000	Cell signaling technology	8242T
Rabbit Anti-Nrf2	1:1,000	Proteintech	16396-1-AP
Rabbit anti-Bcl-2	1:1,000	Cell signaling technology	3498T
Rabbit anti-Bax	1:1,000	Cell signaling technology	2772T
Rabbit anti-cleaved Caspase-3	1:5,000	Abcam	ab214430
Rabbit Anti-AKT	1:1,000	Proteintech	10176-2-AP
Mouse Anti-pAKT	1:5,000	Proteintech	66444-1-Ig
Rabbit Anti-GAPDH	1:10000	Proteintech	10494-1-AP
Rabbit anti-histone H3	1:2000	Cell signaling technology	4499T
For immunofluorescence analysis			
Rabbit anti-NF-κB p65	1:500	Cell signaling technology	8242T

All the animals were randomly assigned five groups with ten mice in each group. RUT and OME were prepared as a stock solution in 0.5% carboxymethyl cellulose sodium (CMC-Na) and diluted to the appropriate dosage or concentration. In the first 3 days, RUT of 450 and 900 μg/kg were administered intragastrically to RUT low dose group and RUT high dose group, respectively. OME group were administered omeprazole 20 mg/kg, while normal control group and model group were given the vehicle (0.5% CMC-Na). On the third day, 2 h after each group administration, normal control group received normal saline while other groups intragastrically received ethanol (10 ml/kg) instead. The animals were deprived of food for 24 h before the experiments but allowed free access to water and placed in wire cages to avoid interference from litter and feces. Finally, the animals were sacrificed after 2 h and their serum and gastric tissues were harvested for the further studies.

Macroscopic Assessment of Mucosal Lesions

Stomachs were removed and expanded along the larger curvature and rinsed thoroughly in saline solution. Then two observers who unaware of the treatment measured the lesion size with a vernier caliper and a magnifying glass, and calculated the ulcer index (UI) according to the Guth standard (Guth et al., 1979): no lesion (score 0), epithelial lesion or the lesion <1 mm (score 1), 1 mm ≤ lesion < 2 mm (score 2), 2 mm ≤ lesion <3 mm (score 3), 3 mm ≤ lesion <4 mm (score 4), 4 mm ≤ lesion (score segmentally), and twice for width > 1 mm. The scores were relative values, and the average UI of each group was obtained by dividing the total scores by the number of animals. The inhibition effect (%) of each protective material was calculated by using the following formula:

$$\text{Ulcer inhibition}\% = (\text{UI in model} - \text{UI in test}) \times 100/\text{UI in model}$$

Histological Analysis

Gastric tissues were excised and fixed in 10% buffered formalin for more than 48 h. After dehydrating in gradient alcohol and embedding in paraffin, three or four paraffin-embedded sections (4–5 μm thick) were prepared and stained with hematoxylin and eosin (H&E) for histological evaluation. Then the pathological changes in the gastric tissues were observed under a Nikon microscope (Nikon Instruments Inc., Japan) and analyzed by NIS-Elements (version F 4.0, Japan) software.

Determinations of GSH, SOD, CAT, MDA, MPO, TNF-α, IL-6, IL-1β Levels

Blood samples were collected and centrifuged at 3,000 rpm for 10 min, and then the serum samples were stored at −80°C until analysis. Gastric tissues were homogenized with cold saline and centrifuged at 12,000 rpm at 4°C for 10 min, and the supernatant of the homogenate was collected and stored at −80°C. The serum levels of SOD, GSH and the tissue levels of CAT, MDA, MPO, TNF-α, IL-6, IL-1β were measured (Liu et al., 2010; Yang et al., 2019). In brief, according to the manufacturer's protocols, the level of SOD were tested by water-soluble tetrazolium-1 (WST-1) method, the final color was read at 450 nm. Then we used ammonium molybdate method to measure the change of CAT at 405 nm and the protein level was detected by BCA Protein Assay kit (Beijing Solarbio Science & Technology Co., Ltd. Beijing, China), because ammonium molybdate can stop decomposition of H_2O_2 by CAT and form a yellow complex with remaining H_2O_2. Based on the principle that GSH can react with dithiodinitrobenzoic acid (DTNB), we quantitatively determined the content of GSH in serum by colorimetry at 405 nm. Additionally, the MDA activity were detected by thiobarbituric acid (TBA) method, the final color was detected at 450, 532, and 600 nm. According to the capability of MPO contained in neutrophils to reduce the hydrogen peroxide, we quantitatively detected the content of MPO at 460 nm to determine the number of neutrophils. For TNF-α, IL-6, IL-1β, we used enzyme-linked immune sorbent assay (ELISA) to implement. The detection operations of all these experiments

TABLE 2 | Primers sequences for RT-PCR.

Gene	Sense primer (5′-3′)	Antisense primer (5′-3′)
NF-κB p65	TCCAGGCTCCTGTTCGAGTCTC	CGGTGGCGATCATCTGTGTCTG
PI3K	CTGAGAACGCCACCGCCTTG	TCCACCACGACTTGACACATTAGC
Nrf2	GTAGATGACCATGAGTCGCTTGCC	CTTGCTCCATGTCCTGCTCTATGC
Nqo1	AGGCTGCTGTAGAGGCTCTGAAG	GCTCAGGCGTCCTTCCTTATATGC
HO-1	ACCGCCTTCCTGCTCAACATTG	CTCTGACGAAGTGACGCCATCTG
Bcl-2	TCCTTCCAGCCTGAGAGCAACC	TCACGACGGGTAGCGACGAGAG
Bax	CGTGAGCGGCTGCTTGTCTG	ATGGTGAGCGAGGCGGTGAG
β-actin	ATCACTATTGGCAACGAGCGGTTC	CAGCACTGTGTTGGCATAGAGGTC

Quantitative RT-PCR Analyses

The mRNA expressions of NF-κB, PI3K, Nrf2, Nqo1, HO-1, Bcl-2, and Bax in the gastric tissue were detected by quantitative reverse transcription polymerase chain reaction (RT-PCR). According to the manufacturer's protocol, total RNA was isolated from about 40 mg frozen gastric tissues of each group using Trizol reagent (Life Technologies, CA, United States). The RNA concentration was measured at 260 and 280 nm on a spectrophotometer (Purity (A260/A280) was considered qualified within the threshold of 1.8–2.2). Hereafter, RNA (2 μg) was reverse-transcribed using a RevertAid First Strand cNDA Synthesis Kit (Thermo Fisher Scientific, MA, United States). The program setting was: incubate for 5 min at 25°C followed by 60 min at 42°C and terminate the reaction by heating at 70°C for 5 min, and the obtained cDNA was stored at −20°C for subsequent PCR reactions. At last, 2 μL cDNA and SYBR™ Select Master Mix (Applied Biosystem, CA, United States) was used and then PCR amplification was carried out by ABI 7500 Real Time PCR machine (Applied Biosystems Inc., Carlsbad, CA, United States), running 45 cycles at 95°C for 5 s and 60°C for 60 s. The method recommended in Minimum Information for the Publication of Quantitative Real-Time PCR Experiments (MIQE) was strictly followed (Bustin et al., 2009). The data was calculated through $2^{-\triangle\triangle CT}$ method with β-actin as an endogenous reference. **Table 2** listed the primers used in this study.

Western Blot Analysis

Mice gastric tissue (50 mg) was homogenized and lysed in ice-cold radio immunoprecipitation assay (RIPA) lysis buffer containing 1% phenylmethylsulfonyl fluoride (PMSF), phosphatase inhibitor and protease inhibitor cocktail. Subsequently, the samples were centrifuged at 10,000 g and 4°C for 10 min. After centrifugation, the supernatant was collected and subjected to BCA Protein Assay kit (Beijing Solarbio Science & Technology Co., Ltd. Beijing, China) to measure protein concentration. In addition, nuclear and cytoplasmic extraction were performed using a nuclear extraction kit (Beijing Solarbio Science & Technology Co., Ltd., Beijing, China) to detect the presence of NF-κB and Nrf2 in nuclear and cytoplasmic proteins. Specifically, according to the manufacturer's instructions, 20 mg gastric tissue homogenate was vortexed at high speed for 15 s in 100 μl cytoplasmic protein extraction reagent containing 1% PMSF and then ice bath for 10 min. Subsequently, the samples were vortexed again for 10 s and centrifuge at 15,000 g at 4°C for 10 min. The resulting supernatant was cytoplasmic protein, whereas the precipitate was nuclear protein. Later, the supernatant was separated completely and 50 ul nuclear protein extraction reagent was added into the nuclear protein. The supernatant containing nucleoprotein was obtained by the same method. Similarly, their protein concentration was determined by BCA Protein Assay kit. The samples were denatured with reducing Laemmli SDS sample buffer and soaked in water at 95°C for 5 min. For Western blot analysis, the same amount of protein from all lysates of each sample was separated by 10–12% sodium dodecyl sulfate-polyacrylamide gel electrophoresis (SDS-PAGE), and then transferred onto the polyvinylidene fluoride (PVDF) membranes. Then immunodetection was carried out using corresponding primary antibodies (**Table 1**) in a solution of 5% bovine serum albumin (BSA), Tris-buffered saline (TBS), and 0.05% Tween 20 overnight at 4°C after blocked in BSA at room temperature for 2 h. GAPDH was used as the control for total and cytosolic protein extract, while Histone H3 was the control for nuclear protein extract. After incubation with the appropriate secondary antibodies at room temperature for 2 h, the membranes were washed 3 times in TBST (TBS with Tween 20), and the immunoreactive protein was measured using a chemiluminescence system. All Western blot studies were repeated three times.

Immunofluorescence Analysis

In order to further verify that RUT reversed ethanol-induced NF-κB translocation from the cytoplasm to the nucleus, immunofluorescence analysis was performed. After deparaffinization and dehydration in gradient alcohol, gastric tissue paraffin sections were placed in ethylenediaminetetraacetic acid (EDTA) for antigen retrieval. Then the sections were washed three times with phosphate-buffered saline (PBS) and blocked with 1% BSA for 30 min at room temperature. Subsequently, sections were incubated with anti-NF-κB p65 antibody (1:500, **Table 1**) in a solution of 5% BSA and PBS at 4°C overnight in a damp box. After washed three times the next day, the sections were incubated with the appropriate secondary antibody for 1 h at room temperature. Later, 4,6-diamidino-2-phenylindole (DAPI) was used to stain nuclei and images were taken with a confocal microscope (NIKON Eclipse C1, Nikon Instruments Inc., Japan)

(at the top of the left column, continuing from previous page:) were carried out on Synergy Hybrid Reader (Biotek, Winooski, VT, United States).

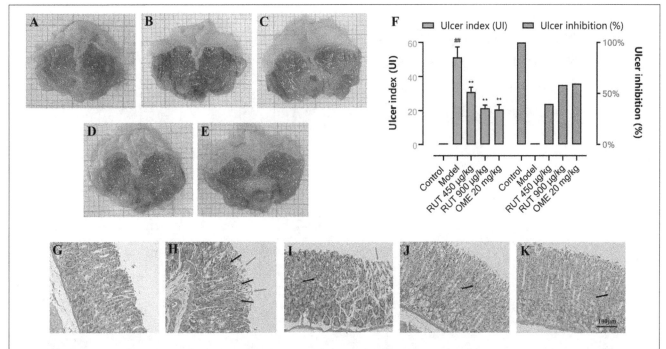

FIGURE 2 | Effect of RUT on ethanol-induced gastric mucosa injury in mice in different groups. Note: **(A–E)** Macroscopic representative images; **(F)** Ulcer index and ulcer inhibition; **(G–K)** Microscopic representative images (H&E stained, ×200 magnification; Scare bar: 100 μm. Blue →: loss of gastric epithelial cells; Black →: hemorrhagic injury; Yellow →: vascular congestion; Green →: edema; Red →: inflammatory cells infiltration). **(A,G)** Normal control group; **(B,H)** Model group; **(C,I)** RUT 450 μg/kg group; **(D,J)** RUT 900 μg/kg group; **(E,K)** OME 20 mg/kg group. Values are expressed as mean ± SD (n = 8). #$p < 0.05$ and ##$p < 0.01$ when compared with the control group. *$p < 0.05$ and **$p < 0.01$ when compared with the model group.

and analyzed by NIKON DS-U3 (Nikon Instruments Inc., Japan). Finally, we use Image-Pro Plus (version 6.0, Media Cybemetics, INC., Rockville, MD, United States) to measure and inregrate the optical density and total per area for a statistical analysis of Immunofluorescence staining.

Statistical Analysis

The experimental data were expressed as mean ± standard deviation (SD), and analyzed with the SPSS software program (Version 24.0, SPSS Inc., Chicago, IL, United States). Differences between groups were evaluated by one-way analysis of variance (ANOVA). Statistical analysis was performed using the GraphPad Prism Software (Version 8.0.1, California, United States). A value of $p < 0.05$ was considered statistically significant, and a value of $p < 0.01$ was considered highly significant.

RESULTS

Effect of RUT on Gross Evaluation of the Gastric Mucasa in Mice

Acute gastric mucosal injury was induced by intragastric administration of absolute ethanol. **Figure 2** shows that no visible lesions developed in the normal control group. The RUT groups or OME group showed extensively reduced gastric injury compared with the model group, which showed

severe gastric mucosal damage appearing as glandular area hyperemia, mucosal edema accompanied by dot and linear hemorrhage necrosis.

Then, in order to reflect the effect of RUT on ethanol stimulation, we used the Guth standard to quantitatively assess the gastric lesions and calculate ulcer inhibition rate. As shown in **Figure 2F**, the model group indicated by an average UI of 51.25 ± 6.09 ($p < 0.01$). However, pre-treatment with RUT at doses of 450 and 900 μg/kg or omeprazole (20 mg/kg) produced a significant reduction in the percentage of UI (by 39.76, 58.28 and 59.75%, respectively) when compared to the model group ($p < 0.01$).

Effect of Rutaecarpine on Histopathological Assessment of Gastric Damage

In order to evaluate the protective effect of RUT on the stomach in microscopic conditions, we conducted histopathological analysis. **Figures 2G–K** shows the histopathological alterations in gastric specimens of different experimental groups. The normal control group showed normal histological structures of the mucosa, submucosa as well as the muscularis. Serious damage of gastric mucosa was found in the submucosa of the model group, and the superficial gastric epithelium was disrupted and exfoliated. Moreover, vascular congestion, edema and inflammatory cells infiltration were also observed. It was clear that the gastric mucosa damages were attenuated with omeprazole or RUT demonstrated by the integrity of superficial gastric epithelium and improvement of

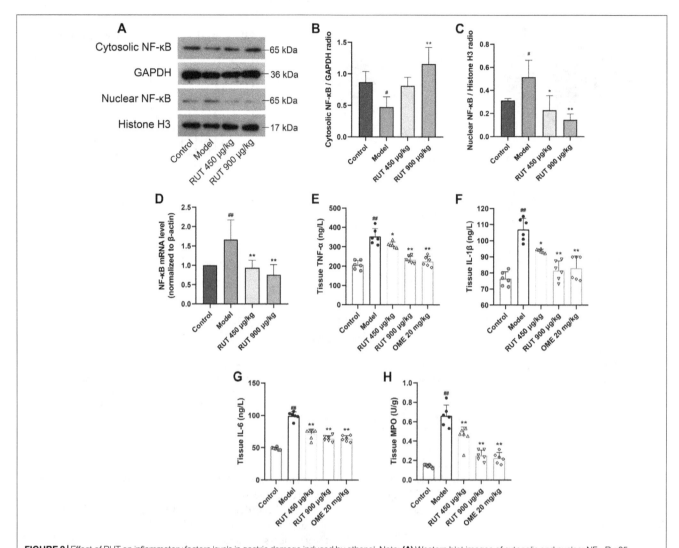

FIGURE 3 | Effect of RUT on inflammatory factors levels in gastric damage induced by ethanol. Note: **(A)** Western blot images of cytosolic and nuclear NF-κB p65; **(B)** Cytosolic NF-κB p65 protein level; **(C)** Nuclear NF-κB p65 protein level; **(D)** NF-κB p65 mRNA level; **(E)** Tissue TNF-α level; **(F)** Tissue IL-1β level; **(G)** Tissue IL-6 level; **(H)** Tissue MPO level. Values are expressed as mean ± SD (n = 6). #$p < 0.05$ and ##$p < 0.01$ when compared with the control group. *$p < 0.05$ and **$p < 0.01$ when compared with the model group.

hemorrhagic injury, edema and inflammatory infiltration Notably, the pretreatment of mice with 900 µg/kg of RUT conferred the most gastroprotection.

Effect of Rutaecarpine on Gastric NF-κB Activation and Its Downstream Inflammatory Cytokines Levels

Next, we assessed the variation of inflammatory factors in gastric mucosa aiming at exploring the intervene of RUT on inflammation. As revealed in **Figure 3**, the inflammatory disturbances were evaluated by monitoring the NF-κB nuclear translocation and alterations in its downstream signals. In terms of results, ethanol intake leaded to a sharp increase in NF-κB expression and nuclear translocation compared with control group (**Figures 3A–D**). Meanwhile, it also upregulated the level of some proinflammatory cytokines, such as TNF-α, IL-

1β, IL-6 as well as MPO (**Figures 3E–H**). While performance of RUT pretreatment attenuated the expression and nuclear translocation of NF-κB. In addition, RUT reversed the level of TNF-α, IL-1β, IL-6 and MPO effectively, which is consistent with the results after OME processing. We also additionally used immunofluorescence to analyze the nuclear translocation of NF-κB, and the result also verified the previous results (**Figure 4**). All of which prove that the anti-inflammatory effect of RUT can relieve gastric mucosal damage.

Effect of Rutaecarpine on Ethanol-Triggered Oxidative Stress and Antioxidant Enzumes Activity

Then, we explored the stimulation of oxidative stress in the gastric mucosa by monitoring changes in antioxidants and lipid peroxidation levels. Exposure to ethanol presented a high level

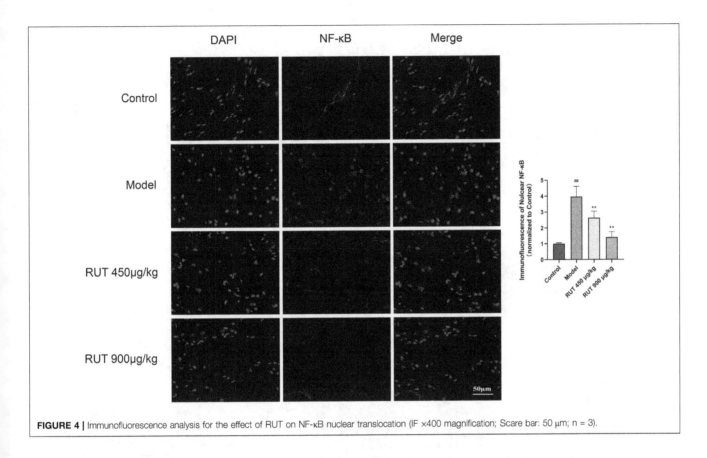

FIGURE 4 | Immunofluorescence analysis for the effect of RUT on NF-κB nuclear translocation (IF ×400 magnification; Scare bar: 50 μm; n = 3).

of lipid peroxidation, which was indicated by the increase of MDA (**Figure 5I**). In addition, the intake of ethanol significantly inhibited the activity and nuclear translocation of the antioxidant element Nrf2 (**Figures 5A–D**), accompanied by a decrease in its downstream signals levels, such as Nqo1, HO-1, SOD, CAT and GSH (**Figures 5E–H**), of which the levels of SOD, CAT and GSH were the same as those after OME treatment. RUT obviously offsets these oxidation distortions as proved by the reversal of the levels of these factors. Therefore, these results indicated that the involvement of RUT antioxidation activity for the restoration of gastric damages partly.

Effect of Rutaecarpine on Apoptosis Factors Levels and PI3K/AKT Pathway

At last, for effect of RUT on apoptosis, we measured the production of apoptotic signals and the activation of the PI3K/AKT pathway. It could be clearly observed that ethanol triggered gastric apoptosis as proved by the pronounced reduction in the level of Bcl-2 (**Figures 6A–C**) and the increase in the level of Bax (**Figures 6A,D,E**), and Caspase 3 (**Figures 6A,F**) when compared with the normal control group. In addition, ethanol inhibited the activity of PI3K/AKT pathway significantly. It is worth noting that RUT counteracted these mutations as demonstrated by the decline of Bax and restoration of Bcl-2. And Caspase 3 maintained its previous level after OME treatment. Besides, RUT restored the mRNA expression of PI3K and protein expression of pAKT. These results demonstrate that RUT

plays a considerable role in ameliorating the apoptosis situation in gastric mucosa and activating PI3K/AKT pathway, which is implicated in RUT gastroprotective effects.

DISCUSSION

GU is a multifactorial gastrointestinal disease, of which alcohol is the biggest contributing factor (Das and Banerjee, 1993). In this previous study, due to the functional and anatomical similarity to the human stomach, the mice were chosen as the model and administered ethanol intragastrically to simulate human GUs caused by excessive drinking. Additionally, in several frequently used models, such as ethanol, pylorus ligation, non-steroidal anti-inflammatory drugs (NSAIDs) and stress-induced GU, the ethanol model is one of the widely used experimental models, which is similar to lots of characteristics of human acute peptic ulcer disease (Deding et al., 2016; Li et al., 2018). However, the mechanism of ethanol damage to gastric mucosa is not completely clear. Previous studies have shown that it is related to the direct damage of gastric epithelial cells (Zhao et al., 2009) and mucus layer (da Silva et al., 2018), or the indirect damage such as the influence of gastric mucosal hemodynamics (Kawano and Tsuji, 2020), infiltration of leukocytes and ensued inflammatory (Li et al., 2017) and oxidative stress (Loguercio et al., 2009; Salaspuro, 2011) and apoptosis distortion (Arab et al., 2019). Thus, this present study focused on the forthputting of

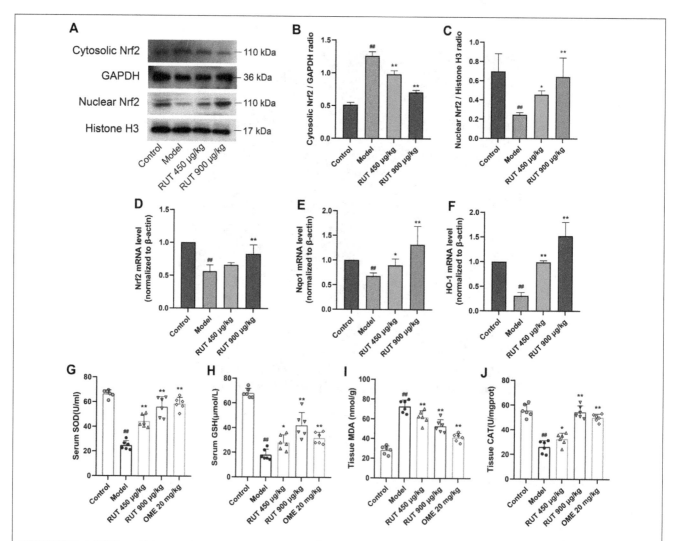

FIGURE 5 | Effect of RUT on oxidative stress factors levels in gastric damage induced by ethanol. Note: **(A)** Western blot images of cytosolic and nuclear Nrf2; **(B)** Cytosolic Nrf2 protein level; **(C)** Nuclear Nrf2 protein level; **(D)** Nrf2 mRNA level; **(E)** Nqo1 mRNA level; **(F)** HO-1 mRNA level; **(G)** Serum SOD level; **(H)** Serum GSH level; **(I)** Tissue MDA level. Values are expressed as mean ± SD (n = 6). #$p < 0.05$ and ##$p < 0.01$ when compared with the control group. *$p < 0.05$ and **$p < 0.01$ when compared with the model group.

RUT to treat ethanol-induced gastric injury through anti-inflammatory, anti-oxidation and anti-apoptosis.

In term of our results, ethanol intake could trigger severe inflammation in stomach, accompanied by activation of the NF-κB pathway and up-regulation of its downstream signal, such as TNF-a, IL-1B, IL-6 and MPO. These findings are in line with previous researches (Raish et al., 2018; Yeo et al., 2018;). In fact, NF-κB is expressed in almost all cells and performs a nonnegligible role in the pathogenesis of GU. Four transcript variants encoding different isoforms have been found including NF-κB p65/p105/p50/p52. In this article, we detected NF-κB p65 due to its contribution to inflammation. Many pro-inflammatory stimuli and ROS can lead to the activation of NF-κB through the phosphorylation of inhibitors of κB (IκBs) by the IκB kinase (IKK) complex (Akanda et al., 2018; Chen et al., 2001; Arab et al., 2019). Afterwards, free NF-κB translocates into the nucleus and consequently results in the transcriptional activation of a variety of pro-inflammatory mediators, such as TNF-α, IL-1β and IL-6 and MPO (Mitsuyama et al., 2006). Interestingly, RUT mitigated the gastric damage by inhibiting the NF-κB pathway, and then suppressed downstream proinflammatory elements. These correlates were consistent with mitigation of leukocyte infiltration. It is undoubtedly an efficacious strategy for the treatment of GU to ameliorate the aberration of these inflammatory pathological factors. In fact, RUT has pronounced anti-inflammatory capabilities in a variety of disease models according to the reports (Li et al., 2019a; Li et al., 2019b; Luo et al., 2020), which also corroborates our results from the side.

It is familiar that in addition to inflammation, the excessive generation of ROS also affects oxidative stress, which leads to altering the endogenous antioxidant defense system, including SOD and GSH (Arunachalam et al., 2019). The main source of ROS in ethanol-damaged gastric tissue is infiltration of activated

Rutaecarpine Ameliorates Ethanol-Induced Gastric Mucosal Injury in Mice by Modulating Genes...

43

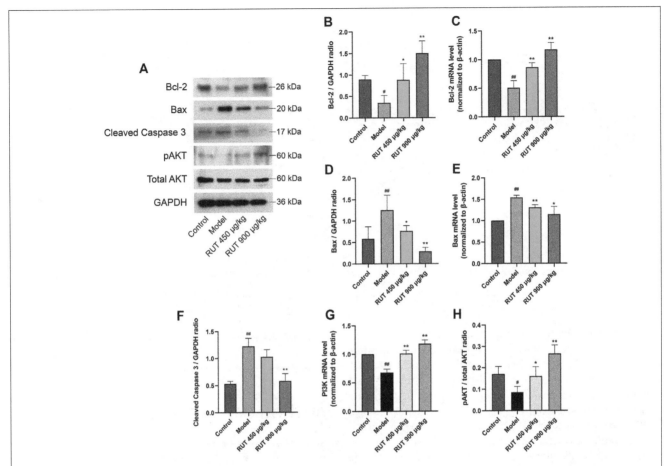

FIGURE 6 | Effect of RUT on apoptosis factors levels and PI3K pathway in gastric damage induced by ethanol. Note: **(A)** Western blot images of Bcl-2, Bax, pAKT and total AKT; **(B)** Bcl-2 protein level; **(C)** Bcl-2 mRNA level; **(D)** Bax protein level; **(E)** Bax mRNA level; **(F)** Tissue Caspase 9 level; **(G)** Caspase 3 mRNA level; **(H)** Tissue Caspase 3 level; **(I)** PI3K mRNA level. **(J)** pAKT protein level; Values are expressed as mean ± SD (n = 6). #$p < 0.05$ and ##$p < 0.01$ when compared with the control group. *$p < 0.05$ and **$p < 0.01$ when compared with the model group.

neutrophils, which MPO is a crucial indicator of neutrophil infiltration in ulcer-induced injuries (Arab et al., 2015; Paulrayer et al., 2017). Lipid peroxidation is consequence of ROS reaction against cell membrane and produces significant levels of MDA, which leads to oxidative gastric damage (Yu et al., 2017). The present findings indicated that the application of ethanol indulged MDA and significantly inhibited the production of the Nrf2. These changes prevented transcription factor Nrf2 from serving as a sensor to regulate the expression of antioxidant enzymes (HO-1 and Nqo1) driven by antioxidant response elements (ARE) in response to oxidative stimulation. The observations were consistent with previous researches (Nguyen et al., 2009; Itoh et al., 2010). Interestingly, our results show that RUT remarkably reverses the redox induced by ethanol. A good explanation for inhibiting oxidative stress was the observed remission of neutrophil infiltration and the decrease of membrane lipid peroxidation level. Ample evidence demonstrated the antioxidants plays a central role in process of GU (Kwiecien et al., 2002; Raish et al., 2018; Mohan, et al., 2020). Our data validated the restoration of Nrf2 along with the prototypical Nrf2 target genes (HO-1 and Nqo1) and the replenish of crucial antioxidation elements (SOD, CAT and GSH) in the wake of RUT treatment. All of data suggest the potential prospects of RUT in treating GU through anti-oxidation.

Numerous studies demonstrated that apoptosis also goes hand in hand with the occurrence of GU, and the continuous excessive production of apoptosis will destroy the integrity of gastric mucosa and eventually induce gastric mucosa dysfunction (Liu et al., 2020). Mechanistically, our data indicated ethanol intake made the anti-apoptosis gene Bcl-2 down-regulated markedly driven by ROS and pro-inflammatory signals. In this circumstance, the restriction to the apoptotic protein Bax was limited, which in turn leaded to the mitochondrial escape of cytochrome C and subsequently activated Caspase 9 and Caspase 3. This is consistent with previous studies (Raish et al., 2018; Xie et al., 2020). After receiving RUT, it could be clearly observed that the anti-apoptosis capacity of gastric mucosa was enhanced, manifested in the recovery of BCL-2 level and the control of Bax and Caspase 3. Actually, previous studies have demonstrated the latent anti-apoptosis activity (Li et al., 2019a; Li et al., 2019b; Han et al., 2019). And our data strongly indicated that RUT could partly participate in the palliation of the damage caused by ethanol though anti-apoptosis.

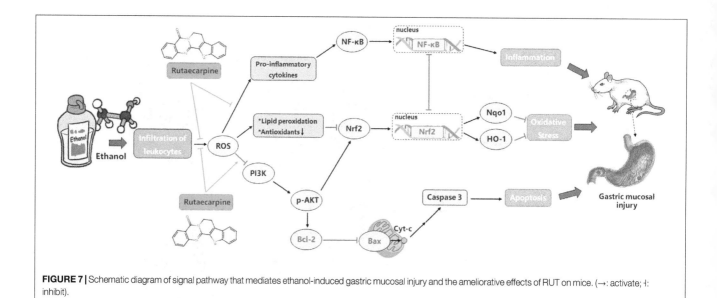

FIGURE 7 | Schematic diagram of signal pathway that mediates ethanol-induced gastric mucosal injury and the ameliorative effects of RUT on mice. (→: activate; ⊣: inhibit).

The present findings also revealed that ethanol inhibited PI3K/AKT pathway, which is consistent with previous literature (Zhang et al., 2019). In fact, the activation of PI3K/AKT pathway is essential for cell resistance to oxidation and apoptosis (Arab et al., 2019; Cao et al., 2020). Our data suggest that the activation of AKT phosphorylation promoted by RUT was associated with the Nrf2 and Bcl-2 up-regulation and in turn to the down-regulation of Bax.

In summary, inflammation, oxidative stress and apoptosis are closely related to the occurrence of GU. The excessive production of ROS released inflammation and apoptosis signals, and inhibited antioxidant elements to promote the continuous production of oxidative stress. Our findings clearly revealed that RUT augments cellular anti-inflammation, antioxidant and anti-apoptosis defense capacities, thereby protecting cells from ethanol damage. The potential mechanism seems to be related to the induction of antioxidant and anti-apoptosis enzymes synthesis by activating Nrf2 and Bcl-2 through PI3K/AKT-dependent pathway, and to the inhibition of NFKB pathway and inflammation signals. **Figure 7** showed their complex relationship. These findings indicate that RUT might be a potential therapeutic agent for GU.

AUTHOR CONTRIBUTIONS

SR and YZ conceived the project and wrote the manuscript. SR performed main part of the experiments, with contributions from YW, RW, SW, and JW. TY, XC, SW, MJ, HL, and MW contributed to the data collection and analysis. YZ participated in the project design as well as manuscript draft preparation and revision. All authors read and approved the final manuscript.

ACKNOWLEDGMENTS

This research was financially supported by the National Key Research and Development Program (No. 2018YFC1704500).

REFERENCES

Ahmad, S. S., Sinha, M., Ahmad, K., Khalid, M., and Choi, I. (2020). Study of Caspase 8 inhibition for the management of Alzheimer's disease: a molecular docking and dynamics simulation. *Molecules* 25 (9), 2071. doi:10.3390/molecules25092071

Akanda, M. R., Kim, I. S., Ahn, D., Tae, H. J., Nam, H. H., Choo, B. K., et al. (2018). Anti-inflammatory and gastroprotective roles of Rabdosia inflexa through downregulation of pro-inflammatory cytokines and MAPK/NF-κB signaling pathways. *Int. J. Mol. Sci.* 19 (2), 584. doi:10.3390/ijms19020584

Arab, H. H., Salama, S. A., Omar, H. A., Arafa, e., and Maghrabi, I. A. (2015). Diosmin protects against ethanol-induced gastric injury in rats: novel anti-ulcer actions. *PloS One* 10 (3), e0122417. doi:10.1371/journal.pone.0122417

Arab, H. H., Salama, S. A., Eid, A. H., Kabel, A. M., and Shahin, N. N. (2019). Targeting MAPKs, NF-κB, and PI3K/AKT pathways by methyl palmitate ameliorates ethanol-induced gastric mucosal injury in rats. *J. Cell. Physiol.* 234 (12), 22424–22438. doi:10.1002/jcp.28807

Arunachalam, K., Damazo, A. S., Pavan, E., Oliveira, D. M., Figueiredo, F. F., Machado, M., et al. (2019). Cochlospermum regium (Mart. ex Schrank) Pilg.: evaluation of chemical profile, gastroprotective activity and mechanism of action of hydroethanolic extract of its xylopodium in acute and chronic experimental models. *J. Ethnopharmacol.* 233, 101–114. doi:10.1016/j.jep.2019.01.002

Bustin, S. A., Benes, V., Garson, J. A., Hellemans, J., Huggett, J., Kubista, M., et al. (2009). The MIQE guidelines: minimum information for publication of quantitative real-time PCR experiments. *Clin. Chem.* 55 (4), 611–622. doi:10.1373/clinchem.2008.112797

Cao, W. Q., Zhai, X. Q., Ma, J. W., Fu, X. Q., Zhao, B. S., Zhang, P., et al. (2020). Natural borneol sensitizes human glioma cells to cisplatin-induced apoptosis by triggering ROS-mediated oxidative damage and regulation of MAPKs and PI3K/AKT pathway. *Pharm. Biol.* 58 (1), 72–79. doi:10.1080/13880209.2019.1703756

Chen, F., Castranova, V., and Shi, X. (2001). New insights into the role of nuclear factor-kappaB in cell growth regulation. *Am. J. Pathol.* 159 (2), 387–397. doi:10.1016/s0002-9440(10)61708-7

da Silva, D. M., Martins, J., de Oliveira, D. R., Florentino, I. F., da Silva, D., Dos Santos, F., et al. (2018). Effect of allantoin on experimentally induced gastric ulcers: pathways of gastroprotection. *Eur. J. Pharmacol.* 821, 68–78. doi:10.1016/j.ejphar.2017.12.052

Das, D. and Banerjee, R. K. (1993). Effect of stress on the antioxidant enzymes and gastric ulceration. *Mol. Cell. Biochem.* 125 (2), 115–125. doi:10.1007/BF00936440

Deding, U., Ejlskov, L., Grabas, M. P., Nielsen, B. J., Torp-Pedersen, C., and Bøggild, H. (2016). Perceived stress as a risk factor for peptic ulcers: a register-based cohort study. *BMC Gastroenterol.* 16 (1), 140. doi:10.1186/s12876-016-0554-9

Fukuma, Y., Sakai, E., Komaki, S., Nishishita, K., Okamoto, K., and Tsukuba, T. (2018). Rutaecarpine attenuates osteoclastogenesis by impairing macrophage colony stimulating factor and receptor activator of nuclear factor κ-B ligand-stimulated signalling pathways. *Clin. Exp. Pharmacol. Physiol.* 45 (8), 863–865. doi:10.1111/1440-1681.12941

Guth, P. H., Aures, D., and Paulsen, G. (1979). Topical aspirin plus HCl gastric lesions in the rat. Cytoprotective effect of prostaglandin, cimetidine, and probanthine. *Gastroenterology* 76 (1), 88–93. doi:10.1016/s0016-5085(79)80133-x

Han, M., Hu, L., and Chen, Y. (2019). Rutaecarpine may improve neuronal injury, inhibits apoptosis, inflammation and oxidative stress by regulating the expression of ERK1/2 and Nrf2/HO-1 pathway in rats with cerebral ischemia-reperfusion injury. *Drug Des. Dev. Ther.* 13, 2923–2931. doi:10.2147/DDDT.S216156

Huang, X. F., Dong, Y. H., Wang, J. H., Ke, H. M., Song, G. Q., and Xu, D. F. (2020). Novel PDE5 inhibitors derived from rutaecarpine for the treatment of Alzheimer's disease. *Bioorg. Med. Chem. Lett.* 30 (9), 127097. doi:10.1016/j.bmcl.2020.127097

Itoh, K., Mimura, J., and Yamamoto, M. (2010). Discovery of the negative regulator of Nrf2, Keap1: a historical overview. *Antioxid. Redox signal.* 13 (11), 1665–1678. doi:10.1089/ars.2010.3222

Jeon, D. B., Shin, H. G., Lee, B. W., Jeong, S. H., Kim, J. H., Ha, J. H., et al. (2020). Effect of heat-killed *Enterococcus faecalis* EF-2001 on ethanol-induced acute gastric injury in mice: protective effect of EF-2001 on acute gastric ulcer. *Hum. Exp. Toxicol.* 39 (5), 721–733. doi:10.1177/0960327119899987

Jia, S. j., and Hu, C. P. (2010). Pharmacological effects of rutaecarpine as a cardiovascular protective agent. *Molecules* 15: 1873–81. doi:10.3390/molecules15031873

Jin, S. W., Hwang, Y. P., Choi, C. Y., Kim, H. G., Kim, S. J., Kim, Y., et al. (2017). Protective effect of rutaecarpine against t-BHP-induced hepatotoxicity by upregulating antioxidant enzymes via the CaMKII-AKT and Nrf2/ARE pathways. *Food Chem. Toxicol.* 100, 138–148. doi:10.1016/j.fct.2016.12.031

Kawano, S. and Tsuji, S. (2000). Role of mucosal blood flow: a conceptional review in gastric mucosal injury and protection. *J. Gastroenterol. Hepatol.* 15 (Suppl. l), D1–D6. doi:10.1046/j.1440-1746.2000.02142.x

Khan, M., Khundmiri, S., Khundmiri, S. R., Al-Sanea, M. M., and Mok, P. L. (2018). Fruit-Derived polysaccharides and terpenoids: recent update on the gastroprotective effects and mechanisms. *Front. Pharmacol.* 9, 569. doi:10.3389/fphar.2018.00569

Kwiecień, S., Brzozowski, T., and Konturek, S. J. (2002). Effects of reactive oxygen species action on gastric mucosa in various models of mucosal injury. *J. Physiol. Pharmacol.* 53 (1), 39–50.

Lee, S. J., Ahn, H., Nam, K. W., Kim, K. H., and Mar, W. (2012). Effects of rutaecarpine on hydrogen peroxide-induced apoptosis in murine hepa-1c1c7 cells. *Biomol. Ther.* 20 (5), 487–491. doi:10.4062/biomolther.2012.20.5.487

Lee, Y. B., Yu, J., Choi, H. H., Jeon, B. S., Kim, H. K., Kim, S. W., et al. (2017). The association between peptic ulcer diseases and mental health problems: a population-based study: a STROBE compliant article. *Medicine* 96 (34), e7828. doi:10.1097/MD.0000000000007828

Li, W., Wang, Y., Wang, X., Zhang, H., He, Z., Zhi, W., et al. (2017). Gastroprotective effect of esculin on ethanol-induced gastric lesion in mice. *Fundam. Clin. Pharmacol.* 31 (2), 174–184. doi:10.1111/fcp.12255

Li, Q., Hu, X., Xuan, Y., Ying, J., Fei, Y., Rong, J., et al. (2018). Kaempferol protects ethanol-induced gastric ulcers in mice via pro-inflammatory cytokines and NO. *Acta Biochim. Biophys. Sin.* 50 (3), 246–253. doi:10.1093/abbs/gmy002

Li, Y., Zhang, G., Chen, M., Tong, M., Zhao, M., Tang, F., et al. (2019a). Rutaecarpine inhibited imiquimod-induced psoriasis-like dermatitis via inhibiting the NF-κB and TLR7 pathways in mice. *Biomed. Pharmacother.* 109, 1876–1883. doi:10.1016/j.biopha.2018.10.062

Li, Z., Yang, M., Peng, Y., Gao, M., and Yang, B. (2019b). Rutaecarpine ameliorated sepsis-induced peritoneal resident macrophages apoptosis and inflammation responses. *Life Sci.* 228, 11–20. doi:10.1016/j.lfs.2019.01.038

Liu, S. H., Ma, K., Xu, X. R., and Xu, B. (2010). A single dose of carbon monoxide intraperitoneal administration protects rat intestine from injury induced by lipopolysaccharide. *Cell Stress Chaperones*, 15 (5), 717–727. doi:10.1007/s12192-010-0183-0

Liu, R., Hao, Y. T., Zhu, N., Liu, X. R., Kang, J. W., Mao, R. X., et al. (2020a). The gastroprotective effect of small molecule oligopeptides isolated from Walnut (*Juglans regia* L.) against ethanol-induced gastric mucosal injury in rats. *Nutrients* 12 (4), 1138. doi:10.3390/nu12041138

Liu, X. Q., Jin, J., Li, Z., Jiang, L., Dong, Y. H., Cai, Y. T., et al. (2020b). Rutaecarpine derivative Cpd-6c alleviates acute kidney injury by targeting PDE4B, a key enzyme mediating inflammation in cisplatin nephropathy. *Biochem. Pharmacol.* 180, 114132. doi:10.1016/j.bcp.2020.114132

Liu, Y., Fu, Y. Q., Peng, W. J., Yu, Y. R., Wu, Y. S., Yan, H., et al. (2016). Rutaecarpine reverses the altered Connexin expression pattern induced by oxidized low-density Lipoprotein in monocytes. *J. Cardiovasc. Pharmacol.* 67 (6), 519–525. doi:10.1097/FJC.0000000000000372

Loguercio, C., Tuccillo, C., Federico, A., Fogliano, V., Del Vecchio Blanco, C., and Romano, M. (2009). Alcoholic beverages and gastric epithelial cell viability: effect on oxidative stress-induced damage. *J. Physiol. Pharmacol.* 60 (Suppl. 7), 87–92. PMID: 20388950. Available at: https://pubmed.ncbi.nlm.nih.gov/20388950/

Luo, J., Wang, X., Jiang, X., Liu, C., Li, Y., Han, X., et al. (2020). Rutaecarpine derivative R3 attenuates atherosclerosis via inhibiting NLRP3 inflammasome-related inflammation and modulating cholesterol transport. *FASEB J.* 34 (1), 1398–1411. doi:10.1096/fj.201900903RRR

Ma, J., Chen, L., Fan, J., Cao, W., Zeng, G., Wang, Y., et al. (2019). Dual-targeting Rutaecarpine-NO donor hybrids as novel anti-hypertensive agents by promoting release of CGRP. *Eur. J. Med. Chem.* 168, 146–153. doi:10.1016/j.ejmech.2019.02.037

Mitsuyama, K., Tsuruta, O., Matsui, Y., Harada, K., Tomiyasu, N., Suzuki, A., et al. (2006). Activation of c-Jun N-terminal kinase (JNK) signalling in experimentally induced gastric lesions in rats. *Clin. Exp. Immunol.* 143 (1), 24–29. doi:10.1111/j.1365-2249.2005.02959.x

Mohan, S., Hobani, Y. H., Shaheen, E., Abou-Elhamd, A. S., Abdelhaleem, A., Alhazmi, H. A., et al. (2020). Ameliorative effect of Boesenbergin A, a chalcone isolated from *Boesenbergia rotunda* (Fingerroot) on oxidative stress and inflammation in ethanol-induced gastric ulcer *in vivo*. *J. Ethnopharmacol.* 261, 113104. doi:10.1016/j.jep.2020.113104

Nguyen, T., Nioi, P., and Pickett, C. B. (2009). The Nrf2-antioxidant response element signaling pathway and its activation by oxidative stress. *J. Biol. Chem.* 284 (20), 13291–13295. doi:10.1074/jbc.r900010200

Paulrayer, A., Adithan, A., Lee, J. H., Moon, K. H., Kim, D. G., Im, S. Y., et al. (2017). Aronia melanocarpa (Black Chokeberry) reduces ethanol-induced gastric damage via regulation of HSP-70, NF-κB, and MCP-1 signaling. *Int. J. Mol. Sci.* 18 (6), 1195. doi:10.3390/ijms18061195

Piao, X., Li, S., Sui, X., Guo, L., Liu, X., Li, H., et al. (2018). 1-Deoxynojirimycin (DNJ) ameliorates indomethacin-induced gastric ulcer in mice by affecting NF-kappaB signaling pathway. *Front. Pharmacol.* 9, 372. doi:10.3389/fphar.2018.00372

Raish, M., Ahmad, A., Ansari, M. A., Alkharfy, K. M., Aljenoobi, F. I., Jan, B. L., et al. (2018). Momordica charantia polysaccharides ameliorate oxidative stress, inflammation, and apoptosis in ethanol-induced gastritis in mucosa through NF-kB signaling pathway inhibition. *Int. J. Biol. Macromol.* 111, 193–199. doi:10.1016/j.ijbiomac.2018.01.008

Salaspuro, M. (2011). Acetaldehyde and gastric cancer. *J. Dig. Dis.* 12 (2), 51–59. doi:10.1111/j.1751-2980.2011.00480.x

Søreide, K., Thorsen, K., Harrison, E. M., Bingener, J., Møller, M. H., Ohene-Yeboah, M., et al. (2015). Perforated peptic ulcer. *Lancet* 386 (10000), 1288–1298. doi:10.1016/s0140-6736(15)00276-7 |

Sung, J. J., Tsoi, K. K., Ma, T. K., Yung, M. Y., Lau, J. Y., and Chiu, P. W. (2010). Causes of mortality in patients with peptic ulcer bleeding: a prospective cohort study of 10,428 cases. *Am. J. Gastroenterol.* 105 (1), 84–89. doi:10.1038/ajg.2009.507

Surbala, L., Singh, C. B., Devi, R. V., and Singh, O. J. (2020). Rutaecarpine exhibits anti-diabetic potential in high fat diet-multiple low dose streptozotocin induced type 2 diabetic mice and *in vitro* by modulating hepatic glucose homeostasis. *J. Pharmacol. Sci.* 143 (4), 307–314. doi:10.1016/j.jphs.2020.04.008

Tian, K. M., Li, J. J., and Xu, S. W. (2019). Rutaecarpine: a promising cardiovascular protective alkaloid from Evodia rutaecarpa (Wu Zhu Yu). *Pharmacol. Res.* 141, 541–550. doi:10.1016/j.phrs.2018.12.019

Wallace, J. L. (2008). Prostaglandins, NSAIDs, and gastric mucosal protection: why doesn't the stomach digest itself?. *Physiol. Rev.* 88 (4), 1547–1565. doi:10.1152/physrev.00004.2008

Xie, L., Guo, Y. L., Chen, Y. R., Zhang, L. Y., Wang, Z. C., Zhang, T., et al. (2020). A potential drug combination of omeprazole and patchouli alcohol significantly normalizes oxidative stress and inflammatory responses against gastric ulcer in ethanol-induced rat model. *Int. Immunopharmacol.* 85, 106660. doi:10.1016/j.intimp.2020.106660

Yang, S., Wang, H., Yang, Y., Wang, R., Wang, Y., Wu, C., et al. (2019). Baicalein administered in the subacute phase ameliorates ischemia-reperfusion-induced brain injury by reducing neuroinflammation and neuronal damage. *Biomed. Pharmacother.* 117, 109102. doi:10.1016/j.biopha.2019.109102

Yeo, D., Hwang, S. J., Kim, W. J., Youn, H. J., and Lee, H. J. (2018). The aqueous extract from Artemisia capillaris inhibits acute gastric mucosal injury by inhibition of ROS and NF-kB. *Biomed. Pharmacother.* 99, 681–687. doi:10.1016/j.biopha.2018.01.118

Yu, T., Yang, Y., Kwak, Y. S., Song, G. G., Kim, M. Y., Rhee, M. H., et al. (2017). Ginsenoside Rc from Panax ginseng exerts anti-inflammatory activity by targeting TANK-binding kinase 1/interferon regulatory factor-3 and p38/ATF-2. *J. Ginseng Res.* 41 (2), 127–133. doi:10.1016/j.jgr.2016.02.001

Zhang, Z., Wen, H., Weng, J., Feng, L., Liu, H., Hu, X., et al. (2019). Silencing of EPCAM suppresses hepatic fibrosis and hepatic stellate cell proliferation in mice with alcoholic hepatitis via the PI3K/AKT/mTOR signaling pathway. *Cell Cycle* 18 (18), 2239–2254. doi:10.1080/15384101.2019.1642067

Zhang, Y., Yan, T., Sun, D., Xie, C., Wang, T., Liu, X., et al. (2020). Rutaecarpine inhibits KEAP1-NRF2 interaction to activate NRF2 and ameliorate dextran sulfate sodium-induced colitis. *Free Radic. Biol. Med.* 148, 33–41. doi:10.1093/abbs/gmp014

Zhao, W., Zhu, F., Shen, W., Fu, A., Zheng, L., Yan, Z., et al. (2009). Protective effects of DIDS against ethanol-induced gastric mucosal injury in rats. *Acta Biochim. Biophys. Sin.* 41 (4), 301–308. doi:10.1093/abbs/gmp014

Zhao, Z., Gong, S., Wang, S., and Ma, C. (2015). Effect and mechanism of evodiamine against ethanol-induced gastric ulcer in mice by suppressing Rho/NF-кБ оатжхачǎ *Int. Immunopharmacol.* 28 (1), 588–595. doi:10.1016/j.intimp.2015.07.030

5

Intrahepatic T$_H$17/T$_{Reg}$ Cells in Homeostasis and Disease—It's All About the Balance

Hannah K. Drescher[1*†], Lea M. Bartsch[1*†], Sabine Weiskirchen[2] and Ralf Weiskirchen[2]

[1] Division of Gastroenterology, Massachusetts General Hospital and Harvard Medical School, Boston, MA, United States,
[2] Institute of Molecular Pathobiochemistry, Experimental Gene Therapy and Clinical Chemistry (IFMPEGKC), University Hospital, RWTH Aachen, Aachen, Germany

*Correspondence:
Hannah K. Drescher
hdrescher@mgh.harvard.edu
Lea M. Bartsch
lbartsch1@mgh.harvard.edu

†These authors have contributed equally to this work

Both acute and chronic hepatic inflammation likely result from an imbalance in the T$_H$1/T$_H$2 cell response and can lead to liver fibrosis and end-stage liver disease. More recently, a novel CD4+ T helper cell subset was described, characterized by the production of IL-17 and IL-22. These T$_H$17 cells 50were predominantly implicated in host defense against infections and in autoimmune diseases. Interestingly, studies over the last 10 years revealed that the development of T$_H$17 cells favors pro-inflammatory responses in almost all tissues and there is a reciprocal relationship between T$_H$17 and T$_{Reg}$ cells. The balance between T$_H$17 and T$_{Reg}$ cells is critical for immune reactions, especially in injured liver tissue and the return to immune homeostasis. The pathogenic contribution of T$_H$17 and T$_{Reg}$ cells in autoimmunity, acute infection, and chronic liver injury is diverse and varies among disease etiologies. Understanding the mechanisms underlying T$_H$17 cell development, recruitment, and maintenance, along with the suppression of T$_{Reg}$ cells, will inform the development of new therapeutic strategies in liver diseases. Active manipulation of the balance between pathogenic and regulatory processes in the liver may assist in the restoration of homeostasis, especially in hepatic inflammation.

Keywords: T$_H$17 cells, T$_{Reg}$ cells, T$_H$17/T$_{Reg}$ balance, liver, autoimmune diseases, viral infection

INTRODUCTION

CD4 T cells play a central role in mediating the host immune response to pathogens and in autoimmunity, cancer, and chronic inflammation. They maintain and enhance CD8 T cell responses, interact with B cells to induce antibody development, regulate the function of monocytes/macrophages, and orchestrate the immune response to pathogens. CD4+ T cells also modulate immune homeostasis by suppressing pro-inflammatory immune responses, build immunologic memory, and control autoimmunity (Zhu et al., 2010). These functions are achieved through the differentiation of naïve CD4+ T cells into subsets of effector, memory, and regulatory T cells.

T cell activation and differentiation rely on different stimuli, and differentiation is initiated by a cognate antigen presented by specialized antigen-presenting cells (APCs) or other immune cells. Fragmented antigens are presented on major histocompatibility complex 2 (MHC-2) molecules and recognized by the T cell receptor (TCR). Various co-stimulatory receptors and cytokines are essential for T cell activation and determine the direction of T cell differentiation.

Distinct subpopulations of CD4 T cells originating from a common precursor were first described in 1986: in mouse T cell clones, Mosmann and Coffman found that two types of T helper cells could be distinguished by their cytokine production, lymphokine activity, and transcription factor and surface marker expression (Mosmann et al., 1986). The authors defined type 1 T helper cells (T_H1) by their secretion of interferon-γ (IFN-γ), interleukin-2 (IL-2) and tumor necrosis factor-α (TNF-α). Type 2 T helper cells (T_H2) were characterized by the expression of IL-4, IL-5, and IL-13. Interestingly, the cytokines secreted by each mature T helper cell subset directly antagonize the development and differentiation of the corresponding opposite T helper cell subtype, thereby sustaining lineage-specific immune responses.

This profile has since been refined. Intensive studies of the complex cytokine milieu and transcription factor networks involved in the differentiation of CD4 T helper cell subsets originating from the same naïve CD4 T cell precursor identified many more T helper cell subsets. The potentially distinct T cell lineages include not only T_H1, T_H2, T_H17, and peripheral regulatory T cells (pT_{Reg}) cells, but also T_H9, T_H22, regulatory type 1 (Tr1), and follicular helper T cells (T_{FH}) (Saravia et al., 2019). CD4+ T cell lineages are now understood to be a plastic and flexible network. One CD4+ subset cannot differentiate from only one distinct precursor cell, but rather

differentiates from different subsets depending on the environmental milieu (**Figure 1**).

In this review, we discuss developmental differences between T_H17 and T_{Reg} cells and their roles in health and disease, with a focus on liver disease. The fragile balance between these two cell types was recently found to play a crucial role in maintaining immune homeostasis. A shift of this balance drives pro-inflammatory immune responses, especially in chronic inflammatory diseases, cancer and autoimmunity. Here, we highlight the intrahepatic effects of this balance in acute and chronic inflammation as well as in liver cancer and autoimmunity.

T_H17 CELLS IN HEALTH AND DISEASE

A T helper cell subset of IL-17 producing T_H17 cells defends against fungal and extracellular bacterial infection and are integral in tissue inflammation and autoimmune diseases (Tesmer et al., 2008). While it was first believed that these cells are an inflammatory subset within the T_H1 lineage, it was later determined that T_H17 cells are an independent T helper cell lineage (Aarvak et al., 1999).

T_H17 Cell Development

The discovery of a new T helper cell subset with pro-inflammatory properties, referred to as T_H17 cells because of their expression of IL-17A, revolutionized the understanding of the adaptive immune system in the early 2000s (Park et al., 2005). T_H17 cell differentiation in secondary lymphoid organs

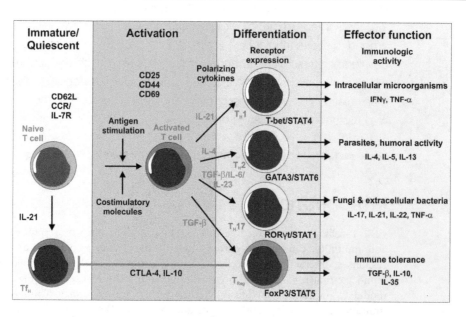

FIGURE 1 | After activation of the T cell receptor by antigen stimulation and co-stimulation, immature CD4+ naïve T cells proliferate and can differentiate into different effector T cells depending on the cytokine milieu. IL-21 stimulation promotes the T_H1 subpopulation accompanied with T-bet/STAT4 expression and effector function against intracellular pathogens. T_H2 cell populations develop after IL-4 stimulation with GATA3/STAT6 upregulation and supporting anti-parasite immune response and humoral activity. TGF-β in the presence of pro-inflammatory cytokines promotes T_H17 cell differentiation. T_H17 cells support the immune response against fungi and extracellular bacteria, whereas T_{Reg} cells have an immune tolerant function by producing anti-inflammatory cytokines and inhibiting T_{FH} function. Although these specific cytokines are important for CD4+ T cell subpopulation development, the differentiation is a plastic and flexible network.

depends on an inflammatory cytokine milieu consisting of IL-23, TGF-β, IL-6, IL-1β, and IL-21 to activate the expression of the lineage-specific transcription factor RORγt, fostering T_H17 cell generation. The role of RORγt was described by Ivanov et al. in 2006, who found this transcription factor to be expressed by IL-17 producing T helper cells in the lamina propria; in RORγt-deficient mice, IL-17+ cells were absent (Ivanov et al., 2006).

T_H17 cells expand in the periphery and at the tissue site of inflammation and secrete a distinct group of effector molecules such as IL-17A, IL-17F, IL-21, IL-22, and IL-6 and express IL-23 receptor (IL-23R) on their surface (Bettelli et al., 2006; Mangan et al., 2006). Human T_H17 cells originate from a CD161+ (the human equivalent to NK1.1) precursor in the thymus and umbilical cord blood and express CCR4 and CCR6 but not CXCR3 (Cosmi et al., 2008; Maggi et al., 2010).

Autocrine- and paracrine-derived TGF-β plays an interesting role during T_H17 cell polarization. During the induction of RORγt expression, TGF-β synergizes with IL-6. TGF-β and IL-6 typically have opposing effects, but in this setting these proteins amplify the maturation of T_H17 cells. In an autocrine amplification loop, TGF-β is further able to synergize with IL-21, which is predominantly produced by T_H17 cells. This synergy promotes and enhances T_H17 cell differentiation and pro-inflammatory immune responses (Gutcher et al., 2011). High concentrations of TGF-β in the absence of pro-inflammatory cytokines can lead to the inhibition of RORγt expression.

TGF-β can also induce the surface expression of IL-23R on differentiating T_H17 cells, along with IL-6/IL-21, making the cells responsive to the inflammatory cytokine IL-23. IL-23 is a member of the IL-12 cytokine family and is mainly produced by APCs. It enhances the activation of STAT3, which together with RORγt stabilizes T_H17 cell function. Therefore, IL-23 is not only important for T_H17 cell generation and thereby the activation and maintenance of inflammatory responses at the tissue site of inflammation, but also promotes persistent chronic inflammation by supporting the proliferation of T_H17 cells within the activated memory T cell pool (Aggarwal et al., 2003; Zhou et al., 2007; McGeachy et al., 2009).

In 2007, McGeachy et al. and Korn et al. described "classical" and "alternative" modes of T_H17 cell activation that were further supported by a study from Ghoreschi et al. in 2010 (Korn et al., 2007; McGeachy et al., 2007; Ghoreschi et al., 2010). The different modes are driven by the availability of IL-23 and TGF-β. "Classical" T_H17 cells, which arise from naïve CD4 T cells in the presence of TGF-β and IL-6 and the relative lack of IL-23, act through nonpathogenic expression of IL-10. Absence of expression of the TGF-β RII prevents the formation of T_H17 cells that mediate the development of experimental autoimmune encephalomyelitis (EAE) (Veldhoen et al., 2006). The idea of a nonpathogenic T_H17 cell subtype is further underlined by the fact that in homeostasis, T_H17 cells are present in the intestine without detrimental effects. "Alternative" T_H17 cells mature in the presence of IL-23 and are the pathogenic T_H17 subtype. Overall, the development of T_H17 cells is driven by a complex equilibrium of cytokine milieu, which influences many fine-tuning processes and a spectrum of effector functions.

The secretion of cytokines from either terminally differentiated T_H1 (IFN-γ) or T_H2 (IL-4) cells antagonizes the expansion of other T helper cell subtypes to sustain a lineage-specific immune response during infection. The differentiation of T_H17 cells is negatively regulated by IFN-γ and IL-4 via the inhibition of IL-23 and by T_{Reg} cells via retinoic acid and IL-2. Opposingly, IL-17 and IL-23 hamper the development of T_H1 cells (Harrington et al., 2005; Nakae et al., 2007). Interestingly, another IFN-γ and IL-4 independent pathway controls the development of T_H17 cells. This process is driven by an additional member of the IL-12 family, IL-27. Like IL-12 and IL-23, IL-27 is secreted by APCs and acts independently of IFN-γR, IL-6R, and T-Bet but requires STAT1. Batten et al. and Stumhofer et al. found that a lack of IL-27 signaling lead to an increase in T_H17 cells in autoimmune encephalomyelitis and chronic encephalitis (Batten et al., 2006; Stumhofer et al., 2006).

Unlike T_H1 and T_H2 cells, T_H17 cells have an unstable cytokine memory and convey a surprising capacity of late-stage plasticity in their polarization status to adapt to a changing microenvironment. Because T_H17 cells express low levels of IL-12R, they influence a phenotype shift after IL-12 stimulation that downregulates IL-17 and makes the cells susceptible to polarizing into a T_H1-, but not a T_H2-, like phenotype (Lee et al., 2009). This plasticity and the synergy between T_H1 and T_H17 cells is important for host defense mechanisms, as shown in a mouse model of *Mycobacterium tuberculosis* infection in which an early T_H17 immune response recruited T_H1 cells to the site of inflammation and promoted the development of T cell memory (Khader et al., 2007). It can also be a driving mechanism in autoimmunity and cancer.

T_H17 Cells in Host Defense and Autoimmunity

Until 1996, it was assumed that autoimmune diseases are the consequence of a dysregulation of T_H1 responses. A study by Ferber et al. showed that loss of IFN-γ did not prevent the development of EAE but rather worsened disease progression (Ferber et al., 1996). Based on those findings, Oppmann and colleagues described IL-23 as new cytokine secreted by dendritic cells (DCs) that can induce the production of IFN-γ and IL-17 (Oppmann et al., 2000). Antibody-mediated blockade of IL-23 and generation of IL-23 deficient mice highlighted its involvement in the development of Crohn's disease, psoriasis, EAE, and collagen-induced arthritis and the experimental animals either showed delayed and reduced disease severity or never developed autoimmune disease (Cua et al., 2003; Murphy et al., 2003; Mannon et al., 2004; Krueger et al., 2007). Clinical trials using monoclonal antibodies interfering with IL-12 and IL-23, such as ustekinumab, showed promising results in the improvement of psoriasis and psoriatic arthritis symptoms. In chronic ulcerative colitis patients, blockade of the interaction of IL-12 and IL-23 and their specific receptors on T_H1 and T_H17 cells also showed beneficial effects (Sands et al., 2019). Other antibodies, such as secukinumab, specifically targeting IL-17A were also highly effective in psoriasis patients (Sanford and McKeage, 2015).

Additionally, blockade of IL-17 or the loss of the regulatory mediators RORγt and IL-6 resulted in comparable outcomes *via* a lack of infiltration of T_H17 cells into the tissue sites of inflammation, pointing to a crucial role for these cells in the development and progression of autoimmune diseases. Finally, experiments performing an adoptive transfer of T_H17 cells clearly showed that these cells, but not T_H1 cells, modulate autoimmune conditions in mice. This finding was supported in human patients with multiple sclerosis, rheumatoid arthritis, and psoriasis, in whom increased levels of IL-17 and IL-23 were observed (Ziolkowska et al., 2000; Cho et al., 2004; Vaknin-Dembinsky et al., 2006). Although an increasing body of evidence points to a dominant role of T_H17 cells as inducers of autoimmunity, it is important to note that T_H1 cells are also crucial in the development of autoimmunity. Each target tissue of inflammation actively participates in the formation of a site-specific cytokine milieu through its cellular composition.

The gut is an especially interesting organ to investigate the plasticity of T_H17 cells. In homeostasis, the intestine is the primary site of T_H17 cell differentiation, and the gut microbiota heavily influences its regulation. The TCR of intestinal T_H17 cells has a distinct specificity for antigens coming from segmented filamentous bacteria, suggesting that these bacteria are critical for the induction of gut-resident T_H17 maturation (Huber et al., 2012). The function of these cells under non-pathogenic conditions is to protect against microbial invasion and maintain intestinal barrier function as well as to maintain other barrier sites of the body such as the lung epithelium or the skin. Non-pathogenic characteristics of these cells can specifically be found in the small intestine, where they limit inflammation in response to bacterial or parasitic infections *via* the secretion of IL-10. The fragile and complexly controlled phenotype of T_H17 cells can easily shift to an activated state in which cells attain pathogenicity and induce tissue inflammation that often leads to autoimmunity in the intestine and in other distant organs (Wu et al., 2010). In Peyer's Patches, T_H17 cells transition into a phenotype similar to T_{FH} cells producing IL-21 and Bcl-6 that can induce the production of IgA antibodies by germinal center B cells (Hirota et al., 2013). Upon bacterial infection in the colon, T_H17 cells can transform into cells producing IL-17 and IFN-γ simultaneously in an IL-23 dependent manner and further develop into a TH1-like cell type. Transferring this cell type can lead to a T_H17/T_H1 cell-induced transfer-colitis (Morrison et al., 2013; Harbour et al., 2015).

In humans, T cells expressing IL-17 and IFN-γ were found in peripheral blood and the gut lamina propria of patients with inflammatory bowel disease (Globig et al., 2014). T_H17/T_H1 cells are present at the organ site of inflammatory responses in different models of autoimmune diseases, such as in the colon in chronic colitis or as revealed by single-cell RNA-sequencing analysis in experimental autoimmune encephalitis (EAE), which serves as model for human multiple sclerosis (Neurath et al., 2002; Gaublomme et al., 2015). Hirota and colleagues demonstrated that these cells derive from T_H17 rather than from T_H1 cells (Hirota et al., 2011). This was further supported by a study from Bettelli **et al.** who showed that animals deficient for the transcription factor T-bet were protected against the development of EAE (Bettelli et al., 2004).

These findings suggest that T cells expressing IL-17 and IFN-γ, also known as double producers, are highly pathogenic and predominantly involved in autoimmune diseases and tissue inflammation. However, it is not fully understood whether the production of IFN-γ by T_H17 cells serves to limit T_H17 cell-induced inflammation or rather promotes inflammation.

REGULATORY T CELLS (T_{REG}) IN HEALTH AND DISEASE

T_{Reg} Development

Regulatory T cells (T_{Reg}) balance host defense against foreign pathogens, foster immune tolerance, and orchestrate immune homeostasis. The two main T_{Reg} subsets are natural T_{Reg} cells (nT_{Reg}), which provide central tolerance against self-antigens, and peripheral T_{Reg} cells (pTReg), which develop extrathymically from conventional T cells and recognize non-self-antigens (Sakaguchi, 2004). T cells maintain peripheral tolerance by regulating inflammatory responses against the microbiota, commensals, and pathogens (Hadis et al., 2011; Lathrop et al., 2011) (**Figure 2**).

Natural T_{Reg} Development

nT_{Regs} develop during the neonatal period during thymocyte maturation (Liston et al., 2008). Stable nT_{Reg} development requires a complex network of antigen presenting cells (APCs) and 1) TCR-dependent recognition of self-antigens, 2) cytokine stimulation (IL-2, IL-15, and IL-7), and 3) other costimulatory signals (Bayer et al., 2005). The TCR repertoire of nT_{Reg} cells varies from the effector T cell repertoire with only minor overlap (Wong et al., 2007). The recognition affinity of self-antigens by nT_{Reg} cells is crucial for nT_{Reg} development and must fall between positive and negative selection (Maloy and Powrie, 2001). In addition to affinity to the MHC self-antigen complex, the expression level on the APC is important for optimal nT_{Reg} maturation. Cytokine stimulation by IL-2, IL-15, and IL-7 promote nT_{Reg} development, function, and homeostasis (Vang et al., 2008). Costimulatory signals through CD28 stimulation are also essential to maintain nT_{Reg} survival and to avoid defective nT_{Reg} development (Tai et al., 2005). Thus, costimulatory signals function as expansion, rather than as selective, signals.

During thymic differentiation of nT_{Reg} cells, immature single-positive CD4+ T cells express the IL-2 receptor α chain (CD25) (Setoguchi et al., 2005). CD25 has high IL-2 affinity, is continuously expressed on T_{Reg} cells, and benefits T_{Reg} responsiveness in comparison to effector cells when IL-2 concentrations are low. CD25 deficiency is related to defective T_{Reg} development, function, and an imbalanced immune system (Goudy et al., 2013). After differentiation, nT_{Reg} cells stabilize their lineage specific transcription factor forkhead box protein 3 (FOXP3) and gain suppressive functions (Fontenot et al., 2017).

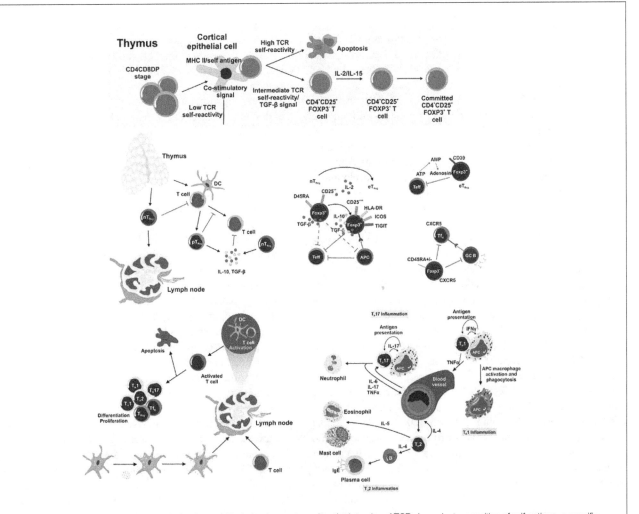

FIGURE 2 | Natural T_{Reg} cells (nT_{Reg}) maturate in the thymus. Their development requires the interplay of TCR-dependent recognition of self-antigen, a specific cytokine milieu (including TGF-β, IL-2, IL-7, IL-15) and the presence of co-stimulatory factors. They then infiltrate into the periphery. In the lymph node, T cells encounter a specific antigen from antigen presenting cells and become activated. Depending on the strength of the TCR binding and the presence or absence of co-stimulatory factors, cells either differentiate and proliferate into effector cells or undergo apoptosis. Peripheral T_{Reg} (pT_{Reg}) cells develop predominately in the periphery from naïve CD4+ T cells. However, nT_{Reg} and pT_{Reg} cells share the lineage markers CD25 and FoxP3 which are highly expressed in effector T_{Reg} cells (eT_{Reg}). eT_{Reg} cells suppress antigen presenting cells (APC) and effector T cells (T_{eff}) and are thereby very efficient in inhibiting the pro-inflammatory immune response. Furthermore, T_{Reg} cells express CD39 on the cell surface to convert extracellular ATP (eATP) to adenosine and prevent a pro-inflammatory immune response. Follicular helper T (T_{FH}) cells suppress the germinal center B cell reaction. Importantly, T_{Reg}s also inhibit T_{eff} in the circulation. T_H17 cells secret pro-inflammatory cytokines and attract neutrophils to the inflammation site, while T_H1 cells promote macrophage development and function and T_H2 cells lead to plasma, eosinophil, and mast cell differentiation and generate a pro-inflammatory immune response.

They further exhibit a specific CpG hypomethylation at three conserved non-coding DNA sequences (CNS) at the FOXP3 promotor, influencing the overall transcriptional activity of the cell (Toker et al., 2013). These epigenetic modifications are obligatory for T_{Reg} lineage stability, because they influence the activity of central signaling pathways like NF-κB, NFAT, STAT5, mTOR, and the binding of transcription factors to the FOXP3 promotor (Zheng et al., 2010). Further, T_{Reg}-specific demethylation regions (TSDRs) contribute to a specific demethylation signature abundant in T_{Reg} function-defining genes (e.g., CTLA-4, IL-2RA, IKzf4) which regulate the overall transcriptional activity, development, and function of T_{Reg} cells.

Although FOXP3 is interrelated with T_{Reg} function, its expression is not exclusive for T_{Reg} cells as it can be transiently upregulated in activated T cells and likewise several T_{Reg} specific genes are FOXP3 independent. However, FOXP3 is necessary but not sufficient to induce T_{Reg} cells (Hill et al., 2007).

Peripheral T_{Reg} Development

In contrast to nT_{Reg} cells, pT_{Reg} cells develop in the peripheral tissue from naïve CD4+ T cells across the lifespan of an individual. pT_{Reg} cells also have a slightly different TCR repertoire and prevent an overwhelming immune response from occurring in response to microbiota, commensals, and pathogens (Hadis et al., 2011; Lathrop et al., 2011). pT_{Reg} and nT_{Reg} cells share the expression of the lineage defining molecules CD25 and FOXP3. Although, the frequency of pT_{Reg} cells is low, their percentage can be enriched in different tissues under inflammatory conditions (Curotto de Lafaille et al., 2008). Like nT$_{Reg}$ cells, the promotion of pT$_{Reg}$ differentiation is driven by TCR signaling, TGF-β, and IL-2 and costimulatory signals (Chen et al., 2003). The importance of TGF-β signaling was demonstrated in mice, when TGF-β deficiency prevented pT$_{Reg}$ differentiation and FOXP3 stabilization (Marie et al., 2005) suggesting that specific demethylation at the FOXP3 promotor is important for pT$_{Reg}$ differentiation, function, and lineage stability (Takimoto et al., 2010).

pT$_{Reg}$ development can differ by tissue. The process is highly induced in the intestine because of the special immune demands at this site. Primarily, mucosal DCs support pT$_{Reg}$ development by producing TGF-β and retinoic acid (Coombes et al., 2007). The latter supports FOXP3 stabilization by CNS1 (Mucida et al., 2009). In addition, pT$_{Reg}$ differentiation is enhanced by metabolites produced by the microbiota in the intestine, along with chromatin structure and FOXP3 stabilization facilitated by short chain fatty acids (Arpaia et al., 2013). Fascinatingly, a high percentage of the pT$_{Reg}$ population in the intestine co-expresses RORγt and FOXP3 while preserving the overall epigenetic and genetic signature and function of T$_{Reg}$ cells (Yang et al., 2016).

The peripheral FOXP3+ cell population is very heterogenous and can be divided into different subpopulations according to FOXP3, CD25, and CD45RA expression profiles reflecting their activation, cytokine expression, and manifestation of epigenetic changes. CD45RA^{+}FOXP3^{low}CD25^{low} are defined as resting or naïve T$_{Reg}$ cells. CD45RA^{-}FOXP3^{high}CD25^{high} are described as effector T$_{Reg}$ cells (eT$_{Reg}$), and CD45RA^{-}FOXP3^{low}CD25^{low} cells are non T$_{Reg}$ cells and represent activated conventional T cells. The CD45RA^{+}FOXP3^{low}CD25^{low} subpopulation is further characterized by the expression of naïve T cell markers, the majority of which express CD31, a thymic emigrant marker, and the TSDR is widely conserved. The CD45RA^{-}FOXP3^{high}CD25^{high} subpopulation, in contrast, exhibits a highly suppressive and proliferative capacity and is profoundly demethylated (Miyara et al., 2009).

The Role of T$_{Reg}$ Cells in Immune Homeostasis and Inflammation

T$_{Reg}$ cells balance the immune response in homeostasis and inflammation. These cells orchestrate the immune response of effector T cells (T$_{eff}$) and initiate anti-inflammatory mechanisms.

Basic Mechanism of T$_{Reg}$ Function

T$_{Reg}$ cells influence the immune response by producing anti-inflammatory cytokines such as IL-10 and TGF-β. IL-10 has a potent immunosuppressive function by inhibiting the production of pro-inflammatory chemokines and cytokines and establishing immune balance in response to a pathogen, autoimmune disease, and allergy (O'Garra et al., 2004). IL-10 directly inhibits co-stimulation *via* CD28 and ICOS and indirectly by the downregulation of co-stimulatory molecules on APCs (Taylor et al., 2007). In addition, IL-10 produced by T$_{Reg}$ cells orchestrates antibody production in allergies from IgE toward IgG4. IgG4 and IL-10 production is upregulated in a course of allergen-specific immunotherapies and inhibits IgE-mediated anaphylaxis (Epp et al., 2018).

Interestingly, T$_{Regs}$ producing TGF-β may not be required for complete T$_{Reg}$ function and influence overall T$_{Reg}$ differentiation (Piccirillo, 2008). Numerous studies revealed the importance of TGF-β mediated T$_{Reg}$ function and the upregulation of TGF-β to amend their suppressive function. TGF-β represses the cytolytic function of effector CD8+ cells by downregulating cytolytic genes (e.g., Fas ligand, perforin, granzyme A, B and IFN-γ) in autoimmune diseases and cancer (Thomas and Massague, 2005). In addition, TGF-β produced by T$_{Reg}$ cells inhibits natural killer cell function and contributes to the overall anti-inflammatory effects of TGF-β (Cortez et al., 2017). Furthermore, T$_{Reg}$-mediated TGF-β can suppress naïve T cell activation and differentiation and can function as a self-regulating stimulus to maintain T$_{Reg}$ development (Tran, 2012). Although the role of TGF-β in direct suppressive T$_{Reg}$ function remains controversial, this cytokine seems important but not obligatory.

Another anti-inflammatory cytokine that complements the inhibitory repertoire of T$_{Reg}$ cells is IL-35. IL-35 plays a suppressive role in autoimmune diseases, allergies, and cancer models. In addition to T$_{Reg}$ cells, IL-35 is secreted by B$_{Reg}$ cells and CD8+ cells. Thus, this cytokine prevents effector T cell expansion, cytokine production, and T$_H$17 differentiation (Collison et al., 2007; Niedbala et al., 2007). IL-35 also supports T$_{Reg}$ and B$_{Reg}$ expansion and activation by influencing the immune response in autoimmunity (Dambuza et al., 2017). In sum, cytokines fundamentally contribute to suppressive T$_{Reg}$ function.

T$_{Reg}$ cells express various inhibitory receptors on the cell surface. One of the most important and well-studied inhibitory receptors is the cytotoxic T lymphocyte antigen-4 (CTLA-4), which is functionally and structurally related to CD28 and can bind B7 with a 50–100-fold higher affinity. CTLA-4 is upregulated in activated and exhausted T cells but continuously expressed on T$_{Reg}$ cells and supports their inhibitory function. By binding to B7, CTLA-4 inhibits T cell activation, proliferation, and cytokine production including IL-2 (Krummel and Allison, 1996). CTLA-4 further leads to the removal of costimulatory receptors on APCs (Sansom, 2015). A defect in CTLA-4 function, for example by non-sense mutation in the gene encoding CTLA-4, leads to defective T$_{Reg}$ function and is accompanied by complex autoimmune disorder and immunodeficiency in humans. Interestingly, patients had a higher T$_{Reg}$ abundancy but decreased CTLA-4 expression on the T$_{Reg}$ cell surface. Patients with the inherited heterozygous loss of function mutation develop systemic autoimmune disorders like type 1 diabetes, autoimmune thyroid disease, systemic lupus erythematosus, and inflammatory bowel disease (Kuehn et al., 2014; Schubert et al., 2014).

T$_{Reg}$ cells also express the inhibitory receptors programmed cell death protein 1 (PD-1) and lymphocyte-activation gene function 3 (LAG-3). PD-1 and FOXP3 work collaboratively to maintain immune tolerance, with PD-1 important to maintaining the activation balance between effector T cells and T$_{Reg}$ cells (Zhang B. et al., 2016). In a course of anti-PD-1 therapy in cancer, PD-1+ T$_{Reg}$ cells were amplified and mediated cancer growth (Kamada et al., 2019). LAG-3 contributes to immunosuppressive T$_{Reg}$ function in a tumor environment and promotes maternal tolerance during pregnancy (Camisaschi et al., 2010; Zhang and Sun, 2020). Hence, LAG-3 inhibits DC maturation and function. Thus, inhibitory receptors play a fundamental role in T_{Reg} function but remain poorly understood.

In addition to cytokines and inhibitory receptors, T_{Reg} cells use metabolic disruption to influence the immune response. IL-2 is one of the most important cytokines for T cell expansion and is mandatory for T_{Reg} function and differentiation (Davidson et al., 2007). T_{Reg} cells express the high-affinity IL-2 receptor CD25 on their surface and could have a metabolic advantage in comparison to effector T cells, especially in a milieu where the IL-2 concentration is low. Accordingly, cytokine deprivation by T_{Reg} cells induced apoptosis in effector T cells (Pandiyan et al., 2007). In contrast, IL-2 consumption was not required for T_{Reg} suppression (Oberle et al., 2007). Nevertheless, modern low-dose IL-2 therapies in various diseases could demonstrate a preferential T_{Reg} expansion and thereby have a positive effect on patient outcome (Hartemann et al., 2013; Matsuoka et al., 2013; He et al., 2016).

T_{Reg} cells use the membrane-bound ectonucleotidases CD73 and CD39 to generate adenosine from extracellular ATP to influence the immune response. Extracellular ATP usually promotes inflammation, whereas adenosine leads to anti-inflammatory effects. CD39 is abundant on T_{Reg} cells, whereas CD73 is intracellularly enriched in human T_{Reg} cells and upregulated after T_{Reg} activation (Schuler et al., 2014). T_{Reg} cells are sensitive to extracellular ATP, and the upregulation of CD39 is accompanied by remission of inflammatory bowel disease (Gibson et al., 2015). Thus, CD39 signaling is primarily a mechanism to suppress $T_{H}17$ function and development. Adenosine leads to CTLA-4 and PD-1 upregulation in T_{Reg} cells and promotes T_{Reg} suppression of DC function (Ring et al., 2015).

The first indication that cytolytic mechanisms play a role in T_{Reg} function came from studies of granzyme B. In particular, granzyme B is upregulated in activated T_{Reg} cells and mediates suppression of B cell function, and granzyme B deficiency reduces T_{Reg} suppression. Granzyme B-expressing T_{Reg} cells are enriched in human colorectal cancer and potent suppressors of effector T cells. Further, T_{Reg} cells protect themselves from granzyme B-mediated killing by upregulating serine protease inhibitor 6 (Azzi et al., 2013; Sun et al., 2020).

T_{Reg} Function in Autoimmunity

Defects in molecules important for T_{Reg} function can lead to autoimmune diseases, underlying the importance of T_{Reg} effector proteins in pathophysiology. For example, the inherited IPEX syndrome (X-linked autoimmune syndrome immunodysregulation polyendocrinopathy enteropathy X-linked) is caused by different loss of function mutations in the FOXP3 gene. These defects can further lead to the development of autoimmune diseases like diabetes type 1, autoimmune colitis, or hepatitis (Le Bras and Geha, 2006). IL-2RA mutations cause a phenotype similar to IPEX syndrome and CD25 deficiency can increase the vulnerability to viral infection (Goudy et al., 2013). In addition to these monogenetic T_{Reg} diseases, T_{Reg} dysfunction appears in other immune deficient syndromes. Autoimmune diseases like type 1 diabetes, multiple sclerosis, systemic lupus erythematosus,

myasthenia gravis, and rheumatoid arthritis are associated with altered T_{Reg} quantity or quality (Wakabayashi et al., 2006; Lapierre et al., 2013).

The direction of T_{Reg} alteration is controversial. Different studies show either an increase or decrease in T_{Reg} cell numbers based on the stage of the disease and the heterogeneous use of T_{Reg}-defining molecules. In addition, as explained above, T_{Reg} defining molecules can be upregulated after general T cell activation in humans (Pillai et al., 2007). Nevertheless, T_{Reg} cells are an important target for therapy of autoimmune diseases and remission can partly reverse the defective T_{Reg} function (Hartemann et al., 2013; Humrich et al., 2015; Rosenzwajg et al., 2015; He et al., 2016). Treatment with tocilizumab in patients with rheumatoid arthritis, for example, increased T_{Reg} frequency and restored T_{Reg} function (Kikuchi et al., 2015). Another therapeutic approach is the adoptive transfer of *in vitro*-expanded T_{Reg} cells. This strategy was beneficial in mouse models and is now being tested in humans (Morgan et al., 2005; Mathew et al., 2018).

Tumor tissue is especially challenging for the immune system. T_{Reg} cells impair the immune response against tumor antigens by effector T cells that evolve from potential self-reactive cells. In general, a T_{Reg}-enriched tumor tissue with decreased abundance of CD8+ cells is associated with poor prognosis, metastasis, and reduced survival (Mougiakakos et al., 2010). Tumor-infiltrating T_{Reg} cells are primarily effector T_{Reg} cells (CD45RA-FOXP3highCD25high), which are active and proliferative. Furthermore, these cells differ in the expression of activation markers, T_{Reg} markers, and inhibitory receptors on their cell surface. Tumor-infiltrating T_{Reg} cells also express several chemokine receptors such as CCR4 and CCR8 (De Simone et al., 2016). In the tumor, T_{Reg} cells interact with immune cells, cancer cells, and fibroblasts to influence tumor immunity. Tumor-associated fibroblasts promote tumor progression and positively regulate T_{Reg} function and frequency (Kato et al., 2018). Furthermore, T_{Reg} cells and cancer cells bidirectionally support their growth and function. Immunosuppressive T_{Reg} function enables tumor progression, while cancer cells secrete TGF-β, IDO, and COX-2 to promote T_{Reg} trafficking and differentiation (Costa et al., 2018). Adenosine is produced by cancer cells and T_{Reg} cells and functions as a mediator, encouraging cancer cell growth, angiogenesis, and metastasis (Chimote et al., 2018). In addition to cancer cell effects, T_{Reg} cells have a tremendous impact on tumor-infiltrating immune cells. They reciprocally promote nonclassical monocytes, B_{Reg} differentiation, and MDSCs trafficking to create an immunosuppressive cell composition. Furthermore, T_{Reg} cells inhibit proinflammatory immune cells such as NK cells and cytotoxic lymphocytes to prevent an effective anti-tumor immune response (Chang et al., 2016; Sarhan et al., 2018). Modern immunotherapies use anti-CTLA-4 and anti-PD-1, which mainly target the T_{Reg} immune response (Ha et al., 2019).

An important cell subpopulation that balances the immune response in the course of pathogen infection and vaccination are follicular regulatory T cells (T_{FR}). T_{FR} cells affect the humoral immune response by influencing B cell maturation in the germinal center (GC). During this process, B cells undergo somatic hypermutation to establish a high affinity and effective humoral immune response. This development is supported by T_{FH} cells and is tightly regulated by T_{FR} to prevent autoimmunity and an imbalanced immune response (Wollenberg et al., 2011). T_{FR} influence T_{FH} frequency and function and in addition B cells directly by inhibiting their activation. Interestingly, T_{FR} express a distinct TCR repertoire for foreign antigens and potential self-antigens. T_{FR} resemble T_{FH} cells in CXCR5, ICOS, and BCL-6 expression but T_{FR} also express CD28, FOXP3, and Blimp1 (Chung et al., 2011). T_{FR} cells differentiate from CD25 +FOXP3+ cells and function as an effector T_{Reg} subpopulation (Linterman et al., 2011). CTLA-4 is the most important mode of T_{FR}-mediated immune cell regulation, but PD-1 also contributes to full T_{FR} function (Sage et al., 2014). T_{FR} and T_{FH} influence one another reciprocally, and the interaction can be influenced by the microenvironment. In a recently published study, different adjuvants balanced T_{FR} frequency and function during vaccination (Bartsch et al., 2020). The T_{FR} function was affected by IL-6 signaling and the altered T_{FR} cell frequency influenced antibody glycosylation and the overall humoral immune response (Bartsch et al., 2020).

In addition to the GC reaction, T_{FR} can be detected in the blood even at low frequency. Circulating T_{FR} cells have a memory-like phenotype and fine tune the secondary response to an antigen by influencing reactivation of DCs to GC and cytokine production, antibody class-switching, and B cell activation (Sage et al., 2014). T_{FR} dysfunction can be associated with autoimmune diseases, graft versus host reactions, and allergies (He et al., 2013). Overall, T_{Reg} cells play an important role in orchestrating the immune response in health and disease.

THE T_H17/T_{REG} CELL BALANCE IN THE LIVER

The liver is an immunogenetic organ exposed to a variety of antigens and pathogens from the digestive tract and is essential to building an effective immune response. Interestingly, and in contrast to the blood, the CD4/CD8 ratio is reversed in the liver (Doherty and O'Farrelly, 2000). The liver is naturally enriched with innate immune cells, namely, macrophages (Kupffer cells), natural killer (NK) cells, and NK T cells. Especially during fibrogenesis, infiltrating monocytes are important for continuous inflammation and the activation of extracellular matrix producing hepatic stellate cells (HSCs). The adaptive immune system also plays a critical role in these processes. The intrahepatic T_{Reg} frequency can differ from 1% to 5% among all intrahepatic lymphocytes (Oo et al., 2012). The expression of IL-17RA was observed on parenchymal and non-parenchymal cells including hepatocytes, HSCs, Kupffer cells, and endothelial cells, all of which exacerbate inflammatory reactions upon injury. In two different mouse models of hepatic fibrosis (bile duct ligation and carbon tetrachloride), the deletion of IL-17A, IL-23, and IL-17RA inhibited HSC activation and fibrosis development. This finding implies a direct functional link between IL-17A mediated stimulation of HSCs by activation of STAT3-dependent

signaling (Meng et al., 2012). Further, isolation experiments in primary liver-resident cells revealed IL-17 production and IL-17 signal transmission by almost all liver-resident cell types. Kupffer cells especially express high levels of IL-17 and show significant upregulation of IL-17 and IL-1β upon stimulation. mRNA expression of IL-17RA and IL-17RC could additionally be found in hepatocytes, Kupffer cells, HSCs, and liver endothelial cells. Despite IL-17RA expression, hepatocytes and liver endothelial cells do not express IL-17 themselves (Zenewicz et al., 2007). Another study using a cell transplantation model pointed to a direct interaction between HSCs and T_{Reg} cells. Jiang et al. found that upon transplantation, HSCs in allogeneic recipients convey the selective expansion of $CD4^+CD25^+FoxP3^+$ cells in an IL-2-dependent fashion to protect parenchymal cells from rejection (Jiang et al., 2008).

In contrast, CD4+ and CD8+ T cells, NK T cells, γδT cells, neutrophils, and macrophages do express IL-17 in the liver. The equilibrium of T_H17 and T_{Reg} cells is regulated not only by differentiation but also at the epigenetic level. Interestingly, recent studies show that in the presence of IL-1β, IL-2, IL-21, and IL-23, IL-17 producing cells can also develop from T_{Reg} cells due to a differentiation switch that removes their suppressive function (Koenen et al., 2008; Deknuydt et al., 2009).

T_{Reg} and T_H17 cells are also often significantly increased in chronic inflammatory liver diseases and are important to balance the persisting pro-inflammatory immune response. Interestingly, a reciprocal relationship between T_H17 and T_{Reg} cells exists in their differentiation as in their effector function (**Figure 3**).

T_{Reg} and T_H17 cells can co-express the lineage defining transcription factors RORγt and FOXP3. Environmental conditions such as the tissue-specific cytokine milieu at the site of infection can influence this expression and influence the balance by fostering either T_{Reg} or T_H17 cell development by simultaneous inhibition of the other cell type. TGF-β, for example, is required for the differentiation of both subsets; the absence or presence of proinflammatory cytokines defines whether a T_H17 or T_{Reg} cell develops (Yang et al., 2008; Hammerich et al., 2011). In contrast, T_H17 cells express IL-10 receptor α, which can convey a T_{Reg}-induced decrease in T_H17 cells in an IL-10-dependent manner (Huber et al., 2011). Recent studies point to a delicate balance between T_H17 and T_{Reg} cells crucial to maintaining tissue homeostasis. In addition to IL-6, other factors such as retinoic acid, rapamycin, or cytokines (e.g., IL-2 and IL-27) influence this balance significantly. T_{Reg} cells are assigned a decisive role in hepatic immunity. Results obtained in mouse models of acute and chronic liver disease also point to a major involvement of T_H17 and T_{Reg} cells in a variety of human inflammatory liver diseases. For example, in a cancer milieu, glucose consumption by tumor cells preferentially promotes T_{Reg} differentiation and decreases T_H17 cell development thereby supporting the immune escape strategy of tumor cells. Another important ubiquitous environmental condition during chronic and acute infection is hypoxia. Hypoxia can induce the hypoxia inducible factor 1α (HIF-1α) as an adaptive mechanism of the cells to low oxygen concentration. HIF-1α stabilization supports RORγt and IL-17 production while targeting FOXP3 to

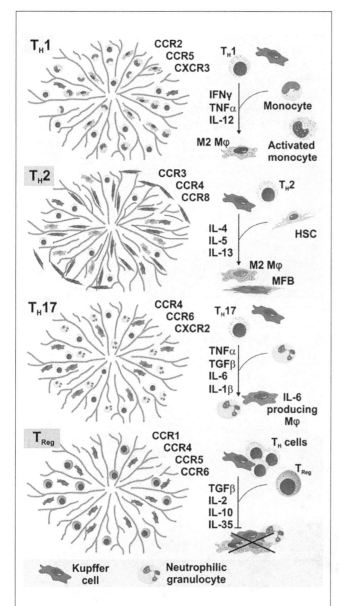

FIGURE 3 | In acute and chronic liver diseases, T cells are crucial to either initiate, maintain, or terminate pro-inflammatory immune responses. Different T cell subpopulations develop, expand, and function based on a distinct cytokine milieu influenced by the presence of different types of immune cells. Different CD4+ cells recognize certain chemokine receptors within the liver and are thereby attracted by different cell types and stimuli to infiltrate the liver tissue. The differentiation of these subsets requires a specific cytokine milieu generated by non-parenchymal cells (e.g. monocytes) or parenchymal cells [e.g., hepatic stellate cells (HSCs)]. T_H1 cell cells promote alternatively activated macrophage development (M2), whereas T_H2 cells additionally promote liver myofibroblast (MFB) activation. T_H17 cells leads to the recruitment of neutrophils, granulocytes, and macrophages to the site of inflammation to induce and sustain a pro-inflammatory immune response. Regulatory T (T_{Reg}) cells and follicular T (T_{FH}) cells prevent the pro-inflammatory immune response of several parenchymal and non-parenchymal cells within the liver tissue in course of an inflammatory immune response.

proteasomal degradation. Manipulation of the balance between pathogenic and regulatory processes in the liver are believed to allow the focused restoration of homeostasis especially during hepatic inflammation.

The detailed analysis of T_H17 cells in human liver remains difficult because the cell frequency is low and cells can only be analyzed after their *in vitro* activation with phorbol 12-myristate 13-acetate (PMA) and ionomycin. This *in vitro* activation is interesting but must be critically considered because the extent to which it reflects the *in vivo* situation and cell status upon isolation is unknown.

Autoimmune Diseases

One example of specific immune change in the liver is autoimmune hepatitis (AIH). Although the cause of AIH is not fully understood, T cell mediated liver tissue destruction is involved and AIH could be associated with genetic and environmental alterations. AIH leads to chronic liver inflammation, circulating autoantibodies, and elevated liver enzymes (Tait et al., 1989). Zhao et al. showed that patients with AIH have increased serum levels of IL-17 and IL-23 together with an increased frequency of T_H17 cells in the liver compared to controls. Furthermore, the frequency and function of T_{Reg} cells in the blood was decreased (Ferri et al., 2010). By analyzing the T cell composition in the liver, it was demonstrated that the total T_{Reg} number was not altered in AIH patients. In contrast, these patients displayed higher hepatic expression of the T_H17-related cytokines IL-17, IL-23, IL-6, and RORγt. *In vitro* experiments showed that IL-17 induces IL-6 *via* MAPK signaling in hepatocytes, which in turn stimulates T_H17 cell differentiation and infiltration in a positive feedback loop (Zhao et al., 2011). These results are supported by a retrospective study of 100 AIH patients. In addition to elevated serum levels of IL-17, IL-6, IL-21, and TNF-α, an increased frequency of T_H17 cells was observed. Pro-inflammatory cytokines were positively correlated with liver injury, whereas IL-10 was negatively regulated with autoantibodies (An, 2019). Likewise, T_{Reg} cells from AIH patients had decreased CD39 expression and functionally failed to prevent T_H17 accumulation mediated by extracellular ATP (Grant et al., 2014). Remission in AIH patients was associated with restored T cell balance, and the infusion of ex vivo expanded T_{Reg} cells was beneficial in a murine model (Lapierre et al., 2013). In sum, the balance of T_{Reg} and T_H17 composition at the site of inflammation and T_{Reg} function is critical in AIH pathomechanisms.

Primary biliary cirrhosis (PBC) is a chronic cholestatic liver disease characterized by the loss of immune self-tolerance leading to the chronic injury of biliary epithelial cells. Ninety percent of affected patients are women older than 40 years. The importance of the T_H17/T_{Reg} balance in disease progression of primary biliary cirrhosis (PBC) is evident when considering that a knockout for CD25 (IL-2Rα) in mice serves as an animal model for this disease. Mice spontaneously develop autoantibodies caused by a loss of function of T_{Reg} cells and acquire biliary duct damage similar to that observed in PBC patients (Wakabayashi et al., 2006). Deficiency of functional T_{Reg} cells leads to elevated T_H17 cell numbers in the liver and elevated IL-17 levels in these mice compared to wildtype controls. A possible explanation might be the missing repressive function of IL-2 during T_H17 cell differentiation. In line with the results obtained in mice, patients suffering from liver fibrosis due to PBC show a higher frequency of T_H17 cells in blood than healthy control patients. Liver biopsy samples of PBC patients point to a dislocation of these cells around the portal tracts (Shi et al., 2015). Patients with cirrhosis secondary to PBC displayed an even higher infiltration of T_H17 cells into liver tissue (Tan et al., 2013). However, the exact mechanisms that cause an induction of T_H17 cells in livers of IL-2RA knockout animals remain elusive.

Primary sclerosing cholangitis (PSC) is another chronic-inflammatory liver disease with an unknown pathogenesis. Similar to PBC, PSC can lead to liver fibrosis and obliteration of intra-and extrahepatic bile ducts. PSC is often associated with chronic ulcerative colitis, and there is no effective treatment (Hirschfield et al., 2013). Patients with also have a decreased peripheral T_{Reg} frequency with epigenetic changes. Furthermore, a decrease in T_{Reg} numbers was associated with an IL-2RA gene polymorphism and lead to reduced T_{Reg} function (Sebode et al., 2014), (**Figure 4**).

Acute Liver Injury

Mouse models of acute liver injury were used to further investigate the role of T_H17 cells in the liver. In the concanavalin A- (ConA-) model of acute T cell induced hepatitis, IL-1- deficient animals were challenged and knockout mice developed less severe injury

with higher T_{Reg} numbers compared to wildtype mice (Nagata et al., 2008). However, these results are controversial; another study found in the same model that IL-17-deficient mice seemed to develop a comparable level of liver injury after ConA-treatment (Zenewicz et al., 2007). In another interesting mouse model of drug-induced liver injury (halothane injection intraperitoneally), mice had increased serum levels of IL-17. After the administration of an IL-17 neutralizing antibody serum, liver enzymes AST and ALT had significantly decreased levels, with a downregulation of inflammatory cytokines such as TNF-α. These beneficial effects could be directly reversed by the application of recombinant IL-17 (Kobayashi et al., 2009).

Viral Infection

The T_{Reg}/T_H17 balance is essential for an effective immune response and at the same time preventing excessive liver injury during viral infection. Thus, the liver is affected by several viruses, and some of them lead to persistent infection and can cause liver cirrhosis, organ failure, and cancer. During acute hepatitis A virus (HAV) infection, serum IL-17 levels are correlated with liver injury, and liver resident and circulating T_{Reg} frequencies are negatively linked to elevation of ALT and AST (Choi et al., 2015).

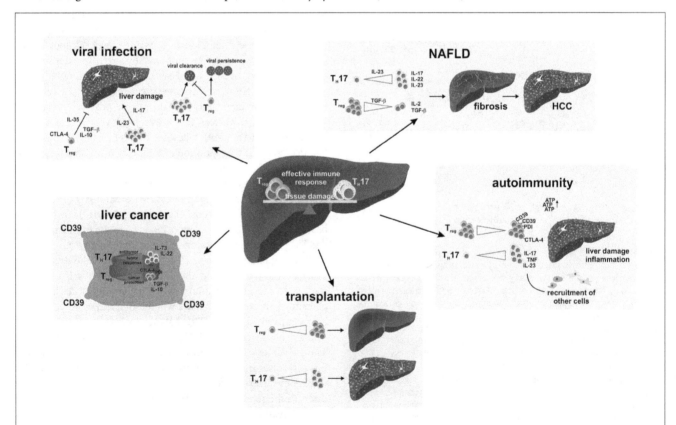

FIGURE 4 | A reciprocal relationship exists between T_H17 and T_{Reg} cells. Their balance is found to be important in the persistence or recovery from liver injury. A shift of the balance to a more dominant T_H17 cell response favors pro-inflammatory reactions and persisting damage. In viral infections, T_H17 are especially important for viral clearance but at the same time cause liver damage. T_{Reg} cell on the other hand prevent liver damage but also trigger viral persistence by strengthening the anti-inflammatory immune response. An imbalance of the T_H17/T_{Reg} milieu to a dominant T_H17 cell response favors disease development and progression in NAFLD. In autoimmune diseases a T_{Reg} cell responses have beneficial effects in regards to self-tolerance, restore immune homeostasis and are even proposed as a treatment option in acute and chronic transplant rejection reactions. In a tumor environment T_{Reg} cells support tumor cells from being targeted by the immune system and hence promote tumor growth and metastasis.

The major problem in persistent viral infection is a failure of the T cell response involving T cell exhaustion due to persistent antigen presentation. T_{Reg} cells also play a role in the immunopathology of persistent viral infection. It was demonstrated that liver sinusoidal endothelial cells (LSEC) are potent enough to promote T_{Reg} differentiation by the continuous induction of FOXP3 in conventional T cells, although all liver cells were able to induce T_{Reg} differentiation. T_{Reg} stabilization did not require inflammation but did require TGF-β, which is abundant on the LSEC cell membrane. Experimentally, LSEC-induced T_{Reg} cells expressed FOXP3 and had efficient inhibitory functions on effector T cells *in vitro* and *in vivo* (Carambia et al., 2014). Antigen presentation on LSECs and thereby an early T_{Reg} development in a course of sub-infectious viral infection of hepatotropic viruses, e.g., chronic hepatitis C virus (HCV), can support ineffective virus clearance and chronic infection (Park et al., 2013). In contrast, virus-specific $T_{H}17$ cells were correlated with liver injury and inflammation, but $T_{H}17$ quantity could not be linked to effective viral clearance. Furthermore, IL-23 and IL-17 levels in HCV-infected patients were elevated, and IL-23 therapy was reported to modulate the antiviral response by preferentially promoting $T_{H}17$ immune cells (Meng et al., 2016). In a course of HCV infection, T_{Reg} cells were mainly found in necro-inflammatory liver areas to inhibit the effector CD8 T cell response, which is the main cause of liver damage in HCV and hepatitis B virus (HBV) infection. Isolated T_{Reg} cells from HCV-infected patients suppressed virus-specific CD8+ cells, whereas the depletion of T_{Reg} cells increased their proliferation. Furthermore, TCR analysis demonstrated that the effective T_{Reg} population during chronic HCV infection is heterogeneous and consists of nT_{Reg} and pT_{Reg} cells (Losikoff et al., 2012). In comparing the T_{Reg} cells of patients who spontaneously resolved the infection and patients with persistent infection, core virus-specific T_{Reg} cells were primarily found in patients with chronic HCV infection. They inhibit the virus-specific T cell response by producing IL-10 and IL-35 (Langhans et al., 2010). Furthermore, several studies investigated a positive correlation between T_{Reg} quantity and function with chronic HCV progression (Cabrera et al., 2004; Ebinuma et al., 2008). $T_{H}17$ cells on the other hand are enriched in livers of patients with chronic HCV infection mainly driven by Tim-3, which leads to a differential regulation of IL-12 and IL-23 (Wang et al., 2013).

The $T_{Reg}/T_{H}17$ balance also plays an important role in chronic HBV infection. T_{Reg} cells inhibit the antiviral response of effector T cells (Yan et al., 2014). The frequency of circulating T_{Reg} cells is differently described in chronic HBV infection, but there are some indications that the T_{Reg} frequency is increased in severe chronic HBV infection. Furthermore, T_{Reg} frequencies could be positively correlated with viral load, HBeAg (Hepatitis B envelope Antigen), and HBsAg (Hepatitis B surface Antigen) (Manigold and Racanelli, 2007; TrehanPati et al., 2011). Patients with a predominant $T_{H}17$ response have high plasma viral loads. Especially in HBV infection and HBV-induced cirrhosis, IL-17+ cells increase with cirrhosis stage and the HBcAg (Hepatitis B core Antigen) mediates $T_{H}17$ cell responses by an IL-17R-induced activation of monocytes/macrophages. This effect leads to the production of elevated levels of pro-inflammatory cytokines such as IL-6, TNF-α, IL-12, and IL-23 (Sun et al., 2012). Further, the elevation of T_{Reg} and T_{FR} cells in chronically HBV infected patients associated with elevated IL-10 and TGF-β levels in comparison to healthy individuals (Liu et al., 2020). T_{Reg} differentiation was thereby promoted by TGF-β production of hepatic stellate cells and activation of Notch signaling during chronic inflammation. In a course of antiviral response, $T_{H}17$ cells increased in quantity accompanied with an increase in viral load (Ichikawa et al., 2011; Yan et al., 2014). In addition, in course of antiviral therapy, PD-1 expression decreased on $T_{H}17$ cells and other effector T cells, indicating an improved T cell exhaustion; however, PD-1 was not present on T_{Reg} cells (Wei et al., 2013). The $T_{H}17/T_{Reg}$ balance is critical in the development of liver cirrhosis in chronically-infected patients. An imbalance in $T_{H}17/T_{Reg}$ cells was thereby an independent predictive factor for decompensated liver cirrhosis (Lan et al., 2019). In addition, Yang et al. demonstrated that IL-35 is responsible to balance the T_{Reg} and $T_{H}17$ balance in acute and chronic HBV infection by preferentially increasing virus-specific T_{Reg} cells and the prevention of $T_{H}17$ cell differentiation (Yang et al., 2019). In conclusion, T_{Reg} and $T_{H}17$ cells contribute to the immune response during viral liver infection and the optimal balance is important for an effective antiviral immune response and prevention of complications (**Figure 4**).

Alcoholic and Nonalcoholic Steatohepatitis (ASH and NASH)

Patients with alcoholic steatohepatitis (ASH) show a direct correlation between the severity of inflammation and the amount of liver damage. The degradation of ethanol mediated by cytochrome P450 2E1 (CYP2E1) is associated with various inflammatory responses within the liver. The immune response leads to the production of reactive oxygen species (ROS) and TNF-α and the infiltration of immune cells. T cells infiltrating into the liver secrete high levels of pro-inflammatory cytokines, thereby attracting neutrophils to the tissue site of inflammation. Neutrophil recruitment could be closely linked to the prominence of $T_{H}17$ cells. This in turn leads to increased IL-17 serum levels in ASH patients, which could be directly linked to progressive liver damage. Further, the number of T_{Reg} cells decreases in the blood of these patients (Lemmers et al., 2009).

Nonalcoholic steatohepatitis (NASH) is related to metabolic syndrome. This condition has become the most common cause of chronic liver disease and will likely be the main cause for liver transplantations within the next decade (Younossi et al., 2019). Patients with non-alcoholic fatty liver disease (NAFLD) have a high risk to progress from simple steatosis to more advanced disease stages such as NASH, cirrhosis, and hepatocellular cancer (HCC). The exact mechanisms of the pathogenesis of NASH are poorly understood. However, the role of the activation of the adaptive immune system *via* a $T_{H}17$-mediated immune responses is becoming evident.

Targeting the balance between $T_{H}17$ and T_{Reg} cells is a relatively new approach and currently topic of many research studies. The lack of available human tissue samples makes it difficult to investigate this as a potential new treatment option.

Nevertheless, recent studies in mice and few data from humans indicate a decisive role of CD4+ T cells in the progression from NAFLD to NASH up to HCC development (Hammerich et al., 2011; Rau et al., 2016). A key mechanism within this process is a strong infiltration of neutrophils together with an increased IL-6 signaling and T_H17 accumulation (Hubscher, 2006). This further leads to a depolarization of the intrahepatic CD4+ cell response to a more T_H17 cell-driven reaction; at the same time, T_{Reg} cell activity is suppressed (Gomes et al., 2016; Rau et al., 2016). Although the total T_{Reg} number of circulating and intrahepatic T_{Reg} cells is not altered, the overall T_H17/T_{Reg} balance is shifted to a more dominant pro-inflammatory immune response.

The majority of data on T_H17 cells in NASH is limited to mice. Different mouse models for diet-induced nonalcoholic steatohepatitis, such as the methionine-choline deficient-diet (MCD-diet) and the widely used high fat diet (HFD) model, can lead to steatohepatitis and subsequent fibrosis. Disease development and progression in these models is accompanied with an increase in T_{Reg} cell numbers at early disease stages in which only steatosis is present, and shifts significantly to a more dominant T_H17 cell-driven response at later time points when steatohepatitis and beginning fibrosis are present. In the liver fibrosis CCL4 mouse model, increased IL-17 levels led to an elevated collagen1α1 expression in HSCs triggered by STAT3 signaling (Meng et al., 2012). Gomes et al. showed in 2016 that the excess of nutrients leads to the expression of the factor unconventional prefoldin RPB5 interactor (URI) in liver of mice treated with different steatohepatitis-inducing diets. URI promoted HCC development *via* a shift of the CD4+ T cell composition during NASH and NASH-HCC development. The overexpression of human URI in mouse hepatocytes led to spontaneous development of steatohepatitis, which could be strengthened by feeding steatohepatitis-inducing diets (CD-HFD) or MCD. Disease was accompanied by increased IL-17 and T_H17 cells in blood and liver. Mice with a heterozygous, hepatocyte-specific deficiency for URI were protected from the development of steatohepatitis together with decreased numbers of T_H17 cells. Inhibiting the differentiation of T_H17 cells through the blockade of RORγt lead to an improved in lipid metabolism, insulin resistance, and HCC development. The application of recombinant IL-17 in wildtype mice induced steatohepatitis, the infiltration of neutrophils to white adipose tissue, and led to an increased number of T_H17 cells.

Interestingly, data from human NASH patients correlated with the expression of URI with high IL-17 levels and hepatic steatosis (Gomes et al., 2016). Another study points to overall diminished CD4+ T cell numbers in NASH, and that this reduction is an essential factor in the progression from NASH to HCC development (Ma et al., 2016). The observed changes in the T helper cell profile during NASH development can be caused either by a depolarization of CD4+ T cells to a T_H17 cell phenotype, or by a relative shift of the CD4+ T cell composition in the liver due to depletion of other T helper cell subsets, or driven by an altered infiltration of distinct CD4+ T cell subsets.

A study from Rau et al. in 2016 showed that the progression from NAFLD to NASH is directly correlated with an increased frequency in T_H17 cells in blood and liver of NAFLD and NASH patients together with an altered T_H17/T_{Reg} balance depicted by an increased T_H17/T_{Reg} cell ratio in both compartments (Rau et al., 2016). In visceral adipose tissue and subcutaneous adipose tissue of morbid obese patients, an increase in the mRNA expression of IL-17 was found compared to normal weight patients. The same patients also showed increased numbers of T_H17 cells in both adipose tissues and peripheral blood mononuclear cells (PBMCs), while T_{Reg} cell numbers were decreased due to impaired survival of these cells (McLaughlin et al., 2014). A recent study published in April 2020 further points to the direct relationship between liver and adipose tissue in regulating the T_H17/T_{Reg} balance. Van Herck and colleagues demonstrated that mice fed a high-fat high-fructose diet displayed an increase in T_H17 cells in both compartments, with a simultaneous decrease in T_{Reg} cells. After removing the steatohepatitis-inducing diet, the disruption in the T_H17/T_{Reg} balance persisted. The administration of an IL-17 neutralizing antibody subsequently decreased the pro-inflammatory immune response in the liver (Van Herck et al., 2020). NASH is further closely related to the development of HCC. The involvement of TH17 cells in tumor formation and patient survival was recently described as influencing the prevention of apoptosis in tumor cells induced by T_H17 cells due to IL-17 promoting angiogenesis and an IL-23 driven tumor growth (Langowski et al., 2006; Zhang et al., 2009). Understanding the role of T_H17/T_{Reg} balance and targeting it therapeutically is an interesting approach for the treatment of NASH (**Figure 4**).

Liver Fibrosis and Hepatocellular Carcinoma

Chronic liver disease changes and impairs organ structure and function. Liver disease leads to tissue replacement and scaring subsequently leading to liver fibroses and cirrhosis. Several studies describe the importance of T_H17 and T_{Reg} cells in this process. Although the exact role of T_{Reg} cells in liver fibrogenesis is not fully understood, T_{Reg} cells support liver fibrosis by influencing metalloproteinases activation (Zhang X. et al., 2016). T_H17 cells further signal on non-lymphoid cells such as endothelial cells, fibroblasts, and keratinocytes inducing the production of inflammatory cytokines such as IL-6, GM-CSF, IL-1, TGF-β, TNF-α, and MCP-1 to attract immune cells thereby promoting pro-inflammatory immune responses. IL-17 receptor signaling further activates the expression of antimicrobial peptides and matrix metalloproteinases, whereas the latter are important for the degradation of scar tissue during infection (Bettelli et al., 2008). In patients with more severe liver cirrhosis, an increased frequency of circulating T_{Reg} cells, but a decreased T_{Reg}/T_H17 ratio was positively correlated with disease progression (Li et al., 2012). More particularly, the abundant expression of TGF-β and IL-6 in the liver, which both favor the differentiation of T_H17 cells, points to a major contribution of these cells during this process. Liver cirrhosis is one of the major risk factors for the development of HCC. Thus, 80%–90% of HCC develop in the course of chronic inflammation (Refolo et al., 2020). HCC is associated with a poor prognosis, is hard to detect, is aggressive, and has limited therapeutic options. T_{Reg} and T_H17 cells were increased in tumor tissue in comparison to the surrounding liver tissue. Not only high intra-tumoral T_{Reg} frequencies and a decreased T_H17 quantity but also CD39 expressed by tumor cells and T_{Reg} cells facilitated HCC growth, metastasis, and poor prognosis by mainly affecting T_H17 function and differentiation (Bettini et al., 2012). T_{Reg} cell depletion, however, negatively influenced HCC growth (Cany et al., 2011). Interestingly, high IL-17 and IL-17R expression in the tumor tissue and elevated circulating T_H17 cells are also associated with poor survival and early HCC recurrence. Sorafenib is currently used in HCC treatment and targets varies kinases expressed in T_{Reg} cells. This therapy negatively affects the T_{Reg} frequency, which can be correlated to overall improved survival (Voron et al., 2014). To improve the overall survival of HCC patients, new therapeutic approaches are essential. A defect in T cell function is described and immunotherapies are potential effective treatment strategies. One possibility could be checkpoint inhibition. PD-1 upregulation for example can be detected in circulating T_{Reg} cells in HCC patients, supporting the overall immune dysregulation. Therefore, anti PD-1 is a promising strategy. This therapy reverses the T_{Reg} mediated inhibition of T_H17 cells and other effector T cells (Langhans et al., 2010) (**Figure 4**).

Liver Transplantation

Liver transplantation is in many cases the only possibility to cure end-stage liver disease. The short-term outcome has significantly improved, but chronic organ rejection and the side effects of immunosuppressive therapy remain a concern. The optimal immunosuppressive treatment to prevent organ rejection and toxicity and at the same time avoid opportunistic infections must be tightly balanced and will vary between individuals. The state of optimal immunotherapy, called operational tolerance, is difficult to achieve, and most patients require a life-long therapy with numerous side effects. Thus, new therapeutic approaches following liver transplantation are urgently needed.

T_{Reg} cells play a leading role in averting the cause of graft-versus-host disease (GvHD) which leads to organ rejection. T_{Reg}/T_H17 balance plays a fundamental role in rejection pathogenesis (Wang et al., 2019), and T_H17 cells were found to be elevated during acute and chronic organ rejection. In addition, the pro-inflammatory cytokine milieu during organ rejection can induce RORγt and IL-17 expression in T_{Reg} cells. Thus, T_{Reg} cells seem to contribute to organ rejection. Indeed, an early decrease in T_{Reg} frequency is a risk factor for suspected acute and biopsy proven acute rejection (Han et al., 2020). In addition, CD39 expression in the transplanted liver tissue influences the T_{Reg} and T_H17 immune response and thereby organ rejection and GvHD (Yoshida et al., 2015). Adoptive T_{Reg} transfer was protective in mice, and currently several clinical trials are testing the efficiency and safety in humans (Romano et al., 2017). Another study tested the T_{Reg} therapy in patients 6–12 months after liver transplantation and demonstrated an increase in circulating T_{Reg} cells and reduced anti-donor T cell response (Sanchez-Fueyo et al., 2020). Although the long-term effects are not evaluated, T_{Reg} therapy could be a promising therapeutic approach. In contrast to the beneficial effects, in transplant patients with HCV infection, early high levels of T_{Reg} cells and T_H1 cells after liver transplantation are associated with severe recurrent HCV infection (Ghazal et al., 2019).

In addition to T cell-mediated organ rejection, danger associated molecular patterns (DAMPs) play an important role in triggering sterile inflammation in the liver after organ transplantation. Sterile inflammation could be detected in different solid organs after implantation, and sterile inflammation influences the transplant tolerance and chronic rejection. A recently published study described the correlation between elevated DAMPs and acute postoperative multi-organ dysfunction (Nagakawa et al., 2020). In sum, several studies implicate the contribution of sterile inflammation in acute and chronic organ rejection and are reviewed elsewhere (Braza et al., 2016) (**Figure 4**).

CONCLUSION

T_H17 and T_{Reg} cells are essential in orchestrating the intrahepatic immune response in health and disease. Under homeostatic conditions their balance must be tightly regulated to have an effective immune response and to prevent tissue damage. In the course of several diseases, their balance is shifted. Especially in the liver, the T_H17/T_{Reg} response is tremendously important. An overwhelming T_H17 response, for example in NASH, can promote the inflammatory state of disease and is associated with disease progression. On the other hand, T_{Reg} cells prevent the anti-tumoral immune response in HCC and promote metastasis and cancer growth. Furthermore, both cell subsets can be beneficial in different liver diseases settings. Thus, T_H17 cells are necessary for effective pathogen clearance in the liver and T_{Reg} cells are important to coordinate the immune response in autoimmunity and after liver transplantation. Most of the findings on the role of T_H17 and T_{Reg} cells were generated in mice. The importance of investigating their influence in humans is highlighted in several disease settings. Many studies demonstrate the necessity of investigating the function and quantity of these cells in liver tissue specifically, as circulating cells may not reflect intrahepatic conditions. In addition to altered function and quantities in liver diseases, T_H17/T_{Reg} cell balance could be a therapeutic target in disease settings.

Future studies should investigate the function of T_H17 and T_{Reg} cells in liver tissue and review their balance. Furthermore, different signals that might influence T_H17/T_{Reg} cells, especially in the liver, must be analyzed to fully understand the liver-specific pathomechanism and to inform a liver-specific therapy.

AUTHOR CONTRIBUTIONS

Conceptualization: HD and LB. Writing—original draft preparation: HD, LB, and RW. Visualization: SW. funding acquisition: HD, LB, and RW. All authors contributed to the article and approved the submitted version.

REFERENCES

Aarvak, T., Chabaud, M., Miossec, P., and Natvig, J. B. (1999). IL-17 is produced by some proinflammatory Th1/Th0 cells but not by Th2 cells. *J. Immunol.* 162 (3), 1246–1251.

Aggarwal, S., Ghilardi, N., Xie, M. H., de Sauvage, F. J., and Gurney, A. L. (2003). Interleukin-23 promotes a distinct CD4 T cell activation state characterized by the production of interleukin-17. *J. Biol. Chem.* 278 (3), 1910–1914. doi: 10.1074/jbc.M207577200

An, J. (2019). Expression and significance of Th17 cells and related factors in patients with autoimmune hepatitis. *Comb. Chem. High Throughput Screen* 22 (4), 232–237. doi: 10.2174/1386207322666190402160455

Arpaia, N., Campbell, C., Fan, X., Dikiy, S., van der Veeken, J., deRoos, P., et al. (2013). Metabolites produced by commensal bacteria promote peripheral regulatory T-cell generation. *Nature* 504 (7480), 451–455. doi: 10.1038/nature12726

Azzi, J., Skartsis, N., Mounayar, M., Magee, C. N., Batal, I., Ting, C., et al. (2013). Serine protease inhibitor 6 plays a critical role in protecting murine granzyme B-producing regulatory T cells. *J. Immunol.* 191 (5), 2319–2327. doi: 10.4049/jimmunol.1300851

Bartsch, Y. C., Eschweiler, S., Leliavski, A., Lunding, H. B., Wagt, S., Petry, J., et al. (2020). IgG Fc sialylation is regulated during the germinal center reaction upon immunization with different adjuvants. *J. Allergy Clin. Immunol.* 146 (3), 652–666.e11. doi: 10.1016/j.jaci.2020.04.059

Batten, M., Li, J., Yi, S., Kljavin, N. M., Danilenko, D. M., Lucas, S., et al. (2006). Interleukin 27 limits autoimmune encephalomyelitis by suppressing the development of interleukin 17-producing T cells. *Nat. Immunol.* 7 (9), 929–936. doi: 10.1038/ni1375

Bayer, A. L., Yu, A., Adeegbe, D., and Malek, T. R. (2005). Essential role for interleukin-2 for CD4(+)CD25(+) T regulatory cell development during the neonatal period. *J. Exp. Med.* 201 (5), 769–777. doi: 10.1084/jem.20041179

Bettelli, E., Sullivan, B., Szabo, S. J., Sobel, R. A., Glimcher, L. H., and Kuchroo, V. K. (2004). Loss of T-bet, but not STAT1, prevents the development of experimental autoimmune encephalomyelitis. *J. Exp. Med.* 200 (1), 79–87. doi: 10.1084/jem.20031819

Bettelli, E., Carrier, Y., Gao, W., Korn, T., Strom, T. B., Oukka, M., et al. (2006). Reciprocal developmental pathways for the generation of pathogenic effector TH17 and regulatory T cells. *Nature* 441 (7090), 235–238. doi: 10.1038/nature04753

Bettelli, E., Korn, T., Oukka, M., and Kuchroo, V. K. (2008). Induction and effector functions of T(H)17 cells. *Nature* 453 (7198), 1051–1057. doi: 10.1038/nature07036

Bettini, M., Castellaw, A. H., Lennon, G. P., Burton, A. R., and Vignali, D. A. (2012). Prevention of autoimmune diabetes by ectopic pancreatic beta-cell expression of interleukin-35. *Diabetes* 61 (6), 1519–1526. doi: 10.2337/db11-0784

Braza, F., Brouard, S., Chadban, S., and Goldstein, D. R. (2016). Role of TLRs and DAMPs in allograft inflammation and transplant outcomes. *Nat. Rev. Nephrol.* 12 (5), 281–290. doi: 10.1038/nrneph.2016.41

Cabrera, R., Tu, Z., Xu, Y., Firpi, R. J., Rosen, H. R., Liu, C., et al. (2004). An immunomodulatory role for CD4(+)CD25(+) regulatory T lymphocytes in hepatitis C virus infection. *Hepatology* 40 (5), 1062–1071. doi: 10.1002/hep.20454

Camisaschi, C., Casati, C., Rini, F., Perego, M., De Filippo, A., Triebel, F., et al. (2010). LAG-3 expression defines a subset of CD4(+)CD25(high)Foxp3(+) regulatory T cells that are expanded at tumor sites. *J. Immunol.* 184 (11), 6545–6551. doi: 10.4049/jimmunol.0903879

Cany, J., Tran, L., Gauttier, V., Judor, J. P., Vassaux, G., Ferry, N., et al. (2011). Immunotherapy of hepatocellular carcinoma: is there a place for regulatory T-lymphocyte depletion? *Immunotherapy* 3 (4 Suppl), 32–34. doi: 10.2217/imt.11.29

Carambia, A., Freund, B., Schwinge, D., Heine, M., Laschtowitz, A., Huber, S., et al. (2014). TGF-beta-dependent induction of CD4(+)CD25(+)Foxp3(+) Tregs by liver sinusoidal endothelial cells. *J. Hepatol.* 61 (3), 594–599. doi: 10.1016/j.jhep.2014.04.027

Chang, A. L., Miska, J., Wainwright, D. A., Dey, M., Rivetta, C. V., Yu, D., et al. (2016). CCL2 Produced by the glioma microenvironment is essential for the recruitment of regulatory T cells and myeloid-derived suppressor cells. *Cancer Res.* 76 (19), 5671–5682. doi: 10.1158/0008-5472.CAN-16-0144

Chen, W., Jin, W., Hardegen, N., Lei, K. J., Li, L., Marinos, N., et al. (2003). Conversion of peripheral CD4+CD25- naive T cells to CD4+CD25+ regulatory T cells by TGF-beta induction of transcription factor Foxp3. *J. Exp. Med.* 198 (12), 1875–1886. doi: 10.1084/jem.20030152

Chimote, A. A., Balajthy, A., Arnold, M. J., Newton, H. S., Hajdu, P., Qualtieri, J., et al. (2018). A defect in KCa3.1 channel activity limits the ability of CD8(+) T cells from cancer patients to infiltrate an adenosine-rich microenvironment. *Sci. Signal* 11 (527), eaaq1616. doi: 10.1126/scisignal.aaq1616

Cho, M. L., Yoon, C. H., Hwang, S. Y., Park, M. K., Min, S. Y., Lee, S. H., et al. (2004). Effector function of type II collagen-stimulated T cells from rheumatoid arthritis patients: cross-talk between T cells and synovial fibroblasts. *Arthritis Rheum.* 50 (3), 776–784. doi: 10.1002/art.20106

Choi, Y. S., Lee, J., Lee, H. W., Chang, D. Y., Sung, P. S., Jung, M. K., et al. (2015). Liver injury in acute hepatitis A is associated with decreased frequency of regulatory T cells caused by Fas-mediated apoptosis. *Gut* 64 (8), 1303–1313. doi: 10.1136/gutjnl-2013-306213

Chung, Y., Tanaka, S., Chu, F., Nurieva, R.II, Martinez, G. J., Rawal, S., et al. (2011). Follicular regulatory T cells expressing Foxp3 and Bcl-6 suppress germinal center reactions. *Nat. Med.* 17 (8), 983–988. doi: 10.1038/nm.2426

Collison, L. W., Workman, C. J., Kuo, T. T., Boyd, K., Wang, Y., Vignali, K. M., et al. (2007). The inhibitory cytokine IL-35 contributes to regulatory T-cell function. *Nature* 450 (7169), 566–569. doi: 10.1038/nature06306

Coombes, J. L., Siddiqui, K. R., Arancibia-Carcamo, C. V., Hall, J., Sun, C. M., Belkaid, Y., et al. (2007). A functionally specialized population of mucosal CD103+ DCs induces Foxp3+ regulatory T cells via a TGF-beta and retinoic acid-dependent mechanism. *J. Exp. Med.* 204 (8), 1757–1764. doi: 10.1084/jem.20070590

Cortez, V. S., Ulland, T. K., Cervantes-Barragan, L., Bando, J. K., Robinette, M. L., Wang, Q., et al. (2017). SMAD4 impedes the conversion of NK cells into ILC1-like cells by curtailing non-canonical TGF-beta signaling. *Nat. Immunol.* 18 (9), 995–1003. doi: 10.1038/ni.3809

Cosmi, L., De Palma, R., Santarlasci, V., Maggi, L., Capone, M., Frosali, F., et al. (2008). Human interleukin 17-producing cells originate from a CD161+CD4+ T cell precursor. *J. Exp. Med.* 205 (8), 1903–1916. doi: 10.1084/jem.20080397

Costa, A., Kieffer, Y., Scholer-Dahirel, A., Pelon, F., Bourachot, B., Cardon, M., et al. (2018). Fibroblast heterogeneity and immunosuppressive environment in human breast cancer. *Cancer Cell* 33 (3), 463–479 e410. doi: 10.1016/j.ccell.2018.01.011

Cua, D. J., Sherlock, J., Chen, Y., Murphy, C. A., Joyce, B., Seymour, B., et al. (2003). Interleukin-23 rather than interleukin-12 is the critical cytokine for autoimmune inflammation of the brain. *Nature* 421 (6924), 744–748. doi: 10.1038/nature01355

Curotto de Lafaille, M. A., Kutchukhidze, N., Shen, S., Ding, Y., Yee, H., and Lafaille, J. J. (2008). Adaptive Foxp3+ regulatory T cell-dependent and -independent control of allergic inflammation. *Immunity* 29 (1), 114–126. doi: 10.1016/j.immuni.2008.05.010

Dambuza, I. M., He, C., Choi, J. K., Yu, C. R., Wang, R., Mattapallil, M. J., et al. (2017). IL-12p35 induces expansion of IL-10 and IL-35-expressing regulatory B cells and ameliorates autoimmune disease. *Nat. Commun.* 8 (1), 719. doi: 10.1038/s41467-017-00838-4

Davidson, T. S., DiPaolo, R. J., Andersson, J., and Shevach, E. M. (2007). Cutting Edge: IL-2 is essential for TGF-beta-mediated induction of Foxp3+ T regulatory cells. *J. Immunol.* 178 (7), 4022–4026. doi: 10.4049/jimmunol.178.7.4022

De Simone, M., Arrigoni, A., Rossetti, G., Gruarin, P., Ranzani, V., Politano, C., et al. (2016). Transcriptional landscape of human tissue lymphocytes unveils uniqueness of tumor-infiltrating T regulatory cells. *Immunity* 45 (5), 1135–1147. doi: 10.1016/j.immuni.2016.10.021

Deknuydt, F., Bioley, G., Valmori, D., and Ayyoub, M. (2009). IL-1beta and IL-2 convert human Treg into T(H)17 cells. *Clin. Immunol.* 131 (2), 298–307. doi: 10.1016/j.clim.2008.12.008

Doherty, D. G., and O'Farrelly, C. (2000). Innate and adaptive lymphoid cells in the human liver. *Immunol. Rev.* 174, 5–20. doi: 10.1034/j.1600-0528.2002.017416.x

Ebinuma, H., Nakamoto, N., Li, Y., Price, D. A., Gostick, E., Levine, B. L., et al. (2008). Identification and in vitro expansion of functional antigen-specific

CD25+ FoxP3+ regulatory T cells in hepatitis C virus infection. *J. Virol.* 82 (10), 5043–5053. doi: 10.1128/JVI.01548-07

Epp, A., Hobusch, J., Bartsch, Y. C., Petry, J., Lilienthal, G. M., Koeleman, C. A. M., et al. (2018). Sialylation of IgG antibodies inhibits IgG-mediated allergic reactions. *J. Allergy Clin. Immunol.* 141 (1), 399–402 e398. doi: 10.1016/j.jaci.2017.06.021

Ferber, I. A., Brocke, S., Taylor-Edwards, C., Ridgway, W., Dinisco, C., Steinman, L., et al. (1996). Mice with a disrupted IFN-gamma gene are susceptible to the induction of experimental autoimmune encephalomyelitis (EAE). *J. Immunol.* 156 (1), 5–7.

Ferri, S., Longhi, M. S., De Molo, C., Lalanne, C., Muratori, P., Granito, A., et al. (2010). A multifaceted imbalance of T cells with regulatory function characterizes type 1 autoimmune hepatitis. *Hepatology* 52 (3), 999–1007. doi: 10.1002/hep.23792

Fontenot, J. D., Gavin, M. A., and Rudensky, A. Y. (2017). Pillars article: Foxp3 programs the development and function of CD4+CD25+ regulatory T cells. *Nat. Immunol.* 2003. 4, 330–336. *J. Immunol.* 198 (3), 986–992. doi: 10.1038/ni904

Gaublomme, J. T., Yosef, N., Lee, Y., Gertner, R. S., Yang, L. V., Wu, C., et al. (2015). Single-cell genomics unveils critical regulators of Th17 cell pathogenicity. *Cell* 163 (6), 1400–1412. doi: 10.1016/j.cell.2015.11.009

Ghazal, K., Morales, O., Barjon, C., Dahlqvist, G., Aoudjehane, L., Ouaguia, L., et al. (2019). Early high levels of regulatory T cells and T helper 1 may predict the progression of recurrent hepatitis C after liver transplantation. *Clin. Res. Hepatol. Gastroenterol.* 43 (3), 273–281. doi: 10.1016/j.clinre.2018.10.005

Ghoreschi, K., Laurence, A., Yang, X. P., Tato, C. M., McGeachy, M. J., Konkel, J. E., et al. (2010). Generation of pathogenic T(H)17 cells in the absence of TGF-beta signalling. *Nature* 467 (7318), 967–971. doi: 10.1038/nature09447

Gibson, D. J., Elliott, L., McDermott, E., Tosetto, M., Keegan, D., Byrne, K., et al. (2015). Heightened expression of CD39 by regulatory T lymphocytes Is associated with therapeutic remission in inflammatory bowel disease. *Inflammation Bowel. Dis.* 21 (12), 2806–2814. doi: 10.1097/MIB.00 00000000000566

Globig, A. M., Hennecke, N., Martin, B., Seidl, M., Ruf, G., Hasselblatt, P., et al. (2014). Comprehensive intestinal T helper cell profiling reveals specific accumulation of IFN-gamma+IL-17+coproducing CD4+ T cells in active inflammatory bowel disease. *Inflammation Bowel. Dis.* 20 (12), 2321–2329. doi: 10.1097/MIB.0000000000000210

Gomes, A. L., Teijeiro, A., Buren, S., Tummala, K. S., Yilmaz, M., Waisman, A., et al. (2016). Metabolic inflammation-associated IL-17A causes non-alcoholic steatohepatitis and hepatocellular carcinoma. *Cancer Cell* 30 (1), 161–175. doi: 10.1016/j.ccell.2016.05.020

Goudy, K., Aydin, D., Barzaghi, F., Gambineri, E., Vignoli, M., Ciullini Mannurita, S., et al. (2013). Human IL2RA null mutation mediates immunodeficiency with lymphoproliferation and autoimmunity. *Clin. Immunol.* 146 (3), 248–261. doi: 10.1016/j.clim.2013.01.004

Grant, C. R., Liberal, R., Holder, B. S., Cardone, J., Ma, Y., Robson, S. C., et al. (2014). Dysfunctional CD39(POS) regulatory T cells and aberrant control of T-helper type 17 cells in autoimmune hepatitis. *Hepatology* 59 (3), 1007–1015. doi: 10.1002/hep.26583

Gutcher, I., Donkor, M. K., Ma, Q., Rudensky, A. Y., Flavell, R. A., and Li, M. O. (2011). Autocrine transforming growth factor-beta1 promotes in vivo Th17 cell differentiation. *Immunity* 34 (3), 396–408. doi: 10.1016/j.immuni.2011.03.005

Ha, D., Tanaka, A., Kibayashi, T., Tanemura, A., Sugiyama, D., Wing, J. B., et al. (2019). Differential control of human Treg and effector T cells in tumor immunity by Fc-engineered anti-CTLA-4 antibody. *Proc. Natl. Acad. Sci. U.S.A.* 116 (2), 609–618. doi: 10.1073/pnas.1812186116

Hadis, U., Wahl, B., Schulz, O., Hardtke-Wolenski, M., Schippers, A., Wagner, N., et al. (2011). Intestinal tolerance requires gut homing and expansion of FoxP3+ regulatory T cells in the lamina propria. *Immunity* 34 (2), 237–246. doi: 10.1016/j.immuni.2011.01.016

Hammerich, L., Heymann, F., and Tacke, F. (2011). Role of IL-17 and Th17 cells in liver diseases. *Clin. Dev. Immunol.* 2011, 345803. doi: 10.1155/2011/345803

Han, J. W., Joo, D. J., Kim, J. H., Rha, M. S., Koh, J. Y., Park, H. J., et al. (2020). Early reduction of regulatory T cells is associated with acute rejection in liver transplantation under tacrolimus-based immunosuppression with basiliximab induction. *Am. J. Transplant.* 20 (8), 2058–2069. doi: 10.1111/ajt.15789

Harbour, S. N., Maynard, C. L., Zindl, C. L., Schoeb, T. R., and Weaver, C. T. (2015). Th17 cells give rise to Th1 cells that are required for the pathogenesis of colitis. *Proc. Natl. Acad. Sci. U.S.A.* 112 (22), 7061–7066. doi: 10.1073/pnas.1415675112

Harrington, L. E., Hatton, R. D., Mangan, P. R., Turner, H., Murphy, T. L., Murphy, K. M., et al. (2005). Interleukin 17-producing CD4+ effector T cells develop via a lineage distinct from the T helper type 1 and 2 lineages. *Nat. Immunol.* 6 (11), 1123–1132. doi: 10.1038/ni1254

Hartemann, A., Bensimon, G., Payan, C. A., Jacqueminet, S., Bourron, O., Nicolas, N., et al. (2013). Low-dose interleukin 2 in patients with type 1 diabetes: a phase 1/2 randomised, double-blind, placebo-controlled trial. *Lancet Diabetes Endocrinol.* 1 (4), 295–305. doi: 10.1016/S2213-8587(13)70113-X

He, J. S., Meyer-Hermann, M., Xiangying, D., Zuan, L. Y., Jones, L. A., Ramakrishna, L., et al. (2013). The distinctive germinal center phase of IgE+ B lymphocytes limits their contribution to the classical memory response. *J. Exp. Med.* 210 (12), 2755–2771. doi: 10.1084/jem.20131539

He, J., Zhang, X., Wei, Y., Sun, X., Chen, Y., Deng, J., et al. (2016). Low-dose interleukin-2 treatment selectively modulates CD4(+) T cell subsets in patients with systemic lupus erythematosus. *Nat. Med.* 22 (9), 991–993. doi: 10.1038/nm.4148

Hill, J. A., Feuerer, M., Tash, K., Haxhinasto, S., Perez, J., Melamed, R., et al. (2007). Foxp3 transcription-factor-dependent and -independent regulation of the regulatory T cell transcriptional signature. *Immunity* 27 (5), 786–800. doi: 10.1016/j.immuni.2007.09.010

Hirota, K., Duarte, J. H., Veldhoen, M., Hornsby, E., Li, Y., Cua, D. J., et al. (2011). Fate mapping of IL-17-producing T cells in inflammatory responses. *Nat. Immunol.* 12 (3), 255–263. doi: 10.1038/ni.1993

Hirota, K., Turner, J. E., Villa, M., Duarte, J. H., Demengeot, J., Steinmetz, O. M., et al. (2013). Plasticity of Th17 cells in Peyer's patches is responsible for the induction of T cell-dependent IgA responses. *Nat. Immunol.* 14 (4), 372–379. doi: 10.1038/ni.2552

Hirschfield, G. M., Karlsen, T. H., Lindor, K. D., and Adams, D. H. (2013). Primary sclerosing cholangitis. *Lancet* 382 (9904), 1587–1599. doi: 10.1016/S0140-6736(13)60096-3

Huber, S., Gagliani, N., Esplugues, E., O'Connor, W. Jr., Huber, F. J., Chaudhry, A., et al. (2011). Th17 cells express interleukin-10 receptor and are controlled by Foxp3(-) and Foxp3+ regulatory CD4+ T cells in an interleukin-10-dependent manner. *Immunity* 34 (4), 554–565. doi: 10.1016/j.immuni.2011.01.020

Huber, S., Gagliani, N., and Flavell, R. A. (2012). Life, death, and miracles: Th17 cells in the intestine. *Eur. J. Immunol.* 42 (9), 2238–2245. doi: 10.1002/eji.201242619

Hubscher, S. G. (2006). Histological assessment of non-alcoholic fatty liver disease. *Histopathology* 49 (5), 450–465. doi: 10.1111/j.1365-2559.2006.02416.x

Humrich, J. Y., von Spee-Mayer, C., Siegert, E., Alexander, T., Hiepe, F., Radbruch, A., et al. (2015). Rapid induction of clinical remission by low-dose interleukin-2 in a patient with refractory SLE. *Ann. Rheum. Dis.* 74 (4), 791–792. doi: 10.1136/annrheumdis-2014-206506

Ichikawa, S., Mucida, D., Tyznik, A. J., Kronenberg, M., and Cheroutre, H. (2011). Hepatic stellate cells function as regulatory bystanders. *J. Immunol.* 186 (10), 5549–5555. doi: 10.4049/jimmunol.1003917

Ivanov, I. I., McKenzie, B. S., Zhou, L., Tadokoro, C. E., Lepelley, A., Lafaille, J. J., et al. (2006). The orphan nuclear receptor RORgammat directs the differentiation program of proinflammatory IL-17+ T helper cells. *Cell* 126 (6), 1121–1133. doi: 10.1016/j.cell.2006.07.035

Jiang, G., Yang, H. R., Wang, L., Wildey, G. M., Fung, J., Qian, S., et al. (2008). Hepatic stellate cells preferentially expand allogeneic CD4+ CD25+ FoxP3+ regulatory T cells in an IL-2-dependent manner. *Transplantation* 86 (11), 1492–1502. doi: 10.1097/TP.0b013e31818bfd13

Kamada, T., Togashi, Y., Tay, C., Ha, D., Sasaki, A., Nakamura, Y., et al. (2019). PD-1(+) regulatory T cells amplified by PD-1 blockade promote hyperprogression of cancer. *Proc. Natl. Acad. Sci. U.S.A.* 116 (20), 9999–10008. doi: 10.1073/pnas.1822001116

Kato, T., Noma, K., Ohara, T., Kashima, H., Katsura, Y., Sato, H., et al. (2018). Cancer-associated fibroblasts affect intratumoral CD8(+) and FoxP3(+) T cells via IL6 in the tumor microenvironment. *Clin. Cancer Res.* 24 (19), 4820–4833. doi: 10.1158/1078-0432.CCR-18-0205

Khader, S. A., Bell, G. K., Pearl, J. E., Fountain, J. J., Rangel-Moreno, J., Cilley, G. E., et al. (2007). IL-23 and IL-17 in the establishment of protective pulmonary

CD4+ T cell responses after vaccination and during Mycobacterium tuberculosis challenge. *Nat. Immunol.* 8 (4), 369–377. doi: 10.1038/ni1449

Kikuchi, J., Hashizume, M., Kaneko, Y., Yoshimoto, K., Nishina, N., and Takeuchi, T. (2015). Peripheral blood CD4(+)CD25(+)CD127(low) regulatory T cells are significantly increased by tocilizumab treatment in patients with rheumatoid arthritis: increase in regulatory T cells correlates with clinical response. *Arthritis Res. Ther.* 17, 10. doi: 10.1186/s13075-015-0526-4

Kobayashi, E., Kobayashi, M., Tsuneyama, K., Fukami, T., Nakajima, M., and Yokoi, T. (2009). Halothane-induced liver injury is mediated by interleukin-17 in mice. *Toxicol. Sci.* 111 (2), 302–310. doi: 10.1093/toxsci/kfp165

Koenen, H. J., Smeets, R. L., Vink, P. M., van Rijssen, E., Boots, A. M., and Joosten, I. (2008). Human CD25highFoxp3pos regulatory T cells differentiate into IL-17-producing cells. *Blood* 112 (6), 2340–2352. doi: 10.1182/blood-2008-01-133967

Korn, T., Bettelli, E., Gao, W., Awasthi, A., Jager, A., Strom, T. B., et al. (2007). IL-21 initiates an alternative pathway to induce proinflammatory T(H)17 cells. *Nature* 448 (7152), 484–487. doi: 10.1038/nature05970

Krueger, G. G., Langley, R. G., Leonardi, C., Yeilding, N., Guzzo, C., Wang, Y., et al. (2007). A human interleukin-12/23 monoclonal antibody for the treatment of psoriasis. *N. Engl. J. Med.* 356 (6), 580–592. doi: 10.1056/NEJMoa062382

Krummel, M. F., and Allison, J. P. (1996). CTLA-4 engagement inhibits IL-2 accumulation and cell cycle progression upon activation of resting T cells. *J. Exp. Med.* 183 (6), 2533–2540. doi: 10.1084/jem.183.6.2533

Kuehn, H. S., Ouyang, W., Lo, B., Deenick, E. K., Niemela, J. E., Avery, D. T., et al. (2014). Immune dysregulation in human subjects with heterozygous germline mutations in CTLA4. *Science* 345 (6204), 1623–1627. doi: 10.1126/science.1255904

Lan, Y. T., Wang, Z. L., Tian, P., Gong, X. N., Fan, Y. C., and Wang, K. (2019). Treg/Th17 imbalance and its clinical significance in patients with hepatitis B-associated liver cirrhosis. *Diagn. Pathol.* 14 (1), 114. doi: 10.1186/s13000-019-0891-4

Langhans, B., Braunschweiger, I., Arndt, S., Schulte, W., Satoguina, J., Layland, L. E., et al. (2010). Core-specific adaptive regulatory T-cells in different outcomes of hepatitis C. *Clin. Sci. (Lond)* 119 (2), 97–109. doi: 10.1042/CS20090661

Langowski, J. L., Zhang, X., Wu, L., Mattson, J. D., Chen, T., Smith, K., et al. (2006). IL-23 promotes tumour incidence and growth. *Nature* 442 (7101), 461–465. doi: 10.1038/nature04808

Lapierre, P., Beland, K., Yang, R., and Alvarez, F. (2013). Adoptive transfer of ex vivo expanded regulatory T cells in an autoimmune hepatitis murine model restores peripheral tolerance. *Hepatology* 57 (1), 217–227. doi: 10.1002/hep.26023

Lathrop, S. K., Bloom, S. M., Rao, S. M., Nutsch, K., Lio, C. W., Santacruz, N., et al. (2011). Peripheral education of the immune system by colonic commensal microbiota. *Nature* 478 (7368), 250–254. doi: 10.1038/nature10434

Le Bras, S., and Geha, R. S. (2006). IPEX and the role of Foxp3 in the development and function of human Tregs. *J. Clin. Invest.* 116 (6), 1473–1475. doi: 10.1172/JCI28880

Lee, Y. K., Turner, H., Maynard, C. L., Oliver, J. R., Chen, D., Elson, C. O., et al. (2009). Late developmental plasticity in the T helper 17 lineage. *Immunity* 30 (1), 92–107. doi: 10.1016/j.immuni.2008.11.005

Lemmers, A., Moreno, C., Gustot, T., Marechal, R., Degre, D., Demetter, P., et al. (2009). The interleukin-17 pathway is involved in human alcoholic liver disease. *Hepatology* 49 (2), 646–657. doi: 10.1002/hep.22680

Li, J., Qiu, S. J., She, W. M., Wang, F. P., Gao, H., Li, L., et al. (2012). Significance of the balance between regulatory T (Treg) and T helper 17 (Th17) cells during hepatitis B virus related liver fibrosis. *PloS One* 7 (6), e39307. doi: 10.1371/journal.pone.0039307

Linterman, M. A., Pierson, W., Lee, S. K., Kallies, A., Kawamoto, S., Rayner, T. F., et al. (2011). Foxp3+ follicular regulatory T cells control the germinal center response. *Nat. Med.* 17 (8), 975–982. doi: 10.1038/nm.2425

Liston, A., Nutsch, K. M., Farr, A. G., Lund, J. M., Rasmussen, J. P., Koni, P. A., et al. (2008). Differentiation of regulatory Foxp3+ T cells in the thymic cortex. *Proc. Natl. Acad. Sci. U. S. A.* 105 (33), 11903–11908. doi: 10.1073/pnas.0801506105

Liu, C., Xu, L., Xia, C., Long, Y., Liu, C., Lu, S., et al. (2020). Increased proportion of functional subpopulations in circulating regulatory T cells in patients with chronic hepatitis B. *Hepatol. Res.* 50 (4), 439–452. doi: 10.1111/hepr.13472

Losikoff, P. T., Self, A. A., and Gregory, S. H. (2012). Dendritic cells, regulatory T cells and the pathogenesis of chronic hepatitis C. *Virulence* 3 (7), 610–620. doi: 10.4161/viru.21823

Ma, C., Kesarwala, A. H., Eggert, T., Medina-Echeverz, J., Kleiner, D. E., Jin, P., et al. (2016). NAFLD causes selective CD4(+) T lymphocyte loss and promotes hepatocarcinogenesis. *Nature* 531 (7593), 253–257. doi: 10.1038/nature16969

Maggi, L., Santarlasci, V., Capone, M., Peired, A., Frosali, F., Crome, S. Q., et al. (2010). CD161 is a marker of all human IL-17-producing T-cell subsets and is induced by RORC. *Eur. J. Immunol.* 40 (8), 2174–2181. doi: 10.1002/eji.200940257

Maloy, K. J., and Powrie, F. (2001). Regulatory T cells in the control of immune pathology. *Nat. Immunol.* 2 (9), 816–822. doi: 10.1038/ni0901-816

Mangan, P. R., Harrington, L. E., O'Quinn, D. B., Helms, W. S., Bullard, D. C., Elson, C. O., et al. (2006). Transforming growth factor-beta induces development of the T(H)17 lineage. *Nature* 441 (7090), 231–234. doi: 10.1038/nature04754

Manigold, T., and Racanelli, V. (2007). T-cell regulation by CD4 regulatory T cells during hepatitis B and C virus infections: facts and controversies. *Lancet Infect. Dis.* 7 (12), 804–813. doi: 10.1016/S1473-3099(07)70289-X

Mannon, P. J., Fuss, I. J., Mayer, L., Elson, C. O., Sandborn, W. J., Present, D., et al. (2004). Anti-interleukin-12 antibody for active Crohn's disease. *N. Engl. J. Med.* 351 (20), 2069–2079. doi: 10.1056/NEJMoa033402

Marie, J. C., Letterio, J. J., Gavin, M., and Rudensky, A. Y. (2005). TGF-beta1 maintains suppressor function and Foxp3 expression in CD4+CD25+ regulatory T cells. *J. Exp. Med.* 201 (7), 1061–1067. doi: 10.1084/jem.20042276

Mathew, J. M., V. J, H., LeFever, A., Konieczna, I., Stratton, C., He, J., et al. (2018). A phase I clinical trial with ex vivo expanded recipient regulatory T cells in living donor kidney transplants. *Sci. Rep.* 8 (1), 7428. doi: 10.1038/s41598-018-25574-7

Matsuoka, K., Koreth, J., Kim, H. T., Bascug, G., McDonough, S., Kawano, Y., et al. (2013). Low-dose interleukin-2 therapy restores regulatory T cell homeostasis in patients with chronic graft-versus-host disease. *Sci. Transl. Med.* 5 (179), 179ra143. doi: 10.1126/scitranslmed.3005265

McGeachy, M. J., Bak-Jensen, K. S., Chen, Y., Tato, C. M., Blumenschein, W., McClanahan, T., et al. (2007). TGF-beta and IL-6 drive the production of IL-17 and IL-10 by T cells and restrain T(H)-17 cell-mediated pathology. *Nat. Immunol.* 8 (12), 1390–1397. doi: 10.1038/ni1539

McGeachy, M. J., Chen, Y., Tato, C. M., Laurence, A., Joyce-Shaikh, B., Blumenschein, W. M., et al. (2009). The interleukin 23 receptor is essential for the terminal differentiation of interleukin 17-producing effector T helper cells in vivo. *Nat. Immunol.* 10 (3), 314–324. doi: 10.1038/ni.1698

McLaughlin, T., Liu, L. F., Lamendola, C., Shen, L., Morton, J., Rivas, H., et al. (2014). T-cell profile in adipose tissue is associated with insulin resistance and systemic inflammation in humans. *Arterioscler. Thromb. Vasc. Biol.* 34 (12), 2637–2643. doi: 10.1161/ATVBAHA.114.304636

Meng, F., Wang, K., Aoyama, T., Grivennikov, S. I., Paik, Y., Scholten, D., et al. (2012). Interleukin-17 signaling in inflammatory, Kupffer cells, and hepatic stellate cells exacerbates liver fibrosis in mice. *Gastroenterology* 143 (3), 765–776.e3. doi: 10.1053/j.gastro.2012.05.049

Meng, P., Zhao, S., Niu, X., Fu, N., Su, S., Wang, R., et al. (2016). Involvement of the interleukin-23/interleukin-17 axis in chronic hepatitis C virus infection and its treatment responses. *Int. J. Mol. Sci.* 17 (11). doi: 10.3390/ijms17071070

Miyara, M., Yoshioka, Y., Kitoh, A., Shima, T., Wing, K., Niwa, A., et al. (2009). Functional delineation and differentiation dynamics of human CD4+ T cells expressing the FoxP3 transcription factor. *Immunity* 30 (6), 899–911. doi: 10.1016/j.immuni.2009.03.019

Morgan, M. E., Flierman, R., van Duivenvoorde, L. M., Witteveen, H. J., van Ewijk, W., van Laar, J. M., et al. (2005). Effective treatment of collagen-induced arthritis by adoptive transfer of CD25+ regulatory T cells. *Arthritis Rheum.* 52 (7), 2212–2221. doi: 10.1002/art.21195

Morrison, P. J., Bending, D., Fouser, L. A., Wright, J. F., Stockinger, B., Cooke, A., et al. (2013). Th17-cell plasticity in Helicobacter hepaticus-induced intestinal inflammation. *Mucosal. Immunol.* 6 (6), 1143–1156. doi: 10.1038/mi.2013.11

Mosmann, T. R., Cherwinski, H., Bond, M. W., Giedlin, M. A., and Coffman, R. L. (1986). Two types of murine helper T cell clone. I. Definition according to profiles of lymphokine activities and secreted proteins. *J. Immunol.* 136 (7), 2348–2357.

Mougiakakos, D., Johansson, C. C., Trocme, E., All-Ericsson, C., Economou, M. A., Larsson, O., et al. (2010). Intratumoral forkhead box P3-positive regulatory T cells predict poor survival in cyclooxygenase-2-positive uveal melanoma. *Cancer* 116 (9), 2224–2233. doi: 10.1002/cncr.24999

Mucida, D., Pino-Lagos, K., Kim, G., Nowak, E., Benson, M. J., Kronenberg, M., et al. (2009). Retinoic acid can directly promote TGF-beta-mediated Foxp3(+) Treg cell conversion of naive T cells. *Immunity* 30 (4), 471–472; author reply 472-473. doi: 10.1016/j.immuni.2009.03.008

Murphy, C. A., Langrish, C. L., Chen, Y., Blumenschein, W., McClanahan, T., Kastelein, R. A., et al. (2003). Divergent pro- and antiinflammatory roles for IL-23 and IL-12 in joint autoimmune inflammation. *J. Exp. Med.* 198 (12), 1951–1957. doi: 10.1084/jem.20030896

Nagakawa, K., Soyama, A., Hidaka, M., Adachi, T., Ono, S., Hara, T., et al. (2020). Elevated plasma levels of mitochondria-derived damage-associated molecular patterns during liver transplantation: predictors for postoperative multi-organ dysfunction syndrome. *Tohoku J. Exp. Med.* 250 (2), 87–93. doi: 10.1620/tjem.250.87

Nagata, T., McKinley, L., Peschon, J. J., Alcorn, J. F., Aujla, S. J., and Kolls, J. K. (2008). Requirement of IL-17RA in Con A induced hepatitis and negative regulation of IL-17 production in mouse T cells. *J. Immunol.* 181 (11), 7473–7479. doi: 10.4049/jimmunol.181.11.7473

Nakae, S., Iwakura, Y., Suto, H., and Galli, S. J. (2007). Phenotypic differences between Th1 and Th17 cells and negative regulation of Th1 cell differentiation by IL-17. *J. Leukoc. Biol.* 81 (5), 1258–1268. doi: 10.1189/jlb.1006610

Neurath, M. F., Weigmann, B., Finotto, S., Glickman, J., Nieuwenhuis, E., Iijima, H., et al. (2002). The transcription factor T-bet regulates mucosal T cell activation in experimental colitis and Crohn's disease. *J. Exp. Med.* 195 (9), 1129–1143. doi: 10.1084/jem.20011956

Niedbala, W., Wei, X. Q., Cai, B., Hueber, A. J., Leung, B. P., McInnes, I. B., et al. (2007). IL-35 is a novel cytokine with therapeutic effects against collagen-induced arthritis through the expansion of regulatory T cells and suppression of Th17 cells. *Eur. J. Immunol.* 37 (11), 3021–3029. doi: 10.1002/eji.200737810

Oberle, N., Eberhardt, N., Falk, C. S., Krammer, P. H., and Suri-Payer, E. (2007). Rapid suppression of cytokine transcription in human CD4+CD25 T cells by CD4+Foxp3+ regulatory T cells: independence of IL-2 consumption, TGF-beta, and various inhibitors of TCR signaling. *J. Immunol.* 179 (6), 3578–3587. doi: 10.4049/jimmunol.179.6.3578

Oo, Y. H., Banz, V., Kavanagh, D., Liaskou, E., Withers, D. R., Humphreys, E., et al. (2012). CXCR3-dependent recruitment and CCR6-mediated positioning of Th-17 cells in the inflamed liver. *J. Hepatol.* 57 (5), 1044–1051. doi: 10.1016/j.jhep.2012.07.008

Oppmann, B., Lesley, R., Blom, B., Timans, J. C., Xu, Y., Hunte, B., et al. (2000). Novel p19 protein engages IL-12p40 to form a cytokine, IL-23, with biological activities similar as well as distinct from IL-12. *Immunity* 13 (5), 715–725. doi: 10.1016/S1074-7613(00)00070-4

O'Garra, A., Vieira, P. L., Vieira, P., and Goldfeld, A. E. (2004). IL-10-producing and naturally occurring CD4+ Tregs: limiting collateral damage. *J. Clin. Invest.* 114 (10), 1372–1378. doi: 10.1172/JCI23215

Pandiyan, P., Zheng, L., Ishihara, S., Reed, J., and Lenardo, M. J. (2007). CD4 +CD25+Foxp3+ regulatory T cells induce cytokine deprivation-mediated apoptosis of effector CD4+ T cells. *Nat. Immunol.* 8 (12), 1353–1362. doi: 10.1038/ni1536

Park, H., Li, Z., Yang, X. O., Chang, S. H., Nurieva, R., Wang, Y. H., et al. (2005). A distinct lineage of CD4 T cells regulates tissue inflammation by producing interleukin 17. *Nat. Immunol.* 6 (11), 1133–1141. doi: 10.1038/ni1261

Park, S. H., Veerapu, N. S., Shin, E. C., Biancotto, A., McCoy, J. P., Capone, S., et al. (2013). Subinfectious hepatitis C virus exposures suppress T cell responses against subsequent acute infection. *Nat. Med.* 19 (12), 1638–1642. doi: 10.1038/nm.3408

Piccirillo, C. A. (2008). Regulatory T cells in health and disease. *Cytokine* 43 (3), 395–401. doi: 10.1016/j.cyto.2008.07.469

Pillai, V., Ortega, S. B., Wang, C. K., and Karandikar, N. J. (2007). Transient regulatory T-cells: a state attained by all activated human T-cells. *Clin. Immunol.* 123 (1), 18–29. doi: 10.1016/j.clim.2006.10.014

Rau, M., Schilling, A. K., Meertens, J., Hering, I., Weiss, J., Jurowich, C., et al. (2016). Progression from nonalcoholic fatty liver to nonalcoholic steatohepatitis is marked by a higher frequency of Th17 cells in the liver and an increased Th17/resting regulatory T cell ratio in peripheral blood and in the liver. *J. Immunol.* 196 (1), 97–105. doi: 10.4049/jimmunol.1501175

Refolo, M. G., Messa, C., Guerra, V., Carr, B. I., and D'Alessandro, R. (2020). Inflammatory Mechanisms of HCC Development. *Cancers (Basel)* 12 (3), 641. doi: 10.3390/cancers12030641

Ring, S., Pushkarevskaya, A., Schild, H., Probst, H. C., Jendrossek, V., Wirsdorfer, F., et al. (2015). Regulatory T cell-derived adenosine induces dendritic cell migration through the Epac-Rap1 pathway. *J. Immunol.* 194 (8), 3735–3744. doi: 10.4049/jimmunol.1401434

Romano, M., Tung, S. L., Smyth, L. A., and Lombardi, G. (2017). Treg therapy in transplantation: a general overview. *Transpl. Int.* 30 (8), 745–753. doi: 10.1111/tri.12909

Rosenzwajg, M., Churlaud, G., Mallone, R., Six, A., Derian, N., Chaara, W., et al. (2015). Low-dose interleukin-2 fosters a dose-dependent regulatory T cell tuned milieu in T1D patients. *J. Autoimmun.* 58, 48–58. doi: 10.1016/j.jaut.2015.01.001

Sage, P. T., Paterson, A. M., Lovitch, S. B., and Sharpe, A. H. (2014). The coinhibitory receptor CTLA-4 controls B cell responses by modulating T follicular helper, T follicular regulatory, and T regulatory cells. *Immunity* 41 (6), 1026–1039. doi: 10.1016/j.immuni.2014.12.005

Sakaguchi, S. (2004). Naturally arising CD4+ regulatory t cells for immunologic self-tolerance and negative control of immune responses. *Annu. Rev. Immunol.* 22, 531–562. doi: 10.1146/annurev.immunol.21.120601.141122

Sanchez-Fueyo, A., Whitehouse, G., Grageda, N., Cramp, M. E., Lim, T. Y., Romano, M., et al. (2020). Applicability, safety, and biological activity of regulatory T cell therapy in liver transplantation. *Am. J. Transplant.* 20 (4), 1125–1136. doi: 10.1111/ajt.15700

Sands, B. E., Sandborn, W. J., Panaccione, R., O'Brien, C. D., Zhang, H., Johanns, J., et al. (2019). Ustekinumab as induction and maintenance therapy for ulcerative colitis. *N. Engl. J. Med.* 381 (13), 1201–1214. doi: 10.1056/NEJMoa1900750

Sanford, M., and McKeage, K. (2015). Secukinumab: first global approval. *Drugs* 75 (3), 329–338. doi: 10.1007/s40265-015-0359-0

Sansom, D. M. (2015). IMMUNOLOGY. Moving CTLA-4 from the trash to recycling. *Science* 349 (6246), 377–378. doi: 10.1126/science.aac7888

Saravia, J., Chapman, N. M., and Chi, H. (2019). Helper T cell differentiation. *Cell Mol. Immunol.* 16 (7), 634–643. doi: 10.1038/s41423-019-0220-6

Sarhan, D., Hippen, K. L., Lemire, A., Hying, S., Luo, X., Lenvik, T., et al. (2018). Adaptive NK cells resist regulatory T-cell suppression driven by IL37. *Cancer Immunol. Res.* 6 (7), 766–775. doi: 10.1158/2326-6066.CIR-17-0498

Schubert, D., Bode, C., Kenefeck, R., Hou, T. Z., Wing, J. B., Kennedy, A., et al. (2014). Autosomal dominant immune dysregulation syndrome in humans with CTLA4 mutations. *Nat. Med.* 20 (12), 1410–1416. doi: 10.1038/nm.3746

Schuler, P. J., Saze, Z., Hong, C. S., Muller, L., Gillespie, D. G., Cheng, D., et al. (2014). Human CD4+ CD39+ regulatory T cells produce adenosine upon co-expression of surface CD73 or contact with CD73+ exosomes or CD73+ cells. *Clin. Exp. Immunol.* 177 (2), 531–543. doi: 10.1111/cei.12354

Sebode, M., Peiseler, M., Franke, B., Schwinge, D., Schoknecht, T., Wortmann, F., et al. (2014). Reduced FOXP3(+) regulatory T cells in patients with primary sclerosing cholangitis are associated with IL2RA gene polymorphisms. *J. Hepatol.* 60 (5), 1010–1016. doi: 10.1016/j.jhep.2013.12.027

Setoguchi, R., Hori, S., Takahashi, T., and Sakaguchi, S. (2005). Homeostatic maintenance of natural Foxp3(+) CD25(+) CD4(+) regulatory T cells by interleukin (IL)-2 and induction of autoimmune disease by IL-2 neutralization. *J. Exp. Med.* 201 (5), 723–735. doi: 10.1084/jem.20041982

Shi, T., Zhang, T., Zhang, L., Yang, Y., Zhang, H., and Zhang, F. (2015). The distribution and the fibrotic role of elevated inflammatory Th17 cells in patients with primary biliary cirrhosis. *Med. (Baltimore)* 94 (44), e1888. doi: 10.1097/MD.0000000000001888

Stumhofer, J. S., Laurence, A., Wilson, E. H., Huang, E., Tato, C. M., Johnson, L. M., et al. (2006). Interleukin 27 negatively regulates the development of interleukin 17-producing T helper cells during chronic inflammation of the central nervous system. *Nat. Immunol.* 7 (9), 937–945. doi: 10.1038/ni1376

Sun, H. Q., Zhang, J. Y., Zhang, H., Zou, Z. S., Wang, F. S., and Jia, J. H. (2012). Increased Th17 cells contribute to disease progression in patients with HBV-associated liver cirrhosis. *J. Viral. Hepat.* 19 (6), 396–403. doi: 10.1111/j.1365-2893.2011.01561.x

Sun, B., Liu, M., Cui, M., and Li, T. (2020). Granzyme B-expressing treg cells are enriched in colorectal cancer and present the potential to eliminate autologous T conventional cells. *Immunol. Lett.* 217, 7–14. doi: 10.1016/j.imlet.2019.10.007

Tai, X., Cowan, M., Feigenbaum, L., and Singer, A. (2005). CD28 costimulation of developing thymocytes induces Foxp3 expression and regulatory T cell differentiation independently of interleukin 2. *Nat. Immunol.* 6 (2), 152–162. doi: 10.1038/ni1160

Tait, B., Mackay, I. R., Board, P., Coggan, M., Emery, P., and Eckardt, G. (1989). HLA A1, B8, DR3 extended haplotypes in autoimmune chronic hepatitis. *Gastroenterology* 97 (2), 479–481. doi: 10.1016/0016-5085(89)90088-7

Takimoto, T., Wakabayashi, Y., Sekiya, T., Inoue, N., Morita, R., Ichiyama, K., et al. (2010). Smad2 and Smad3 are redundantly essential for the TGF-beta-mediated regulation of regulatory T plasticity and Th1 development. *J. Immunol.* 185 (2), 842–855. doi: 10.4049/jimmunol.0904100

Tan, Z., Qian, X., Jiang, R., Liu, Q., Wang, Y., Chen, C., et al. (2013). IL-17A plays a critical role in the pathogenesis of liver fibrosis through hepatic stellate cell activation. *J. Immunol.* 191 (4), 1835–1844. doi: 10.4049/jimmunol.1203013

Taylor, A., Akdis, M., Joss, A., Akkoc, T., Wenig, R., Colonna, M., et al. (2007). IL-10 inhibits CD28 and ICOS costimulations of T cells via src homology 2 domain-containing protein tyrosine phosphatase 1. *J. Allergy Clin. Immunol.* 120 (1), 76–83. doi: 10.1016/j.jaci.2007.04.004

Tesmer, L. A., Lundy, S. K., Sarkar, S., and Fox, D. A. (2008). Th17 cells in human disease. *Immunol. Rev.* 223, 87–113. doi: 10.1111/j.1600-065X.2008.00628.x

Thomas, D. A., and Massague, J. (2005). TGF-beta directly targets cytotoxic T cell functions during tumor evasion of immune surveillance. *Cancer Cell* 8 (5), 369–380. doi: 10.1016/j.ccr.2005.10.012

Toker, A., Engelbert, D., Garg, G., Polansky, J. K., Floess, S., Miyao, T., et al. (2013). Active demethylation of the Foxp3 locus leads to the generation of stable regulatory T cells within the thymus. *J. Immunol.* 190 (7), 3180–3188. doi: 10.4049/jimmunol.1203473

Tran, D. Q. (2012). TGF-beta: the sword, the wand, and the shield of FOXP3(+) regulatory T cells. *J. Mol. Cell Biol.* 4 (1), 29–37. doi: 10.1093/jmcb/mjr033

TrehanPati, N., Kotillil, S., Hissar, S. S., Shrivastava, S., Khanam, A., Sukriti, S., et al. (2011). Circulating Tregs correlate with viral load reduction in chronic HBV-treated patients with tenofovir disoproxil fumarate. *J. Clin. Immunol.* 31 (3), 509–520. doi: 10.1007/s10875-011-9509-7

Vaknin-Dembinsky, A., Balashov, K., and Weiner, H. L. (2006). IL-23 is increased in dendritic cells in multiple sclerosis and down-regulation of IL-23 by antisense oligos increases dendritic cell IL-10 production. *J. Immunol.* 176 (12), 7768–7774. doi: 10.4049/jimmunol.176.12.7768

Van Herck, M. A., Vonghia, L., Kwanten, W. J., Jule, Y., Vanwolleghem, T., Ebo, D., et al. (2020). Diet reversal and immune modulation show key role for liver and adipose tissue T cells in murine non-alcoholic steatohepatitis. *Cell Mol. Gastroenterol. Hepatol.* 10 (3), 467–490. doi: 10.1016/j.jcmgh.2020.04.010

Vang, K. B., Yang, J., Mahmud, S. A., Burchill, M. A., Vegoe, A. L., and Farrar, M. A. (2008). IL-2, -7, and -15, but not thymic stromal lymphopoeitin, redundantly govern CD4+Foxp3+ regulatory T cell development. *J. Immunol.* 181 (5), 3285–3290. doi: 10.4049/jimmunol.181.5.3285

Veldhoen, M., Hocking, R. J., Flavell, R. A., and Stockinger, B. (2006). Signals mediated by transforming growth factor-beta initiate autoimmune encephalomyelitis, but chronic inflammation is needed to sustain disease. *Nat. Immunol.* 7 (11), 1151–1156. doi: 10.1038/ni1391

Voron, T., Marcheteau, E., Pernot, S., Colussi, O., Tartour, E., Taieb, J., et al. (2014). Control of the immune response by pro-angiogenic factors. *Front. Oncol.* 4, 70. doi: 10.3389/fonc.2014.00070

Wakabayashi, K., Lian, Z. X., Moritoki, Y., Lan, R. Y., Tsuneyama, K., Chuang, Y. H., et al. (2006). IL-2 receptor alpha(-/-) mice and the development of primary biliary cirrhosis. *Hepatology* 44 (5), 1240–1249. doi: 10.1002/hep.21385

Wang, J. M., Shi, L., Ma, C. J., Ji, X. J., Ying, R. S., Wu, X. Y., et al. (2013). Differential regulation of interleukin-12 (IL-12)/IL-23 by Tim-3 drives T(H)17 cell development during hepatitis C virus infection. *J. Virol.* 87 (8), 4372–4383. doi: 10.1128/JVI.03376-12

Wang, K., Song, Z. L., Wu, B., Zhou, C. L., Liu, W., and Gao, W. (2019). The T-helper cells 17 instead of Tregs play the key role in acute rejection after pediatric liver transplantation. *Pediatr. Transplant.* 23 (3), e13363. doi: 10.1111/petr.13363

Wei, F., Zhong, S., Ma, Z., Kong, H., Medvec, A., Ahmed, R., et al. (2013). Strength of PD-1 signaling differentially affects T-cell effector functions. *Proc. Natl. Acad. Sci. U.S.A.* 110 (27), E2480–E2489. doi: 10.1073/pnas.1305394110

Wollenberg, I., Agua-Doce, A., Hernandez, A., Almeida, C., Oliveira, V. G., Faro, J., et al. (2011). Regulation of the germinal center reaction by Foxp3+ follicular regulatory T cells. *J. Immunol.* 187 (9), 4553–4560. doi: 10.4049/jimmunol.1101328

Wong, J., Obst, R., Correia-Neves, M., Losyev, G., Mathis, D., and Benoist, C. (2007). Adaptation of TCR repertoires to self-peptides in regulatory and nonregulatory CD4+ T cells. *J. Immunol.* 178 (11), 7032–7041. doi: 10.4049/jimmunol.178.11.7032

Wu, H. J., Ivanov, I. I., Darce, J., Hattori, K., Shima, T., Umesaki, Y., et al. (2010). Gut-residing segmented filamentous bacteria drive autoimmune arthritis via T helper 17 cells. *Immunity* 32 (6), 815–827. doi: 10.1016/j.immuni.2010.06.001

Yan, Z., Zhou, J., Zhang, M., Fu, X., Wu, Y., and Wang, Y. (2014). Telbivudine decreases proportion of peripheral blood CD4+CD25+CD127low T cells in parallel with inhibiting hepatitis B virus DNA. *Mol. Med. Rep.* 9 (5), 2024–2030. doi: 10.3892/mmr.2014.2042

Yang, X. O., Nurieva, R., Martinez, G. J., Kang, H. S., Chung, Y., Pappu, B. P., et al. (2008). Molecular antagonism and plasticity of regulatory and inflammatory T cell programs. *Immunity* 29 (1), 44–56. doi: 10.1016/j.immuni.2008.05.007

Yang, B. H., Hagemann, S., Mamareli, P., Lauer, U., Hoffmann, U., Beckstette, M., et al. (2016). Foxp3(+) T cells expressing RORgammat represent a stable regulatory T-cell effector lineage with enhanced suppressive capacity during intestinal inflammation. *Mucosal. Immunol.* 9 (2), 444–457. doi: 10.1038/mi.2015.74

Yang, L., Jia, S., Shao, X., Liu, S., Zhang, Q., Song, J., et al. (2019). Interleukin-35 modulates the balance between viral specific CD4(+)CD25(+)CD127(dim/-) regulatory T cells and T helper 17 cells in chronic hepatitis B virus infection. *Virol. J.* 16 (1), 48. doi: 10.1186/s12985-019-1158-0

Yoshida, O., Dou, L., Kimura, S., Yokota, S., Isse, K., Robson, S. C., et al. (2015). CD39 deficiency in murine liver allografts promotes inflammatory injury and immune-mediated rejection. *Transpl. Immunol.* 32 (2), 76–83. doi: 10.1016/j.trim.2015.01.003

Younossi, Z., Tacke, F., Arrese, M., Chander Sharma, B., Mostafa, I., Bugianesi, E., et al. (2019). Global Perspectives on Nonalcoholic Fatty Liver Disease and Nonalcoholic Steatohepatitis. *Hepatology* 69 (6), 2672–2682. doi: 10.1002/hep.30251

Zenewicz, L. A., Yancopoulos, G. D., Valenzuela, D. M., Murphy, A. J., Karow, M., and Flavell, R. A. (2007). Interleukin-22 but not interleukin-17 provides protection to hepatocytes during acute liver inflammation. *Immunity* 27 (4), 647–659. doi: 10.1016/j.immuni.2007.07.023

Zhang, Y. H., and Sun, H. X. (2020). Immune checkpoint molecules in pregnancy: Focus on regulatory T cells. *Eur. J. Immunol.* 50 (2), 160–169. doi: 10.1002/eji.201948382

Zhang, J. P., Yan, J., Xu, J., Pang, X. H., Chen, M. S., Li, L., et al. (2009). Increased intratumoral IL-17-producing cells correlate with poor survival in hepatocellular carcinoma patients. *J. Hepatol.* 50 (5), 980–989. doi: 10.1016/j.jhep.2008.12.033

Zhang, B., Chikuma, S., Hori, S., Fagarasan, S., and Honjo, T. (2016). Nonoverlapping roles of PD-1 and FoxP3 in maintaining immune tolerance in a novel autoimmune pancreatitis mouse model. *Proc. Natl. Acad. Sci. U.S.A.* 113 (30), 8490–8495. doi: 10.1073/pnas.1608873113

Zhang, X., Feng, M., Liu, X., Bai, L., Kong, M., Chen, Y., et al. (2016). Persistence of cirrhosis is maintained by intrahepatic regulatory T cells that inhibit fibrosis resolution by regulating the balance of tissue inhibitors of metalloproteinases and matrix metalloproteinases. *Transl. Res.* 169, 67–79 e61-62. doi: 10.1016/j.trsl.2015.10.008

Zhao, L., Tang, Y., You, Z., Wang, Q., Liang, S., Han, X., et al. (2011). Interleukin-17 contributes to the pathogenesis of autoimmune hepatitis through inducing hepatic interleukin-6 expression. *PloS One* 6 (4), e18909. doi: 10.1371/journal.pone.0018909

Zheng, Y., Josefowicz, S., Chaudhry, A., Peng, X. P., Forbush, K., and Rudensky, A. Y. (2010). Role of conserved non-coding DNA elements in the Foxp3 gene in regulatory T-cell fate. *Nature* 463 (7282), 808–812. doi: 10.1038/nature08750

Zhou, L., Ivanov, I. I., Spolski, R., Min, R., Shenderov, K., Egawa, T., et al. (2007). IL-6 programs T(H)-17 cell differentiation by promoting sequential engagement of the IL-21 and IL-23 pathways. *Nat. Immunol.* 8 (9), 967–974. doi: 10.1038/ni1488

Zhu, J., Yamane, H., and Paul, W. E. (2010). Differentiation of effector CD4 T cell populations (*). *Annu. Rev. Immunol.* 28, 445–489. doi: 10.1146/annurev-immunol-030409-101212

Ziolkowska, M., Koc, A., Luszczykiewicz, G., Ksiezopolska-Pietrzak, K., Klimczak, E., Chwalinska-Sadowska, H., et al. (2000). High levels of IL-17 in rheumatoid arthritis patients: IL-15 triggers in vitro IL-17 production via cyclosporin A-sensitive mechanism. *J. Immunol.* 164 (5), 2832–2838. doi: 10.4049/jimmunol.164.5.2832

6

Tpl2 Protects Against Fulminant Hepatitis Through Mobilization of Myeloid-Derived Suppressor Cells

Jing Xu [1,2], Siyu Pei [2], Yan Wang [2], Junli Liu [2], Youcun Qian [2], Mingzhu Huang [3*], Yanyun Zhang [1,2*] and Yichuan Xiao [2*]

[1] The First Affiliated Hospital of Soochow University, Institutes for Translational Medicine, State Key Laboratory of Radiation Medicine and Protection, Key Laboratory of Stem Cells and Medical Biomaterials of Jiangsu Province, Medical College of Soochow University, Soochow University, Suzhou, China, [2] CAS Key Laboratory of Tissue Microenvironment and Tumor, Shanghai Institute of Nutrition and Health, Shanghai Institutes for Biological Sciences, University of Chinese Academy of Sciences, Chinese Academy of Sciences, Shanghai, China, [3] Department of Medical Oncology, Fudan University Shanghai Cancer Center, Shanghai, China

*Correspondence:
Mingzhu Huang
mingzhuhuang0718@163.com
Yanyun Zhang
yyzhang@sibs.ac.cn
Yichuan Xiao
ycxiao@sibs.ac.cn

Myeloid derived suppressor cells (MDSC) in the liver microenvironment protects against the inflammation-induced liver injury in fulminant hepatitis (FH). However, the molecular mechanism through which MDSC is recruited into the inflamed liver remain elusive. Here we identified a protein kinase Tpl2 as a critical mediator of MDSC recruitment into liver during the pathogenesis of *Propionibacterium acnes*/LPS-induced FH. Loss of Tpl2 dramatically suppressed MDSC mobilization into liver, leading to exaggerated local inflammation and increased FH-induced mortality. Mechanistically, although the protective effect of Tpl2 for FH-induced mortality was dependent on the presence of MDSC, Tpl2 neither directly targeted myeloid cells nor T cells to regulate FH pathogenesis, but functioned in hepatocytes to mediate the induction of MDSC-attracting chemokine CXCL1 and CXCL2 through modulating IL-25 (also known as IL-17E) signaling. As a consequence, increased MDSC in the inflamed liver specifically restrained the local proliferation of infiltrated pathogenic CD4$^+$ T cells, and thus protected against the inflammation-induced acute liver failure. Together, our findings established Tpl2 as a critical mediator of MDSC recruitment and highlighted the therapeutic potential of Tpl2 for the treatment of FH.

Keywords: hepatitis, myeloid-derive suppressor cells (MDSCs), TPL2, IL-25, chemokine

INTRODUCTION

Fulminant hepatitis (FH) is a dreaded disease characterized by rapid development of hepatocellular dysfunction, leading to the failure of hepatic regeneration (1). Published studies have shown that the pathogenesis of FH is associated with huge liver infiltration of immune cells, which secrete a large number of pro-inflammatory cytokines and thus induce acute inflammatory necrosis of hepatocytes (2, 3). The bacterial infection has been considered as a key factor that contribute to the development of FH pathology (4). Indeed, mice injected with heat-killed *Propionibacterium acnes* followed by lipopolysaccharide (LPS), one of the most commonly used FH animal models, phenocopy the inflammatory infiltration in hepatic parenchyma and finally lead to the acute liver failure (5–8). Although the pathogenesis of FH has been extensively investigated, there is no proper therapeutic strategies for this disease, leading to high mortality if there is no supportive management and/or liver transplantation (9).

Myeloid derived suppressor cells (MDSC) are a heterogeneous group of immune cells derived from bone marrow and have been implicated to play important immunosuppressive and protective roles in human hepatitis, hepatocellular carcinoma or various mouse hepatitis models through different mechanism. For example, MDSC inhibited T cell proliferation and IFN-γ production in chronic HCV patients (10), and suppressed NK cell function during the pathogenesis of human hepatocellular carcinoma (11). In hepatitis mouse models, MDSC also exhibited immunosuppressive function through inhibiting the T cells proliferation, activation and secretion of pro-inflammatory cytokines, and thus protected against hepatic inflammation and fibrosis through different mechanisms (12–14). Therefore, increasing the number of MDSC in the liver may help to inhibit the occurrence of local inflammation of the liver and protect against FH. Indeed, administration of IL-25 dramatically prevented and reverses acute liver damage through promoting the recruitment of the MDSC into liver in FH mouse (15).

IL-25, also known as IL-17E, belongs to IL-17 cytokine family, and was initially found to be highly expressed in T helper (Th) 2 cells and promote the proliferation of Th2 cells and eosinophils (16–18). In addition, it has been reported that IL-25 exhibited inhibitory effect of the proliferation of Th1 and Th17 cells and further suppressed the occurrence of autoimmune diseases in mice (19, 20). However, it is not clear how IL-25 initiates the signal pathway to mediate MDSC recruitment into liver during FH pathogenesis. Published study has identified that IL-25 can bind to the heterodimer receptor composed of IL-17RA and IL-17RB, which then recruit Act1 to activate downstream NF-κB and MAPK (21–23), suggesting a similarity with IL-17A-induced signaling pathway. Our previous study has demonstrated that the serine/threonine protein kinase Tpl2 is a key component in regulating the IL-17A signaling pathway, in which the activated Tpl2 directly bound to and phosphorylated TAK1 and further induce the activation of downstream NF-κB and MAPK (24, 25). Based on the similarity of IL-17A- and IL-25-induced signaling and the critical protective role of IL-25 in FH, we speculated that Tpl2 may also regulated the FH pathogenesis through modulation of IL-25 signaling.

In the present study, we found that Tpl2 protected against FH-induced acute liver injury and mouse mortality. Loss of Tpl2 in hepatocytes suppressed IL-25-induced chemokine CXCL1/2 expression, which impaired the recruitment of MDSC into the liver, leading to promoted proliferation of liver-infiltrating CD4+ T cells and enhanced FH pathology.

RESULTS

Tpl2 Protected Against P. acne/LPS-Induced FH

To investigate the *in vivo* role of Tpl2 during FH pathogenesis, we induced a FH model by intravenously injecting the mice with heat-killed *P. acnes* and followed by LPS. In this model, only *P. acnes* priming is not lethal for the mice, and *P. acnes* priming plus LPS injection 7 days later will strongly induce acute liver damage, leading to FH-related mortality. However,

P. acnes priming-induced liver inflammation is necessary and the reason for the mortality after LPS injection in this FH model (6, 7). As shown in **Figure 1A**, low dose of *P. acnes*/LPS priming provoked a non-lethal moderate hepatitis in wild-type (hereafter termed WT) mice. In contrast, *Tpl2*-deficient mice that induced with FH by using the same dose of *P. acnes*/LPS developed a much severer disease, leading to 86% lethality within 8 h (**Figure 1A**). Consistently, we observed the increased production of serum aspartate aminotransferase (AST) and higher ratio of AST/aminotransferase (ALT) levels, which is a hallmark of hepatitis-induced liver failure, in *Tpl2*-deficient mice accordingly (**Figure 1B**). In addition, histological analysis showed that there was more inflammatory infiltration observed in the *Tpl2*-deficient liver tissues on day 7 after *P. acnes* priming (**Figures 1C,D**). These results collectively suggested an important beneficial role of Tpl2 in protecting *P. acnes*/LPS-driven acute liver damage.

Tpl2 Deficiency Increased the Liver Infiltration of Pathogenic CD4+ T Cells

The exaggerated FH in *Tpl2*-deficient mice promoted us to examine the cellular mechanism by which Tpl2 protect against liver failure during FH pathogenesis. We firstly examined the peripheral immune activation after *P. acnes* priming, and the results revealed that *Tpl2*-deficient and WT control mice had similar frequencies and absolute numbers of CD4+ T cells, CD8+ T cells, CD11c+ dendritic cells, B220+ B cells and CD4+Foxp3+ regulatory T cells (Treg) in the spleens 7 days after challenged with *P. acnes* (**Figures 2A–D**). In addition, the frequencies and absolute numbers of IFN-γ- and TNF-α-producing T helper (Th)1 CD4+ T cells in the spleens were also comparable between the WT and *Tpl2*-deficient mice (**Figures 2E,F**). These data suggested Tpl2 does not affect peripheral immune activation during FH pathogenesis.

It is known that *P. acnes* priming promoted the liver infiltration of CD4+ T cells, which contributed to the inflammation-induced liver injury (8). Although the frequencies and absolute cell numbers of CD4+ T cells in the spleens or peripheral blood were comparable in WT and *Tpl2*-deficient mice during *P. acnes*-primed process (**Figures 2G–J**), loss of Tpl2 dramatically increased the frequencies and absolute numbers of CD4+ T cells in the livers as compared with that in WT liver, whereas didn't affect the liver infiltration of CD8+ T cells, dendritic cells, B cells and Treg cells at day 7 after *P. acnes* priming (**Figures 3A–E**). Since the Th1 cells are the major pathogenic contributor of *P. acnes*-induced liver injury (26), we next examined the TNF-α and IFN-γ production among the infiltrated CD4+ T cells. Interestingly, *Tpl2* deficiency didn't affect the ability of liver-infiltrating CD4+ T cells to produce TNF-α and IFN-γ, as reflected by comparable frequencies of IFN-γ- and TNF-α-producing Th1 cells in the inflamed livers of WT and *Tpl2*-deficient mice (**Figures 3F,G**). However, the absolute cell numbers of the pathogenic Th1 cells were dramatically increased in the inflamed livers of *Tpl2*-deficient mice (**Figures 3F,G**). Moreover, *Tpl2* deficiency gradually increased the liver infiltration of CD4+ T cells, notably

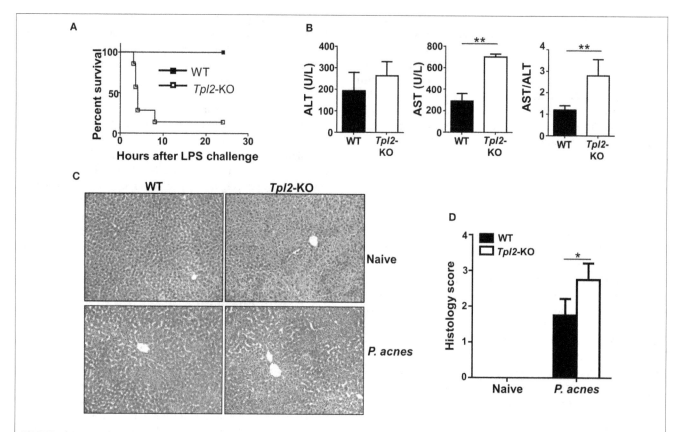

FIGURE 1 | *Tpl2* deficiency exaggerated *P. acnes*/LPS-induced FH. WT and *Tpl2*-KO mice were injected with 0.5 mg *P. acnes* suspended in 200 µl of phosphate-buffered saline (PBS), and then 1 µg of LPS in 200 µl of PBS was injected on day 7 to induce fulminant hepatitis (FH). **(A)** Cumulative survival rates of WT and *Tpl2*-KO mice were analyzed (*n* = 7 mice/group) after LPS injection. **(B)** Serum levels of aminotransferase (ALT), aspartate aminotransferase (AST) and the AST/ALT ratios (*n* = 5 mice per group) were measured on day 7 after *P. acnes* priming. **(C)** H&E staining showing the representative inflammatory infiltration in the livers of WT and *Tpl2*-KO mice that injected with *P. acnes* at day 7. The liver sections from WT and *Tpl2*-KO naive mice were stained as negative controls (magnification, ×200). **(D)** Semiquantitative analysis of inflammatory conditions in the livers from WT and *Tpl2*-KO naive and *P. acnes*-primed mice. Results are mean ± SD from three independent experiments. Two-tailed Student's *t*-tests were performed. *$P < 0.05$; **$P < 0.01$.

at day 5 and 7 after *P. acnes* priming (**Figures 3H,I**). These data collectively suggested Tpl2 may inhibited the liver infiltration of CD4$^+$ T cells during *P. acnes*-induced liver injury.

Tpl2 Specifically Restricted the Proliferation of Liver-Infiltrating CD4$^+$ T Cells

To confirm the pathogenic role of liver-infiltrating CD4$^+$ T cells after *P. acnes* priming in the FH model, we injected different dose of *P. acnes* and examined the survival rate and liver infiltration of CD4$^+$ T cells. The results revealed that after challenged with a single shot of same dose of LPS, higher dose of *P. acnes* priming dramatically increased the mouse mortality rate as compared with that primed with lower dose of *P. acnes* (**Figure 4A**). As expected, higher dose of *P. acnes* priming significantly increased the infiltration of CD4$^+$ T cells in the livers, along with decreased frequencies of liver infiltration of MDSC (**Figures 4B,C**), which is known to restrain the local inflammation in inflamed liver microenvironment through inhibiting T cell proliferation (15, 27). Therefore, we speculated that Tpl2 may regulate the proliferation of liver-infiltrating

CD4$^+$ T cells, and then injected bromodeoxyuridine (BrdU), a synthetic nucleoside that could be incorporated into newly synthesized DNA to monitor the cell proliferation, into WT or *Tpl2*-deficient mice before *P. acnes* priming. The flow cytometric analysis revealed that *Tpl2* deficiency specifically increased the frequencies of BrdU$^+$ CD4$^+$ T cells that isolated from the inflamed livers, whereas the frequencies of BrdU$^+$ CD4$^+$ T cells were comparable in the spleens between WT and *Tpl2*-deficient mice after *P. acnes* priming (**Figures 4D,E**), suggesting Tpl2 may indirectly regulate the proliferation of CD4$^+$ T cells in the inflamed liver microenvironment. Indeed, Tpl2 is dispensable for the *in vitro* CD4$^+$ T cell proliferation, as characterized by comparable proliferation rate of naïve WT and *Tpl2*-deficient CD4$^+$ T cells upon the stimulation of anti-CD3 plus anti-CD28 antibodies (**Figure 4F**).

To further exclude the possibility that Tpl2 may directly function in CD4$^+$ T cell to regulate FH pathogenesis, we adoptively transferred WT or *Tpl2*-deficient CD4$^+$ T cells into T cell-deficient *Rag1*-KO mice, which were then induced the FH model by injecting *P. acnes*/LPS. Expectedly, the FH-induced mortality rates are comparable in recipient *Rag1*-KO

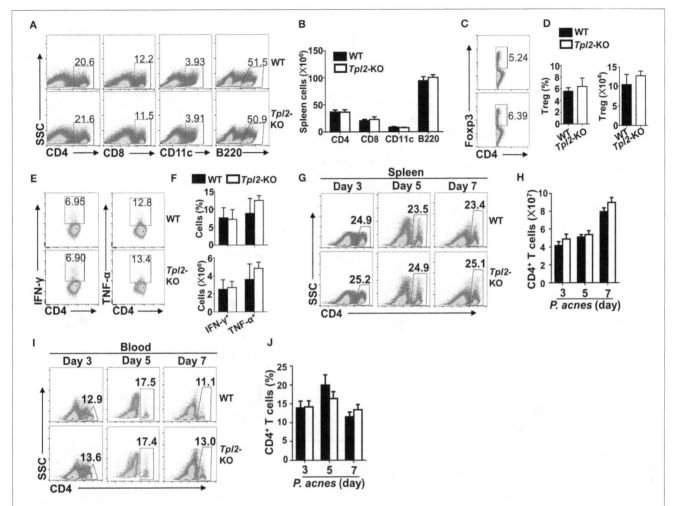

FIGURE 2 | Tpl2 didn't affect peripheral immune activation during FH pathogenesis. The splenic cells or peripheral blood immune cells were isolated from *P. acnes*-primed WT and *Tpl2*-KO mice at day 3, 5, and 7 as described in Materials and methods (*n* = 4 mice/group), and subjected for flow cytometry analysis. **(A–F)** Flow cytometry analysis of the frequencies and absolute numbers of CD4+ T cells, CD8+ T cells, B220+ B cells, CD11c+ dendritic cells **(A,B)**, CD4+Foxp3+ Treg cells **(C,D)**, and IFN-γ- and TNF-α-producing pathogenic Th1 cells **(E,F)** in the spleens of WT and *Tpl2*-KO mice at day 7 after *P. acnes* priming. Data are presented as representative plots of the frequencies of immune cell subpopulations **(A,C,E)** and a summary graph of the cell frequencies or absolute cell numbers **(B,D,F)**. **(G–J)** Flow cytometry analysis of the frequencies and absolute numbers of CD4+ T cells in the spleens **(G,H)** or peripheral blood **(I,J)** of WT and *Tpl2*-KO mice at day 3, 5, and 7 after *P. acnes* priming. Data are presented as representative plots of the frequencies of immune cell subpopulations **(G,I)** and a summary graph of the cell frequencies or absolute cell numbers **(H,J)**. Results are mean ± SD from three independent experiments.

mice that either transferred with WT or *Tpl2*-deficient CD4+ T cells (**Figure 4G**). Collectively, these results suggested that Tpl2 specifically restricted the proliferation of liver-infiltrating CD4+ T cells through an indirect mechanism during FH pathogenesis.

Tpl2 Mediated the Recruitment of MDSC Into Liver

Considering the indirect function of Tpl2 in regulating CD4+ T cell proliferation, we examined the infiltration status of MDSC in inflamed liver. In contrast to the increased infiltrating rate of CD4+ T cells in inflamed liver (**Figures 3H,I**), *Tpl2* deficiency gradually decreased the frequencies and absolute numbers of liver-infiltrating CD11b+Gr-1+ MDSC, notably at day 5 and 7 after *P. acnes* priming, as compared with that of WT mice (**Figures 5A,B**). The immunofluorescence analysis also confirmed the decreased infiltration of MDSC in the

hepatic parenchyma of *Tpl2*-KO mice at day 7 after *P. acnes* priming (**Figure 5C**). However, loss of Tpl2 neither altered the frequencies and absolute numbers of MDSC in the spleens nor affected the peripheral distribution of MDSC in the circulation system during *P. acnes*-primed process (**Figures 5D–G**). In addition, *in vitro* proliferation assay revealed that *Tpl2*-deficient MDSC exhibited similar ability as WT MDSC to suppress either WT or *Tpl2*-deficient T cell proliferation after cocultured with CD4+ T cell that stimulated with anti-CD3 plus anti-CD28 antibodies (**Figures 5H,I**). These data suggested that *Tpl2* deficiency suppressed the liver recruitment of MDSC without affecting their immunosuppressive function.

We next examined whether the impaired liver recruitment of MDSC contributed to the enhanced mortality in *Tpl2*-deficient FH mice. To this end, we specifically deleted the MDSC by injection of anti-Ly-6G neutralizing antibody

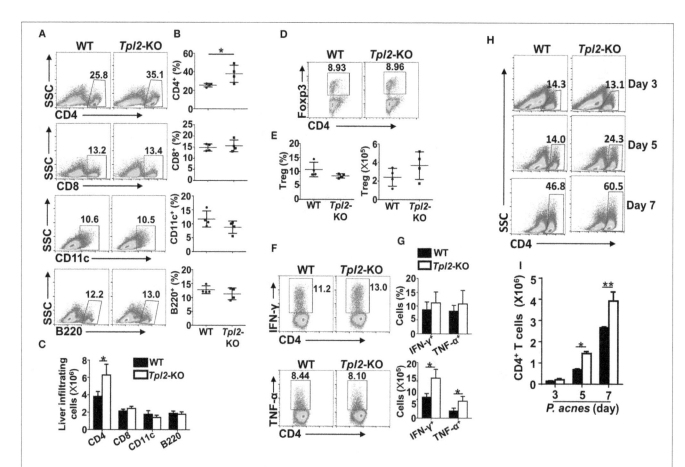

FIGURE 3 | Tpl2 reduced liver infiltration of pathogenic CD4+ T cells. Liver-infiltrating immune cells were isolated from *P. acnes*-primed WT and *Tpl2*-KO mice at day 3, 5, and 7 as described in Materials and methods (*n* = 4 mice/group). **(A–G)** Flow cytometry analysis of the frequencies and absolute numbers of CD4+ and CD8+ T cells, B220+ B cell, CD11c+ dendritic cells **(A–C)**, CD4+Foxp3+ Treg cells **(D,E)**, and IFN-γ- and TNF-α-producing pathogenic Th1 cells **(F,G)** in the livers of WT and *Tpl2*-KO mice at day 7 after *P. acnes* priming. Data are presented as representative plots of the frequencies of immune cell subpopulations **(A,D,F)** and a summary graph of the frequencies and absolute cell numbers **(B,C,E,G)**. **(H,I)** Flow cytometry analysis of the frequencies and absolute numbers of CD4+ T cells in the livers of WT and *Tpl2*-KO mice at day 3, 5, and 7 after *P. acnes* priming. Data are presented as representative plots of the frequencies of immune cell subpopulations **(H)** and a summary graph of the absolute cell numbers **(I)**. Results are mean ± SD from three independent experiments. Two-tailed Student's *t*-tests were performed. *P < 0.05; **P < 0.01.

(**Supplementary Figures 1A,B**), and challenged mice with *P. acnes*/LPS to induce FH. As expected, *in vivo* MDSC depletion dramatically increased the mortality rate of WT FH mice, and largely abolished the difference of the survival rate between WT and *Tpl2*-deficient mice that injected with *P. acnes*/LPS (**Figure 5J**). These results collectively established Tpl2 as a critical mediator of MDSC mobilization into liver to protect inflammation-induced liver injury during FH pathogenesis.

Tpl2 Functioned in Liver-Resident Cells to Protect Against FH

To figure out which type of cells *in vivo* was directly targeted by Tpl2 to protect against FH-induced liver failure, we generated the mixed bone marrow (BM) chimeric mice by reconstituting the lethally irradiated WT mice with WT or *Tpl2*-deficient BM, which were then challenged with *P. acnes*/LPS to induce FH. Unexpectedly, *Tpl2*-deficient BM reconstituted chimeric mice were totally resistant to FH-induced death (**Figure 6A**), suggesting that *Tpl2* deficiency in myeloid cells (including

macrophages and MDSC) does not contribute to the aggregation of FH-induced mortality. However, when reconstituting the WT BM into lethally irradiated WT or *Tpl2*-deficient mice, we found that WT BM failed to induce FH-mediated death in WT recipient mice, whereas dramatically promoted the mortality rate of *Tpl2*-deficient recipient mice (**Figure 6B**). These data collectively suggested that Tpl2 didn't target myeloid cells, but functioned in liver-resident cells to protect against FH pathology.

Next, we examined the proinflammatory cytokine and chemokine induction in the livers at the early priming phase of FH model. After 3 days of *P. acnes* challenge, the expression of Th1 cytokine genes *Ifng* and *Tnf* in the *Tpl2*-deficient inflamed livers were much higher than that in WT livers (**Figure 6C**), which suggested that the increased liver infiltration of pathogenic Th1 cells as shown in **Figure 3G** may contribute to the enhanced expression of these pro-inflammatory genes. Accordingly, the expression of MDSC-attracting chemokine genes *Cxcl1* and *Cxcl2* were dramatically suppressed in the *Tpl2*-deficient livers as compared with that in WT livers (**Figure 6C**). In addition, the

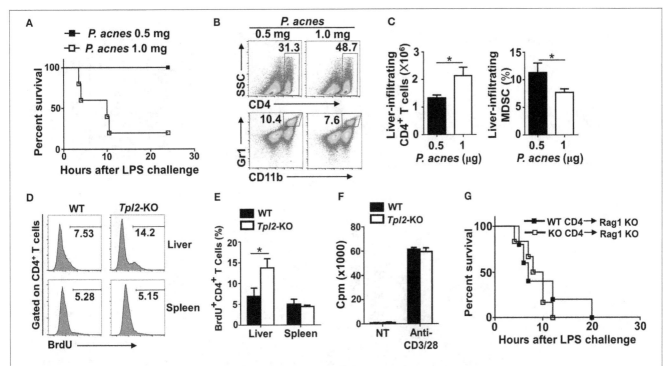

FIGURE 4 | *Tpl2* deficiency specifically inhibited the proliferation of liver-infiltrated CD4$^+$ T cells. **(A)** Cumulative survival analysis of WT C57BL/6 mice ($n = 5$ mice/group) that were injected with 0.5 or 1.0 mg *P. acnes* suspended in 200 μl of phosphate-buffered saline (PBS), and then with 1 μg of LPS in 200 μl of PBS at day 7 to induce fulminant hepatitis (FH). **(B,C)** Flow cytometry analysis of the frequencies and absolute numbers of CD4$^+$ and Gr-1$^+$CD11b$^+$ MDSC in the livers of WT C57BL/6 mice at day 7 after different dose of *P. acnes* priming. Data are presented as representative plots of the frequencies of immune cell subpopulations **(B)** and a summary graph of the frequencies or absolute cell numbers **(C)**. **(D,E)** Flow cytometry analysis of CD4$^+$ T cell proliferation in the spleens and livers of WT and *Tpl2*-KO mice at day 7 after *P. acnes* priming ($n = 4$ mice/group). Data are presented as a representative histogram **(D)** and a summary bar graph **(E)** showing the frequencies of proliferating BrdU$^+$ CD4$^+$ T cells. **(F)** Proliferation of WT and *Tpl2*-KO CD4$^+$ T cells in the absence (NT) or presence of anti-CD3/CD28 antibodies, then assessed by [^{3}H] thymidine incorporation. **(G)** Cumulative survival rates of age- and sex-matched *Rag1*-KO mice that adoptively transferred with WT and *Tpl2*-KO CD4$^+$ T cells and then subjected to *P. acnes*/LPS-mediated FH induction ($n = 5$ mice/group). Results are mean ± SD from three independent experiments. Two-tailed Student's *t*-tests were performed. *$P < 0.05$.

expression of the genes that encoding DC-recruiting chemokine MIP-1α (6) and other two MDSC-attracting chemokine CCL17 and CCL19 (15) were not affected in the livers of *P. acnes*-primed *Tpl2*-deficient mice (**Supplementary Figures 1C,D**). Moreover, the enzyme-linked immunosorbent assay confirmed that *Tpl2* ablation inhibited *P. acnes*-induced CXCL1 chemokine protein production in the liver parenchyma as compared with that in WT livers (**Figure 6D**). Together, these results suggested that Tpl2 directly functioned in liver-resident cells, but not in peripheral immune cells, to mediate MDSC recruitment, and thus protect against FH pathology.

Tpl2 Regulated IL-25 Signaling in Hepatocytes

Published study has suggested that IL-25 is highly produced in both human and mouse livers, and it is critical for the liver recruitment of MDSC in D-Gal/LPS-induced FH mouse model (15). In addition, we have previously demonstrated that Tpl2 mediates the activation of signaling pathway induced by IL-17A, which belongs to the same IL-17 family as IL-25 (24, 25). Therefore, we speculated that Tpl2 may potentially modulates IL-25 signaling in the liver-resident cells to regulate FH pathogenesis. To test this hypothesis, we firstly examined

the IL-25 production in the livers, and found that there is no significant difference of IL-25 levels in the liver homogenates between WT and *Tpl2*-deficient mice that were either under physiological condition or challenged with *P. acnes* (**Figure 7A**), suggesting Tpl2 is dispensable for the IL-25 secretion in the liver tissue. In addition, we observed that IL-25 production in the livers of *P. acnes*-primed mice were comparable with that of naïve mice (**Figure 7A**), which is different from the D-Gal/LPS-induced FH model that IL-25 levels are decreased in the livers of FH mice (15). Next, we generated the *Tpl2*/*Il25* double knockout mice and examined the potential *in vivo* link between Tpl2 and IL-25. Expectedly, IL-25 deletion under WT or *Tpl2*-KO background both dramatically increased the mortality rate of FH mice, and suppressed the expression of MDSC-recruiting chemokine genes *Cxcl1* and *Cxcl2* in *P. acnes*-primed livers (**Figures 7B,C**), implying IL-25 is also critical for the liver recruitment of MDSC and thus protect against *P. acnes*/LPS-induced FH. Interestingly, *Tpl2*/*Il25* double knockout mice didn't further exaggerated the disease severity of *P. acnes*/LPS-induced FH when compared with *Tpl2*-deficient mice, as reflected by comparable mortality rate of these two strains of FH mice (**Figure 7B**), suggesting Tpl2-mediated prevention of FH is indeed through IL-25 signaling.

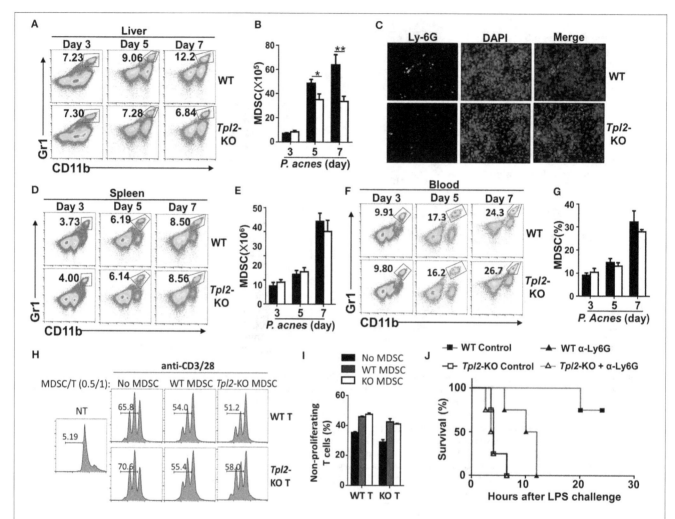

FIGURE 5 | Tpl2 mediated the liver recruitment of MDSC during FH pathogenesis. **(A,B,D–G)** Flow cytometric analysis of Gr-1⁺CD11b⁺ MDSC in the livers **(A,B)** or spleens **(D,E)** or peripheral blood **(F,G)** of WT and *Tpl2*-KO mice at day 3, 5, and 7 after *P. acnes* priming (n = 4 mice/group). Data are presented as representative plots **(A,D,F)** and summary bar graph **(B,E,G)** showing the absolute numbers or frequencies of MDSC. **(C)** Immunofluorescence images showing the infiltrated MDSC by using the anti-Ly6G antibody in the liver sections obtained from WT and *Tpl2*-KO mice at day 7 after *P. acnes* priming (magnification, ×200). **(H,I)** Flow cytometry analysis of the proliferation of WT CD4⁺ T cells that labeled with CFSE, and then cocultured with WT or *Tpl2*-KO MDSC at the indicated ratio in the absence (NT) or presence of anti-CD3/28 antibodies for 72 h. Data are presented representative histograms **(H)** and bar graph **(I)**. **(J)** Cumulative survival rates of WT and *Tpl2*-KO mice that injected with anti-Ly6G antibody (200 μg/mouse, three times) to deplete in vivo MDSC or control antibody, and then subjected to *P. acnes*/LPS-mediated FH induction (n = 4 mice/group). Results are mean ± SD from three independent experiments. Two-tailed Student's t-tests were performed. *P < 0.05; **P < 0.01.

Next, we examined the cellular source of CXCL1 and CXCL2 in the *P. acnes*-primed livers. The results revealed that *Tpl2* deficiency didn't affect the expression of *Cxcl1* and *Cxcl2* in *P. acnes*-primed liver CD11b⁺F4/80⁺GR-1⁻ kuffer cells and macrophages (**Supplementary Figure 1E**). However, loss of Tpl2 or IL-25 both significantly suppressed these two genes' expression in the hepatocytes that isolated from *P. acnes*-primed livers (**Figure 7D**). In addition, the RNA sequencing analysis showed that the expression of *Cxcl1*, *Cxcl2*, and other IL-25-response genes are dramatically decreased in IL-25-stimulated *Tpl2*-deficient primary mouse hepatocytes as compared with that of WT cells (**Supplementary Figures 2A–D**, **Figure 7E**). Moreover, the quantitative PCR resulted also confirmed that Tpl2 is indispensable for the constitutively and IL-25-induced expression of *Cxcl1* and *Cxcl2* in primary mouse hepatocytes

(**Figure 7F**). Collectively, these results suggested that Tpl2 mediated IL-25 signaling in hepatocyte to protect against FH.

DISCUSSION

FH is a life-threatening disease and liver transplantation is the only definitive treatment for the acute liver injury. However, the obvious side-effects of transplantation, such as donor shortage, immune rejection, detrimental effect of immunosuppressive drugs, etc., suggested an urgent to develop novel therapeutic strategies (1, 9, 28). Recently, accumulating evidences suggested that MDSC is critical to maintain the immunosuppressive niche in inflamed liver during the pathogenesis of various kinds of human hepatitis and related mouse models, and

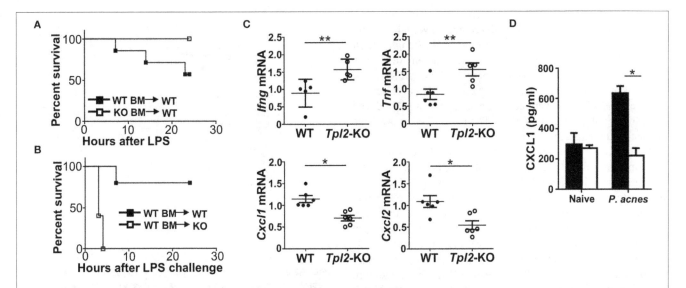

FIGURE 6 | Tpl2 functioned in liver-resident cells to protect against FH. **(A,B)** Cumulative survival rates of the lethally irradiated bone marrow (BM) chimeric WT mice that reconstituted with WT or *Tpl2*-KO BM **(A)** or the BM chimeric WT or *Tpl2*-KO mice that reconstituted with WT BM **(B)**, and then subjected to *P. acnes*/LPS-mediated FH induction (*n* = 7 or 5 mice/group). **(C)** QPCR analysis to determine the relative mRNA expression level of proinflammatory genes in livers of WT and *Tpl2*-KO mice at day 3 after *P. acnes* priming (*n* = 6 mice/group). Data were normalized to a reference gene, *Actb*. **(D)** Enzyme-linked immunosorbent assay of CXCL1 cytokine secretion in the supernatants of liver homogenates from WT and *Tpl2*-KO naïve or *P. acnes*-primed mice at day 3 (*n* = 4). Results are mean ± SD from three independent experiments. Two-tailed Student's *t*-tests were performed. *P < 0.05; **P < 0.01.

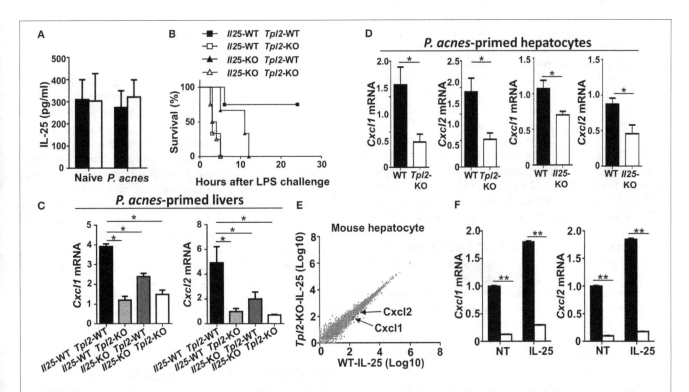

FIGURE 7 | Tpl2 regulated IL-25 signaling in hepatocytes. **(A)** Enzyme-linked immunosorbent assay showing IL-25 cytokine secretion in the supernatants of liver homogenates from WT and *Tpl2*-KO naïve or *P. acnes*-primed mice at day 3 (*n* = 3 or 4). **(B)** Cumulative survival rates of WT, *Tpl2*-KO, *Il25*-KO, *Tpl2/Il25* double knockout mice that subjected to *P. acnes*/LPS-mediated FH induction (*n* = 3 or 4 mice/group). **(C,D)** QPCR analysis of *Cxcl1* and *Cxcl2* genes' expression of livers **(C)** or hepatocytes **(D)** in WT, *Tpl2*-KO, *Il25*-KO, *Tpl2/Il25* double knockout mice at day 3 after *P. acnes* priming (*n* = 6 mice/group). **(E)** Scatter diagram showing the RNA-sequencing analysis of the gene expression pattern in WT and *Tpl2*-KO primary hepatocytes that stimulated by IL-25 for 8 h. The blue dots indicated the IL-25-induced up- or down-regulated genes, and the red dots indicated the down-regulation of *Cxcl1* and *Cxcl2* in *Tpl2*-KO hepatocytes. **(F)** QPCR determining the relative mRNA expression level of *Cxcl1* and *Cxcl2* in WT and *Tpl2*-KO hepatocytes that left untreated (NT) or stimulated with IL-25 for 8 h. Data were normalized to a reference gene, *Actb*. Results are mean ± SD from three independent experiments. Two-tailed Student's *t*-tests were performed. *P < 0.05; **P < 0.01.

increased infiltration of MDSC effectively attenuated the liver inflammation and protected FH-induced acute liver failure (10–15, 27). However, the molecular mechanism through which driving MDSC mobilization into inflamed liver remain elusive. Here we identified the protein kinase Tpl2 as an essential mediator to mobilize MDSC into liver during FH pathogenesis, and thus Tpl2 effectively protected the mice against FH-induced acute liver failure and mortality. Therefore, Tpl2 may have therapeutic potential for the treatment of FH.

Tpl2 is a protein kinase that was initially identified as protooncogene due to the tumor promoting function of its C-terminal truncation (29, 30). The expression of Tpl2 is universal and it is found to expressed in both innate and adaptive immune cells and in diverse tissues, including the liver, lung, and intestines (30–33). The immune-regulatory function of Tpl2 is largely attributed to its activation of the MEK/ERK pathway in toll-like receptor (TLR), interleukin-1 receptor (IL-1R), or tumor necrosis factor receptor (TNFR) signaling (34, 35). In addition, Tpl2 also modulate the activation of p38, JNK, protein kinase B, and mammalian target of rapamycin in a context-dependent manner (25, 36). We previously found that Tpl2 functions in astrocytes to mediate IL-17A-induced chemokine (*Cxcl1/2*) expression through promoting TAK1 phosphorylation and its downstream NF-κB, p38, and JNK activation, whereas ERK activation is not affected (24). Therefore, it is not surprising we found in the present study that Tpl2 functioned in hepatocyte to modulate *Cxcl1/2* expression, which then modulated the recruitment of MDSC into liver during FH pathogenesis. A recent study has suggested that Tpl2 exhibited neutrophil intrinsic function to mediate the trafficking of this type of immune cells (37), so it is also possible that Tpl2 may functioned directly in MDSC to promote its liver mobilization in FH mice. However, the increased mortality was only observed in Tpl2 germline knockout FH mice or *Tpl2*-deficient recipient chimeric FH mice that adoptively transferred with WT BM, but not in the WT recipient chimeric FH mice that adoptively transferred with either WT or *Tpl2*-deficient BM, suggesting the liver MDSC mobilization during FH pathogenesis is not attributed to the direct intrinsic function of Tpl2 in MDSC, but in hepatocytes.

Although IL-25 is one of the IL-17 family protein, there is no functional similarity of IL-25 as compared with the pro-inflammatory IL-17A (16, 17). For example, IL-25 augments type 2 immune responses and promote the airway inflammation of patients with asthma (38). A recent study suggested that IL-25 is highly expressed in both human and mouse liver, and plays a critical function in maintaining the homeostasis and limiting local inflammation through recruiting the immunosuppressive MDSC (15). Nevertheless, the molecular mechanism through which IL-25 recruit MDSC into liver is not clear. Our present study provided a Tpl2 link between IL-25 and MDSC mobilization, and established Tpl2 as a key mediator of IL-25-induced signaling that contribute to the MDSC recruitment. In addition, during *P. acnes*/LPS-induced FH pathogenesis, Tpl2 seemed specifically mediate IL-25-induced expression of CXCL1/2, but not affected the induction of CCL17, a previously reported MDSC-attracting chemokine that could be induced

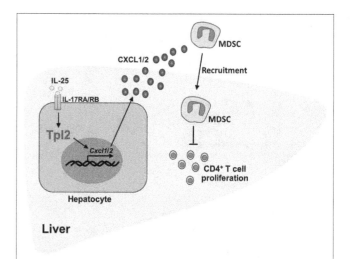

FIGURE 8 | The working model of Tpl2 in protecting against fulminant hepatitis. During the pathogenesis of *P. acnes*/LPS-induced FH, high levels of IL-25 in the liver microenvironment activated the signaling pathway mediated by IL-17RA/IL-17RB heterodimer receptor in hepatocytes, which were induced the expression of *Cxcl1/2* on a Tpl2-dependent manner. Increased CXCL1/2 production promoted the liver recruitment of the immunosuppressive MDSC, which further impaired the proliferation of liver-infiltrated pathogenic CD4⁺ T cells, and finally suppressed the inflammation-induced acute liver injury.

by IL-25 administration in D-Gal/LPS-induced FH mice (15), suggesting Tpl2 modulated IL-25-induced chemokine expression in a context-dependent manner.

Our previously study has suggested that Tpl2 critically regulate IL-17A-induced signaling in astrocytes to mediate autoimmune inflammation, here we also demonstrated that Tpl2 is a key modulator in IL-25-induced signaling in hepatocyte to restrain hepatitis. This functional controversy may be due to Tpl2 regulates the function of different cells upon different stimulus, and suggest Tpl2 have a dual role in promoting or restraining inflammatory processes in a context-dependent manner.

In conclusion, our findings demonstrated that Tpl2 effectively attenuated the severity of acute liver injury and increased the survival rate of FH mice. Mechanistically, Tpl2 functioned in hepatocytes to mediate IL-25-induced CXCL1/2 chemokines, which promoted the recruitment of MDSC to suppress Th1-mediated local inflammation, resulting in the amelioration of FH (**Figure 8**). Our data not only highlighted a novel function of Tpl2 in mediating IL-25 signaling, but also raised the possibility to develop Tpl2-based therapeutic strategies against this dreaded disease.

MATERIALS AND METHODS

Mice

Tpl2-deficient mice (C57BL/6 background) were described as previously (24). The *Tpl2*⁺/⁻ mice were bred to generate age-matched *Tpl2*⁻/⁻ (*Tpl2*-KO) and *Tpl2*⁺/⁺ (WT) mice. The *Il25*-defcient mice (C57BL/6 background) were provided by Dr. Y. Qian (Shanghai Institutes for Biological Sciences, Chinese Academy of Sciences). In some experiments, *Tpl2*⁻/⁻ mice were crossed with $Il25^{-/-}$ mice to generate $Tpl2^{+/-}Il25^{+/-}$ mouse, which were then bred to generate age-matched $Tpl2^{+/+}Il25^{+/+}$, $Tpl2^{-/-}Il25^{+/+}$, $Tpl2^{+/+}Il25^{-/-}$, and $Tpl2^{-/-}Il25^{-/-}$ mice. $Rag1^{-/-}$ mice (NM-KO-00069) were purchased from Shanghai Model Organisms Center. Mice were maintained in a specific pathogen-free facility, and all animal experiments were in accordance with protocols approved by the institutional Biomedical Research Ethics Committee, Shanghai Institutes for Biological Sciences, Chinese Academy of Sciences.

Induction of FH Mouse Model

For the induction of FH model, the age- and sex-matched mice were intravenously injected with 0.5 mg of heat-killed *P. acnes* suspended in 200 μl of phosphate-buffered saline (PBS) and after 7 days mice were injected intravenously with 1 μg of LPS and were monitored the survival rate. In some experiments, the WT and *Tpl2*-deficient mice were intravenously injected with 200 μg anti-Ly6G antibody for 3 times to deplete MDSC *in vivo*, or the *Rag1*-KO mice were adoptively transferred with WT or *Tpl2*-deficient CD4$^+$ T cells, or the lethally irradiated mice that were reconstituted with WT or *Tpl2*-deficient bone marrows, and then these mice were injected with *P. acnes*/LPS to induce FH and were monitored the survival rate.

Antibodies and Reagents

APC conjugated anti-mouse CD4 (17-0041-83), PB conjugated anti-mouse CD4 (48-0042-82), PE-cy7 conjugated anti-mouse CD8 (25-0081-82), APC-cy7 conjugated anti-mouse CD11b (47-0112-82), PB conjugated anti-mouse CD11c (48-0114-82), PerCP conjugated anti-mouse Ly6G (46-9668-82), FITC conjugated anti-mouse B220 (11-0452-85), PE conjugated anti-mouse CD45 (12-0451-83), APC conjugated anti-mouse IFNγ (17-7311-82), PE conjugated anti-mouse TNFα (12-7321-82), PE-cy7 conjugated anti-mouse CD25 (25-0251-82), APC conjugated anti-mouse Foxp3 (17-5773-82), PE conjugated anti-mouse CD44 (12-0441-83), FITC conjugated anti-mouse CD62L (11-0621-86), anti-mouse CD3 (16-0031-86), and anti-mouse CD28 (16-0281-86) antibodies were purchased from eBioscience. BrdU Flow Kits (559619) were purchased from BD Biosciences. Anti-mouse Ly6G (BE0075) antibody was purchased from Bioxcell. Alexa Fluor 488-conjugated anti-Rat IgG secondary antibody (A-21210) was from Thermo Fisher. Mouse anti-CD4 (L3T4, 130-049-201) and mouse anti-Ly-6G (130-092-332) Micro Beads were purchased from Miltenyi Biotec. Murine IL-25 (1399) were purchased from R&D. Lipopolysaccharides (LPS, L3129) were purchased from Sigma. *P. acnes* were prepared as previously described (7).

Flow Cytometry

The infiltrated immune cells from WT and *Tpl2*-deficient inflamed livers were prepared through 33% Percoll gradient as previously described (6). The collected liver-infiltrated immune cells or splenic cell suspensions were stained with the indicated antibodies and were subjected to flow cytometry analyses as previously described by using a Beckman Gallios flow cytometer (39). For the intracellular staining of TNF-α, IFN-γ, and Foxp3, the cells were fixed and permeabilized by fixation/permeabilization buffer (Thermo Fisher) before staining these antibodies, and then detected by flow cytometer. The absolute numbers of splenic and liver-infiltrating immune cells subpopulations were calculated based on their frequencies and the total number of isolated splenic and liver immune cells, and the data were presented as the average numbers of immune cell subpopulations per one spleen or liver of one mouse.

Histology and Immunofluorescence Analysis

Liver specimens were fixed in 4% paraformaldehyde and paraffin-embedded. Deparaffinized sections (8 μm) were stained with hematoxylin and eosin. Semiquantitative analysis of the status of liver inflammation was performed in a blinded manner as previously described (40). Briefly, the H&E stained liver slides were scored by a pathologist in a "blinded fashion" to determine the degree of inflammatory condition as follows: 0 = no infiltration, 1 = minimal/slight infiltration, 2 = moderate infiltration, 3 = severe infiltration. For immunofluorescence staining, the frozen sections (10 μm) from liver specimens were incubated with rat anti-mouse Ly6G (BE0075, Bioxcell) and were then labeled with Alexa Fluor 488-conjugated rabbit anti-rat IgG (A21210, Invitrogen), and the nuclei were stained by using DAPI (28718-90-3, Sangon Biotech).

Bone Marrow Chimeras

The bone marrow cells were prepared from WT or *Tpl2*-deficient mice and adoptively transferred into lethally irradiated (^{137}Cs, γ-ray, 950 rad) WT or *Tpl2*-deficient mice (around 7-week-old; 10^7 cells/mouse) as previously described (41). The lethal-dose irradiation would eliminate the bone marrow and peripheral immune cells without affecting the radioresistant liver-resident cells, and the bone marrow chimeric mice would thus have their peripheral immune system reconstituted. After 8 weeks, the chimeric mice were applied for the indicated experiments.

Mouse Hepatocyte Isolation

The mouse primary hepatocytes were prepared as previously described (42). In brief, the livers were sequentially perfused with Earle's balanced salt solutions (EBSS) without Ca$^+$ and Mg$^+$ containing EGTA, EBSS with Ca$^+$ and Mg$^+$ containing Hepes, EBSS with Ca$^+$ and Mg$^+$ containing Hepes and Collagenase IV, and the liver cells were squeezed out to obtain cell suspension in DMEM medium, which were then applied for centrifugation over a mixture of 9 ml Percoll, 1 ml 10 × EBSS and 10 ml DMEM. The precipitated hepatocytes were suspended and cultured with DMEM complete medium in a collagen-coated culture dish. Cell viability was determined by using Trypan blue exclusion assay.

In vivo BrdU Incorporation

Seven days after *P. acnes* priming, 2 mg BrdU (559619, BD) in 200 μl PBS was intraperitoneally injected into WT or *Tpl2*-deficient mice. The mice were sacrificed 2 h after the BrdU administration, and the immune cell suspensions from livers or spleens were prepared for flow cytometric analysis.

T Cell Proliferation Assay

The WT CD4$^+$ T cells were purified by MACS sorting and were labeled with $5\,\mu M$ CFSE. The labeled cells were then seeded in the anti-CD3/CD28 antibodies-pre-coated plates and cocultured with MDSCs that isolated from WT or *Tpl2*-deficient bone marrow at the indicated ratio for 72 h. The cell proliferation was then determined by flow cytometry. In some experiment, WT or *Tpl2*-deficient CD4$^+$ T cells were seeded in anti-CD3/CD28 antibodies-pre-coated plates with 3 replicates and cultured for a total 72 h. The cell proliferation was recorded based on the [^{3}H] thymidine labeling 8 h before examination.

RNA-Seq Analysis

Total RNA isolated from WT and *Tpl2*-KO hepatocytes stimulated with IL-25 were subjected to RNA-sequencing analysis. RNA sequencing was performed by BGI Tech Solutions. Transcriptomic reads from the RNA-Seq experiments were mapped to a reference genome (build mm 10) by using Bowtie. Gene expression levels were quantified by using the RSEM software package. Significant genes were defined by the *p*-value and false discovery rate of cutoff of 0.05 and fold changes ≥ 1.5. Differentially expressed genes were analyzed by the IPA and DAVID bioinformatics platform.

Quantitative RT-PCR

Liver tissues or cell samples were homogenized in Trizol reagent (Invitrogen). The cDNA was synthesized from 500 ng of extracted total RNA using M-MLV Reverse Transcriptase kit (Takara) according to the manufacturer's instructions. Quantitative PCR was performed with SYBR-Green premix ExTaq (Roche) and detected by a Real-time PCR System by using gene-specific primers. Gene expression was assessed in triplicate and normalized to a reference gene, β-actin. The gene-specific PCR primers are listed in **Supplementary Table 1**.

Quantification and Statistical Analysis

Statistical analyses were measured by GraphPad Software. Except where otherwise indicated, all the presented data are representative results of at least three independent repeats. Data are presented as mean $\pm$ SD, and the *P*-values were determined by two-tailed Student's *t*-tests. The *P*-values <0.05 were considered statistically significant.

ETHICS STATEMENT

This study was carried out in accordance with the recommendations of animal protocols that approved by Biomedical Research Ethics Committee, Shanghai Institutes for Biological Sciences, Chinese Academy of Sciences. The protocol was approved by the Biomedical Research Ethics Committee, Shanghai Institutes for Biological Sciences, Chinese Academy of Sciences.

AUTHOR CONTRIBUTIONS

JX designed and performed the experiments, prepared the figures, and wrote part of the manuscript. SP, YW, and JL contributed to part of the experiments. YQ provided the *Il25*-deficient mice. MH and YZ supervised the work and contributed to data analysis. YX designed and supervised the work, prepared the figures, and wrote the manuscript.

FUNDING

We thank Dr. Shao-Cong Sun (Department of Immunology, MD Anderson Cancer Center, The University of Texas) for providing the *Tpl2*-deficient mice. This research was supported by the grants from the National Natural Science Foundation of China (81770567 and 81571545), the National Key R&D Program of China (2018YFA0107201, 2018YFA0902700), the Strategic Priority Research Program of the Chinese Academy of Sciences (XDPB10), the Key Arrangements of the Chinese Academy of Sciences (KFZD-SW-216), the Thousand Young Talents Plan of China, CAS Key Laboratory of Tissue Microenvironment and Tumor.

REFERENCES

Bernal W, Auzinger G, Dhawan A, Wendon J. Acute liver failure. *Lancet.* (2010) 376:190–201. doi: 10.1016/S0140-6736(10)60274-7

Antoniades CG, Berry PA, Wendon JA, Vergani D. The importance of immune dysfunction in determining outcome in acute liver failure. *J Hepatol.* (2008) 49:845–61. doi: 10.1016/j.jhep.2008.08.009

Crispe IN. The liver as a lymphoid organ. *Annu Rev Immunol.* (2009) 27:147–63. doi: 10.1146/annurev.immunol.021908.132629

Rolando N, Harvey F, Brahm J, Philpott-Howard J, Alexander G, Gimson A, et al. Prospective study of bacterial infection in acute liver failure: an analysis of fifty patients. *Hepatology.* (1990) 11:49–53. doi: 10.1002/hep.1840110110

Nakayama Y, Shimizu Y, Hirano K, Ebata K, Minemura M, Watanabe A, et al. CTLA-4Ig suppresses liver injury by inhibiting acquired immune responses in a mouse model of fulminant hepatitis. *Hepatology.* (2005) 42:915–24. doi: 10.1002/hep.20872

Xiao Y, Xu J, Mao C, Jin M, Wu Q, Zou J, et al. 18Beta-glycyrrhetinic acid ameliorates acute Propionibacterium acnes-induced liver injury through inhibition of macrophage inflammatory protein-1alpha. *J Biol Chem.* (2010) 285:1128–37. doi: 10.1074/jbc.M109.037705

Zhang Y, Cai W, Huang Q, Gu Y, Shi Y, Huang J, et al. Mesenchymal stem cells alleviate bacteria-induced liver injury in mice by inducing regulatory dendritic cells. *Hepatology.* (2014) 59:671–82. doi: 10.1002/hep.26670

Zhang Y, Yoneyama H, Wang Y, Ishikawa S, Hashimoto S, Gao JL, et al.

Mobilization of dendritic cell precursors into the circulation by administration of MIP-1alpha in mice. *J Natl Cancer Inst.* (2004) 96:201–9. doi: 10.1093/jnci/djh024

Nemes B, Gelley F, Piros L, Zadori G, Gorog D, Fehervari I, et al. The impact of Milan criteria on liver transplantation for hepatocellular carcinoma: first 15 years' experience of the Hungarian Liver Transplant Program. *Transplant Proc.* (2011) 43:1272–4. doi: 10.1016/j.transproceed.2011.03.077

Cai W, Qin A, Guo P, Yan D, Hu F, Yang Q, et al. Clinical significance and functional studies of myeloid-derived suppressor cells in chronic hepatitis C patients. *J Clin Immunol.* (2013) 33:798–808. doi: 10.1007/s10875-012-9861-2

Hoechst B, Voigtlaender T, Ormandy L, Gamrekelashvili J, Zhao F, Wedemeyer H, et al. Myeloid derived suppressor cells inhibit natural killer cells in patients with hepatocellular carcinoma via the NKp30 receptor. *Hepatology.* (2009) 50:799–807. doi: 10.1002/hep.23054

Cripps JG, Wang J, Maria A, Blumenthal I, Gorham JD. Type 1 T helper cells induce the accumulation of myeloid-derived suppressor cells in the inflamed Tgfb1 knockout mouse liver. *Hepatology.* (2010) 52:1350–9. doi: 10.1002/hep.23841

Jenne CN, Wong CH, Zemp FJ, McDonald B, Rahman MM, Forsyth PA, et al. Neutrophils recruited to sites of infection protect from virus challenge by releasing neutrophil extracellular traps. *Cell Host Microbe.* (2013) 13:169–80. doi: 10.1016/j.chom.2013.01.005

Suh YG, Kim JK, Byun JS, Yi HS, Lee YS, Eun HS, et al. CD11b(+) Gr1(+) bone marrow cells ameliorate liver fibrosis by producing interleukin-10 in mice. *Hepatology.* (2012) 56:1902–12. doi: 10.1002/hep.25817

Sarra M, Cupi ML, Bernardini R, Ronchetti G, Monteleone I, Ranalli M, et al. IL-25 prevents and cures fulminant hepatitis in mice through a myeloid-derived suppressor cell-dependent mechanism. *Hepatology.* (2013) 58:1436–50. doi: 10.1002/hep.26446

Angkasekwinai P, Park H, Wang YH, Wang YH, Chang SH, Corry DB, et al. Interleukin 25 promotes the initiation of proallergic type 2 responses. *J Exp Med.* (2007) 204:1509–17. doi: 10.1084/jem.20061675

Fort MM, Cheung J, Yen D, Li J, Zurawski SM, Lo S, et al. IL-25 induces IL-4, IL-5, and IL-13 and Th2-associated pathologies *in vivo. Immunity.* (2001) 15:985–95. doi: 10.1016/S1074-7613(01)00243-6

Kim MR, Manoukian R, Yeh R, Silbiger SM, Danilenko DM, Scully S, et al. Transgenic overexpression of human IL-17E results in eosinophilia, B-lymphocyte hyperplasia, and altered antibody production. *Blood.* (2002) 100:2330–40. doi: 10.1182/blood-2002-01-0012

Caruso R, Sarra M, Stolfi C, Rizzo A, Fina D, Fantini MC, et al. Interleukin-25 inhibits interleukin-12 production and Th1 cell-driven inflammation in the gut. *Gastroenterology.* (2009) 136:2270–9. doi: 10.1053/j.gastro.2009.02.049

Liu D, Cao T, Wang N, Liu C, Ma N, Tu R, et al. IL-25 attenuates rheumatoid arthritis through suppression of Th17 immune responses in an IL-13-dependent manner. *Sci Rep.* (2016) 6:36002. doi: 10.1038/srep36002

Gu C, Wu L, Li X. IL-17 family: cytokines, receptors and signaling. *Cytokine.* (2013) 64:477–85. doi: 10.1016/j.cyto.2013.07.022

Kang Z, Swaidani S, Yin W, Wang C, Barlow JL, Gulen MF, et al. Epithelial cell-specific Act1 adaptor mediates interleukin-25-dependent helminth expulsion through expansion of Lin(-)c-Kit(+) innate cell population. *Immunity.* (2012) 36:821–33. doi: 10.1016/j.immuni.2012.03.021

Swaidani S, Bulek K, Kang Z, Liu C, Lu Y, Yin W, et al. The critical role of epithelial-derived Act1 in IL-17- and IL-25- mediated pulmonary inflammation. *J Immunol.* (2009) 182:1631–40. doi: 10.4049/jimmunol.182.3.1631

Xiao Y, Jin J, Chang M, Nakaya M, Hu H, Zou Q, et al. TPL2 mediates autoimmune inflammation through activation of the TAK1 axis of IL-17 signaling. *J Exp Med.* (2014) 211:1689–702. doi: 10.1084/jem.20132640

Xiao Y, Sun SC. TPL2 mediates IL-17R signaling in neuroinflammation. *Oncotarget.* (2015) 6:21789–90. doi: 10.18632/oncotarget.4888

Yoneyama H, Harada A, Imai T, Baba M, Yoshie O, Zhang Y, et al. Pivotal role of TARC, a CC chemokine, in bacteria-induced fulminant hepatic failure in mice. *J Clin Invest.* (1998) 102:1933–41. doi: 10.1172/JCI4619

Pallett LJ, Gill US, Quaglia A, Sinclair LV, Jover-Cobos M, Schurich A, et al. Metabolic regulation of hepatitis B immunopathology by myeloid-derived suppressor cells. *Nat Med.* (2015) 21:591–600. doi: 10.1038/nm.3856

Stravitz RT, Kramer DJ. Management of acute liver failure. *Nat Rev Gastroenterol Hepatol.* (2009) 6:542–53. doi: 10.1038/nrgastro.2009.127

Ceci JD, Patriotis CP, Tsatsanis C, Makris AM, Kovatch R, Swing DA, et al. Tpl-2 is an oncogenic kinase that is activated by carboxy-terminal truncation. *Genes Dev.* (1997) 11:688–700. doi: 10.1101/gad.11.6.688

Patriotis C, Makris A, Bear SE, Tsichlis PN. Tumor progression locus 2 (Tpl-2) encodes a protein kinase involved in the progression of rodent T-cell lymphomas and in T-cell activation. *Proc Natl Acad Sci USA.* (1993) 90:2251–5. doi: 10.1073/pnas.90.6.2251

Hedl M, Abraham C. A TPL2 (MAP3K8) disease-risk polymorphism increases TPL2 expression thereby leading to increased pattern recognition receptor- initiated caspase-1 and caspase-8 activation, signalling and cytokine secretion. *Gut.* (2016) 65:1799–811. doi: 10.1136/gutjnl-2014-308922

Chowdhury FZ, Estrada LD, Murray S, Forman J, Farrar JD. Pharmacological inhibition of TPL2/MAP3K8 blocks human cytotoxic T lymphocyte effector functions. *PLoS ONE.* (2014) 9:e92187. doi: 10.1371/journal.pone.0092187

Watford WT, Wang CC, Tsatsanis C, Mielke LA, Eliopoulos AG, Daskalakis C, et al. Ablation of tumor progression locus 2 promotes a type 2 Th cell response in Ovalbumin-immunized mice. *J Immunol.* (2010) 184:105–13. doi:10.4049/jimmunol.0803730

Vougioukalaki M, Kanellis DC, Gkouskou K, Eliopoulos AG. Tpl2 kinase signal transduction in inflammation and cancer. *Cancer Lett.* (2011) 304:80–9. doi: 10.1016/j.canlet.2011.02.004

Perugorria MJ, Murphy LB, Fullard N, Chakraborty JB, Vyrla D, Wilson CL, et al. Tumor progression locus 2/Cot is required for activation of extracellular regulated kinase in liver injury and toll-like receptor-induced TIMP-1 gene transcription in hepatic stellate cells in mice. *Hepatology.* (2013) 57:1238–49. doi: 10.1002/hep.26100

Li X, Acuff NV, Peeks AR, Kirkland R, Wyatt KD, Nagy T, et al. Tumor Progression Locus 2 (Tpl2) activates the Mammalian Target of Rapamycin (mTOR) pathway, inhibits Forkhead Box P3 (FoxP3) expression, and limits Regulatory T Cell (Treg) immunosuppressive functions. *J Biol Chem.* (2016) 291:16802–15. doi: 10.1074/jbc.M116.718783

Acuff NV, Li X, Elmore J, Rada B, Watford WT. Tpl2 promotes neutrophil trafficking, oxidative burst, and bacterial killing. *J Leukoc Biol.* (2017) 101:1325–33. doi: 10.1189/jlb.3A0316-146R

Wang YH, Angkasekwinai P, Lu N, Voo KS, Arima K, Hanabuchi S, et al. IL-25 augments type 2 immune responses by enhancing the expansion and functions of TSLP-DC-activated Th2 memory cells. *J Exp Med.* (2007) 204:1837–47. doi: 10.1084/jem.20070406

Liu J, Huang X, Hao S, Wang Y, Liu M, Xu J, et al. Peli1 negatively regulates noncanonical NF-kappaB signaling to restrain systemic lupus erythematosus. *Nat Commun.* (2018) 9:1136. doi: 10.1038/s41467-018-03530-3

Xiao Y, Xu J, Wang S, Mao C, Jin M, Ning G, et al. Genetic ablation of steroid receptor coactivator-3 promotes PPAR-beta-mediated alternative activation of microglia in experimental autoimmune encephalomyelitis. *Glia.* (2010) 58:932–42. doi: 10.1002/glia.20975

Zhang X, Wang Y, Yuan J, Li N, Pei S, Xu J, et al. Macrophage/microglial Ezh2 facilitates autoimmune inflammation through inhibition of Socs3. *J Exp Med.* (2018) 215:1365–82. doi: 10.1084/jem.20171417

Li D, Cen J, Chen X, Conway EM, Ji Y, Hui L. Hepatic loss of survivin impairs postnatal liver development and promotes expansion of hepatic progenitor cells in mice. *Hepatology.* (2013) 58:2109–21. doi: 10.1002/hep.26601

7

Intestinal Epithelial Cell-Derived Extracellular Vesicles Modulate Hepatic Injury via the Gut-Liver Axis During Acute Alcohol Injury

Arantza Lamas-Paz [1,2†], Laura Morán [1,3†], Jin Peng [4†], Beatriz Salinas [3,5,6,7], Nuria López-Alcántara [1], Svenja Sydor [8], Ramiro Vilchez-Vargas [9], Iris Asensio [3,10], Fengjie Hao [1,2,11], Kang Zheng [1,2,12], Beatriz Martín-Adrados [1,2], Laura Moreno [8,13], Angel Cogolludo [8,13], Manuel Gómez del Moral [2,14], Lars Bechmann [8], Eduardo Martínez-Naves [1,2], Javier Vaquero [3,10], Rafael Bañares [3,10], Yulia A. Nevzorova [1,2,15‡] and Francisco Javier Cubero [1,2*‡]

[1]Department of Immunology, Ophthalmology and ENT, Complutense University School of Medicine, Madrid, Spain, [2]12 de Octubre Health Research Institute (imas12), Madrid, Spain, [3]Servicio de Aparato Digestivo del Hospital General Universitario Gregorio Marañón, Instituto de Investigación Sanitaria Gregorio Marañón (IiSGM), Madrid, Spain, [4]Department of Hepatobiliary Surgery, Nanjing Drum Tower Hospital, The Affiliated Hospital of Nanjing University Medical School, Nanjing, China, [5]Centro Nacional de Investigaciones Cardiovasculares Carlos III, Madrid, Spain, [6]Bioengineering and Aerospace Engineering Department, Universidad Carlos III de Madrid, Madrid, Spain, [7]Centro de Investigación Biomédico en Red de Salud Mental (CIBERSAM), Madrid, Spain, [8]Department of Internal Medicine, University Hospital Knappschaftskrankenhaus, Ruhr-University Bochum, Bochum, Germany, [9]Department of Gastroenterology, Hepatology, and Infectious Diseases, Otto von Guericke University Hospital Magdeburg, Magdeburg, Germany, [10]Centre for Biomedical Research, Network on Liver and Digestive Diseases (CIBEREHD), Madrid, Spain, [11]Department of General Surgery, Hepatobiliary Surgery, Ruijin Hospital, Shanghai Jiao Tong University School of Medicine, Shanghai, China, [12]Department of Anesthesiology, Zhongda Hospital, School of Medicine, Southeast University, Nanjing, China, [13]Department of Pharmacology and Toxicology, Complutense University School of Medicine and Centre for Biomedical Research, Network on Respiratory Diseases (CIBERES), Madrid, Spain, [14]Department of Cell Biology, Complutense University School of Medicine, Madrid, Spain, [15]Department of Internal Medicine III, University Hospital RWTH Aachen, Aachen, Germany

*Correspondence:
Francisco Javier Cubero
fcubero@ucm.es

†These authors have contributed equally to this work and share first authorship
‡These authors have contributed equally to this work and share senior authorship

Binge drinking, i.e., heavy episodic drinking in a short time, has recently become an alarming societal problem with negative health impact. However, the harmful effects of acute alcohol injury in the gut-liver axis remain elusive. Hence, we focused on the physiological and pathological changes and the underlying mechanisms of experimental binge drinking in the context of the gut-liver axis. Eight-week-old mice with a C57BL/6 background received a single dose (p.o.) of ethanol (EtOH) [6 g/kg b.w.] as a preclinical model of acute alcohol injury. Controls received a single dose of PBS. Mice were sacrificed 8 h later. In parallel, HepaRGs and Caco-2 cells, human cell lines of differentiated hepatocytes and intestinal epithelial cells intestinal epithelial cells (IECs), respectively, were challenged in the presence or absence of EtOH [0–100 mM]. Extracellular vesicles (EVs) isolated by ultracentrifugation from culture media of IECs were added to hepatocyte cell cultures. Increased intestinal permeability, loss of

Abbreviations: ADH, alcohol dehydrogenase; ALDH, aldehyde dehydrogenase; BAC, blood alcohol concentration; DLS, dynamic light scattering; EtOH, ethanol; EVs, extracellular vesicles; H&E, hematoxylin and eosin; IF, immunofluorescence; IECs, intestinal epithelial cells; IL-1β, interleukin-1β; KCs, Kupffer cells; LPS, lipopolysaccharides; LW/BW, liver weight vs. body weight; NTA, nanoparticle tracking analysis; ORO, oil red O; qRT-PCR, quantitative real-time PCR; Srebp-1, sterol regulatory binding protein-1; Tnf-α, tumor necrosis factor-alpha; TJs, tight junctions; Tlr-4, toll-like receptor-4; ZO-1, zone occludens-1.

zonula occludens-1 (ZO-1) and MUCIN-2 expression, and alterations in microbiota—increased *Lactobacillus* and decreased Lachnospiraceae species—were found in the large intestine of mice exposed to EtOH. Increased TUNEL-positive cells, infiltration of CD11b-positive immune cells, pro-inflammatory cytokines (e.g., *tlr4*, *tnf*, *il1β*), and markers of lipid accumulation (Oil Red O, *srbep1*) were evident in livers of mice exposed to EtOH, particularly in females. *In vitro* experiments indicated that EVs released by IECs in response to ethanol exerted a deleterious effect on hepatocyte viability and lipid accumulation. Overall, our data identified a novel mechanism responsible for driving hepatic injury in the gut-liver axis, opening novel avenues for therapy.

Keywords: hepatocytes, intestinal epithelial cells, extracellular vesicles, alcohol (EtOH), gut-liver axis

INTRODUCTION

Alcohol abuse is a leading cause of liver-related morbidity and mortality, which has become a global problem due to the financial burden on society and the healthcare system (Dolganiuc and Szabo, 2009; Gao and Bataller, 2011). While the adverse effects of long-term chronic alcohol abuse have been widely studied, the underlying mechanisms of short-term binge and sporadic drinking, also termed acute alcohol-derived tissue injury, remain elusive.

Binge drinking refers to an excessive consumption of large amounts of alcohol in a very short period of time, in which increases the blood alcohol concentration (BAC) levels to at least 0.08 g/dl (Ventura-Cots et al., 2017). The National Institute on Alcohol Abuse and Alcoholism defines binge drinking as a consume of four (women) or five (men) standard drinks per day within 2 h at least once during Binge drinking refers to excessive consumption of large amounts of alcohol in a short period of time, in which the (BAC) levels increase to at least 0.08 g/dl (Ventura-Cots et al., 2017). The National Institute on Alcohol Abuse and Alcoholism defines binge drinking as the consumption of four (women) or five (men) standard drinks per day within 2 h at least once during the past 30 days (Ventura-Cots et al., 2017). However, the standard drink varies significantly from country to country from 7.9 g of alcohol in the United Kingdom to 14 g in the United States or 19.75 g in Japan (Dolganiuc and Szabo, 2009).

Noticeably, the rate of alcohol absorption depends on several factors, including the amount and concentration of alcohol ingested and physiological factors determined by gender (Cederbaum, 2012; Kim et al., 2015; Griswold et al., 2018). Furthermore, sex differences such as body fat, body water, levels of alcohol dehydrogenase (ADH), and hormones affect the hepatic metabolism of alcohol (Gill, 2000; Naugler et al., 2007; Griswold et al., 2018; Lamas-Paz et al., 2018).

Upon acute alcohol injury, alterations of the intestinal epithelial barrier occur at multiple levels including tight junctions (TJs), between gut epithelial cells, production of mucin, recruitment and activation of inflammatory cells to the intestinal wall. In addition, the composition of the gut microbiome changes as a result of alcohol consumption. These result in increased translocation of microbial product from the gut to the liver via the portal circulation. Besides increased levels of lipopolysaccharides, other microbial components may also reach the liver where in the liver sinusoids Kupffer cells and other

recruited immune cells become activated and produce large amounts of pro-inflammatory cytokines (e.g., TNF, IL-1β), which further increase gut permeability, thus fueling inflammation in the gut and favoring the development of liver disease (Szabo, 2015; Gao et al., 2019).

Emerging evidence showed that EVs are important contributors to the coordinated signaling events between the gut and the liver (Bui et al., 2018), a bidirectional axis linking the biliary tract, the portal vein, and the systemic circulation (Tripathi et al., 2018).

In the present study, we aimed to evaluate the underlying mechanisms driving acute alcohol injury *in vitro* and in female and male mice in the context of the gut-liver axis.

MATERIALS AND METHODS

Cell Culture and Cell Viability

HepaRG cells (BioPredict International, Rennes, France) were seeded following the supplier's protocol, and Caco-2 cells, a human intestinal cell line widely used as a model of the intestinal barrier, were cultured in Dulbecco's modified Eagle's medium (Gibco, Rockville, MD) containing 20% heat-inactivated FBS, 1% penicillin/streptomycin, and 2 mM L-glutamine (ICN Pharmaceuticals, Costa Mesa, CA). Once HepaRGs or Caco-2 cells reached approximately 85% confluence, starving was performed for 4 h, and cells were challenged with EtOH [0–100 mM] (Panreac AppliChem, Darmstadt, Germany) for another 24 h. Cells were kept at 37°C in an atmosphere with 5% CO_2. Pictures of cells were taken in an optical microscope (DMIL LED, Leica, Wetzlar, Germany) connected to a camera (Leica MC170HD, Leica). Cell viability was determined by CCK8 (Merck, Munich, Germany) following the manufacturer's instructions. After fixing the cells with 4% PFA, cell death and lipid accumulation were tested by TUNEL (Roche, Rotkreuz, Switzerland) and oil red O (ORO) (Merck), respectively, as previously described (Cubero et al., 2015; Liao et al., 2019).

Animal Model of Acute Alcohol Injury

Healthy C57BL/6J mice purchased from ENVIGO (Valencia, Spain) were bred and maintained in the Animal Facility of the Faculty of Biology at UCM, Madrid, in a temperature-controlled room with 12 h light/dark cycles and allowed food and water *ad libitum*. For our study, we used female and male 8 week-old mice.

Animal studies were approved by the local authority (Consejería de Medio Ambiente, Administración Local y Ordenación del Territorio; PROEX-154/16).

Acute alcohol injury was performed by oral gavage. Briefly, mice ($n = 8$–10/group) were fasted overnight for 12 h. In the morning, they were fed with a dose of 30% EtOH (gavage of 6 g/kg b.w.) (Pruett et al., 2020) using a gavage needle (Kent Scientific, Torrington, CT). Mice fed with PBS instead of EtOH served as controls. All animals were sacrificed at 8 h after the EtOH challenge using an overdose of isoflurane (Solvet, Segovia, Spain) inhalation.

Intestinal Permeability *In Vivo*

Isothiocyanate conjugated dextran (FITC-dextran, molecular mass 4.0 kDa) (TdBCons, Uppsala, Sweden) was dissolved in PBS at a concentration of 200 mg/ml and administrated to 12 h fasted mice (10 ml/kg body weight) using a gavage needle (Kent Scientific). After 4 h, mice were sacrificed by an overdose of isoflurane (Solvet) inhalation. Concentration of FITC was determined in serum by fluorometry with an excitation of 485 nm and an emission wavelength of 528 nm using serially diluted FITC-dextran (0, 125, 250, 500, 1,000, 2,000, 4,000, 6,000, 8,000, 10,000 ng/ml) as standards.

Histological and Morphological Analyses

Livers from mice were harvested, fixed with 4% PFA, and embedded in paraffin for histological evaluation using hematoxylin and eosin (H&E), performed by Dr Juana Flores, an experienced pathologist (School of Veterinary, UCM). Photomicrographs of stained sections were randomly taken in a ×20 magnification in an optical microscope (Nikon Eclipse Ci, Tokyo, Japan), and ORO-positive areas were quantified using free NIH Image/J software (National Institutes of Health, Bethesda, MD).

Immunofluorescence Staining

Liver and colon from each mouse were preserved in cassettes in Tissue-Tek (Sakura Finetek U.S.A, Torrance, CA) at −80 C. Immunostainings for ZO-1 (Invitrogen, Paisley, FL), MUCIN-2 (Santa Cruz, Dallas, TX), TUNEL (Roche), and CD11b (BD, Madrid, Spain) were performed as previously described (Liao et al., 2019). Anti-mouse and anti-rabbit Alexa Fluor 488 (Invitrogen) were used as secondary antibodies.

Quantitative Real-Time Polymerase Chain Reaction

Total RNA was purified from liver tissue using Trizol reagent (Invitrogen). Total RNA [1 μg] was used to synthesize cDNA using Super Script first Stand Synthesis System (Invitrogen) and was resuspended in 100 μl of RNAse-free water (Merck). Quantitative real-time PCR was performed using SYBR Green Reagent (Invitrogen) by the Genomics and Proteomics Facility (School of Biology, UCM). The mRNA expression of *il1β*, *Srebp1*, *Tlr4*, *Tnf*, and *Gapdh* expression was studied (**Supplementary Table S1**). Relative gene expression was normalized to the expression of *Gapdh*. Primer sequences are provided upon request.

Microbiota Analysis

DNA was extracted from foecal content as previously described (Sydor et al., 2020). All samples were resampled to the minimum sequencing depth of 17719 reads using phyloseq package (Mcmurdie and Holmes, 2013) and returning 2,167 phylotypes (**Supplementary Figure S2**).

Biochemical Measurements

Serum transaminases in blood and cell's supernatant were analyzed in the Central Laboratory Facility at the Gregorio Marañón Research Health Institute at Madrid (iISGM) using automated analyzers. For the evaluation of intrahepatic triglycerides, liver samples were homogenized in a specific Tris buffer (10 mM Tris, 2 mM EDTA, 0.25 M sucrose, and pH 7.5) and successively processed using a commercial colorimetric kit (Human Diagnostics, Wiesbaden), according to the manufacturer's instructions.

Isolation of Extracellular Vesicles

For *in vivo* experiments, blood from the cava vein was collected in 1.1 ml serum gel polypropylene microtubes (Sarstedt, Barcelona). Serum was obtained by centrifugation at 12,000 g for 10 min at 4°C. Serum was then centrifuged using a Microliter Centrifuge Z233 MK-2 (Hermle, Wehingen, Germany) at 10,000 g during 30 min. Then, the supernatant was ultracentrifuged twice at 100,000 g using a Hitachi micro ultracentrifuge CS150FNX (Hitachi, Tokyo, Japan) with an S5AA2 rotor in 1.5 ml Eppendorf tubes (Fisher Scientific, Madrid, Spain) during 75 min each. Finally, the pellet containing EVs was resuspended in 50 μl of PBS. Samples were measured by dynamic light scattering (Malvern Instruments, United Kingdom). Next, recollected samples were filtered through 0.44 μm filters, and the obtained sample was diluted 1:10 for nanoparticle tracking analysis (NTA).

For *in vitro* tests, supernatants were collected from cultures of Caco-2 and HepaRG cells treated with EtOH [0–100 mM]. EVs were isolated from supernatants using ultracentrifugation. Briefly, the culture supernatant was centrifuged at 2,000 g and 10,000 g for 20 and 30 min, respectively, to remove cellular debris and larger vesicles. The resultant supernatant was ultracentrifuged twice at 100,000 g for 75 min. The pellet was resuspended in 50 μl of PBS and stored at −80°C. Free EVs medium was prepared by ultracentrifugation of 10% FBS for 16 h on a Hitachi micro ultracentrifuge CS150FNX (Hitachi, Japan).

Experiments With Extracellular Vesicles

HepaRG cells were cultured with EVs isolated from the supernatant of Caco-2 cells previously treated with EtOH [0–100 mM] and diluted into EVs-free medium. Controls were challenged with EVs-free medium. Twenty-four hours later, cells were washed and fixed with 4% PFA. Cell viability, cell death, and lipid deposition were then evaluated.

Nanoparticle Tracking Analysis

The number and size of EVs were quantified and characterized using NTA with the Nanosight NS300 instrument equipped with a 405 nm green laser and an sCMOS high sensitivity camera with NTA (Malvern Instruments). Particles were recorded in five different 60-s videos. The data were analyzed using NTA software SOPs v3.4, following the manufacturer's instructions.

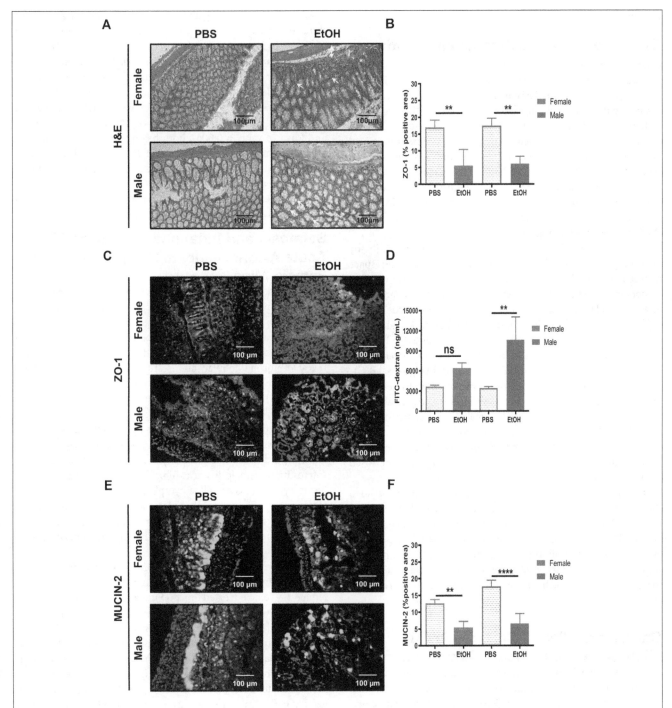

FIGURE 1 | Acute alcohol injury disrupts the gut intestinal barrier in female and male mice. **(A)** Representative H&E staining was performed in paraffin colon sections of female and male mice treated with EtOH [6 g/kg] or PBS (n = 5–7/group). **(B)** Quantification of the ZO-1 positive area was performed and graphed (n = 4/group). **(C)** ZO-1 immunofluorescence staining was performed in colons of male and female mice. **(D)** FITC-dextran levels in serum from female and male mice was quantified as a measure of intestinal permeability (n = 3–4/group). **(E)** MUCIN-2 immunofluorescence staining was performed in colons of female and male mice. **(F)** Quantification of the MUCIN-2 positive area was done and graphed (n = 4–5/group; **p < 0.01, ****p < 0.0001). In female mice, arrows mark mixed inflammation; double arrow, oedema in submucosa and a star, degeneration of crypt basal cells. In male mice, arrows mark mild hypertrophy in Goblet cells.

Statistical Analysis

All statistical analyses consisted of One-Way ANOVA followed by Tukey post-hoc test using GraphPad Prism version 8.0 software (San Diego, CA). A $p < 0.05$ was considered statistically significant. Data were expressed as mean ± SD of the mean (SEM).

RESULT

Experimental Acute Alcohol Injury Induces Gut Dysbiosis

The gut mucosa is particularly susceptible to alcohol-induced tissue injury (Molina and Nelson, 2018). Thus, we first focused on evaluating the impact of binge alcohol drinking via the circulatory system in the large intestine. Histopathological evaluation of experimental acute alcohol injury revealed mixed inflammation in the colon, oedema in the submucosa, and cellular degeneration of crypt basal cells in colons of female mice exposed to acute alcohol injury (**Figure 1A**). In contrast, male-EtOH treated colon displayed mild hypertrophy in Goblet cells (**Figure 1A**). No relevant findings were observed in mice challenged with PBS (**Figure 1A**).

Since acute alcohol exposure induces gut permeability by disrupting not only the epithelial cells, but also the space between them that is controlled by (TJs) (Fanning and Anderson, 2009), we next evaluated whether changes in intestinal TJs that result in leaky gut occurred during experimental acute alcohol injury in female and male mice. Interestingly, the expression of zonula occludens-1 (ZO-1) was significantly decreased in colons of female and, to a bigger extent, of male mice, compared with PBS-fed animals (**Figures 1B,C**).

Next, we used the FITC-dextran gavage method to determine the impact of acute alcohol injury on intestinal permeability *in vivo*. Compared with PBS-treated animals, intestinal permeability tended to increase in female mice and was significantly increased in male mice exposed to EtOH (**Figure 1D**). Altogether, these results indicated that experimental acute alcohol injury increased intestinal permeability in mice.

The intestinal mucous layer prevents direct contact between the intestinal epithelium and bacteria by avoiding its way through. The major component of the intestinal mucous layer is MUCIN-2, which is secreted by Goblet cells (Van Der Sluis et al., 2006). Immunofluorescent staining of MUCIN-2 revealed thinner layers in the large intestine of EtOH-treated female and, to a bigger extent, male mice, compared with PBS-treated animals (**Figures 1E,F**).

Characterization of Changes in Gut Microbiota During Acute Alcohol Injury

Overwhelming evidence has shown that changes in the intestinal microbiome might contribute to alcohol-associated intestinal inflammation and permeability (Sarin et al., 2019). Therefore, foecal microbiota from all experimental groups was analyzed (**Supplementary Figures S1A,B**). No difference in gut microbiota composition was found between female or male mice treated with either PBS or EtOH (p value = 0.049). Principal coordinates analysis (**Supplementary Figure S1A**) revealed that six phylotypes, four of them belonging to the phylum Firmicutes, trended to increase under acute ethanol consumption. On the contrary, 12 phylotypes, seven belonging also to Firmicutes, trended to diminished in EtOH-treated mice. Especially Phy1 and Phy5 (both belonging to the family

Erysipelotrichaceae) together with Phy2 (*Lactobacillus* sp.) were observed in more abundance in EtOH-treated mice, while Phy3 (*Turicibacter* sp.), Phy7 (*Bifidobacterium pseudolongum*), and Phy9 (*Lactobacillus johnsonii* or *acidophilus*) were observed in less abundances in EtOH-treated mice (**Supplementary Figure S1B**). Mann-Whitney test detected statistically significant differences between EtOH-treated and PBS-treated mice in three phylotypes. Phy2 (p value = 0.006) and Phy5 (p value = 0.006), both belonging to *Lactobacillus* sp., increased the relative abundance in EtOH-treated mice, while Phy63 (p value = 0.03), belonging to Lachnospiraceae, diminished in EtOH-treated mice.

Altogether, these results suggest that experimental acute alcohol-derived tissue injury triggers gut dysbiosis.

Steatosis and Inflammation Induced by Acute Alcohol Injury Is More Pronounced in Female Mice

The disruption of the intestinal barrier during alcohol exposure is related to liver injury (Sambrotta et al., 2014; Roychowdhury et al., 2019). Since experimental binge EtOH exposure impaired intestinal barrier integrity, we subsequently investigated the effects of acute alcohol injury on the liver. Light microscopy revealed normal lobular architecture with sinusoidal hepatic cords and typical liver architecture in PBS-treated mice (**Figure 2A**). In contrast, the structure of the hepatic lobules was disordered in mice with acute alcohol injury, with noticeable swelling around the central vein. The cytoplasm was translucent, exhibiting ballooning degeneration, some extent of hepatocellular necrosis, and visible inflammatory cell infiltration (CD11b[+] cells). Interestingly, female livers exhibited extensive degeneration of hepatocytes (eosinophil cytoplasm) and nuclear lysis (**Figure 2A**). In line with these data, the LW/BW ratio of EtOH-treated female mice was significantly higher compared with PBS-treated mice (**Figure 2B; Supplementary Figure S2A,B**).

Next, serum markers of liver damage were evaluated. ALT levels were increased in male EtOH-treated mice compared with female or vehicle-treated mice (**Figure 2C**). ALP–a marker of cholestasis–was elevated in male mice after acute alcohol injury, while a tendency toward increased ALP was observed in female mice compared with PBS-treated animals (**Figure 2D**). Alcohol triggers hepatocyte cell death; thus, we investigated cell death in the liver using TUNEL. The percentage of TUNEL-positive cells increased after acute alcohol injury in female livers and, to a lesser extent, in male mice. In contrast, no relevant cell death was found in PBS-treated mice (**Figures 2E,F**).

Ethanol is metabolized in the liver by hepatocytes, being a primary inducer of liver injury and hepatic steatosis (Diehl et al., 1988; Ji et al., 2006; Kwon et al., 2014; Steiner and Lang, 2017). The staining of neutral lipids with ORO staining indicated an increase of lipid accumulation in livers of female and, to a lesser extent, of male mice, challenged with experimental acute alcohol injury (**Figures 3A,B**). Moreover, quantification of hepatic triglycerides showed an increase in both female and male animals, and activation of srebp-1, associated with increased

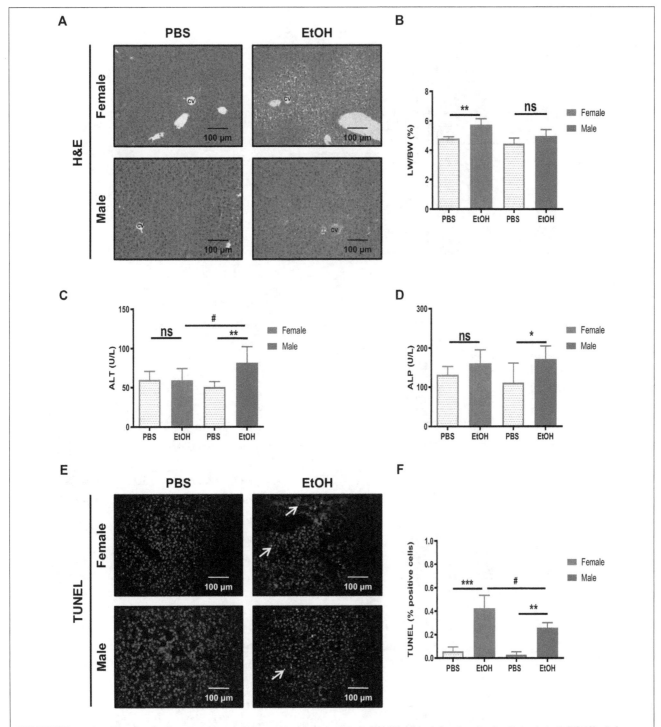

FIGURE 2 | Binge ethanol exposure to mice causes changes in liver architecture and cell death. **(A)** H&E staining in female and male mice treated with EtOH [6 g/kg] or PBS performed in paraffin liver sections (n = 6–8/group). **(B)** Liver-to-body weight (LW/BW) ratio in female and male mice after acute alcohol injury (n = 5–8/group). Serum **(C)** ALT and **(D)** ALP levels in female and male mice (n = 7–8/group). **(E)** TUNEL staining was performed in liver cryosections of female and male mice. **(F)** Quantification of TUNEL positive cells was done and graphed (n = 3/group;*p < 0.05, ***p < 0.001, #p < 0.05).

expression of lipogenic genes, was also induced by EtOH predominantly in female mice (**Figures 3C,D**).

Since immune infiltration and inflammation are characteristic of alcohol-induced liver injury, quantification of CD11b-positive cells and markers of inflammation, including *tnf-α*, *il1β*, and *tlr4*, were also evaluated. The number of CD11b positive cells was increased in female livers (**Figure 3E**), in agreement with the upregulation of mRNA transcripts for *tnf-α*, *il1β*, and *tlr4* observed in female mice (**Figures 3F–H**). In summary, our data suggest that female mice are more sensitive to liver injury

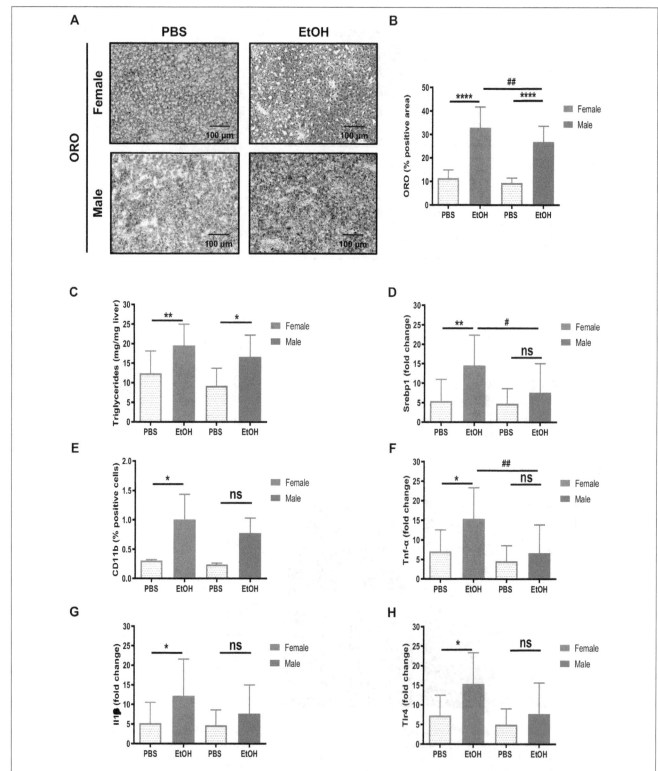

FIGURE 3 | Hepatic lipid accumulation and inflammation are characteristic of female mice. **(A)** ORO staining performed in liver cryosection of female and male C57BL/6J mice treated with EtOH [6 g/kg] or PBS. **(B)** Quantification of lipid droplets by ORO positive area was done and graphed (n = 5–6/group). **(C)** Quantification of hepatic triglycerides was done and graphed (n = 8/group). **(D)** *Srbp-1* mRNA expression was determined by qPCR and normalized to the amount of GAPDH in the liver of female and male mice (n = 5–8/group). **(E)** Quantification of CD11b positive cells was done and graphed (n = 3/group). **(F)** *Tnf-α*, **(G)** *Il1β*, and **(H)** *Tlr4* mRNA expression determined by qPCR and normalized to the amount of *gapdh* in liver of female and male mice (n = 4–10/group; *p < 0.05, ****p < 0.0001, #p < 0.05, ##p < 0.01).

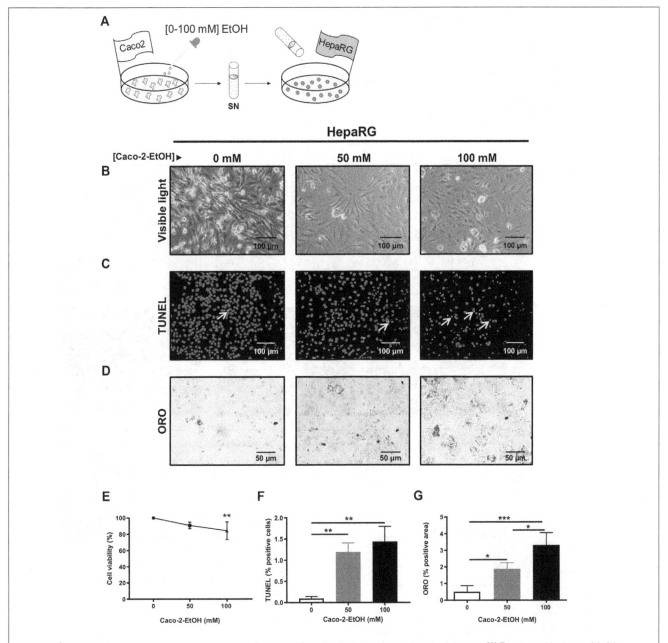

FIGURE 4 | HepaRG cells challenged with supernatant from EtOH-treated Caco-2 cells displayed exacerbated cell damage. **(A)** Experimental *in vitro* model of the effect of acute alcohol injury on intestinal epithelial permeability and on liver injury: cultures of HepaRG cells were exposed to the supernatant from Caco-2 cells that had been previously treated with different concentrations of EtOH [0–100 mM]. **(B)** HepaRG cells exposed to the supernatant of Caco-2 cells treated with EtOH [0–100 mM] showed by visible light (*n* = 4/group). **(C)** TUNEL staining was performed in HepaRG cells exposed to the supernatant of Caco-2 cells treated with EtOH [0–100 mM]. **(D)** Oil Red O (ORO) staining was performed in HepaRG cells exposed to the supernatant of Caco-2 cells treated with EtOH [0–100 mM]. **(E)** Cell viability of HepaRG cells challenged with supernatant from EtOH-treated Caco-2 cells determined by CCK8 (*n* = 6/group). **(F)** Quantification of TUNEL positive cells HepaRG cells exposed to supernatant from EtOH-treated Caco-2 cells (*n* = 3/group). **(G)** Quantification of lipid droplets by ORO positive area in HepaRG cells exposed to supernatant from EtOH-treated Caco-2 cells (%) (*n* = 3–4/group; *$p < 0.05$, ***$p < 0.001$).

due to acute alcohol injury in terms of steatosis and inflammation.

Assessment of Acute Alcohol Injury-Derived Damage in an *In Vitro* Model

In order to reproduce an *in vitro* model of the intestinal epithelial barrier, Caco-2 cells were plated and regularly monitored visually using a light microscope. First, Caco-2 cells were challenged with EtOH [0–100 mM], which caused cytoplasmic retractions, cell shrinkage, and cell death. High EtOH concentrations evidenced loss of cell-cell contact and detachment after 24 h EtOH exposure as observed under the visible light (**Supplementary Figure S3A,B**). Cell viability tested by CCK8 showed decreased cell viability along with increasing concentrations of EtOH (**Supplementary Figure**

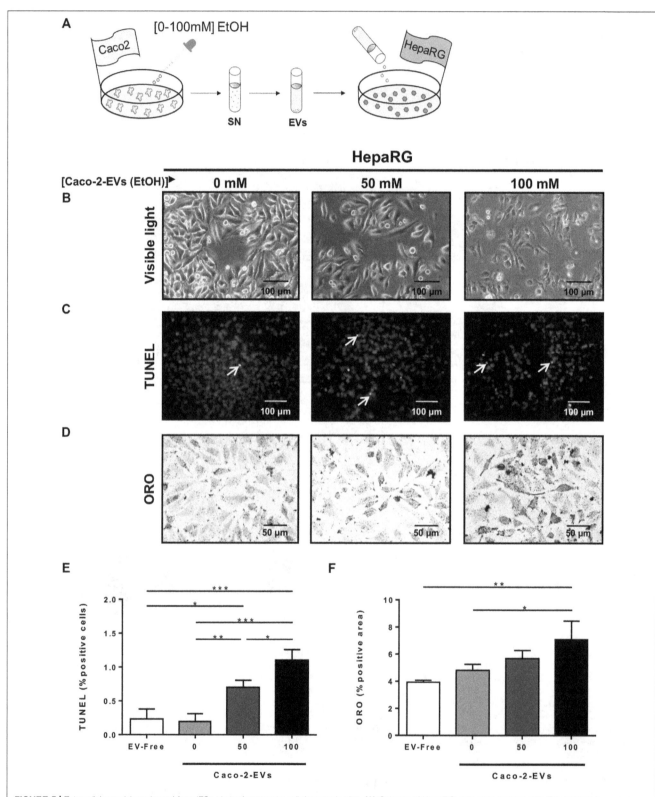

FIGURE 5 | Extracellular vesicles released from IECs trigger hepatocyte cell damage *in vitro*. **(A)** Cultures of HepaRG cells were treated with EVs isolated by ultracentrifugation from the supernatant of Caco-2 cells previously exposed to different concentrations of EtOH [0–100 mM]. **(B)** Morphology analysis of HepaRG cells by visible light. **(C)** TUNEL staining was performed in HepG2 cells exposed to EVs from EtOH-pretreated Caco-2-cells. **(D)** ORO staining performed in HepaRG cells challenged with EVs from EtOH-pretreated Caco-2-cells. **(E)** Quantification of TUNEL positive HepaRG cells after challenge with EVs isolated from the supernatant of Caco-2 cells previously treated with different concentrations of EtOH [0–100 mM] (*n* = 3/group). **(F)** Quantification of lipid droplets by ORO positive area in HepaRG cells challenged with EVs isolated from the supernatant of Caco-2 cells previously treated with different concentrations of EtOH [0–100 mM] (*n* = 3/group; *p* < 0.05, ***p* < 0.001).

S3C). These data were corroborated using TUNEL staining, which also showed an elevation of the number of Caco-2 TUNEL-positive cells with increasing concentrations of alcohol (**Supplementary Figure S3B,D**).

As an *in vitro* model of hepatocytes, we also used the well-characterized HepaRG hepatocyte human cell line to understand the effect of alcohol exposure in the liver. HepaRG cells were challenged by exposure to EtOH [0–100]. The loss of cell architecture was evident with a concentration of 50 mM EtOH (**Supplementary Figure S3A**). Cell viability assay revealed a decrease of alive cells proportionally associated with increasing concentrations of EtOH (**Supplementary Figure S3B,C**). Moreover, TUNEL staining also confirmed that the number of dead HepaRG cells increased after exposure to EtOH (**Supplementary Figures S3D**). Besides, lipid deposition evaluated by ORO staining showed higher lipid accumulation with increasing EtOH concentrations (**Supplementary Figures S3C,F**).

Intestinal Epithelial Cells Secrete Factors That Modulate Hepatocyte Injury During Acute Alcohol Injury

To replicate the effect of acute ethanol-derived injury on intestinal epithelial permeability and its impact on liver cell injury, 85% confluent HepaRG cells cultured in 12-well plates were challenged with 1 ml of supernatant from Caco-2 cells treated with EtOH [0–100 mM] (**Figure 4A**). The viability of HepaRG cells decreased at the higher concentrations of EtOH in the Caco-2 supernatant (**Figures 4B,E**), and these data correlated with the percentage of TUNEL positive cells (**Figures 4C,F**). Increased lipid accumulation, as assessed by ORO staining, was also found in HepaRG cells challenged with the supernatant of EtOH-treated Caco-2 cells (**Figures 4D,G**). These data indicate that the release of mediators from (IECs) might be responsible for hepatocyte injury during acute alcohol injury.

Extracellular Vesicles Released From Intestinal Epithelial Cells Trigger Hepatocyte Damage *In Vitro*

It has been well-documented that the release of EVs, produced under pathological conditions, might be responsible for cell damage. To understand whether the release of EVs by IECs might trigger liver damage during acute alcohol injury, we tested this hypothesis by isolating EVs from our *in vitro* model of the intestinal epithelial barrier.

Cell cultures of differentiated hepatocytes were exposed to EVs treated with EtOH [0–100 mM] (**Figure 5A**). HepaRG cells changed the morphology and lost the polarity when challenged with EVs from EtOH-pretreated Caco-2 cells (**Figure 5B**).

Concomitant with these changes, the cell viability of HepaRG cells decreased, as observed by the increase of positive TUNEL cells after *in vitro* acute alcohol injury (**Figures 5C,E**). Next, we measured lipid deposition in hepatocytes in response to EVs released by EtOH-pretreated Caco-2 cells. Interestingly, EVs from EtOH-pretreated Caco-2 cells caused an increase in lipid deposition of differentiated hepatocytes (**Figures 5D,F**), suggesting a possible role for EVs released by IECs in liver damage during acute alcohol injury.

Characterization of Extracellular Vesicles During Acute Alcohol Injury *In Vitro* and *In Vivo*

EVs were isolated from the supernatant of Caco-2 cells exposed to EtOH [0–100 mM] and from serum extracted from the portal vein of mice challenged to experimental acute alcohol injury, respectively, using a sequential ultracentrifugation method. Dynamic Light Scattering analysis showed the size distribution by intensity, confirming the existence of different populations of EVs (**Supplementary Table S2**), and NTA validated the morphology, size, and concentration of EVs in the diverse experimental groups (**Figure 6** and **Supplementary Figures S5B–D**). Although the concentration of particles was significantly increased to $2.34\,E^9 \pm 1.14\,E^8$ and $2.9\,E^9 \pm 5.82\,E^8$ particles/ml in the supernatant of Caco-2 cells exposed to 50 and 100 mM EtOH, respectively, compared with the control group $1.17\,E^9 \pm 2.31\,E^8$ (**Figure 6A**), no differences were found in the size of EVs upon EtOH exposure (**Figure 6B**).

Next, we measured the number of particles in serum extracted from mice subjected to experimental acute alcohol injury. While no differences were found in the number of particles/ml between PBS and EtOH-treated animals, the concentration of particles was $1.12\,E^9 \pm 1.40\,E^8$ and $1.59\,E^9 \pm 2.00\,E^8$ in EtOH-fed male and female mice, respectively, compared with PBS-injected male and female mice $1.30\,E^9 \pm 1.61\,E^8$ and $1.80\,E^9 \pm 3.99\,E^8$. These results might indicate a tendency toward a reduced particle concentration in male animals after acute alcohol exposure (**Figure 6C**). NTA showed mean particle size of 90 nm in serum samples consistent with the size of exosomes (**Figure 6D**).

DISCUSSION

Scientific research on alcohol abuse has traditionally focused on the mechanisms of chronic toxicity, given its financial burden and societal costs. More recently, acute alcohol injury has emerged as a social problem since binge drinking is alarmingly increasing both in women and in men (Dolganiuc and Szabo, 2009; Mcketta and Keyes, 2019). However, the mechanisms by which acute alcohol injury affects human health are not fully understood. Thus, there is a need for preclinical and translational studies focused on the effects of binge alcohol drinking.

In the present study, we first used a suitable *in vivo* model for assessing the effects of a single binge episode by administering 6 g/kg b.w. of EtOH to mice, based on previous studies (Carson and Pruett, 1996).

Intestinal barrier function is key to preventing the alcohol-induced inflammation locally and systemically. Goblet cells in the intestinal epithelium produce protective trefoil factors and mucins, which are abundantly core glycosylated and either localized to the cell membrane or secreted into the lumen to form the mucous layer (Shao et al., 2018). Decreased expression

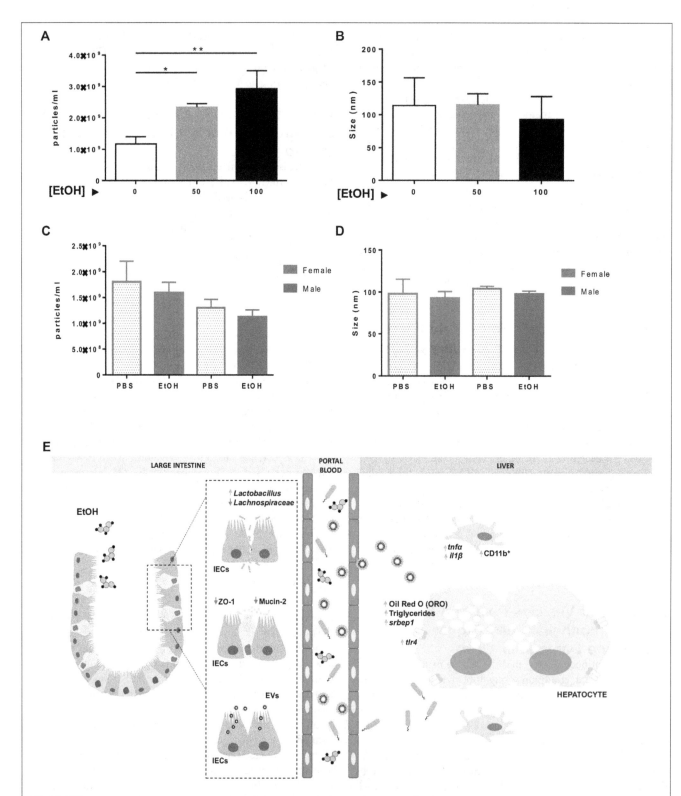

FIGURE 6 | Characterization of extracellular vesicles *in vitro* and *in vivo*. Isolated EVs from the supernatant of Caco-2 cells challenged with different concentrations of EtOH [0–100 mM] were measured by NTA, and **(A)** particles/ml and **(B)** size of EVs were represented. Isolated EVs were extracted from the serum of female and male mice treated with EtOH or PBS, and they were analyzed using NTA. **(C)** Particles/ml and **(D)** size of EVs were graphed (n = 3/group; $^{*}p$ < 0.05, $^{**}p$ < 0.01). **(E)** Schematic representation of the pathophysiological events that occur during acute alcohol exposure. Acute alcohol ingestion triggers damage to the intestinal epithelial barrier. Increased FITC-Dextran, disruption in tight junctions (ZO-1), and loss of mucosa (MUCIN-2) and alteration of the gut microbiota (increased *Lactobacillus* and decreased Lachnospiraceae) indicate damage to the intestinal epithelial barrier and gut dysbiosis. Translocation of microbial bacterial products through the leaky gut causes overexpression of *tlr4* and intestinal-derived inflammation in the liver–presence of CD11b-positive cells, *tnf-α*, and *il1β*, and mild steatosis and lipid accumulation. Our *in vitro* experiments suggest that ethanol triggers the release of EVs by intestinal epithelial cells (IECs), which exert a deleterious effect on hepatocyte viability and lipid accumulation.

of MUCIN-2 protein in the large intestine of female and male mice was observed after acute alcohol exposure. Interestingly, *mucin-2* knockout mice are protected against alcohol feeding-induced dysbiosis (Hartmann et al., 2013), likely due to higher expression of antimicrobial peptides.

Additionally, paracellular permeability in the intestinal epithelium sealed by TJs (Shao et al., 2018) was disrupted in the colon of EtOH-treated female and male mice, in which the loss of ZO-1 was characteristic. These results are in agreement with previous observations reporting that chronic-binge ethanol feeding impaired intestinal TJs (Cresci et al., 2017). Moreover, occludin deficiency increases susceptibility to EOH-induced mucosal dysfunction and liver damage in mice (Mir et al., 2016).

Alcohol ingestion causes intestinal bacterial overgrowth and changes in microbial composition in preclinical models as well as in patients with alcohol use disorder (Sarin et al., 2019). In our study, one alcohol binge increased the *Lactobacillus* phylum and decreased the Lachnospiraceae family. A decrease in *Lactobacillus* species and Lachnospiraceae family has been reported in alcohol consumption/feeding and alcoholic cirrhosis (Bajaj et al., 2012; Sarin et al., 2019). However, *Lactobacillus* species are increased in hepatic steatosis (Jang et al., 2019), which was observed in acute alcohol injury-exposed animals, and bacterial microbiota also change with the progression of alcoholic liver disease. Moreover, in a similar preclinical model that used a lower EtOH dosage (3 g/kg b.w.), Chen and colleagues (2016) reported no changes in intestinal microbiota and relative abundance of *Lactobacillus* and Firmicutes. Moreover, it is very likely that *Lactobacillus* elevation acts to counteract lipid metabolism imbalance as previously reported (Martin et al., 2008). Overall, these data suggest that alterations to the gut mucus layer, together with intestinal hyperpermeability and bacterial overgrowth, trigger bacterial translocation. Therefore, microbial products that reach the liver might contribute to hepatic injury during acute alcohol exposure.

Hepatic steatosis develops acutely in most individuals that consume even moderate amounts of alcohol. Steatosis changes are also seen in rodent models of binge drinking (Massey and Arteel, 2012). Although steatosis is an inert pathology *per se*, it sensitizes the liver to injury caused by a second insult. Binge drinking is a major risk factor for advanced liver disease (Ventura-Cots et al., 2017). Ethanol-treated mice displayed increased hepatic lipid accumulation, and this effect was more noticeable in female animals. This phenomenon was associated with increased immune infiltration (CD11b putative macrophages) and pro-inflammatory mediators of hepatic inflammation (e.g., *tnf-α*, *il1β*), which contribute to alcohol-related liver injury (Kawaratani et al., 2013; Bala et al., 2014; Rocco et al., 2014; Cresci et al., 2017).

Ethanol pre-exposure can prime Kupffer cells to lipopolysaccharides stimulation, resulting in enhanced *tnf-α* release, and binge drinking can impair the immune response via alteration of *tlr4* signaling (Massey and Arteel, 2012; Bala et al., 2014), as observed in our acute alcohol injury model. Moreover, our data demonstrated a significant increase in cell death in EtOH-treated mice, corroborated by elevated serum markers of liver injury (e.g., ALT). In agreement with other publications (Wagnerberger et al., 2013; Cresci et al., 2017), the more pronounced liver damage observed after acute alcohol injury in the liver of female mice may result from increased activation of TLR4-dependent signaling in this gender. However, in-depth studies need to be performed to shed light on the activation of specific molecular mechanisms that might be sex-dependent in the gut-liver axis.

Gender-related differences in total liver (ADH) and aldehyde dehydrogenase activity among different animal species have been observed in many studies. The differential liver injury between female and male animals could be explained by various factors, including the lower activity of class I and II ADH isoenzymes in females (Chrostek et al., 2003). This difference could help explain the fact that after men and women ingest the same dose of alcohol, women have higher BAC levels and increased injury. Corrao and colleagues (1998) reported that the same amount of average alcohol consumption was related to a higher risk of liver cirrhosis in women than in men. In contrast, women displayed slower gastric metabolism. Additionally, the levels of hormones, such as estrogen, might also influence several of the above factors (Wagnerberger et al., 2013).

Next, we sought to mechanistically approach the pathomechanisms underlying acute alcohol injury in the context of the gut-liver axis by modeling our experimental model *in vitro*. First, the effects of EtOH were assessed in Caco-2 cells, a human cell line of IECs. Concomitant with Wang's study (Wang et al., 2014), acute alcohol injury in culture decreased cell viability and exacerbated cell death, even though our results were collected 24 h after challenge (Dolganiuc and Szabo, 2009). Furthermore, EtOH caused changes in cell death and lipid deposition in HepaRGs, a human hepatoma cell line, in a dose-dependent manner, data that agree with previous publications (Tuoi Do et al., 2011). However, these authors observed that exposure to 100 mM ethanol significantly raised caspase 3/7 activity between 48 and 72 h, suggesting that apoptosis might occur later in time in culture. However, *in vivo*, we observed TUNEL-related cell death 8 h after acute ethanol injury. Others reported maximal apoptotic rate levels 4 h after ethanol exposure but TUNEL-positivity from 1 to 9 h (Yun et al., 2014), which might be increased levels of expression of CYP2E1 at these times after acute ethanol-derived tissue injury.

Accumulating evidence supports a role for EVs in regulating hepatic function. The gut-liver axis communication was modeled *in vitro* by challenging HepaRG cells with supernatant of Caco-2 cells. Human HepaRG hepatocytes treated with the supernatant of EtOH-pretreated Caco-2 cells dramatically changed their morphology, increased cell death, and accumulated lipids, as it occurs *in vivo*. This set of results suggested that the release of mediators by IECs may play a crucial role in the initiation and development of liver injury, and thus hepatocyte might uptake EVs as observed in models of viral hepatitis, partial hepatectomy and ischemia-reperfusion injury (Hirsova et al., 2016).

Recent studies pointed to a defined group of biological nanovesicles, namely exosomes or extracellular vesicles, as a key player in modulating the deleterious effects of alcohol in different tissues (Eguchi and Feldstein, 2018). Since our data indicated that EVs might be potential communicating tools in the gut-liver axis, we performed an *in vitro* model whereby EVs secreted by IECs (Caco-2 cells) in response to EtOH were added to HepaRG hepatocytes. EtOH significantly increased the number of nanoparticles released by Caco-2 cells, which were challenged to HepaRG cells. Decreased cell viability and high lipid accumulation were observed in this cell line of human hepatocytes, concomitant with our *in vivo* results.

In parallel, EVs isolated from portal blood of EtOH- and PBS-treated mice were collected and characterized. Our goal was to demonstrate that EVs released specifically by IECs can be used as potential biomarkers of acute alcohol injury. Our data showed a mean size of 90 nm in serum samples consistent with the size of EVs. However, hepatocytes also release EVs that are detected in blood as well, as previously reported (Eguchi et al., 2017), suggesting that the gut-liver axis is a bidirectional communication pathway.

Our results show that mice develop alterations in the gut-liver axis in response to experimental acute alcohol injury. Overall, alterations in the intestinal epithelial barrier associated with increased permeability, a thinner mucous protective layer, and changes in gut microbiota were evident. Interestingly, female mice were more prone to hepatic injury in response to a single binge episode, specifically in markers of steatosis and inflammation. Moreover, we showed that the release of mediators by IECs might have an impact on liver cells during acute alcohol injury, and demonstrated the presence and the effects of EVs both *in vivo* and *in vitro* (**Figure 6E**). These findings further deepen in the mechanisms triggered by acute alcohol exposure and open new therapeutic windows.

ETHICS STATEMENT

Animal studies were approved by the Consejería de Medio Ambiente, Administración Local y Ordenación del Territorio (PROEX-154/16).

AUTHOR CONTRIBUTIONS

AL-P and LM carried out the experiments and drafted the manuscript. JP provided funds for the study. NL-A, FH, and KZ performed experiments. SS, RV-V, and LB performed the microbiota studies. YN contributed to the intellectual work and provided experimental techniques. BM-A, LM-G, and AC contributed with the extracellular vesicles characterization. IA, MG, JV, RB, BM-A, and EM-N conducted experiments and/or provided pivotal intellectual and YN and FJ supervised, and analyzed the experiments, provided the funding and drafted the manuscript

FUNDING

This work was supported by the MINECO Retos SAF2016-78711, SAF2017-87919-R, EXOHEP-CM S2017/BMD-3727, NanoLiver-CM Y2018/NMT-4949, ERAB Ref. EA 18/14, AMMF 2018/117, UCM-25-2019 and COST Action CA17112, the German Research Foundation (SFB/TRR57/P04, SFB 1382-403224013/A02, and DFG NE 2128/2-1). FC and YN are Ramón y Cajal Researchers RYC-2014-15242 and RYC-2015-17438. FC is a Gilead Liver Research 2018. KZ is a recipient of a Chinese Scholarship Council (CSC). BK20170127 from the Natural Science Foundation of Jiangsu Province to JP

REFERENCES

Bajaj, J. S., Ridlon, J. M., Hylemon, P. B., Thacker, L. R., Heuman, D. M., Smith, S., et al. (2012). Linkage of gut microbiome with cognition in hepatic encephalopathy. *Am. J. Physiol. Gastrointest. Liver Physiol.* 302, G168–G175. doi:10.1152/ajpgi.00190.2011

Bala, S., Marcos, M., Gattu, A., Catalano, D., and Szabo, G. (2014). Acute binge drinking increases serum endotoxin and bacterial DNA levels in healthy individuals. *PloS One* 9, e96864. doi:10.1371/journal.pone.0096864

Bui, T. M., Mascarenhas, L. A., and Sumagin, R. (2018). Extracellular vesicles regulate immune responses and cellular function in intestinal inflammation and repair. *Tissue Barriers* 6, e1431038. doi:10.1080/21688370.2018. 1431038

Carson, E. J., and Pruett, S. B. (1996). Development and characterization of a binge drinking model in mice for evaluation of the immunological effects of ethanol. *Alcohol Clin. Exp. Res.* 20, 132–138. doi:10.1111/j.1530-0277.1996. tb01055.x

Cederbaum, A. I. (2012). Alcohol metabolism. *Clin. Liver Dis.* 16, 667–685. doi:10. 1016/j.cld.2012.08.002

Chen, P., Miyamoto, Y., Mazagova, M., Lee, K.-C., Eckmann, L., and Schnabl, B. (2016). Microbiota and alcoholic liver disease. *Alcohol Clin. Exp. Res.* 40, 1791–1792. doi:10.1111/acer.13129

Chrostek, L., Jelski, W., Szmitkowski, M., and Puchalski, Z. (2003). Gender-related differences in hepatic activity of alcohol dehydrogenase isoenzymes and aldehyde dehydrogenase in humans. *J. Clin. Lab. Anal.* 17, 93–96. doi:10. 1002/jcla.10076

Corrao, G., Bagnardi, V., Zambon, A., and Torchio, P. (1998). Meta-analysis of alcohol intake in relation to risk of liver cirrhosis. *Alcohol Alcohol.* 33, 381–392. doi:10.1093/oxfordjournals.alcalc.a008408

Cresci, G. A., Glueck, B., Mcmullen, M. R., Xin, W., Allende, D., and Nagy, L. E. (2017). Prophylactic tributyrin treatment mitigates chronic-binge ethanol-induced intestinal barrier and liver injury. *J. Gastroenterol. Hepatol.* 32, 1587–1597. doi:10.1111/jgh.13731

Cubero, F. J., Zhao, G., Nevzorova, Y. A., Hatting, M., Al Masaoudi, M., Verdier, J., et al. (2015). Haematopoietic cell-derived Jnk1 is crucial for chronic inflammation and carcinogenesis in an experimental model of liver injury. *J. Hepatol.* 62, 140–149. doi:10.1016/j.jhep.2014.08.029

Diehl, A. M., Goodman, Z., and Ishak, K. G. (1988). Alcohollike liver disease in nonalcoholics. *Gastroenterology* 95, 1056–1062. doi:10.1016/0016-5085(88) 90183-7

Dolganiuc, A., and Szabo, G. (2009). *In vitro* and *in vivo* models of acute alcohol exposure. *World J. Gastroenterol.* 15, 1168–1177. doi:10.3748/wjg.15. 1168

Eguchi, A., and Feldstein, A. E. (2018). Extracellular vesicles in non-alcoholic and alcoholic fatty liver diseases. *Liver Res.* 2, 30–34. doi:10.1016/j.livres.2018.01. 001

Eguchi, A., Lazaro, R. G., Wang, J., Kim, J., Povero, D., Willliams, B., et al. (2017). Extracellular vesicles released by hepatocytes from gastric infusion model of alcoholic liver disease contain a MicroRNA barcode that can be detected in blood. *Hepatology* 65, 475–490. doi:10.1002/hep.28838

Fanning, A. S., and Anderson, J. M. (2009). Zonula occludens-1 and -2 are cytosolic scaffolds that regulate the assembly of cellular junctions. *Ann. N. Y. Acad. Sci.* 1165, 113–120. doi:10.1111/j.1749-6632.2009.04440.x

Gao, B., Ahmad, M. F., Nagy, L. E., and Tsukamoto, H. (2019). Inflammatory pathways in alcoholic steatohepatitis. *J. Hepatol.* 70, 249–259. doi:10.1016/j.jhep.2018.10.023

Gao, B., and Bataller, R. (2011). Alcoholic liver disease: pathogenesis and new therapeutic targets. *Gastroenterology* 141, 1572–1585. doi:10.1053/j.gastro.2011.09.002

Gill, J. (2000). The effects of moderate alcohol consumption on female hormone levels and reproductive function. *Alcohol Alcohol.* 35, 417–423. doi:10.1093/alcalc/35.5.417

Griswold, M. G., Fullman, N., Hawley, C., Arian, N., Zimsen, S. R. M., Tymeson, H. D., et al. (2018). Alcohol use and burden for 195 countries and territories, 1990–2016: a systematic analysis for the Global Burden of Disease Study 2016. *Lancet* 392, 1015–1035. doi:10.1016/s0140-6736(18)31310-2

Hartmann, P., Chen, P., Wang, H. J., Wang, L., Mccole, D. F., Brandl, K., et al. (2013). Deficiency of intestinal mucin-2 ameliorates experimental alcoholic liver disease in mice. *Hepatology* 58, 108–119. doi:10.1002/hep.26321

Hirsova, P., Ibrahim, S. H., Verma, V. K., Morton, L. A., Shah, V. H., Larusso, N. F., et al. (2016). Extracellular vesicles in liver pathobiology: small particles with big impact. *Hepatology* 64, 2219–2233. doi:10.1002/hep.28814

Jang, H. R., Park, H.-J., Kang, D., Chung, H., Nam, M. H., Lee, Y., et al. (2019). A protective mechanism of probiotic *Lactobacillus* against hepatic steatosis via reducing host intestinal fatty acid absorption. *Exp. Mol. Med.* 51, 1–14. doi:10.1038/s12276-019-0293-4

Ji, C., Chan, C., and Kaplowitz, N. (2006). Predominant role of sterol response element binding proteins (SREBP) lipogenic pathways in hepatic steatosis in the murine intragastric ethanol feeding model. *J. Hepatol.* 45, 717–724. doi:10.1016/j.jhep.2006.05.009

Kawaratani, H., Tsujimoto, T., Douhara, A., Takaya, H., Moriya, K., Namisaki, T., et al. (2013). The effect of inflammatory cytokines in alcoholic liver disease. *Mediat. Inflamm.* 2013, 495156. doi:10.1155/2013/495156

Kim, I. H., Kisseleva, T., and Brenner, D. A. (2015). Aging and liver disease. *Curr. Opin. Gastroenterol.* 31, 184–191. doi:10.1097/mog.0000000000000176

Kwon, H.-J., Won, Y.-S., Park, O., Chang, B., Duryee, M. J., Thiele, G. E., et al. (2014). Aldehyde dehydrogenase 2 deficiency ameliorates alcoholic fatty liver but worsens liver inflammation and fibrosis in mice. *Hepatology* 60, 146–157. doi:10.1002/hep.27036

Lamas-Paz, A., Hao, F., Nelson, L. J., Vázquez, M. T., Canals, S., Moral, M. G. d., et al. (2018). Alcoholic liver disease: utility of animal models. *World J. Gastroenterol.* 24, 5063–5075. doi:10.3748/wjg.v24.i45.5063

Liao, L., Schneider, K. M., Galvez, E. J. C., Frissen, M., Marschall, H.-U., Su, H., et al. (2019). Intestinal dysbiosis augments liver disease progression via NLRP3 in a murine model of primary sclerosing cholangitis. *Gut* 68, 1477–1492. doi:10.1136/gutjnl-2018-316670

Martin, F. P. J., Wang, Y., Sprenger, N., Yap, I. K. S., Lundstedt, T., Lek, P., et al. (2008). Probiotic modulation of symbiotic gut microbial-host metabolic interactions in a humanized microbiome mouse model. *Mol. Syst. Biol.* 4, 157. doi:10.1038/msb4100190

Massey, V. L., and Arteel, G. E. (2012). Acute alcohol-induced liver injury. *Front. Physiol.* 3, 193. doi:10.3389/fphys.2012.00193

Mcketta, S., and Keyes, K. M. (2019). Heavy and binge alcohol drinking and parenting status in the United States from 2006 to 2018: an analysis of nationally representative cross-sectional surveys. *PLoS Med.* 16, e1002954. doi:10.1371/journal.pmed.1002954

Mcmurdie, P. J., and Holmes, S. (2013). phyloseq: an R package for reproducible interactive analysis and graphics of microbiome census data. *PLoS One* 8, e61217. doi:10.1371/journal.pone.0061217

Mir, H., Meena, A. S., Chaudhry, K. K., Shukla, P. K., Gangwar, R., Manda, B., et al. (2016). Occludin deficiency promotes ethanol-induced disruption of colonic epithelial junctions, gut barrier dysfunction and liver damage in mice. *Biochim. Biophys. Acta Gen. Subj.* 1860, 765–774. doi:10.1016/j.bbagen.2015.12.013

Molina, P. E., and Nelson, S. (2018). Binge drinking's effects on the body. Alcohol research: current reviews vol. 39 (1) (2018):99–109. PMC6104963 PMID: 30557153 ISSN 2168-3492

Naugler, W. E., Sakurai, T., Kim, S., Maeda, S., Kim, K., Elsharkawy, A. M., et al. (2007). Gender disparity in liver cancer due to sex differences in MyD88-dependent IL-6 production. *Science* 317, 121–124. doi:10.1126/science.1140485

Pruett, S., Tan, W., Howell, G. E., 3rd, and Nanduri, B. (2020). Dosage scaling of alcohol in binge exposure models in mice: an empirical assessment of the relationship between dose, alcohol exposure, and peak blood concentrations in humans and mice. *Alcohol* 89, 9–17. doi:10.1016/j.alcohol.2020.03.011

Rocco, A., Compare, D., Angrisani, D., Sanduzzi Zamparelli, M., and Nardone, G. (2014). Alcoholic disease: liver and beyond. *World J. Gastroenterol.* 20, 14652–14659. doi:10.3748/wjg.v20.i40.14652

Roychowdhury, S., Glueck, B., Han, Y., Mohammad, M. A., and Cresci, G. A. M. (2019). A designer synbiotic attenuates chronic-binge ethanol-induced gut-liver injury in mice. *Nutrients* 11, 97. doi:10.3390/nu11010097

Sambrotta, M., Strautnieks, S., Papouli, E., Rushton, P., Clark, B. E., Parry, D. A., et al. (2014). Mutations in TJP2 cause progressive cholestatic liver disease. *Nat. Genet.* 46, 326–328. doi:10.1038/ng.2918

Sarin, S. K., Pande, A., and Schnabl, B. (2019). Microbiome as a therapeutic target in alcohol-related liver disease. *J. Hepatol.* 70, 260–272. doi:10.1016/j.jhep.2018.10.019

Shao, T., Zhao, C., Li, F., Gu, Z., Liu, L., Zhang, L., et al. (2018). Intestinal HIF-1α deletion exacerbates alcoholic liver disease by inducing intestinal dysbiosis and barrier dysfunction. *J. Hepatol.* 69, 886–895. doi:10.1016/j.jhep.2018.05.021

Steiner, J. L., and Lang, C. H. (2017). Alcohol, adipose tissue and lipid dysregulation. *Biomolecules* 7, 16. doi:10.3390/biom7010016

Sydor, S., Best, J., Messerschmidt, I., Manka, P., Vilchez-Vargas, R., Brodesser, S., et al. (2020). Altered microbiota diversity and bile acid signaling in cirrhotic and noncirrhotic NASH-HCC. *Clin. Transl. Gastroenterol.* 11, e00131. doi:10.14309/ctg.0000000000000131

Szabo, G. (2015). Gut-liver axis in alcoholic liver disease. *Gastroenterology* 148, 30–36. doi:10.1053/j.gastro.2014.10.042

Tripathi, A., Debelius, J., Brenner, D. A., Karin, M., Loomba, R., Schnabl, B., et al. (2018). The gut-liver axis and the intersection with the microbiome. *Nat. Rev. Gastroenterol. Hepatol.* 15, 397–411. doi:10.1038/s41575-018-0011-z

Tuoi Do, T. H., Gaboriau, F., Ropert, M., Moirand, R., Cannie, I., Brissot, P., et al. (2011). Ethanol effect on cell proliferation in the human hepatoma HepaRG cell line: relationship with iron metabolism. *Alcohol Clin. Exp. Res.* 35, 408–419. doi:10.1111/j.1530-0277.2010.01358.x

Van Der Sluis, M., De Koning, B. A. E., De Bruijn, A. C. J. M., Velcich, A., Meijerink, J. P. P., Van Goudoever, J. B., et al. (2006). Muc2-deficient mice spontaneously develop colitis, indicating that MUC2 is critical for colonic protection. *Gastroenterology* 131, 117–129. doi:10.1053/j.gastro.2006.04.020

Ventura-Cots, M., Watts, A. E., and Bataller, R. (2017). Binge drinking as a risk factor for advanced alcoholic liver disease. *Liver Int.* 37, 1281–1283. doi:10.1111/liv.13482

Wagnerberger, S., Fiederlein, L., Kanuri, G., Stahl, C., Millonig, G., Mueller, S., et al. (2013). Sex-specific differences in the development of acute alcohol-induced liver steatosis in mice. *Alcohol Alcohol.* 48, 648–656. doi:10.1093/alcalc/agt138

Wang, Y., Tong, J., Chang, B., Wang, B., Zhang, D., and Wang, B. (2014). Effects of alcohol on intestinal epithelial barrier permeability and expression of tight junction-associated proteins. *Mol. Med. Rep.* 9, 2352–2356. doi:10.3892/mmr.2014.2126

Yun, J.-W., Son, M.-J., Abdelmegeed, M. A., Banerjee, A., Morgan, T. R., Yoo, S.-H., et al. (2014). Binge alcohol promotes hypoxic liver injury through a CYP2E1-HIF-1α-dependent apoptosis pathway in mice and humans. *Free Radic. Biol. Med.* 77, 183–194. doi:10.1016/j.freeradbiomed.2014.08.030

8

Rapamycin is Effective for Upper but not for Lower Gastrointestinal Crohn's Disease-Related Stricture

Min Zhong[1,2], Bota Cui[1,2], Jie Xiang[3], Xia Wu[1,2], Quan Wen[1,2], Qianqian Li[1,2] and Faming Zhang[1,2]*

[1]Medical Center for Digestive Diseases, The Second Affiliated Hospital of Nanjing Medical University, Nanjing, China, [2]Key Lab of Holistic Integrative Enterology, Nanjing Medical University, Nanjing, China, [3]Department of Gastroenterology, The Central Hospital of Enshi Autonomous Prefecture, Enshi, China

*Correspondence:
Faming Zhang
fzhang@njmu.edu.cn

Crohn's disease (CD)-related fibrotic stricture remains a clinical challenge because of no effective treatments. This study aimed to evaluate the potential efficacy of rapamycin in patients with CD-related strictures in different locations in gastrointestinal tract. A pilot prospective study on using rapamycin for CD-related stricture was performed from April 2015 to August 2020 in a single center in China. Fifteen patients were enrolled into the study. The clinical efficacy was evaluated by diet score and gastrointestinal obstruction symptoms score. Clinical responses were defined as the ability to tolerate the regular diet with vegetable fiber combined with a reduction of ≥75% in overall target score and a score of less than two points for each item. Three patients discontinued rapamycin for less than 1-month due to intolerance to adverse events, then, 12 patients received ≥1 dose of the rapamycin and provided ≥1 post-baseline target score after baseline were included for intent-to-treat (ITT) analysis. 100% (5/5) of patients with upper gastrointestinal strictures achieved clinical response after using rapamycin. However, no clinical response was observed in those patients with CD lesions in lower gastrointestinal tract. Adverse events occurred in 40% (6/15) of patients. No death or serious opportunistic infections were observed in the present study. This study firstly reported that rapamycin might be effective for CD-related stricture in the upper, but not in lower gastrointestinal tract.

Keywords: Crohn's disease, rapamycin, fibrosis, stricture, inflammatory bowel diseases, duodenum obstruction

INTRODUCTION

Crohn's disease (CD) is a chronic relapsing inflammatory disease that can occur in any segment of the gastrointestinal tract. However, the naturally progressive disease course culminates in stricture formation (Cosnes et al., 2011), often leading to repeated bowel obstruction and surgery (Rieder et al., 2013; Singh et al., 2017). Mostly, strictures are caused by the combination of inflammation and fibrosis, and the intensity of fibrosis is almost impossible to determine (Feakins, 2020). Clinically, CD-related stenosis can be silent or symptomatic. Symptomatic stenosis may manifest as postprandial bloating, or significant intestinal obstruction, causing nausea, vomiting, and abdominal pain. Up till now, the therapy of choice for CD with fibrotic strictures, mainly comprises endoscopic dilation endoscopic stricturotomy and surgery (Kanazawa et al., 2012; Singh et al., 2017; Shen et al., 2020), in conjunction with purely anti-inflammatory therapy. Although endoscopic dilation procedures for stricturing CD are usually technically successful, the majority of patients still required multiple sessions of endoscopic dilation, and some might develop perforation (Kanazawa et al., 2012; Singh et al., 2017). A significant number of patients have to undergo multiple surgeries, with the attendant risk of developing short bowel syndrome and intestinal failure (Rieder et al., 2013). Therefore, there is necessity to explore more effective treatments for patients with CD-related fibrotic stricture.

In recent studies, rapamycin, a serine/THR kinase inhibitor of mammalian target (mTOR), has been reported as potentially effective treatment in limited populations with refractory CD (Massey et al., 2008; Mutalib et al., 2014). Rapamycin has also been reported to inhibit the progression of kidney fibrosis (Chen et al., 2012), cardiac fibrosis (Haller et al., 2016), and pulmonary fibrosis (Xu et al., 2017). A recent study has shown that rapamycin can reduce intestinal fibrosis by inhibiting CX3Cr1+ mTOR/autophagy in mononuclear phagocytes and up-regulating the IL-23/IL-22 axis (Mathur et al., 2019). Based on the consideration on the two facts: the very low incidence of CD patients with upper gastrointestinal fibrotic stricture (Nugent et al., 1989; Van Assche et al., 2004), and the hypothesis on the local anti-fibrosis effect of rapamycin in upper section of small intestine, the present study aimed to evaluate the potential efficacy of rapamycin for patients with CD-related gastrointestinal stricture.

MATERIALS AND METHODS

Study Design and Participants

Patients with CD from the nation came to the Second Affiliated Hospital of Nanjing Medical University for seeking fecal microbiota transplantation based on automatic filtration and washing process and the related delivery, which was called as washed microbiota transplantation (WMT) (Fecal Microbiota Transplantation-standardization Study Group, 2020; Zhang et al., 2020). However, these patients with CD-related strictures were not considered for WMT, but invited to attend the present trial (NCT02675153). The study was approved by the Second Affiliated Hospital of the Nanjing Medical University Institutional Ethical Review Board (2016KY001), and written informed consent was obtained from all patients. Demographics (age, gender) and disease characteristics (disease location, duration, duration of stricture and other CD drug medications) of each patient were noted before the study.

Inclusion and Exclusion Criteria

Inclusion criteria were: (1) Patients ($\geq$18 years of age) with a documented definite diagnosis of CD; and 2) the presence of a clinically symptomatic stricture; and 3) strictures confirmed by endoscopy (passing endoscope with difficulty) or typical image by CT enterography (CTE) or MR enterography (MRE). Patients were excluded: 1) patients who were pregnant, diagnosed with intestinal perforation, complete intestinal obstruction, any signs of dysplasia or malignancy, or use of anti-tumor necrosis factor (TNF) in the last three months; and 2) patients who were not followed up between the inception of medication and any other subsequent treatments.

Procedures and Outcome Measures

Patients were treated with rapamycin (2 mg/day, Sirolimus, Roche) and short-term enteral nutrition. Patients with colitis were also treated with 5-aminosalicylic acid (5-ASA). The intent-to-treat (ITT) population comprised all patients who received $\geq$1 dose of the study drug and provided $\geq$1 post-baseline target score after baseline.

We used a composite score considering all the essential elements including the gastrointestinal obstruction symptoms score and diet score to assess the effectiveness of treatment in clinical practice during follow-up. Response should meet the following three criteria: (a) the ability to tolerate a normal diet (vegetable fiber), with a reduction of $\geq$75% in overall baseline target score and sub-score $\leq$ 2 (**Table 1**); (b) no need for endoscopic dilation or surgery; (c) no severe adverse events or any other reasons leading to rapamycin withdrawal. The primary aim was the rate of clinical response focusing on obstruction after using rapamycin. The follow-up was at least 6 months for patients with unclear efficacy. Patients who prematurely discontinued rapamycin due to severe adverse events or who did not meet clinical response criteria after 6 months medication usage were considered treatment failure. The secondary aim was to evaluate the adverse events during medication usage in all enrolled patients. In this study, new onset of symptoms and the exacerbation of previous symptoms were recorded as adverse events. We also evaluated the primary endpoint was the rate of surgery or ED after rapamycin as the long-term treatment outcomes.

Statistical Analysis

Data were analyzed using IBM SPSS Statistics 23.0.0 (SPSS Inc., Chicago, IL, United States). Continuous variables were expressed using median and interquartile range and tested by Analysis of Variance test. Categorical data were described as number (percentages) and were tested by Chi-square analysis or Fisher's exact test. The paired data were compared using the Paired t test. $p < 0.05$ was indicative of statistical significance.

RESULTS

From April 2015 to August 2020, totally 15 patients were enrolled. The follow-up finished on December 1, 2020. The patient demographics, characteristics of CD, and previous history of drug therapy at the baseline were well balanced between the treatment groups (as shown in **Table 2**) and three of them with lesions in ileum or colon were administered oral 5-ASA simultaneously. One patient in the upper gastrointestinal group and two patients in the lower gastrointestinal group stopped to take the medication within one month because of adverse events (**Table 2**) and did not provide a post-baseline target score. Therefore, 15 patients were included in the safety

TABLE 1 | Definition of each target and scoring method in patients.

Variables	Scoring method
Abdominal pain	0: No abdominal pain
	1–2: Essentially normal
	3–5: Affecting daily life but not sleeping
	6–9: Affecting sleep
Abdominal distention	0: No abdominal distention
	1–2: Essentially normal
	3–5: Affecting daily life but not sleeping
	6–9: Affecting sleep
Diet	0: No dietary restrictions
	1–2: Essentially normal, without nausea and vomiting
	3–5: Regular diet, with nausea and vomiting
	6–8: Fluid diet and enteral nutrition, with nausea and vomiting
	9: Exclusive enteral nutrition or gastrointestinal decompression

TABLE 2 | Characteristics of the patients at baseline.

	All patients (n = 15)	Upper gastrointestinal (n = 6)	Lower gastrointestinal (n = 9)	p value
Age, years, median (IQR)	30 (28.5–38.5)	29 (24.3–30.8)	31 (29–39)	0.358
Male, n (%)	8 (53.3%)	4 (66.7%)	4 (44.4%)	0.608
Family history of CD, n (%)	0 (0.0%)	0 (0.0%)	0 (0.0%)	
Smoking, n (%)				0.604
Current	0 (0.0%)	0 (0.0%)	0 (0.0%)	
Ex-smoker	4 (26.7%)	1 (16.7%)	3 (33.3%)	
Never	8 (73.3%)	5 (83.3%)	6 (66.7%)	
Age at diagnosis, years, median (IQR)	25 (23–29.5)	24 (21.5–28.8)	26 (23–29)	0.852
Months from CD diagnosis to confirm the stricture, months, median (IQR)	35 (13–49)	7 (1.3–21)	46 (35–68)	0.367
Disease duration, years, median (IQR)	9 (4.5–12)	3 (3–7)	12 (10.5–12.5)	0.082
Fistulizing disease, n (%)	5 (33.3%)	2 (33.3%)	3 (33.3%)	
History of gastrointestinal surgery, n (%)	3 (20%)	0 (0.0%)	3 (33.3%)	
History of medications, n (%)				0.556
5-ASA	9 (60%)	3 (50%)	6 (66.7%)	
PPI	2 (13.3%)	2 (33.3%)	0 (0.0%)	
Immunosuppressants	9 (60%)	3e (50%)	6 (66.7%)	
Corticosteroids	8 (53.3%)	4 (66.7%)	4 (44.4%)	
Biological therapy	2 (13.3%)	1 (16.7%)	1 (11.1%)	
Adverse events				0.091
Palpation	2 (13.3%)	0 (0.0%)	2 (22.2%)	
Loss of libido	2 (13.3%)	0 (0.0%)	2 (22.2%)	
Abnormal liver enzymes	1 (6.7%)	0 (0.0%)	1 (11.1%)	
Mouth ulcer	2 (13.3%)	0 (0.0%)	2 (22.2%)	
Headache	1 (6.7%)	0 (0.0%)	1 (11.1%)	
Rash	0 (0.0%)	1 (16.7%)	2 (22.2%)	
Leukopenia	1 (6.7%)	1 (16.7%)	0 (0.0%)	

CD, Crohn's disease; 5-ASA, 5-aminosalicylic acid; PPI, proton pump inhibitors; IQR, inter quartile range.

population and 12 patients were included for in the ITT population (**Table 3**).

Response rate was 41.7% (5/12) in this study. The patients achieved response were all patients with upper gastrointestinal stricture (lesions in stomach and duodenum), but clinical failure was confirmed in all patients with lower lesions. 100% (5/5) of patients with upper gastrointestinal strictures achieved clinical

response within 6 months after using rapamycin, with the mean time of 4.4 months. The overall target score of the patients decreased from the mean of 12.0 at baseline to 1.6 at 4.4 months (Paired t test, $p = 0.005$), with each target ≤2. By contrast, the mean score for patients with lower gastrointestinal lesions dropped to 8.7 at 6 months from 10.0 at baseline (Paired t test, $p = 0.022$). The adverse events as the secondary aim of the

TABLE 3 | Medications and clinical outcomes of patients.

Pt	Classification	5-ASA	Rapa duration (months)	Response (months)	HBI Before	HBI After[a]	Abdominal pain Before	Abdominal pain After[a]	Abdominal distention Before	Abdominal distention After[a]	Diet Before	Diet After[a]
1	A1, L3L4, B2	No	24	Yes (2)	2	0	0	0	5	0	5	2
2	A2, L3L4, B2	Yes	6	Yes (5)	3	0	3	0	5	0	5	0
3	A1, L4, B2	No	24	Yes (5)	2	0	0	0	0	0	6	0
4	A2, L4, B2	No	10	Yes (6)	5	1	6	0	2	0	9	1
5	A2, L4, B2	No	4	Yes (4)	3	0	0	0	5	2	9	3
6	A2, L3, B2	No	12	No	5	1	5	4	2	2	5	5
7	A2, L3, B2	Yes	11	No	5	3	5	2	1	1	6	6
8	A2, L3, B2	No	6	No	5	4	6	5	5	4	6	6
9	A2, L3, B2	Yes	6	No	5	3	3	3	3	3	3	3
10	A2, L2, B2	No	8	No	3	2	0	0	3	2	3	3
11	A2, L2, B2	No	6	No	2	2	0	0	2	2	3	3
12	A2, L3, B2	No	6	No	10	8	6	4	0	0	3	3

Rapa, Rapamycin; HBI, Harvey-Bradshaw Index; A1, ≤16 years; A2, 17–40 years; L2, colonic; L3, ileocolonic; L4, isolated upper gastrointestinal; B2, structuring; 5-ASA, 5-aminosalicylic acid.
[a]*The time that patients achieved response or received rapamycin for 6 months.*

present study occurred in six patients (6/15, 40%) (**Table 2**). No death or serious opportunistic infections were reported.

The median duration of rapamycin in patients with upper gastrointestinal stenosis was 17 (Interquartile range (IQR): 9–24) months. At a median follow-up of 49 (IQR: 42–53.5) months, three of these patients were identified to be in long-term success and have been able to completely cease medication for more than one year without relapse. One case reported clinical improvement on her obstruction in upper gastrointestinal tract after 6 months of rapamycin, but she developed rectovaginal fistula after the cessation of rapamycin for 16 months. Rapamycin was discontinued in four patients with lower gastrointestinal tract stenosis after 6 months, and three of them continued to receive rapamycin for several months of their own volition, with a median duration of 6 (IQR: 6.0–9.5) months. The median time to follow-up was 37 (IQR: 29–46) months in the lower lesions group. One patient underwent surgery 17 months after rapamycin withdrawal, while the others were treated with other immunosuppressive agents after failure of rapamycin treatment.

DISCUSSION

Treatment of CD-related stricture is a clinical challenge, especially the lesions located in upper gastrointestinal tract, and is also a high socio-economic burden due to frequent hospitalizations and surgery (Bodger et al., 2009). Despite advances in anti-inflammatory therapies in recent decades, the incidence of intestinal stenosis in CD has not changed significantly. Inflammation and fibrosis are associated, in most cases, but to different degrees. Although surgery is the choice for fibrotic stenosis, post-operative disease recurrence and re-stricture are common (Rieder et al., 2013). Endoscopic dilatation is relatively safe for patients, but the efficacy is of limited duration (Hassan et al., 2007; Taida et al., 2018). Given the current uncertainties of the medical treatment regarding the

formation and progression of fibrotic strictures, new treatments are welcome.

The efficacy of mTOR inhibitors in the treatment of CD varies from studies (Massey et al., 2008; Reinisch et al., 2008; Mutalib et al., 2014). This pilot case series study explored the efficacy and safety of rapamycin in CD-related strictures. Overall, five patients (100%) with duodenum stricture achieved clinical response after rapamycin treatment, but none of patients with lower gastrointestinal stricture reported improvement. The present findings inspire us to precisely select the clinical application of rapamycin in CD-associated stenosis in duodenum or lesion close to duodenum.

In the present study, we found that Harvey-Bradshaw Index (HBI) could not accurately reflect the changes in the patients with CD-related gastrointestinal stricture. The evaluation based on clinical outcomes, including symptoms and tolerability, might be the better than using imaging changes. Therefore, the gastrointestinal symptoms and diet assessment were used for the clinical evaluation in these patients. We observed that clinical responses were only achieved in patients with upper gastrointestinal stricture by oral rapamycin, but not in patients with lower lesions. In this population, one male teenager with duodenum stricture who underwent repeated endoscopic dilation and percutaneous endoscopic gastrojejunostomy (PEG-J) for exclusive enteral nutrition, remained unresponsive for two years. After two months of treatment with rapamycin, he switched from enteral nutrition via tube to regular taking food by oral with normal diet, and the total score dropped from 10 at baseline to two at two months. He maintained clinical response to rapamycin for two years. Unfortunately, 10 months after withdrawal of rapamycin, gastroscopy revealed the progression of stenosis. Then he was treated with rapamycin again and has maintained response to date. Another patient with upper lesions took rapamycin continuously for only 6 months and developed rectovaginal fistula after stopping the medication. In view of these results, we suggest that rapamycin should be used as a long-term or maintenance therapy to achieve the best treatment response.

The enteral nutrition via tube can solve the nutritional needs of patients and relieve inflammatory bowel stricture in CD (Hu et al., 2014), but it seems not effective on fibrotic stenosis. Therefore, our results suggest that rapamycin may have a role in the treatment of fibrotic strictures. The present study showed a new treatment option for CD related strictures and further studies are expected to investigate the underlying mechanisms of this effect in the future.

An important question is whether rapamycin could prevent or delay surgery in this category of patients. We observed that 11/12 patients (91.7%) initially treated with rapamycin were surgery-free after a median follow-up of more than 3 years. The results may suggest that rapamycin has changed the natural history of the disease and is able to reverse strictures to some extent, which were thought to be non-reversible according to the Lemann Index in some patients with CD (Fiorino et al., 2015). In our study, the most common adverse event was mouth ulcer, and three patients discontinued the treatment due to adverse events within one month. However, adverse events occurred in patients after one month subsided spontaneously, indicating that the severity of adverse reactions may gradually decrease over time.

There were some limitations in the present study. The simple size was small, and the result might not be representative of the general population. In addition, the evaluation based on endoscopy or radiology was not performed for each patient. The benefits and risks of rapamycin for fibrotic strictures in long term should be assessed in randomized controlled trials.

In conclusion, although CD-related fibrotic stricture in upper gastrointestinal tract is rare, we had opportunity to enroll this specific population for this pilot study in China. We first time reported that the rapamycin should be effective in patients with CD-related fibrotic stricture in upper gastrointestinal tract, not those lesions in lower tract. Further case-control studies with appropriate sample and randomization are required to support the use of rapamycin in this specific subpopulation.

ETHICS STATEMENT

The studies involving human participants were reviewed and approved by Second Affiliated Hospital of the Nanjing Medical University Institutional Ethical Review Board (2016KY001). The patients/participants provided their written informed consent to participate in this study.

AUTHOR CONTRIBUTIONS

MZ contributed to clinical data acquisition, analyzed the data and wrote the manuscript. FZ designed the research. XW contributed to clinical data acquisition and manuscript revision. BC, JX, QL, and QW performed the clinical work.

ACKNOWLEDGMENTS

The authors thank all the participants of the study. The authors also thank Cicilia Marcella for her kindly assistance with language improvement.

REFERENCES

Bodger, K., Kikuchi, T., and Hughes, D. (2009). Cost-effectiveness of biological therapy for Crohn's disease: markov cohort analyses incorporating United Kingdom patient-level cost data. *Aliment. Pharmacol. Ther.* 30 (3), 265–274. doi:10.1111/j.1365-2036.2009.04033.x

Chen, G., Chen, H., Wang, C., Peng, Y., Sun, L., Liu, H., et al. (2012). Rapamycin ameliorates kidney fibrosis by inhibiting the activation of mTOR signaling in interstitial macrophages and myofibroblasts. *PLoS One* 7 (3), e33626. doi:10.1371/journal.pone.0033626

Cosnes, J., Gower-Rousseau, C., Seksik, P., and Cortot, A. (2011). Epidemiology and natural history of inflammatory bowel diseases. *Gastroenterology* 140 (6), 1785–1794. doi:10.1053/j.gastro.2011.01.055

Feakins, R. M. (2020). Transmural histology scores in stricturing crohn's disease: seeking to build precision on uncertain foundations. *J. Crohns. Colitis.* 14 (6), 721–723. doi:10.1093/ecco-jcc/jjaa008

Fecal Microbiota Transplantation-standardization Study Group (2020). Nanjing consensus on methodology of washed microbiota transplantation. *Chin. Med. J.* 133 (19), 2330–2332. doi:10.1097/CM9.0000000000000954

Fiorino, G., Bonifacio, C., Allocca, M., Repici, A., Balzarini, L., Malesci, A., et al. (2015). Bowel damage as assessed by the Lemann Index is reversible on anti-TNF therapy for crohn's disease. *J. Crohns. Colitis.* 9 (8), 633–639. doi:10.1093/ecco-jcc/jjv080

Haller, S. T., Yan, Y., Drummond, C. A., Xie, J., Tian, J., Kennedy, D. J., et al. (2016). Rifamycin attenuates cardiac fibrosis in experimental uremic cardiomyopathy by reducing marinobufagenin levels and inhibiting downstream pro-fibrotic signaling. *J. Am. Heart Assoc.* 5 (10). doi:10.1161/JAHA.116.004106

Hassan, C., Zullo, A., De Francesco, V., Ierardi, E., Giustini, M., Pitidis, A., et al. (2007). Systematic review: endoscopic dilatation in Crohn's disease. *Aliment.*

Pharmacol. Ther. 26, (11–12), 1457–1464. doi:10.1111/j.1365-2036.2007.03532.x

Hu, D., Ren, J., Wang, G., Li, G., Liu, S., and Yan, D. (2014). Exclusive enteral nutritional therapy can relieve inflammatory bowel stricture in Crohn's disease. *J. Clin. Gastroenterol.* 48 (9), 790–795. doi:10.1097/MCG.0000000000000041

Kanazawa, A., Yamana, T., Okamoto, K., and Sahara, R. (2012). Risk factors for postoperative intra-abdominal septic complications after bowel resection in patients with Crohn's disease. *Dis. Colon. Rectum.* 55 (9), 957–962. doi:10.1097/DCR.0b013e3182617716

Massey, D. C., Bredin, F., and Parkes, M. (2008). Use of sirolimus (rapamycin) to treat refractory Crohn's disease. *Gut* 57 (9), 1294–1296. doi:10.1136/gut.2008.157297

Mathur, R., Alam, M. M., Zhao, X. F., Liao, Y., Shen, J., Morgan, S., et al. (2019). Induction of autophagy in Cx3cr1(+) mononuclear cells limits IL-23/IL-22 axis-mediated intestinal fibrosis. *Mucosal Immunol.* 12 (3), 612–623. doi:10.1038/s41385-019-0146-4

Mutalib, M., Borrelli, O., Blackstock, S., Kiparissi, F., Elawad, M., Shah, N., et al. (2014). The use of sirolimus (rapamycin) in the management of refractory inflammatory bowel disease in children. *J. Crohns. Colitis.* 8, (12), 1730–1734. doi:10.1016/j.crohns.2014.08.014

Nugent, F. W., and Roy, M. A. (1989). Duodenal Crohn's disease: an analysis of 89 cases. *Am. J. Gastroenterol.* 84, (3), 249–254

Reinisch, W., Panés, J., Lémann, M., Schreiber, S., Feagan, B., Schmidt, S., et al. (2008). A multicenter, randomized, double-blind trial of everolimus versus azathioprine and placebo to maintain steroid-induced remission in patients with moderate-to-severe active Crohn's disease. *Am. J. Gastroenterol.* 103 (9), 2284–2292. doi:10.1111/j.1572-0241.2008.02024.x

Rieder, F., Zimmermann, E. M., Remzi, F. H., and Sandborn, W. J. (2013). Crohn's disease complicated by strictures: a systematic review. *Gut* 62 (7), 1072–1084. doi:10.1136/gutjnl-2012-304353

Shen, B., Kochhar, G., Navaneethan, U., Farraye, F. A,, Schwartz, D. A., Iacucci, M., et al. (2020). Practical guidelines on endoscopic treatment for Crohn's disease strictures: a consensus statement from the global interventional inflammatory bowel disease group. *Lancet Gastroenterol. Hepatol.* 5 (4), 393–405. doi:10.1016/S2468-1253(19)30366-8

Singh, A., Agrawal, N., Kurada, S., Lopez, R., Kessler, H., Philpott, J., et al. (2017). Efficacy, safety, and long-term outcome of serial endoscopic balloon dilation for upper gastrointestinal crohn's disease-associated strictures-A cohort study. *J. Crohns. Colitis.* 11 (9), 1044–1051. doi:10.1093/ecco-jcc/jjx078

Taida, T., Nakagawa, T., Ohta, Y., Hamanaka, S., Okimoto, K., Saito, K., et al. (2018). Long-term outcome of endoscopic balloon dilatation for strictures in patients with crohn's disease. *Digestion* 98 (1), 26–32. doi:10.1159/000486591

Van Assche, G., Geboes, K., and Rutgeerts, P. (2004). Medical therapy for Crohn's disease strictures. *Inflamm. Bowel Dis.* 10 (1), 55–60. doi:10.1097/00054725-200401000-00009

Xu, Y., Tai, W., Qu, X., Wu, W., Li, Z., Deng, S., et al. (2017). Rifamycin protects against paraquat-induced pulmonary fibrosis: activation of Nrf2 signaling pathway. *Biochem. Biophys. Res. Commun.* 490 (2), 535–540. doi:10.1016/j.bbrc.2017.06.074

Zhang, T., Lu, G., Zhao, Z., Liu, Y., Shen, Q., Li, P., et al. (2020). Washed microbiota transplantation vs. manual fecal microbiota transplantation: clinical findings, animal studies and in vitro screening. *Protein cell* 11 (4), 251–266. doi:10.1007/s13238-019-00684-8

9

Inhibition of 5-Lipoxygenase in Hepatic Stellate Cells Alleviates Liver Fibrosis

Shiyun Pu [1,2†], Yanping Li [2†], Qinhui Liu [2], Xu Zhang [3], Lei Chen [1,2], Rui Li [1,2], Jinhang Zhang [1,2], Tong Wu [1,2], Qin Tang [1,2], Xuping Yang [1,2], Zijing Zhang [1,2], Ya Huang [1,2], Jiangying Kuang [1,2], Hong Li [1,2], Min Zou [1], Wei Jiang [4] and Jinhan He [1,2]*

[1]Department of Pharmacy and State Key Laboratory of Biotherapy, West China Hospital, Sichuan University, Chengdu, China, [2]Laboratory of Clinical Pharmacy and Adverse Drug Reaction, West China Hospital, Sichuan University, Chengdu, China, [3]Tianjin Key Laboratory of Metabolic Diseases and Department of Physiology, Tianjin Medical University, Tianjin, China, [4]Molecular Medicine Research Center, West China Hospital of Sichuan University, Chengdu, China

*Correspondence:
Jinhan He
jinhanhe@scu.edu.cn

†These authors have contributed equally to this work

Background and Purpose: Activation of hepatic stellate cells (HSC) is a central driver of liver fibrosis. 5-lipoxygenase (5-LO) is the key enzyme that catalyzes arachidonic acid into leukotrienes. In this study, we examined the role of 5-LO in HSC activation and liver fibrosis.

Main Methods: Culture medium was collected from quiescent and activated HSC for target metabolomics analysis. Exogenous leukotrienes were added to culture medium to explore their effect in activating HSC. Genetic ablation of 5-LO in mice was used to study its role in liver fibrosis induced by CCl_4 and a methionine-choline-deficient (MCD) diet. Pharmacological inhibition of 5-LO in HSC was used to explore the effect of this enzyme in HSC activation and liver fibrosis.

Key Results: The secretion of LTB_4 and LTC_4 was increased in activated vs. quiescent HSC. LTB_4 and LTC_4 contributed to HSC activation by activating the extracellular signal-regulated protein kinase pathway. The expression of 5-LO was increased in activated HSC and fibrotic livers of mice. Ablation of 5-LO in primary HSC inhibited both mRNA and protein expression of fibrotic genes. In vivo, ablation of 5-LO markedly ameliorated the CCl_4- and MCD diet-induced liver fibrosis and liver injury. Pharmacological inhibition of 5-LO in HSC by targeted delivery of the 5-LO inhibitor zileuton suppressed HSC activation and improved CCl_4- and MCD diet-induced hepatic fibrosis and liver injury. Finally, we found increased 5-LO expression in patients with non-alcoholic steatohepatitis and liver fibrosis.

Conclusion: 5-LO may play a critical role in activating HSC; genetic ablation or pharmacological inhibition of 5-LO improved CCl_4-and MCD diet-induced liver fibrosis.

Keywords: liver fibrosis, non-alcoholic steatohepatitis, α-SMA, ERK, zileuton

Abbreviations: ALT, alanine aminotransferase; AST, aspartate aminotransferase; 5-LO, 5-lipoxygenase; 5-HPETE, 5-hydroperoxyeicosatetraenoic acid; NASH, non-alcoholic steatohepatitis; MCD diet, methionine-choline-deficient diet; MCS diet, methionine-choline-supplied diet; CCl_4, carbon tetrachloride; IL, interleukin; HSC, hepatic stellate cell; α-SMA, alpha smooth muscle actin; LTA4, leukotriene A4; LTB4, leukotriene B4; LTC4, leukotriene C_4; TIMP-1/2, tissue inhibitor of metalloproteinase 1/2; TGF-β1, transforming growth factor-β1; PAI-1, plasminogen activator inhibitor 1; Flaps, 5-LO-activating proteins; ERK, extracellular signal-regulated protein kinase; MCP-1, monocyte chemoattractant protein 1; TNF-α, tumor necrosis factor alpha.

INTRODUCTION

Liver fibrosis is a common outcome of chronic liver injury such as chronic hepatotoxicity and non-alcoholic steatohepatitis (NASH) (Yu et al., 2018). If unmanaged, liver fibrosis can advance to cirrhosis and portal hypertension and often requires liver transplantation.

Hepatic stellate cells (HSC) play a key role in the formation of hepatic fibrosis (Higashi et al., 2017). In normal liver, HSC stay quiescent (Ogawa et al., 2007). With injurious stimuli, HSC transdifferentiate from a quiescent to activated state (Puche et al., 2013), becoming proliferative and producing a high amount of α-smooth muscle actin (α-SMA) and collagens (De Minicis et al., 2008). When this extracellular matrix accumulates excessively, it causes a fibrotic outcome and scars on the liver (Wu et al., 2018). The mechanism of HSC activation is not fully understood. Several signaling pathways participate in activating HSC (Woodhoo et al., 2012). Transforming growth factor-β (TGF-β) induces the phosphorylation of Smad2/3, which in turn promotes HSC activation and regulates the expression of fibrotic genes (Feng and Derynck, 2005). Activation of extracellular signal-regulated kinase (ERK) also contributes to HSC activation (Chen et al., 2016; Xie et al., 2017).

Arachidonic acid is the precursor of biologically and clinically important eicosanoids (Harizi et al., 2008). 5-lipoxygenase (5-LO) is the key enzyme that catalyzes arachidonic acid into leukotrienes (Alexander et al., 2011). Upon activation of 5-LO-activating protein (Flap), 5-LO oxidases arachidonic acid to the unstable intermediate 5-hydroperoxyeicosatetraenoic acid (5-HPETE), which is further dehydrated to form leukotriene A4 (LTA$_4$) (Silverman and Drazen, 1999). LTA$_4$ is converted to LTB$_4$ via LTA$_4$ hydrolase enzymes or to LTC$_4$ via LTC$_4$ synthase (Hofmann and Steinhilber, 2013). Both LTB$_4$ and LTC$_4$ are inflammatory lipid mediators that have important effects on the development of allergic rhinitis, bronchial asthma and atherosclerosis (Kowal et al., 2017). Inhibiting 5-LO by an inhibitor such as zileuton or blocking the effect of leukotrienes by their receptor antagonist such as montelukast, have been clinically used for asthma treatment (De Corso et al., 2019).

Recent studies indicated that the 5-LO pathway is associated with fibrosis (Qian et al., 2015; Su et al., 2016). 5-LO is expressed in human dermal fibroblasts, synovial fibroblasts, pulmonary fibroblasts and rat adventitial fibroblasts (Lin et al., 2014; Su et al., 2016). Activation of these cells can be restrained by 5-LO inhibitors (Lin et al., 2014; Su et al., 2016). LTB$_4$ and LTC$_4$ are secreted from lung fibroblasts (Shiratori et al., 1989; Paiva et al., 2010) and contribute to the proliferation and migration of these cells (Hirata et al., 2013). However, the role of 5-LO in HSC activation and liver fibrosis remains unknown.

In this study, we first used metabolomics to reveal that LTB$_4$ and LTC$_4$ are highly secreted during the activation of HSC. Secreted LTB$_4$ and LTC$_4$ promoted HSC activation via an ERK signaling pathway. Ablation or inhibition of 5-LO could suppress HSC activation. In mouse fibrotic models, ablation or targeted inhibition of 5-LO in HSC relieved liver fibrosis and injury. Finally, we found increased expression of 5-LO in liver sections of patients with NASH and fibrosis.

MATERIALS AND METHODS

CCl$_4$- and Methionine-Choline–Deficient Diet-Induced Models of Liver Fibrosis

For CCl$_4$-induced liver fibrosis, 8-week-old C57 BL/6J (WT) and 5-lipoxygenase knockout (5-LO$^{-/-}$) mice received an intraperitoneal (i.p.) injection of CCl$_4$ (1 ml/kg body weight) twice a week. For MCD diet-induced liver fibrosis, WT and 5-LO$^{-/-}$ mice were fed a methionine-choline-supplied (MCS) or MCD diet (TROPHIC Animal Feed High-Tech, China) for 6 weeks. For therapeutic experiments, zileuton loaded in cRGDyK (Cyclo [Arg-Gly-Asp-$_D$Tyr-Lys])-guided liposome (RGD-Lip; 10 mg/kg) or vehicle was given by tail vein injection once every 3 days during the last 4 weeks of CCl$_4$ or MCD diet treatment. All mice were housed at West China Hospital, Sichuan University in accordance with the guidelines of the animal care utilization committee of the institute. Food and water were freely available to mice, except otherwise stated.

Preparation and Characterization of RGD-Lips

Liposome (Lip) were prepared by the thin-film hydration method as described (Li et al., 2019; Zhang et al., 2020). Zileuton-loaded RGD-Lips (RGD-Lip/zileuton) were prepared by adding zileuton to the lipid organic solution before the solvent evaporation. The mean particle size and zeta potential of Lip were measured by dynamic light scattering with the Zetasizer Nano ZS90 instrument (Malvern, United Kingdom). The morphology of Lip was examined by transmission electron microscopy (H-600, Hitachi, Japan) with 2% phosphotungstic acid staining.

Serum Alanine Aminotransferase and Aspartate Aminotransferase Measurement

Serum ALT and AST levels were detected by using commercial kits (BioSino Bio-Technology and Science).

Hydroxyproline Assay

An amount of 50 mg liver tissue was dissolved in acid hydrolysate in glass tube and heated in boiling water bath for 20 min. Hydroxyproline was extracted according to the manufacturer's instructions and measured by using kits (Nanjing Jiancheng Bioengineering Institute).

Histology Analysis

The left lobe of the mouse liver was removed and immediately fixed in 10% neutral-buffered formalin, embedded in paraffin, and sectioned at 4 μm. Liver sections were stained with hematoxylin and eosin (H&E). For picrosirius red staining, liver sections were incubated with 0.1% sirius red in saturated picric acid for 60 min at room temperature. The Sirus Red positive area were detected by Image J. Fibrosis was assessed by picrosirius red staining according to the Ishak fibrosis criteria (Ishak et al., 1995).

Isolation and Culture of HSC

HSC were isolated from livers of WT mice and 5-LO$^{-/-}$ mice via *in situ* collagenase perfusion and underwent differential centrifugation on Optiprep (Sigma) density gradients, as described (Kwon et al., 2014). Isolated HSC were cultured in collagen-coated dishes with DMEM supplemented with 10% fetal bovine serum and antibiotics at 37°C. The purity of HSC was >95% as determined by their typical star-like shape and abundant lipid droplets.

Measurement of Zileuton Concentration in Different Types of Liver Cells

Mice were injected with CCl_4 to cause liver fibrosis and treated with RGD-Lip/zileuton (10 mg/kg) for 4 h. Primary hepatocytes were isolated as described (Chen et al., 2019). The remaining cells were divided into three groups, fixed, perforated and stained with anti-α-SMA (HSC), anti-F4/80 (Kupffer cells) and anti-CD31 antibodies. HSC, Kupffer cells and LSECs were sorted by flow cytometry. Biliary epithelial cells were isolated as previously described (Li et al., 2019). Before extraction, cells were added to 30 μl ddH_2O and underwent repeated freezing and thawing 5 times. A 25-μl aliquot of samples was added to a 1.5-ml polypropylene tube followed by 200 μl methanol. The mixture was vortex-mixed for 5 min and centrifuged at 14,000 rpm for 10 min at room temperature. The top layer was transferred to a new 1.5 ml polypropylene tube and evaporated to vacuum dryness at 37°C. Samples were re-dissolved with 50 μl 80% methanol. The mixture was vortex-mixed for 30 s and centrifuged at 14,000 rpm for 5 min at 4°C. The 40-μl supernatant was transferred to a 250 μl polypropylene autosampler vial and sealed with a Teflon crimp cap. Partially purified cell samples were analyzed by using LC-MS/MS.

Systematic Metabolomic Analysis of Arachidonic Acid in 5-Lipoxygenase Pathway

Serum-free supernatant from primary mouse HSC were collected in an ice bath and extracted by solid-phase extraction. The metabolomics of arachidonic acid were detected and analyzed as described (Zhang et al., 2015).

LTB$_4$ and LTC$_4$ Measurement

Serum-free primary mouse HSC were collected in an ice bath and protected from light. Samples were centrifuged (600 × g, 5 min, 4°C), and with the resulting supernatant, LTB$_4$ and LTC$_4$ levels were determined by using ELISA kits (Cayman Chemical).

Immunofluorescence Staining

Primary HSC were fixed in 4% paraformaldehyde for 15 min, incubated in 0.2% Triton X-100 1×PBS for 15 min for permeabilization of cytomembrane. Antigens in paraffin sections were repaired by microwaving in 0.01 M citrate buffer (pH = 6.0) for 15 min. Both cells and tissue samples were incubated with antibodies in 4°C for 12 h. Immunoreactive compounds were incubated in room temperature for 1 h for conjugating with fluorescence-labeling secondary antibodies. All antibodies used in these experiments are in Supplementary **Supplementary Table S1**.

Western Blot Analysis

Western blot analysis was performed as described (Chen et al., 2019). The antibodies were listed in supplementary **Supplementary Table S1**. The expression of β-tubulin was a loading control. Immunoreactive bands were visualized on nitrocellulose membranes by using fluorescence-conjugated secondary antibodies (LI-COR, United States). The relative density was calculated by the ratio of the density of the protein of interest to β-tubulin.

Real-Time PCR Analyses

Total RNA isolation and PT-PCR was performed as described (Chen et al., 2019). The primers for detected genes are in **Supplementary Table S2**.

Statistical Analysis

Experiments were repeated at least 3 times with similar results. Quantitative results are expressed as the mean ± SEM. Statistical significance was determined by Student's unpaired two-tailed t test or one-way ANOVA multiple comparison test as indicated in legends. $p < 0.05$ was considered statistically significant.

RESULTS

LTB$_4$ and LTC$_4$ were Enriched in Supernatant of A-HSC

To explore the potential role of lipoxygenase pathway in arachidonic acid during HSC activation, we collected cell supernatants from quiescent HSC (q-HSC) and activated HSC (a-HSC, culture activated for 7 days) (Thi Thanh Hai et al., 2018). Among metabolites identified in the lipoxygenase pathway, target metabolomics revealed that LTB$_4$ level was selectively increased in a-HSC (**Supplementary Figure S1**). ELISA further confirmed the increased LTB$_4$ level in the supernatant of a-HSC (**Figure 1A**). Consistently, the level of LTC$_4$, another metabolite of 5-LO, was also increased (**Figure 1B**).

LTB$_4$ and LTC$_4$ Contributed to Activating HSC via Phosphorylation of the ERK Pathway

The high level of LTB$_4$ and LTC$_4$ released by a-HSC prompted us to explore their function in activating HSC. To exclude the influence of endogenous LTB$_4$ and LTC$_4$, we isolated primary HSC from 5-LO$^{-/-}$ mice and added exogenous LTB$_4$ or LTC$_4$ to these cells for 4 days. Treatment with LTB$_4$ or LTC$_4$ significantly increased the expression of fibrotic genes including α-SMA, collagen 1a1 (Col1a1), Col3a1, Col5a1, tissue inhibitor of metalloproteinase 1 (Timp-1) and plasminogen activator inhibitor 1 (PAI-1) (**Figures 1C,D**). On immunofluorescence staining, LTB$_4$ and LTC$_4$ increased α-SMA accumulation in HSC as compared with controls (**Figure 1E**). Western blot analysis

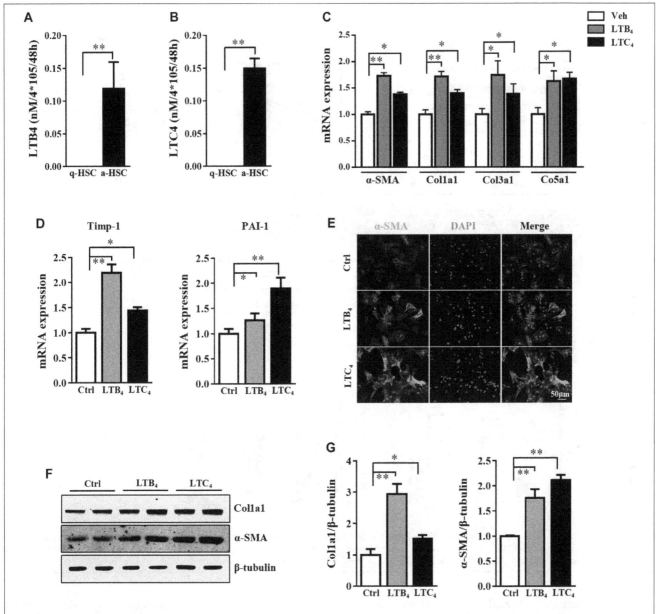

FIGURE 1 | LTB$_4$ and LTC$_4$ levels were elevated during HSC activation and promote HSC activation. **(A,B)** Primary HSC were isolated from wild-type (WT) mice and cultured for 2 days (quiescent HSC [q-HSC]) or 7 days (activated HSC [a-HSC]). ELISA detection of secretion of LTB$_4$ and LTC$_4$ in supernatant from q-HSC or a-HSC. **(C–G)** Primary HSC were isolated from 5-LO$^{-/-}$ mice and cultured in DMEM with high glucose with 10% heat-inactivated fetal bovine serum for 2 days. Cells were co-cultured with vehicle (Veh), LTB$_4$, or LTC$_4$ for 4 days. **(C,D)** qRT-PCR analysis of mRNA levels of fibrotic genes. **(E)** Immunofluorescence analysis of effect of LTB$_4$ or LTC$_4$ treatment on α-SMA expression. **(F,G)** The protein level of α-SMA and Col1a1 protein. Data are mean ± SEM, n = 5, *$p < 0.05$, **$p < 0.01$.

further confirmed that LTB$_4$ and LTC$_4$ elevated the protein levels of α-SMA and Col1a1 (**Figures 1F,G**). Therefore, LTB$_4$ or LTC$_4$ could promote HSC activation. We next explored the signaling pathway conveying the effect of LTB$_4$ or LTC$_4$. LTB$_4$ or LTC$_4$ seemed not to induce the phosphorylation of Smad2/3, a key pathway molecule for TGF-β-induced fibrosis (**Supplementary Figure S2A**). Instead, we found that LTB$_4$ and LTC$_4$ induced phosphorylation of the ERK1 signaling pathway (**Figures 2A,B**). The phosphorylation of ERK is necessary for LTB$_4$- and LTC$_4$-induced fibrosis because PD98059, a mitogen-activated protein kinase inhibitor, abolished their effects (**Figures 2C,D**;

Supplementary Figure S2B). Other MAP kinases, according to p-p38 and p-JNK, were no change after LTB$_4$ or LTC$_4$ administration (**Supplementary Figure S2C**). Therefore, the effect of LTB4 and LTC4 on HSC may be mediated by ERK1 signaling.

5-LO was Upregulated and Promoted HSC Activation

5-LO is the key enzyme in the synthesis of LTB$_4$ and LTC$_4$ (Alexander et al., 2011). We further investigated whether the high

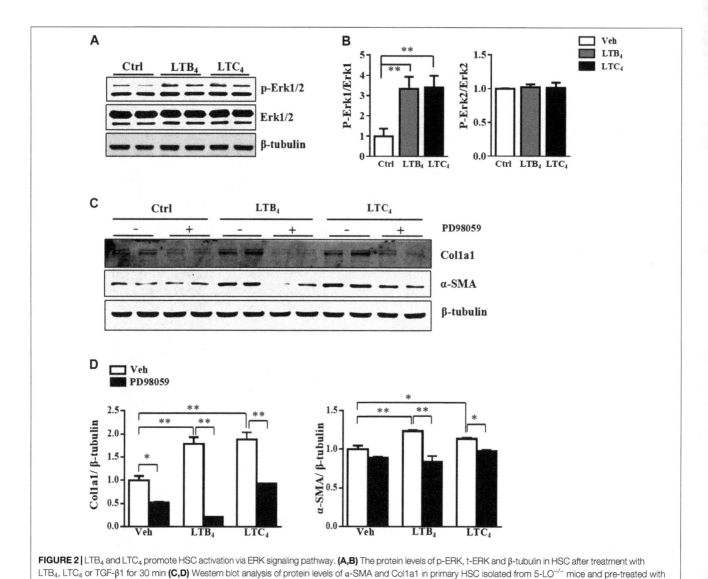

FIGURE 2 | LTB$_4$ and LTC$_4$ promote HSC activation via ERK signaling pathway. **(A,B)** The protein levels of p-ERK, t-ERK and β-tubulin in HSC after treatment with LTB$_4$, LTC$_4$ or TGF-β1 for 30 min **(C,D)** Western blot analysis of protein levels of α-SMA and Col1a1 in primary HSC isolated from 5-LO$^{-/-}$ mice and pre-treated with PD98059 before administration of LTB$_4$ or LTC$_4$. Data are mean ± SEM, n = 5, *$p < 0.05$, **$p < 0.01$.

level of LTB$_4$ and LTC$_4$ released by a-HSC resulted from the increased expression of 5-LO. The mRNA and protein levels of 5-LO were significantly upregulated in a-HSC as compared with q-HSC (**Figures 3A–C**). In contrast, the expression of Flap was not changed by HSC activation (**Figure 3B**). In CCl$_4$-induced liver fibrosis, 5-LO was also significantly increased along with other fibrotic genes (**Figures 3D–F**). Again, Flap expression was not significantly changed (**Figure 3E**). Liver fibrosis occurs during the progression of non-alcoholic steatohepatitis (NASH) (Nasr et al., 2018). Both the mRNA and protein levels of 5-LO were increased in an independent model of MCD diet-induced NASH (Anstee and Goldin, 2006) (**Supplementary Figures S3A–C**). These results suggest that increased 5-LO level may be responsible for the high level of LTB$_4$ and LTC$_4$ in a-HSC.

To further investigate the effect of 5-LO in HSC activation, we isolated primary HSC from wild-type and 5-LO$^{-/-}$ mice, then compared the expression of fibrotic genes after culture activation.

Ablation of 5-LO significantly inhibited the expression of culture-induced fibrotic genes, such as α-SMA, Col1a1, Col3a1, Col5a1, Timp1 and PAI-1 (**Figures 4A,B**), indicating that 5-LO was involved in HSC activation. Inhibition of HSC activation was confirmed by immunofluorescent staining, which showed the expression of α-SMA less detectable in 5-LO$^{-/-}$ HSC (**Figure 4C**). Western blot analysis revealed that ablation of 5-LO suppressed α-SMA and Col1a1 expression (**Figures 4D,E**). The incubation of supernatant from WT a-HSC (WT-CM) was more effective to activate HSC than that from 5-LO$^{-/-}$ a-HSC (5-LO$^{-/-}$-CM) (**Supplementary Figures S4A,B**).

Genetic Ablation of 5-LO Ameliorated CCl$_4$- and MCD Diet-Induced Liver Fibrosis, Inflammation and Hepatic Injury

To explore the *in vivo* function of 5-LO in liver fibrosis, we first exposed WT and 5-LO$^{-/-}$ mice to CCl$_4$ twice a week for 8 weeks

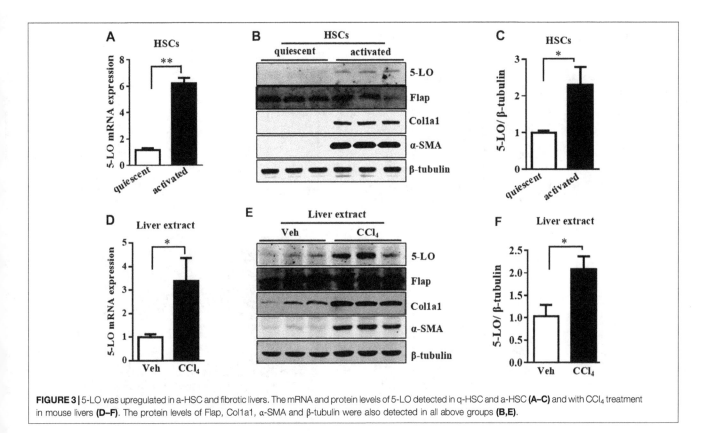

FIGURE 3 | 5-LO was upregulated in a-HSC and fibrotic livers. The mRNA and protein levels of 5-LO detected in q-HSC and a-HSC **(A–C)** and with CCl₄ treatment in mouse livers **(D–F)**. The protein levels of Flap, Col1a1, α-SMA and β-tubulin were also detected in all above groups **(B,E)**.

by intraperitoneal injection. As expected, CCl₄ caused significant hepatic fibrosis as compared with olive oil, as assessed by picrosirius red staining (**Figures 5A,B**). In contrast, 5-LO⁻/⁻ mice showed improved liver fibrosis and decreased hepatic fibrosis scores (**Figure 5C**). Consistently, the level of hydroxyproline was significantly lower in 5-LO⁻/⁻ than WT mice (**Figure 5D**), which suggests that 5-LO deletion conferred resistance to CCl₄-induced hepatic fibrosis. Among the fibrotic markers, α-SMA, collagens, TGF-β1, Timp-1/2 and PAI-1 were greatly suppressed in 5-LO⁻/⁻ mice after CCl₄ treatment (**Figures 5E,F**). The protein levels of α-SMA and Col1a1 were also greatly reduced in 5-LO⁻/⁻ mice with chronic CCl₄ injection (**Figure 5G**). CCl₄ administration showed an increasing serum levels of ALT and AST (**Supplementary Figure S5A**). However, this liver injury was significantly decreased in 5-LO⁻/⁻ mice. Chronic liver injury accelerated the accumulation of inflammatory cells around the vessels (**Supplementary Figure S5B**). Ablation of 5-LO greatly suppressed CCl₄-induced inflammatory cell infiltration (**Supplementary Figures S5B,C**). These results were further supported by the decreased expression of inflammatory genes seen in the liver of 5-LO⁻/⁻ mice (**Supplementary Figure S5D**).

In another independent model of MCD diet-induced NASH, collagen deposition was reduced in livers of 5-LO⁻/⁻ mice along with decreased fibrosis scores and hydroxyproline levels (**Supplementary Figures S6A–D**). Improved liver fibrosis was further confirmed by gene expression and protein analysis. Indeed, 5-LO ablation decreased the mRNA levels of fibrotic genes (α-SMA, Col1a1, Col3a1, Col5a1, TGF-β1, Timp-1/2 and

PAI-1) (**Supplementary Figures S6E,F**) and the protein levels of α-SMA and Col1a1 (**Supplementary Figures S6G,H**). 5-LO ablation was protective in MCD-diet induced liver injury, as indicated by reduced serum levels of ALT and AST and inflammation scores (**Supplementary Figures S7A–C**). Inflammation plays an important role in MCD diet-induced NASH (Locatelli et al., 2014). Consistently, the mRNA levels of inflammatory genes including tumor necrosis factor α (TNF-α), interleukin 1β (IL-1β) and monocyte chemoattractant protein 1 (Mcp-1) were decreased in 5-LO⁻/⁻ mice (**Supplementary Figure S7D**). The hepatic expression of CD68, a marker of macrophages, was also reduced (**Supplementary Figure S7D**). Therefore, 5-LO ablation ameliorated CCl₄- and MCD diet-induced hepatic fibrosis, inflammation and liver injury.

Pharmacological Inhibition of 5-LO by Targeted Delivery Suppressed HSC Activation

The protective effect of 5-LO ablation prompted us to explore whether pharmacological inhibition of 5-LO would have a similar effect in restraining the activation of primary HSC. We used an HSC-specific drug delivery system by modifying sterically stable liposome (Lip) with cRGDyK, a pentapeptide that binds to integrin αvβ3 on the surface of a-HSC (Li et al., 2019). cRGDyK-guided Lip showed high selectivity toward activated but not quiescent HSC, and preferentially accumulated in the fibrotic liver (Li et al., 2019; Zhang et al., 2020). We loaded with zileuton, an

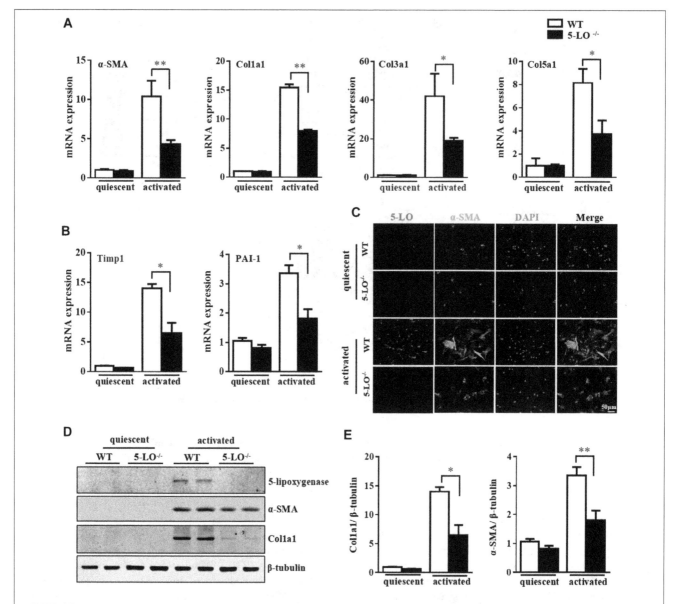

FIGURE 4 | Genetic ablation of 5-LO restrained activation of primary HSC. Primary HSC were isolated from WT and 5-LO $^{-/-}$ mice. **(A,B)** qRT-PCR of mRNA levels of fibrosis genes. **(C)** Immunofluorescence analysis of effect of 5-LO ablation on α-SMA expression. **(D,E)** Western blot analysis of α-SMA and Col1a1 protein levels in q-HSC and a-HSC. Data are mean ± SEM, n = 5, *$p < 0.05$, **$p < 0.01$.

inhibitor of 5-LO, into this delivery system (RGD-Lip/ zileuton). The schematic illustration, particle size, morphology and entrapment efficiency were comparable to regular liposome (**Supplementary Figures S8A,B**, **Supplementary Table S3**). As expected, RGD-Lip/zileuton significantly suppressed the secretion of LTB$_4$ by a-HSC (**Supplementary Figure S9**), which indicates the inhibition of 5-LO. In a-HSC, zileuton delivered by RGD-Lip greatly inhibited the expression of fibrotic genes including α-SMA, Col1a1, Col3a1, Col5a1, Timp-1 and PAI-1 (**Figures 6A,B**). These effects were further confirmed by immunofluorescent staining and western blot analysis (**Figures 6C–E**). Therefore,

pharmacological inhibition of 5-LO suppressed HSC activation.

Targeted Delivery of Zileuton to HSC Is Efficient Against Liver Fibrosis

We then evaluated the *in vivo* therapeutic effect of RGD-Lip/ zileuton in CCl$_4$-and MCD diet-induced liver fibrosis. In this experiment, mice were injected with CCl$_4$ for 4 weeks, then treated with RGD-Lip/zileuton (10 mg/kg) every 3 days (**Supplementary Figure S10A**). RGD-Lip could specifically deliver zileuton to HSC because the concentration of zileuton

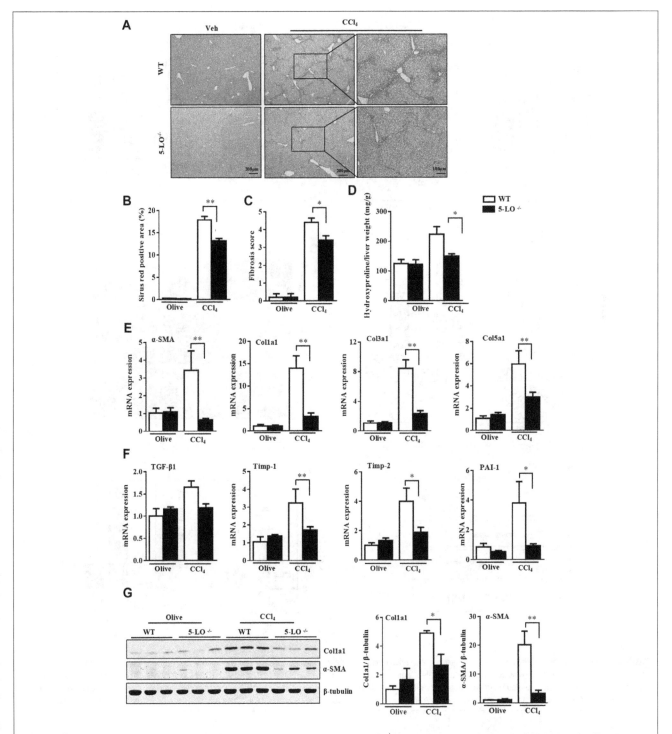

FIGURE 5 | Genetic ablation of 5-LO ameliorated liver fibrosis after CCl_4 injection. WT and 5-LO $^{-/-}$ mice were treated with olive oil or CCl_4 for 8 weeks. Fibrosis stage was assessed by picrosirius red staining **(A,B)** for collagen according to the Ishak criteria **(C)**. **(D)** Detection of hepatic hydroxyproline level. **(E,F)** qRT-PCR analysis of mRNA levels of fibrosis genes in livers of 4 groups. **(G)** Western blot analysis of the protein levels of α-SMA and Col1a1. Data are mean ± SEM, n = 7, *$p < 0.05$, **$p < 0.01$.

in HSC was about 28.99-, 4.71-, 4.67- and 34.01-times higher than that in hepatocytes, Kupffer cells, endothelial cells and biliary epithelial cells, respectively (**Supplementary Figure S10B**). Specific inactivation of 5-LO by RGD-Lip/zileuton in HSC

greatly decreased liver fibrosis as shown by picrosirius red staining and liver hydroxyproline quantification (**Figures 7A–D**). The expression of fibrotic genes such as α-SMA, Col1a1, Col3a1, Col5a1, Timp1 and PAI-1 was also mitigated

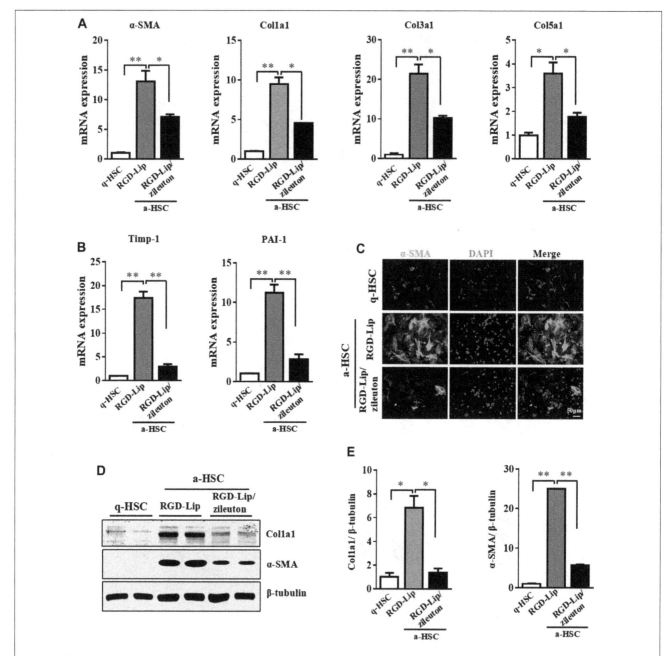

FIGURE 6 | Pharmacological inhibition of 5-LO suppressed activation of HSC. Primary HSC were isolated from WT mice and cultured in DMEM with high glucose and 10% heat-inactivated fetal bovine serum for 2 days (q-HSC) or 7 days (a-HSC). Primary HSC were treated with RGD-Lip or RGD-Lip/zileuton for 48 h **(A,B)** qRT-PCR analysis of effect of RGD-Lip/zileuton treatment on the mRNA expression of fibrotic genes. **(C)** Immunofluorescence analysis of effect of RGD-Lip/zileuton treatment on α-SMA expression. **(D,E)** Western blot analysis of α-SMA and Col1a1 protein levels in q-HSC and a-HSC. Data are mean ± SEM, n = 5, *p < 0.05, **p < 0.01.

(**Figures 6E,F**). Western blot analysis confirmed the reduced protein levels of Col1a1 and α-SMA (**Figures 6G,H**). Targeted inhibition of 5-LO in HSC also alleviated CCl$_4$-induced liver injury and hepatic inflammation (**Supplementary Figures S11A–C**), but did not reduce the accumulation of F4/80 positive cells (**Supplementary Figure S11D**).

The therapeutic effects of RGD-Lip/zileuton were further demonstrated in an MCD diet-induced NASH model (**Supplementary Figure S12**). Specific inactivation of 5-LO

in HSC explicitly alleviated MCD diet-induced liver fibrosis (**Supplementary Figures S13A–D**). Expression of fibrotic genes was suppressed in RGD-Lip/zileuton-treated mice (**Supplementary Figures S13E,F**) and α-SMA and collagen accumulation was reduced (**Supplementary Figures S13G,H**). Targeted delivery of zileuton also relieved liver injury in MCD-induced NASH (**Supplementary Figure S14A**). H&E staining and the expression of proinflammatory genes such as TNF-α and Mcp-1 indicated decreased inflammation in livers of

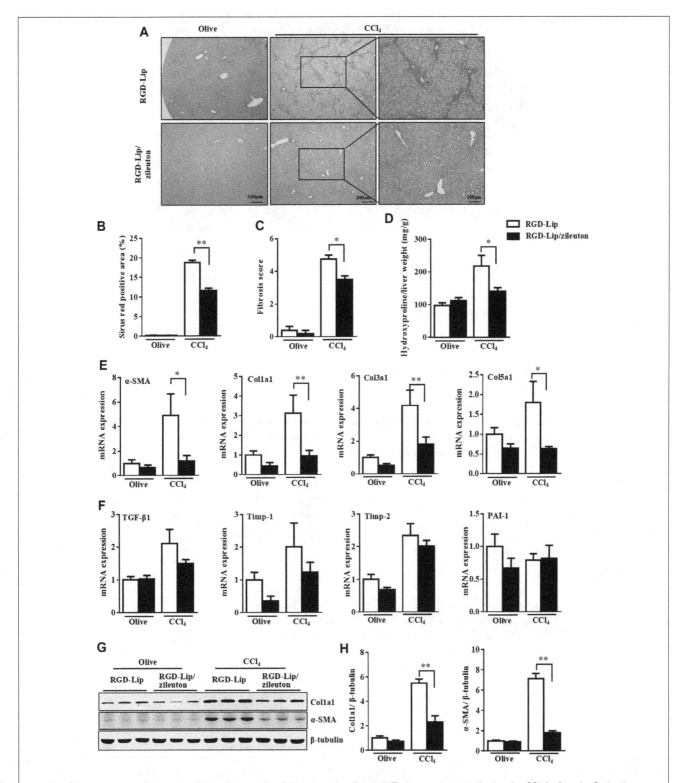

FIGURE 7 | Targeted delivery of zileuton to HSC is efficient against CCl$_4$-induced liver fibrosis. WT mice were treated with olive oil or CCl$_4$ for 8 weeks. During the last 4 weeks, mice given RGD-Lip or RGD-Lip/zileuton (10 mg/kg) every 3 days by tail vein injection. **(A,B)** Liver sections were collected for picrosirius red staining. **(C)** Fibrosis score was assessed for collagen according to the Ishak criteria. **(D)** Detection of hepatic hydroxyproline level. **(E,F)** qRT-PCR analysis of mRNA levels of fibrotic genes in livers of 4 groups. **(G)** Western blot analysis of the protein levels of α-SMA and Col1a1. Data are mean ± SEM, n = 7, *$p < 0.05$, **$p < 0.01$.

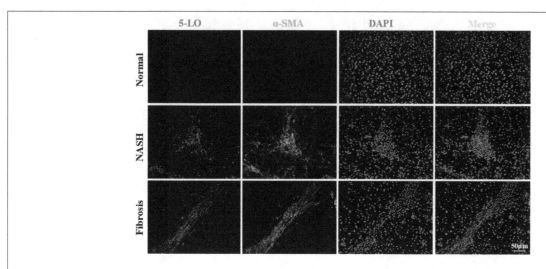

FIGURE 8 | The expression of 5-LO was increased in liver sections of patients with fibrosis. Liver sections were collected from normal individuals or patients with non-alcoholic steatohepatitis or liver fibrosis and were stained with 5-LO and α-SMA. Data are mean ± SEM, n = 3.

RGD-Lip/zileuton-treated mice (**Supplementary Figures S14B–D**).

Increased Expression of 5-LO in Patients with Hepatic Fibrosis

We next determined whether 5-LO expression was changed in patients with NASH or liver fibrosis. The diagnosis of NASH and fibrosis was confirmed by H&E and picrosirius red staining (**Supplementary Figures S15A–C**). As compared with healthy individuals, the expression of 5-LO was increased in liver sections from patients with NASH and fibrosis (**Figure 8**). The expression of 5-LO was largely co-localized in α-SMA-positive cells, which were HSC (**Figure 8**). These results were consistent with 5-LO possibly having a positive role in activation of HSC in rodents.

DISCUSSION

In this study, we found increased secretion of LTB$_4$ and LTC$_4$ in a-HSC. LTB$_4$ and LTC$_4$ contributed to HSC activation via ERK signaling. Elevated LTB$_4$ and LTC$_4$ was likely a result of increased expression of 5-LO during HSC activation. Genetic ablation of 5-LO protected mice against CCl$_4$- and MCD diet-induced fibrosis and liver injury. Pharmacological inhibition of 5-LO in HSC by targeted delivery of zileuton prevented CCl$_4$- and MCD diet-induced liver fibrosis. Finally, we found 5-LO level increased in liver sections of patients with liver fibrosis.

Several reports have suggested that 5-LO may play a role in fibrosis (Titos et al., 2004). 5-LO is expressed in various fibroblast cells, such as pulmonary fibroblasts, human myofibroblasts and skin fibroblasts (Nagy et al., 2011; Xiao et al., 2011) (Su et al., 2016). Titos et al. found 5-LO expressed in Kupffer cells (Titos et al., 2004). Pharmacological inhibition of 5-LO protected mice from CCl$_4$-induced liver fibrosis (Horrillo et al., 2007). However, the following study could not confirm the expression of 5-LO in

Kupffer cells (Takeda et al., 2017). Also, 5-LO expression was detected in HSC isolated from mice and rats (Paiva et al., 2010; Shajari et al., 2015). However, the function of 5-LO in HSC was not known. In our study, we found 5-LO expressed in HSC, and its expression was increased during their activation. With increased expression of 5-LO, the secretion of LTB$_4$ and LTC$_4$ was significantly elevated in a-HSC (**Figures 1A,B; Supplementary Figure S1**). LTB$_4$ and LTC$_4$ promoted HSC activation via ERK1 signaling pathway. This finding was consistent with a previous report of LTB$_4$ and LTC$_4$ leading to pulmonary fibrosis because of stimulating the activation and differentiation of fibroblasts (Hirata et al., 2013). Other lipoxygenases, such as 12-lipoxygenase, was also upregulated in a-HSC compared with q-HSC (Mori et al., 2020). However, we did not found the difference of 12-HETE, a metabolic of arachidonic acid through 12-lipoxygease, in q-HSC and a-HSC supernatant (**Supplementary Figure S1**). The role of 12-lipoxygenase in HSC deserves further study.

Liver fibrosis homeostasis is maintained by the balance of extracellular matrix synthetic machinery, contributing to increased rate of collagen synthesis and activities of the cellular fibrinolytic system. Timp-1 belongs to the Timp family and participates in degrading the extracellular matrix (Iredale, 2007). PAI-1 is a member of the serine protease inhibitor family, the main physiological inhibitor of serine protease, and contributes to the fibrinolytic system (Wang et al., 2007). Several studies have shown that Timp-1 and PAI-1 are key factors modulating fibrolysis and extracellular matrix deposition (Iredale, 2007; Wang et al., 2007). Knockout or pharmacological inhibition of Timp1 and PAI-1 inhibited fibrosis in liver (Parsons et al., 2004). Our in vitro results showed significantly increased expression of Timp-1 and PAI-1 in culture-activated HSC as compared with q-HSC. However, genetic ablation of 5-LO in HSC decreased levels of Timp1 and PAI-1, which may contribute to suppressed extracellular matrix deposition. *In vivo*, 5-LO ablation or pharmacological inhibition reduced the Timp-1 and PAI-1 expression, which helped reduce hydroxyproline level in mouse liver.

Oral treatment or injection of the 5-LO inhibitor zileuton causes systemic pharmacological side effects. Zileuton could increase oxidative stress in hepatocytes and may cause hepatocyte damage (Altumina, 1995). In addition, zileuton treatment was found to increase serum ALT and AST levels (Watkins et al., 2007). These results suggest that systemic zileuton administration may cause drug-induced side effects. cRGD is pentapeptide that binds with high affinity to integrin αV and β3 which are highly expressed in a-HSC (Li et al., 2019). It was also confirmed that cRGD-guided Lips specifically target activated HSC *in vitro* and *vivo* (Li et al., 2019; Zhang et al., 2020). In agreement with a previous report, we found that RGD-Lip-delivered zileuton was highly enriched in HSC but not hepatocytes, Kupffer cells, endothelial cells or biliary cells (**Supplementary Figure S9B**). RGD-Lip/zileuton administration significantly protected mice against CCl_4-and MCD diet-induced liver fibrosis (**Figure 7**; **Supplementary Figure S12**). Therefore, targeted delivery of zileuton to inhibit 5-LO by RGD-Lip may be a promising way to manage liver fibrosis.

Obviously, both CCl_4 and MCD-diet treatments induce inflammation, which were reduced by 5-LO ablation or RGD/Lip-zileuton administration. Horrillo et al. also found that 5-LO inhibitor protected mice from CCl_4-induced liver inflammation (Horrillo et al., 2007). In our study, knockout of 5-LO did reduce the accumulation of F4/80 positive cells in fibrotic liver (**Supplementary Figure S5C**). However, treatment of RGD/Lip-zileuton did not reduce the accumulation of F4/80 positive cells (**Supplementary Figure S11D**). It was reported that activation of HSC mediated immune response (Chou et al., 2011; Chang et al., 2013; Bigorgne et al., 2016). We speculate that the beneficial effect of RGD/Lip-zileuton is more due to reduce in the HSC fibrosis compartment than reduced inflammation in the Kupffer cell compartment. The changes of these inflammatory indicators are related to the decrease of HSC activation.

LTB_4 and LTC_4 were reported as lipid mediators for attracting neutrophils and for lipid accumulation (Lund et al., 2017). Induction of LTB_4 and LTC_4 biosynthesis might cause hepatotoxicity via neutrophil activation (Shiratori et al., 1989; Takeda et al., 2017). 5-LO is the key enzyme that catalyzes arachidonic acid to form LTB_4 and LTC_4 (Alexander et al., 2011). In our study, both deletion of 5-LO and targeted inhibition of 5-LO in HSC protected mice against CCl_4-and MCD diet-induced liver injury, at least in part by reducing LTB_4 and LTC_4 production in the liver.

In summary, we demonstrate that 5-LO inhibition confers resistance to CCl_4- and MCD diet-induced hepatic fibrosis. The protective effect of 5-LO deletion was partially due to decreased level of LTB_4 as well as LTC_4 and reduced activation of HSC. Our data show that 5-LO is critical for liver fibrosis in the setting of supporting HSC activation. 5-LO expression was also increased in HSC in liver sections of patients with fibrosis. Strategies to target inhibition of 5-LO in HSC may be useful for treating liver fibrosis.

ETHICS STATEMENT

Ethical review and approval was not required for the study on human participants in accordance with the local legislation and institutional requirements. Written informed consent for participation was not required for this study in accordance with the national legislation and institutional requirements. The animal study was reviewed and approved by the Animal Care and Utilization Committee of West China Hospital.

AUTHOR CONTRIBUTIONS

Participated in research design: SP, YL and JH. Conducted experiments: SP, YL, QL, XZ, LC, RL, JZ, TW, QT, XY, ZZ, YH, JK, and HL. Performed data analysis: MZ and WJ. Wrote or contributed to the writing of the manuscript: SP, YL, and JH.

ACKNOWLEDGMENTS

The authors thank Miss Huifang Li and Miss Ge Liang from Core Facility of West China Hospital for technical assistance.

REFERENCES

Alexander, S. P., Mathie, A., and Peters, J. A. (2011). Guide to receptors and channels (GRAC), 5th edition. *Br. J. Pharmacol.* 164 (1), S1–S3. doi:10.1111/j.1476-5381.2011.01649_1.x

Altumina, M. M. (1995). Several characteristics of the pulmonary *tuberculosis* course in patients with different degree of diabetes mellitus compensation. *Probl. Tuberk.* 6,15–17.

Anstee, Q. M., and Goldin, R. D. (2006). Mouse models in non-alcoholic fatty liver disease and steatohepatitis research. *Int. J. Exp. Pathol.* 87, 1–16. doi:10.1111/j.0959-9673.2006.00465.x

Bigorgne, A. E., John, B., Ebrahimkhani, M. R., Shimizu-Albergine, M., Campbell, J. S., and Crispe, I. N. (2016). TLR4-Dependent secretion by hepatic stellate cells of the neutrophil-chemoattractant CXCL1 mediates liver response to gut microbiota. *PLoS One* 11, e0151063. doi:10.1371/journal.pone.0151063

Chang, J., Hisamatsu, T., Shimamura, K., Yoneno, K., Adachi, M., Naruse, H., et al. (2013). Activated hepatic stellate cells mediate the differentiation of macrophages. *Hepatol. Res.* 43, 658–669. doi:10.1111/j.1872-034X.2012.01111.x

Chen, L., Liu, Q., Tang, Q., Kuang, J., Li, H., Pu, S., et al. (2019). Hepatocyte-specific Sirt6 deficiency impairs ketogenesis. *J. Biol. Chem.* 294, 1579–1589. doi:10.1074/jbc.RA118.005309

Chen, Q., Chen, L., Kong, D., Shao, J., Wu, L., and Zheng, S. (2016). Dihydroartemisinin alleviates bile duct ligation-induced liver fibrosis and hepatic stellate cell activation by interfering with the PDGF-βR/ERK signaling pathway. *Int. Immunopharm.* 34, 250–258. doi:10.1016/j.intimp.2016.03.011

Chou, H. S., Hsieh, C. C., Yang, H. R., Wang, L., Arakawa, Y., Brown, K., et al. (2011). Hepatic stellate cells regulate immune response by way of induction of myeloid suppressor cells in mice. *Hepatology* 53, 1007–1019. doi:10.1002/hep.24162

De Corso, E., Anzivino, R., Galli, J., Baroni, S., Di Nardo, W., De Vita, C., et al. (2019). Antileukotrienes improve naso-ocular symptoms and biomarkers in patients with NARES and asthma. *Laryngoscope* 129, 551–557. doi:10.1002/lary. 27576

De Minicis, S., Candelaresi, C., Marzioni, M., Saccomano, S., Roskams, T., Casini, A., et al. (2008). Role of endogenous opioids in modulating HSC activity *in vitro* and liver fibrosis *in vivo*. *Gut* 57, 352–364. doi:10.1136/gut.2007.120303

Feng, X. H., and Derynck, R. (2005). Specificity and versatility in tgf-beta signaling through Smads. *Annu. Rev. Cell Dev. Biol.* 21, 659–693. doi:10.1146/annurev. cellbio.21.022404.142018

Harizi, H., Corcuff, J. B., and Gualde, N. (2008). Arachidonic-acid-derived eicosanoids: roles in biology and immunopathology. *Trends Mol. Med.* 14, 461–469. doi:10.1016/j.molmed.2008.08.005

Higashi, T., Friedman, S. L., and Hoshida, Y. (2017). Hepatic stellate cells as key target in liver fibrosis. *Adv. Drug Deliv. Rev.* 121, 27–42. doi:10.1016/j.addr. 2017.05.007

Hirata, H., Arima, M., Fukushima, Y., Sugiyama, K., Tokuhisa, T., and Fukuda, T. (2013). Leukotriene C4 aggravates bleomycin-induced pulmonary fibrosis in mice. *Respirology* 18, 674–681. doi:10.1111/resp.12072

Hofmann, B., and Steinhilber, D. (2013). 5-Lipoxygenase inhibitors: a review of recent patents (2010-2012). *Expert Opin. Ther. Pat.* 23, 895–909. doi:10.1517/ 13543776.2013.791678

Horrillo, R., Planagumà, A., González-Périz, A., Ferré, N., Titos, E., Miquel, R., et al. (2007). Comparative protection against liver inflammation and fibrosis by a selective cyclooxygenase-2 inhibitor and a nonredox-type 5-lipoxygenase inhibitor. *J. Pharmacol. Exp. Therapeut.* 323, 778–786. doi:10.1124/jpet.107. 128264

Iredale, J. P. (2007). Models of liver fibrosis: exploring the dynamic nature of inflammation and repair in a solid organ. *J. Clin. Invest.* 117, 539–548. doi:10. 1172/JCI30542

Ishak, K., Baptista, A., Bianchi, L., Callea, F., De Groote, J., Gudat, F., et al. (1995). Histological grading and staging of chronic hepatitis. *J. Hepatol.* 22, 696–699. doi:10.1016/0168-8278(95)80226-6

Kowal, K., Gielicz, A., and Sanak, M. (2017). The effect of allergen-induced bronchoconstriction on concentration of 5-oxo-ETE in exhaled breath condensate of house dust mite-allergic patients. *Clin. Exp. Allergy* 47, 1253–1262. doi:10.1111/cea.12990

Kwon, H. J., Won, Y. S., Park, O., Chang, B., Duryee, M. J., Thiele, G. E., et al. (2014). Aldehyde dehydrogenase 2 deficiency ameliorates alcoholic fatty liver but worsens liver inflammation and fibrosis in mice. *Hepatology* 60, 146–157. doi:10.1002/hep.27036

Li, Y., Pu, S., Liu, Q., Li, R., Zhang, J., Wu, T., et al. (2019). An integrin-based nanoparticle that targets activated hepatic stellate cells and alleviates liver fibrosis. *J. Contr. Release* 303, 77–90. doi:10.1016/j.jconrel.2019.04.022

Lin, H. C., Lin, T. H., Wu, M. Y., Chiu, Y. C., Tang, C. H., Hour, M. J., et al. (2014). 5-Lipoxygenase inhibitors attenuate TNF-α-induced inflammation in human synovial fibroblasts. *PLoS One* 9, e107890. doi:10.1371/journal.pone.0107890

Locatelli, I., Sutti, S., Jindal, A., Vacchiano, M., Bozzola, C., Reutelingsperger, C., et al. (2014). Endogenous annexin A1 is a novel protective determinant in nonalcoholic steatohepatitis in mice. *Hepatology* 60, 531–544. doi:10.1002/hep. 27141

Lund, S. J., Portillo, A., Cavagnero, K., Baum, R. E., Naji, L. H., Badrani, J. H., et al. (2017). Leukotriene C4 potentiates IL-33-induced group 2 innate lymphoid cell activation and lung inflammation. *J. Immunol.* 199, 1096–1104. doi:10.4049/ jimmunol.1601569

Mori, Y., Kawakami, Y., Kanzaki, K., Otsuki, A., Kimura, H., Kanji, H., et al. (2020). Arachidonate 12S-lipoxygenase of platelet-type in hepatic stellate cells of methionine and choline-deficient diet-fed mice. *J. Biochem.* 168, 455–463. doi:10.1093/jb/mvaa062

Nagy, E., Andersson, D. C., Caidahl, K., Eriksson, M. J., Eriksson, P., Franco-Cereceda, A., et al. (2011). Upregulation of the 5-lipoxygenase pathway in human aortic valves correlates with severity of stenosis and leads to leukotriene-induced effects on valvular myofibroblasts. *Circulation* 123, 1316–1325. doi:10. 1161/CIRCULATIONAHA.110.966846

Nasr, P., Ignatova, S., Kechagias, S., and Ekstedt, M. (2018). Natural history of nonalcoholic fatty liver disease: a prospective follow-up study with serial biopsies. *Hepatol. Commun.* 2, 199 210. doi:10.1002/hep4.1134

Ogawa, T., Tateno, C., Asahina, K., Fujii, H., Kawada, N., Obara, M., et al. (2007). Identification of vitamin A-free cells in a stellate cell-enriched fraction of

normal rat liver as myofibroblasts. *Histochem. Cell Biol.* 127, 161–174. doi:10. 1007/s00418-006-0237-7

Paiva, L. A., Maya-Monteiro, C. M., Bandeira-Melo, C., Silva, P. M., El-Cheikh, M. C., Teodoro, A. J., et al. (2010). Interplay of cysteinyl leukotrienes and TGF-β in the activation of hepatic stellate cells from Schistosoma mansoni granulomas. *Biochim. Biophys. Acta.* 1801, 1341–1348. doi:10.1016/j.bbalip.2010.08.014

Parsons, C. J., Bradford, B. U., Pan, C. Q., Cheung, E., Schauer, M., Knorr, A., et al. (2004). Antifibrotic effects of a tissue inhibitor of metalloproteinase-1 antibody on established liver fibrosis in rats. *Hepatology* 40, 1106–1115. doi:10.1002/hep. 20425

Puche, J. E., Saiman, Y., and Friedman, S. L. (2013). Hepatic stellate cells and liver fibrosis. *Comp. Physiol.* 3, 1473–1492. doi:10.1002/cphy.c120035

Qian, J., Tian, W., Jiang, X., Tamosiuniene, R., Sung, Y. K., Shuffle, E. M., et al. (2015). Leukotriene B4 activates pulmonary artery adventitial fibroblasts in pulmonary hypertension. *Hypertension* 66, 1227–1239. doi:10.1161/ HYPERTENSIONAHA.115.06370

Shajari, S., Laliena, A., Heegsma, J., Tuñón, M. J., Moshage, H., and Faber, K. N. (2015). Melatonin suppresses activation of hepatic stellate cells through RORα-mediated inhibition of 5-lipoxygenase. *J. Pineal Res.* 59, 391–401. doi:10.1111/ jpi.12271

Shiratori, Y., Moriwaki, H., Muto, Y., Onishi, H., Kato, M., and Asano, F. (1989). Production of leukotriene B4 in parenchymal and sinusoidal cells of the liver in rats treated simultaneously with D-galactosamine and endotoxin. *Gastroenterol. Jpn.* 24, 640–645. doi:10.1007/BF02774162

Silverman, E. S., and Drazen, J. M. (1999). The biology of 5-lipoxygenase: function, structure, and regulatory mechanisms. *Proc. Assoc. Am. Phys.* 111, 525–536. doi:10.1046/j.1525-1381.1999.t01-1-99231.x

Su, H. H., Lin, H. T., Suen, J. L., Sheu, C. C., Yokoyama, K. K., Huang, S. K., et al. (2016). Aryl hydrocarbon receptor-ligand axis mediates pulmonary fibroblast migration and differentiation through increased arachidonic acid metabolism. *Toxicology* 370, 116–126. doi:10.1016/j.tox.2016.09.019

Takeda, T., Komiya, Y., Koga, T., Ishida, T., Ishii, Y., Kikuta, Y., et al. (2017). Dioxin-induced increase in leukotriene B4 biosynthesis through the aryl hydrocarbon receptor and its relevance to hepatotoxicity owing to neutrophil infiltration. *J. Biol. Chem.* 292, 10586–10599. doi:10.1074/jbc.M116. 764332

Thi Thanh Hai, N., Thuy, L. T. T., Shiota, A., Kadono, C., Daikuku, A., Hoang, D. V., et al. (2018). Selective overexpression of cytoglobin in stellate cells attenuates thioacetamide-induced liver fibrosis in mice. *Sci. Rep.* 8, 17860. doi:10.1038/ s41598-018-36215-4

Titos, E., Planagumà, A., López-Parra, M., Villamor, N., Miquel, R., Jiménez, W., et al. (2004). 5-Lipoxygenase (5-LO) is involved in kupffer cell survival. Possible role of 5-LO products in the pathogenesis of liver fibrosis. *Comp. Hepatol.* 3 (1), S19. doi:10.1186/1476-5926-2-S1-S19

Wang, H., Zhang, Y., and Heuckeroth, R. O. (2007). PAI-1 deficiency reduces liver fibrosis after bile duct ligation in mice through activation of tPA. *FEBS Lett.* 581, 3098–3104. doi:10.1016/j.febslet.2007.05.049

Watkins, P. B., Dube, L. M., Walton-Bowen, K., Cameron, C. M., and Kasten, L. E. (2007). Clinical pattern of zileuton-associated liver injury: results of a 12-month study in patients with chronic asthma. *Drug Saf.* 30, 805–815. doi:10.2165/ 00002018-200730090-00006

Woodhoo, A., Iruarrizaga-Lejarreta, M., Beraza, N., García-Rodríguez, J. L., Embade, N., Fernández-Ramos, D., et al. (2012). Human antigen R contributes to hepatic stellate cell activation and liver fibrosis. *Hepatology* 56, 1870–1882. doi:10.1002/hep.25828

Wu, X., Zhi, F., Lun, W., Deng, Q., and Zhang, W. (2018). Baicalin inhibits PDGF-BB-induced hepatic stellate cell proliferation, apoptosis, invasion, migration and activation via the miR-3595/ACSL4 axis. *Int. J. Mol. Med.* 41, 1992–2002. doi:10.3892/ijmm.2018.3427

Xiao, R., Yoshida, N., Higashi, Y., Lu, Q. J., Fukushige, T., Kanzaki, T., et al. (2011). Retinoic acids exhibit anti-fibrotic activity through the inhibition of 5-lipoxygenase expression in scleroderma fibroblasts. *J. Dermatol.* 38, 345–353. doi:10.1111/j.1346-8138.2010.00993.x

Xie, Y. X., Liao, R., Pan, L., and Du, C. Y. (2017). ERK pathway activation contributes to the tumor-promoting effects of hepatic stellate cells in hepatocellular carcinoma. *Immunol. Lett.* 188, 116–123. doi:10.1016/j.imlet. 2017.06.009

Yu, J., Hu, Y., Gao, Y., Li, Q., Zeng, Z., Li, Y., et al. (2018). Kindlin-2 regulates hepatic stellate cells activation and liver fibrogenesis. *Cell Death Dis.* 4, 34. doi:10.1038/s41420-018-0095-9

Zhang, J., Li, Y., Liu, Q., Huang, Y., Li, R., Wu, T., et al. (2020). Sirt6 alleviated liver fibrosis by deacetylating conserved lysine 54 on Smad2 in hepatic stellate cells. *Hepatology*. doi:10.1002/hep.31418

Zhang, X., Tan, Z., Wang, Y., Tang, J., Jiang, R., Hou, J., et al. (2015). PTPRO-associated hepatic stellate cell activation plays a critical role in liver fibrosis. *Cell. Physiol. Biochem.* 35, 885–898. doi:10.1159/000369746

10

The Management of Glucocorticoid Therapy in Liver Failure

Ran Xue [1,2] and Qinghua Meng [1*]

[1] Department of Critical Care Medicine of Liver Disease, Beijing You-An Hospital, Capital Medical University, Beijing, China,
[2] Key Laboratory of Carcinogenesis and Translational Research (Ministry of Education), Department of Gastrointestinal Oncology, Peking University Cancer Hospital & Institute, Beijing, China

*Correspondence:
Qinghua Meng
meng_qh@126.com

Liver failure is characterized by rapid progression and high mortality. Excessive systemic inflammation is considered as the trigger of liver failure. Glucocorticoids (GCs) can rapidly suppress excessive inflammatory reactions and immune response. GCs have been applied in the treatment of liver failure since the 1970s. However, until now, the use of GCs in the treatment of liver failure has been somewhat unclear and controversial. New research regarding the molecular mechanisms of GCs may explain the controversial actions of GCs in liver failure. More results should be confirmed in a larger randomized clinical trial; this can aid the discovery of better definitions in terms of treatment schedules according to different clinical settings. Meanwhile, the timing and dosing of GCs in the treatment of liver failure should also be explored.

Keywords: glucocorticoids, liver failure, timing, dosing, mechanism

BACKGROUND

Liver failure is a life-threatening clinical syndrome with heterogeneous etiology that can cause serious disorders, such as coagulation disorders, icteria, hepatic encephalopathy (HE), and ascites (1, 2). Despite significant advances in artificial liver support system (ALSS) and liver transplantation (LT), these techniques are still difficult to apply more widely due to many restrictions, such as the amount of plasma, the limitation of liver donors, and the patient's economic situation, and so the mortality of liver failure is still high (3–5). It is therefore essential to develop more effective therapies for liver failure.

Glucocorticoids (GCs) have been applied to the clinical treatment of liver failure for many years. The first paper on GCs therapy for liver failure was published in the 1960s. Nowadays, many basic and clinical studies have explored the feasibility of GCs treatment in liver failure (6–12), but they remain inconclusive for the application of GCs treatment in liver failure.

THE APPLIED STATUS OF GCS THERAPY IN LIVER FAILURE

Among the different liver diseases, the most authoritative clinical indication of GCs therapy is autoimmune hepatitis (AIH) (7). However, in patients with suspected drug-induced AIH who are undergoing GCs therapy, withdrawal of treatment once the liver injury has resolved should be accompanied by close monitoring (13). A recent report from APASL ACLF Research Consortium Working Party defined the histopathological, clinical spectrum, and role of GCs therapy in patients with AIH-ACLF. It was shown that early stratification to LT or GCs therapy (hepatic encephalopathy in $\geq$F3, MELD$>$27) would improve outcomes and reduce ICU stay in patients with AIH-ACLF (14).

GCs therapy is also recommended as a first-line treatment strategy in patients with severe alcoholic hepatitis, hepatic encephalopathy, or maddrey discriminant function $\geq$32 (6).

Meanwhile, GCs would not increase occurrence of or mortality from bacterial infections in patients with severe alcoholic hepatitis (15). However, a recent meta-analysis showed that it could not determine whether GCs had a positive or negative effect on people with alcoholic liver disease because available data were still insufficient to produce robust results, trials were small, and the included participants differed in severity of disease (16).

Drug-induced liver failure requires evidence of immunopathogenicity to reverse the condition through GCs blocking immune responses. A recent study showed that short-term use of GCs was strongly recommended for severe DILI patients with hyperbilirubinemia (TBil >243 μmol/L) (17). However, Wan et al. found that prednisone was not beneficial for the treatment of severe drug-induced liver injury (18). The newest EASL clinical practice guidelines for drug-induced liver injury consider how GCs are often given when all else fails to procedure results (19). Early trials of GCs therapies, for all forms of ALF, demonstrated limited benefits (10, 20). GCs are also applied to treat drug-induced cholestatic hepatitis, especially in patients with allergic manifestations such as fever, eosinophilia, and rash. Liver injury caused by antiepileptic drugs are commonly related to features of hypersensitivity and may respond to GCs (21).

There exist significant differences in the etiology of liver diseases between the East and West. HBV is the leading cause of chronic liver disease in the Asia-Pacific region, including China and India (2). HBV-activated immune response and immune pathology caused by liver cell inflammation and necrosis are the initiated factors of liver failure. Although a large number of studies reported that GC therapy is effective in liver failure (22, 23), GC therapy is only recommended for the treatment of early stages of liver failure, and there is little evidence to support its effectiveness.

However, with the arrival of nucleoside analogs (NAs), more and more guidelines have recommended NAs to be used in patients with acute exacerbation of chronic HBV infection. The early combined use of NAs and GCs could be a good option to reverse the potential deterioration in patients with HBV-related liver failure. A recent study reported that early combination therapy with corticosteroid and NAs induces rapid resolution of inflammation in ALF due to transient HBV infection (24). It has been shown that with sufficient doses of NAs, GCs cannot affect the replication of HBV (12). However, Huang et al. (12) investigated retrospectively the efficacy of GCs in patients with hepatitis B virus-related acute-on-chronic liver failure (HBV-ACLF). It was indicated that GC treatment did not improve transplant-free survival in patients with HBV-ACLF.

It is not rare for GCs to be abused in the treatment of liver failure as "reduced bilirubin drugs." Therefore, its use in terms

of liver failure therapy should not be exaggerated, although some patients with liver failure can indeed benefit from GCs therapy. As a "double-edged sword," the timing, dosage, and clinical indication of GC therapy are the key points to better definitions in terms of treatment schedules according to different clinical settings in the future.

THE TIMING OF GC THERAPY IN LIVER FAILURE

In the Asia-Pacific region, the most common type of liver failure is HBV-ACLF. The clinical stage of HBV-ACLF can be divided into four stages: early stage of ascending period, late stage of ascending period, platform period, and recovery period. Immune injury is the major event in the early stage of ascending period. The pathogenesis in the late stage of ascending period is involved in ischemia, immune injury, and hypoxia injury (25). During the platform period, body conditions achieve an immunosuppression state.

Endotoxemia is an important factor during the initiation of liver injury. Recent studies have shown that there was an inflammatory cascade in the early period of HBV-ACLF (26, 27). The sooner systemic inflammatory response syndromes (SIRS) occurred, the higher the mortality rate would be. GCs can inhibit inflammation, stabilize the liver cell membrane, and prevent further necrosis of liver cells (28). Therefore, early application of GC therapy can inhibit immune responses. The inhibition of systemic inflammation delays rapid progression and improves the survival rate of patients with ACLF.

Zhao et al. (11) found that patients responding best to GCs were those with less severe liver failure and a higher risk of rapid disease progression, with lower HE grades and MELD scores but extremely high ALT levels. The optimal time of intervention with GCs was within 14 days of the onset of symptoms.

We consider that the efficacy of GC treatment is primarily associated with the timing of GC administration. Meanwhile, the first-time physician, age, basic condition, and complications should also be considered for GC administration. Patients with some specified indicators can benefit more from GC therapy; these could be indicators such as ALT>1,000 U/L, TBIL in the 10~20 × ULN, PTA≥30%, MELD score<28, no obvious signs of infection, hepatic encephalopathy Stage<II, no liver and kidney syndrome trends, as well as overactive immunological responses. However, until now, there has been a lack of accurate quantitative indicators for GC therapy. Therefore, it is particularly important for doctors to accumulate more and more clinical experience.

THE DOSE SELECTION FOR GC THERAPY IN LIVER FAILURE

Today, the ideal choices regarding GC type and does remains inconclusive. Based on current clinical reports, GC dose is generally controlled in 1~2 g/kg/d (methylprednisolone). Kotoh et al. (23) explored the feasibility of large doses of GC treatment for the treatment of liver failure. They divided 34 patients with ALF into two groups; 17 patients were given methylprednisolone

---

Abbreviations: ALF, acute liver failure; GCs, glucocorticoids; HBV, hepatitis B virus; HBV-ACLF, hepatitis B virus-related acute-on-chronic liver failure; HE, hepatic encephalopathy; INF-α, interferon-α; LPS, lipopolysaccharide; SALF, subacute liver failure; SIRS, systemic inflammatory response syndromes; TNF-α, tumor necrosis factor-α.

1,000 mg/d via hepatic artery continuously for 3 days. As a result, 13 patients were cured, 2 patients died, and 2 patients underwent LT without serious complications. Fujiwara et al. (29) discussed the value of high-dose GCs in the treatment of HBV-related liver failure. It was found that the survival rate and liver regeneration in the GC-treated group showed a slim advantage, but there was no statistical difference, while patients with HBV infection and a poor basic condition had an unfavorable prognosis.

When the efficacy of GCs therapy cannot be determined in clinic, it is required that possible side effects of GCs are kept within a controllable range based on the principle of safety. GCs can significantly inhibit the presence of phagocytic cells to the antigen, promote the destruction and disintegration of lymphocytes, and develop the removal of lymphocytes from blood vessels so as to reduce the number of lymphocytes in circulation (30). Small doses of GCs mainly inhibit cellular immunity, while high doses of GCs can suppress humoral immune function by inhibiting B cells and antibody production (31).

The number of liver surface glucocorticoid receptors (GRs) may be reduced in liver failure (27). If greater doses of GCs are given, the GCs cannot play a role during the presence of receptor saturation, but may increase the incidence of side effects of GCs. Therefore, patients with liver failure, especially those with cirrhosis, are not recommended to use high-dose GCs. Although GCs can increase the incidence of infection and upper gastrointestinal bleeding, as well as other complications, the side effects of GCs are controllable. Therefore, it is essential to screen and monitor the side effects during GCs therapy in patients with liver failure.

THE MECHANISM OF THE POTENTIAL BENEFIT OF GC THERAPY IN LIVER FAILURE

The Core Pathogenesis of Liver Failure

Currently, it is widely accepted that "endotoxin-macrophage-cytokine storm" is the core pathogenesis of liver failure, combined with the immune injury as the initial factor in the development of liver failure, especially in the early stage of liver failure (27, 32).

The chemical essence of endotoxin is lipopolysaccharide [LPS, recognized by the pattern-recognition receptor toll-like receptor 4 (TLR4)] (33). With the interaction of LPS-binding proteins, it binds to a variety of cell membranes with receptor CD14, transmitting signals from the outside of the cell to nucleus and stimulating the synthesis and release of cytokines, which involves tumor necrosis factor-α (TNF-α), interferon-α (INF-α), IL-1, and IL-6 and simultaneously induces macrophages to secrete nitric oxide and large amounts of oxygen-free radicals (34–37). The liver cells are injured by delayed type hypersensitivity, oxidative stress, and apoptosis. If the immune response cannot be suspended in time, it would lead to a vicious cycle, resulting in significant liver cell necrosis, apoptosis, and liver failure (38–40). Peripheral blood mononuclear cells (PBMCs) and monocytes from patients with cirrhosis respond stronger to LPS stimulation

(41). Heat shock proteins (HSPs) are well-known as protective proteins that make cells resistant to stress-induced cell damage. However, simultaneous activation of TLR4 by HSPs causes enhanced tissue injury (42).

Immune injury is considered as the first blow in the "triple hit theory" of liver failure, and timely suspension of its excessive immune response may reduce or even reverse its condition (43, 44). As the most commonly used anti-inflammatory and immunosuppressive agents, GCs can inhibit macrophage phagocytosis and antigen treatment and suppress the production of inflammatory cytokines. Therefore, GCs have the theoretical basis for the treatment of liver failure.

The Anti-inflammatory Mechanisms of GCs

Aside from rapid non-genomic effects, GCs exert genomic effects by binding to the glucocorticoid receptor (GR), a member of the nuclear receptor family of transcription factors (45). Upon ligand binding, the GR translocates to the nucleus, where it acts either as a monomeric protein that affects transcription with other transcription factors or as a homodimeric transcription factor, which binds glucocorticoid response elements (GREs) in promoter regions of GC-inducible genes (46). Some reports have clearly showed that GR dimer-dependent transactivation is essential in the anti-inflammatory activities of GR (47–49). GR$^{dim/dim}$ mutant mice were used to show reduced GR dimerization, and hence GC cannot control inflammation (50, 51).

THE POTENTIAL MECHANISM FOR CONTROVERSIAL ACTIONS OF GC THERAPY IN LIVER FAILURE

The Pro-inflammatory Mechanisms of GC

Emerging studies have shown that GCs have a two-way regulation for inflammatory and immune responses (52). The basal state of the immune system and the type of exposure to GCs are significant factors influencing the effects of GCs (53). For instance, while chronic exposure to GCs seems to be immunosuppressive, acute exposure increases the peripheral immune response (54).

It was found that GCs can induce the expression of several innate immune-related genes, including several members of the Toll-like receptor (TLR) family, such as TLR2 and TLR4 (55–57). The activation of TLRs via the repression of NF-κB and AP-1 or via the induction of GC-induced leucine zipper (GILZ) or MKP-1 is a hallmark feature of inflammation (55).

The GR signaling interplays with the TLRs signaling pathway via several mechanisms (58). Hermoso et al. (59) found that dexamethasone increased TNF-α induction of TLR2 through the activation of GR, supporting the existence of positive feedback between the activation of the TLR signaling pathway and GC secretion. Meanwhile, GCs may exert pro-inflammatory actions through interactions with inflammatory cytokines such as TNF-α and acute phase protein serpinA3 (60). Besides, some studies indicated that GCs can work synergistically with pro-inflammatory mediators to enhance the defense mechanisms to ensure removal and clearance of pathogens in the hepatic acute-phase response (58, 61). GC-mediated activation of NLRP3, TLR2, and P2Y2R and the potentiation of LIF and TNF-α regulated pro-inflammatory genes (58, 62). All these results provide a potential explanation for the controversial actions of GC therapy in liver failure. More studies are required to characterize the liver-specific effects of the anti- and pro-inflammatory roles of GR signaling.

GC Resistance (GCR)

There are two types of GCR, inherited or familial GCR and acquired GCR (63). It is accepted that a pro-inflammatory environment can negatively affect GR sensitivity (64, 65). The mechanisms contributing to reduced GC responsiveness are heterogeneous as they involve various cytokines and cell types. The mechanisms of GCR are still unclear. As GCR occurs in many inflammatory diseases, it is widely considered that GCR is a heterogeneous phenomenon with multiple underlying mechanisms (66). Some of these involve problems with the GR protein itself, but many others are independent from GR and involved in mutations in GR-induced genes and problems with chaperones or cofactors (63).

Meanwhile, the down-regulation of the GR protein is associated with GRC, involving many different mechanisms such as reduced transcription and homologous down-regulation (67), GR protein degradation (68), and decreased stability of GR mRNA (the involvement of AUUUA motifs in the $3'$ UTR of GR mRNA) (69). Moreover, post-translational modifications of GR also contribute to a reduced GC response, such as ubiquitination of the GR (Lys-426 within a PEST element) and phosphorylation of the GR (68, 70). Besides, some research also showed miRNAs have a prominent role in the regulation of GR mRNA turnover and the occurrence of GCR (71, 72).

In addition to the non-genomic and genomic actions of GCs, GR signaling also relies on the existence of post-translational modifications (PTMs) and multiple receptor isoforms. GR is transcribed from a single gene, NR3C1; however, alternative splicing of this gene generates GRα and GRβ isoforms (73). The GRβ isoform also participates in the GCR. It was found that up-regulation of the dominant negative GRβ isoform was correlated with GR insensitivity via inhibiting GR-induced transactivation and GR nuclear translocation (74).

The Possible Factors of GC Refractoriness in Liver Failure: Sepsis

Sepsis is a common complication of ACLF, which is an acute systemic inflammatory disease (75). However, GCs are hardly useful in sepsis (63). Thus, sepsis is considered a GCR disease. GCR is an essential problem in sepsis and leads to: lack of transport and removal of bile acids in the liver, resulting in cholestasis; increased production and reduced removal of L-lactate, resulting in lactic acidosis; GCs having no anti-inflammatory effects.

Our previous study proposed that the diagnostic criteria of sepsis are not suitable for patients in HBV-ACLF with sepsis, because patients with underlying chronic liver disease and cirrhosis may have deranged clinical parameters (76). Therefore, it is essential to establish compatible diagnostic criteria for sepsis in patients with ACLF. When sepsis occurred, the serum TBiL level and WBC count elevated significantly while PLT count decreased significantly. We argue that when sepsis occurs during the process of liver failure GCs are not recommended for patients.

CONCLUSIONS AND FUTURE PERSPECTIVES

The idea of using GCs during acute liver failure has circulated for so many years, but, so far, no meaningful work has provided conclusive evidence of its therapeutic efficacy, except in the field of autoimmune etiology. Beyond the east/west demarcation, current data availing GC's use in liver failure revealed benefits that appeared marginal and were no longer present upon adjustment (10), came from evidence recorded in non-randomized studies (22), or were other ones carried out in small groups of patients (23, 24). More results should be confirmed using a larger randomized clinical trial to in order to arrive at better definitions in terms of treatment schedules according to different clinical settings.

Meanwhile, due to the complicated pathophysiology of liver failure, the exploration of immunological manifestations with different etiology and different clinical staging of patients with liver failure is needed urgently. This is a prerequisite for the feasibility and safety of GC applications. With an in-depth study, we can find the accurate timing, dosage, and clinical indicators of GC therapy for the clinical management of liver failure, so that clinicians can make timely treatment options so as to obtain the greatest benefits for patients.

AUTHOR CONTRIBUTIONS

RX wrote this manuscript. QM designed this manuscript.

REFERENCES

Ran X, Zhonghui D, Haixia L, Li C, Hongwei Y, Meixin R, et al. A novel dynamic model for predicting outcome in patients with hepatitis B virus related acute-on-chronic liver failure. *Oncotarget.* (2017) 8:108970–80. doi: 10.18632/oncotarget.22447

Bernal W, Jalan R, Quaglia A, Simpson K, Wendon J, Burroughs A. Acute-on-chronic liver failure. *Lancet.* (2015) 386:1576–87. doi: 10.1016/S0140-6736(15)00309-8

Asrani SK, Simonetto DA, Kamath PS. Acute-on-chronic liver failure. *Clin Gastroenterol Hepatol.* (2015) 13:2128–39. doi: 10.1016/j.cgh.2015.07.008

Blasco-Algora S, Masegosa-Ataz J, Gutiérrez-García ML, Alonso-López S, Fernández-Rodríguez CM. Acute-on-chronic liver failure: pathogenesis, prognostic factors and management. *World J Gastroenterol.* (2015) 21:12125– 40. doi: 10.3748/wjg.v21.i42.12125

Singanayagam A, Bernal W. Update on acute liver failure. *Curr Opin Crit Care.* (2015) 21:134–41. doi: 10.1097/MCC.0000000000000187

Wang F, Wang BY. Corticosteroids or non-corticosteroids:a fresh perspective on alcoholic hepatitis treatment. *Hepatobiliary Pancreat Dis Int.* (2011) 10:458–64. doi: 10.1016/S1499-3872(11)60079-9

Yeoman AD, Westbrook RH, Zen Y, Bernal W, Al-Chalabi T, Wendon JA, et al. Prognosis of acute severe autoimmune hepatitis(AS-AIH): the role of eortieosteroids in modifying outcome. *J Hepatol.* (2014) 61:876– 82. doi: 10.1016/j.jhep.2014.05.021

Yang CH, Wu TS, Chiu CT. Chronic hepatitis B reactivation: a word of caution regarding the use of systemic glueoeortieosteroid therapy. *Br J Dermatol.* (2007) 157:587–90. doi: 10.1111/j.1365-2133.2007.08058.x

Ramachandran J, Sajith KG, Pal S, Rasak JV, Prakash JA, Ramakrishna B. Clinicopathological profile and management of severe autoimmune hepatitis. *Trop Gastmenterol.* (2014) 35:25–31. doi: 10.7869/tg.160

Karkhanis J, Verna EC, Chang MS, Stravitz RT, Schilsky M, Lee WM, et al. acute liver failure study group. steroid use in acute liver failure. *Hepatology.* (2014) 59:612–21. doi: 10.1002/hep.26678

Zhao B, Zhang HY, Xie GJ, Liu HM, Chen Q, Li RF, et al. Evaluation of the efficacy of steroid therapy on acute liver failure. *Exp Ther Med.* (2016) 12:3121–9. doi: 10.3892/etm.2016.3720

Huang C, Yu KK, Zheng JM, Li N. Steroid treatment in patients with acute-on-chronic liver failure precipitated by hepatitis B: A 10-year cohort study in a university hospital in East China. *J Dig Dis.* (2019) 20:38– 44. doi: 10.1111/1751-2980.12691

Björnsson ES, Bergmann O, Jonasson JG, Grondal G, Gudbjornsson B, Olafsson S. Drug-induced autoimmune hepatitis: response to corticosteroids and lack of relapse after cessation of steroids. *Clin Gastroenterol Hepatol.* (2017) 15:1635–6. doi: 10.1016/j.cgh.2017.05.027

Anand L, Choudhury A, Bihari C, Sharma BC, Kumar M, Maiwall R, et al. Flare of autoimmune hepatitis causing acute on chronic liver failure: diagnosis and response to corticosteroid therapy. *Hepatology.* (2018) 70:587– 96. doi: 10.1002/hep.30205

Hmoud BS, Patel K, Bataller R, Singal AK. Corticosteroids and occurrence of and mortality from infections in severe alcoholic hepatitis: a meta-analysis of randomized trials. *Liver Int.* (2016) 36:721–8. doi: 10.1111/liv.12939

Pavlov CS, Varganova DL, Casazza G, Tsochatzis E, Nikolova D, Gluud C. Glucocorticosteroids for people with alcoholic hepatitis. *Cochrane Database Syst Rev.* (2019) 4:CD001511. doi: 10.1002/14651858.CD001511.pub4

Wang PQ, Chen H, Hu XF, Xie QP, Shi J, Lin L, et al. Beneficial effect of corticosteroids for patients with severe drug-induced liver injury. *J Dig Dis.* (2016) 17:618–27. doi: 10.1111/1751-2980.12383

Wan YM, Wu JF, Li YH, Wu HM, Wu XN, Xu Y. Prednisone is not beneficial for the treatment of severe drug-induced liver injury: an observational study (STROBE compliant). *Medicine.* (2019) 98:e15886. doi: 10.1097/MD.0000000000015886

European Association for the Study of the Liver. EASL clinical practice guidelines: drug-induced liver injury. *J Hepatol.* (2019) 70:1222–61. doi: 10.1016/j.jhep.2019.02.014

Tujios SR, Lee WM. Acute liver failure induced by idiosyncratic reaction to drugs: challenges in diagnosis and therapy. *Liver Int.* (2018) 38:6– 14. doi: 10.1111/liv.13535

Björnsson E. Hepatotoxicity associated with antiepileptic drugs. *Acta Neurol Scand.* (2008) 118:281–90. doi: 10.1111/j.1600-0404.2008.01009.x

Zhang XQ, Jiang L, You JP, Liu YY, Peng J, Zhang HY, et al. Efficacy of short- term dexamethasone therapy in acute-on-chronic pre-liver failure. *Hepatol Res.* (2011) 41:46–53. doi: 10.1111/j.1872-034X.2010.00740.x

Kotoh K, Enjoji M, Nakamuta M, Yoshimoto T, Kohjima M, Morizono S, et al. Arterial steroid injection therapy can inhibit the progression of severe acute hepatic failure toward fulminant liver failure. *World J Gastroenterol.* (2006) 12:6678–82. doi: 10.3748/wjg.v12.i41.6678

Fujiwara K, Yasui S, Haga Y, Nakamura M, Yonemitsu Y, Arai M, et al. Early combination therapy with corticosteroid and nucleoside analogue induces rapid resolution of inflammation in acute liver failure due to transient hepatitis B virus infection. *Intern Med.* (2018) 57:1543–52. doi: 10.2169/internalmedicine.9670-17

Zheng YB, Huang ZL, Wu ZB, Zhang M, Gu YR, Su YJ, et al. Dynamic changes of clinical features that predict the prognosis of acute-on-chronic hepatitis B

liver failure: a retrospective cohort study. *Int J Med Sci.* (2013) 10:1658–64. doi: 10.7150/ijms.6415

Xing T, Li L, Cao H, Huang J. Altered immune function of monocytes in different stages of patients with acute on chronic liver failure. *Clin Exp Immunol.* (2007) 147:184–8.

Chen P, Wang YY, Chen C, Guan J, Zhu HH, Chen Z. The immunological roles in acute-on-chronic liver failure: an update. *Hepatobiliary Pancreat Dis Int.* (2019) 18:403–11. doi: 10.1016/j.hbpd.2019.07.003

Ye Y. Three attacks in the development of HBV-related liver failure. *Infect Dis Inform.* (2009) 22:276–9.

Fujiwara K, Yasui S, Okitsu K, Yonemitsu Y, Oda S, Yokosuka O. The requirement for a sufficient period of corticosteroid treatment in combination with nucleoside analogue for severe acute exacerbation of chronic hepatitis B. *J Gastroenterol.* (2010) 45:1255–62. doi: 10.1007/s00535-010-0280-y

Hämäläinen M, Lilja R, Kankaanranta H, Moilanen E. Inhibition of iNOS expression and NO production by anti-inflammatory steroids. Reversal by histone deacetylase inhibitors. *Pulm Pharmacol Ther.* (2008) 21:331– 9. doi: 10.1016/j.pupt.2007.08.003

Lim HY, Müller N, Herold MJ, van den Brandt J, Reichardt HM. Glucocorticoids exert opposing effects on macrophage function dependent on their concentration. *Immunology.* (2007) 122:47–53. doi: 10.1111/j.1365-2567.2007.02611.x

Takeuchi O, Akira S. Pattern recognition receptors and inflammation. *Cell.* (2010) 140:805–20. doi: 10.1016/j.cell.2010.01.022

Jerala R. Structural biology of the LPS recognition. *Int J Med Microbiol.* (2007) 297:353–63. doi: 10.1016/j.ijmm.2007.04.001

Dajani R, Sanlioglu S, Zhang Y, Li Q, Monick MM, Lazartigues E, et al. Pleiotropic functions of TNF-alpha determine distinct IKKbeta-dependent hepatocellular fates in response to LPS. *Am J Physiol Gastrointest Liver Physiol.* (2007) 292:242–52. doi: 10.1152/ajpgi.00043.2006

Nardo B, Montalti R, Puviani L, Pacilè V, Beltempo P, Bertelli R, et al. Portal vein oxygen supply through a liver extracorporeal device to treat acute liver failure in swine induced by subtotal hepatectomy: preliminary data. *Transplant Proc.* (2006) 38:1190–2. doi: 10.1016/j.transproceed.2006.03.057

Radziewicz H, Hanson HL, Ahmed R, Grakoui A. Unraveling the role of PD-1/PD-L interactions in persistent hepatotropic infections: potential for therapeutic application? *Gastroenterology.* (2008) 134:2168– 71. doi: 10.1053/j.gastro.2008.04.012

Zhang Z, Zhang JY, Wherry EJ, Jin B, Xu B, Zou ZS, et al. Dynamic programmed death 1 expression by virus-specific CD8 T cells correlates with the outcome of acute hepatitis B. *Gastroenterology.* (2008) 134:1938– 49. doi: 10.1053/j.gastro.2008.03.037

Tavakoli S, Mederacke I, Herzog-Hauff S, Glebe D, Grün S, Strand D, et al. Peripheral blood dendritic cells are phenotypically and functionally intact in chronic hepatitis B virus (HBV) infection. *Clin Exp Immunol.* (2008) 151:61–70. doi: 10.1111/j.1365-2249.2007.03547.x

Op den Brouw ML, Binda RS, van Roosmalen MH, Protzer U, Janssen HL, van der Molen RG, et al. Hepatitis B virus surface antigen impairs myeloid dendritic cell function: a possible immune escape mechanism of hepatitis B virus. *Immunology.* (2009) 126:280-289. doi: 10.1111/j.1365-2567.2008.02896.x

Xie Q, Shen HC, Jia NN, Wang H, Lin LY, An BY, et al. Patients with chronic hepatitis B infection display deficiency of plasmacytoid dendritic cells with reduced expression of TLR9. *Microbes Infect.* (2009) 11:515– 23. doi: 10.1016/j.micinf.2009.02.008

Gandoura S, Weiss E, Rautou PE, Fasseu M, Gustot T, Lemoine F, et al. Gene- and exon-expression profiling reveals an extensive LPS-induced response in immune cells in patients with cirrhosis. *J Hepatol.* (2013) 58:936– 48. doi: 10.1016/j.jhep.2012.12.025

Rosenberger K, Derkow K, Dembny P, Krüger C, Schott E, Lehnardt S. The impact of single and pairwise Toll-like receptor activation on neuroinflammation and neurodegeneration. *J Neuroinflammation.* (2014) 11:166. doi: 10.1186/s12974-014-0166-7

Zhang Z, Zou ZS, Fu JL, Cai L, Jin L, Liu YJ, et al. Severe dendritic cell perturbation is actively involved in the pathogenesis of acute-on-chronic hepatitis B liver failure. *J Hepatol.* (2008) 49:396–406. doi: 10.1016/j.jhep.2008.05.017

Malhi H, Gores GJ. Cellular and molecular mechanisms of liver injury. *Gastroenterology.* (2008) 134:1641–54. doi: 10.1053/j.gastro.2008.03.002

Scheschowitsch K, Leite J, Assreuy J. New insights in glucocorticoid receptor signaling-more than just a ligand-binding receptor. *Front Endocrinol.* (2017) 8:16. doi: 10.3389/fendo.2017. 00016

Galon J, Franchimont D, Hiroi N, Frey G, Boettner A, Ehrhart-Bornstein M, et al. Gene profiling reveals unknown enhancing and suppressive actions of glucocorticoids on immune cells. *FASEB J.* (2002) 16:61– 71. doi:10.1096/fj.01-0245com

Vandevyver S, Dejager L, Tuckermann J, Libert C. New insights into the anti-inflammatory mechanisms of glucocorticoids: an emerging role for glucocorticoid-receptor-mediated transactivation. *Endocrinology.* (2013) 154:993–1007. doi:10.1210/en.2012-2045

Reichardt HM, Tuckermann JP, Göttlicher M, Vujic M, Weih F, Angel P, et al. Repression of inflammatory responses in the absence of DNA binding by the glucocorticoid receptor. *Embo J.* (2001) 20:7168– 73. doi:10.1093/emboj/20.24.7168

Smoak KA, Cidlowski JA. Mechanisms of glucocorticoid receptor signaling during inflammation. *Mech Ageing Dev.* (2004) 125:697– 706. doi:10.1016/j.mad.2004.06.010

Jewell CM, Scoltock AB, Hamel BL, Yudt MR, Cidlowski JA. Complexhumanglucocorticoid receptor dim mutations define glucocorticoid induced apoptotic resistance in bone cells. *Mol Endocrinol.* (2012) 26:244–56. doi:10.1210/me.2011-1116

Kleiman A, Hubner S, Rodriguez Parkitna JM, Neumann A, Hofer S, Weigand MA, et al. Glucocorticoid receptor dimerization is required for survival in septic shock via suppression of interleukin- 1 in macrophages. *Faseb J.* (2012) 26:722–9. doi: 10.1096/fj.11-1 92112

Cruz-Topete D, Cidlowski JA. One hormone, two actions: anti- and pro-inflammatory effects of glucocorticoids. *Neuroimmunomodulation.* (2015) 22:20–32. doi: 10.1159/000362724

Dhabhar FS. A hassle a day may keep the doctor away: stress and the augmentation of immune function. *Integr Comp Biol.* (2002) 42:556– 64. doi:10.1093/icb/42.3.556

Dhabhar FS. Stress-induced augmentation of immune function–the role of stress hormones, leukocyte trafficking, and cytokines. *Brain Behav Immun.* (2002) 16:785–98. doi:10.1016/S0889-1591(02)00036-3

Chinenov Y, Rogatsky I. Glucocorticoids and the innate immune system: crosstalk with the toll-like receptor signaling network. *Mol Cell Endocrinol.* (2007) 275:30–42. doi:10.1016/j.mce.2007.04.014

Xie Y, Tolmeijer S, Oskam JM, Tonkens T, Meijer AH, Schaaf MJM. Glucocorticoids inhibit macrophage differentiation towards a pro- inflammatory phenotype upon wounding without affecting their migration. *Dis Model Mech.* (2019) 12:dmm037887. doi: 10.1242/dmm.0 37887

Desmet SJ, De Bosscher K. Glucocorticoid receptors: finding the middle ground. *J Clin Invest.* (2017) 127:1136–45. doi:10.1172/JCI88886

Busillo JM, Cidlowski JA. The five Rs of glucocorticoid action during inflammation: ready, reinforce, repress, resolve, and restore. *Trends Endocrinol Metab.* (2013) 24:109–119. doi:10.1016/j.tem.2012.11.005

Hermoso MA, Matsuguchi T, Smoak K, Cidlowski JA. Glucocorticoids and tumor necrosis factor alpha cooperatively regulate toll- like receptor 2 gene expression. *Mol Cell Biol.* (2004) 24:4743– 56. doi:10.1128/MCB.24.11.4743-4756.2004

Lannan EA, Galliher-Beckley AJ, Scoltock AB, Cidlowski JA. Proinflammatory actions of glucocorticoids: glucocorticoids and TNFalpha coregulate gene expression *in vitro* and *in vivo. Endocrinology.* (2012) 153:3701–12. doi:10.1210/en.2012-1020

Langlais D, Couture C, Balsalobre A, Drouin J. Regulatory network analyses reveal genome-wide potentiation of LIF signaling by glucocorticoids and define an innate cell defense response. *PLoS Genet.* (2008) 4:e1000224. doi:10.1371/journal.pgen.1000224

Busillo JM, Azzam KM, Cidlowski JA. Glucocorticoids sensitize the innate immune system through regulation of the NLRP3 inflammasome. *J Biol Chem.* (2011) 286:38703–13. doi:10.1074/jbc.M111.275370

Dendoncker K, Libert C. Glucocorticoid resistance as a major drive in sepsis pathology. *Cytokine Growth Factor Rev.* (2017) 35:85–96. doi:10.1016/j.cytogfr.2017.04.002

Dejager L, Vandevyver S, Petta I, Libert C. Dominance of the strongest: inflammatory cytokines versus glucocorticoids. *Cytokine Growth Factor Rev.* (2014) 25:21–33. doi:10.1016/j.cytogfr.2013.12.006

Van Bogaert T, De Bosscher K, Libert C. Crosstalk between TNF and glucocorticoid receptor signaling pathways. *Cytokine Growth Factor Rev.* (2010) 21:275–86. doi:10.1016/j.cytogfr.2010.04.003

Matsumura Y. Heterogeneity of glucocorticoid resistance in patients with bronchial asthma. *Int J Biomed Sci.* (2010) 6:158–66.

Drouin J, Trifiro MA, Plante RK, Nemer M, Eriksson P, Wrange O. Glucocorticoid receptor binding to a specific DNA sequence is required for hormone-dependent repression of proopiomelanocortin gene transcription. *Mol Cell Biol.* (1989) 9:5305–14. doi:10.1128/MCB.9.12.5305

Wallace AD, Cidlowski JA. Proteasome-mediated glucocorticoid receptor degradation restricts transcriptional signaling by glucocorticoids. *J Biol Chem.* (2001) 276:42714–21. doi:10.1074/jbc.M106033200

Green TL, Leventhal SM, Lim D, Cho K, Greenhalgh DG. A Tri-nucleotide pattern in a 3' UTR segment affects the activity of a human glucocorticoid receptor isoform. *Shock.* (2017) 47:148–57. doi:10.1097/SHK.0000000000000750

Pazdrak K, Straub C, Maroto R, Stafford S, White WI, Calhoun WJ, et al. Cytokine-induced glucocorticoid resistance from eosinophil activation: protein phosphatase 5 modulation of glucocorticoid receptor phosphorylation and signaling. *J Immunol.* (2016) 197:3782–91. doi:10.4049/jimmunol.1601029

Li JJ, Tay HL, Maltby S, Xiang Y, Eyers F, Hatchwell L, et al. MicroRNA-9 regulates steroid-resistant airway hyperresponsiveness by reducing protein phosphatase 2A activity, *J Allergy Clin Immunol.* (2015) 136:462–73. doi:10.1016/j.jaci.2014.11.044

Ledderose C, Möhnle P, Limbeck E, Schütz S, Weis F, Rink J, et al. Corticosteroid resistance in sepsis is influenced by microRNA- 124–induced downregulation of glucocorticoid receptor-α. *Crit Care Med.* (2012) 40:2745–53. doi:10.1097/CCM.0b013e3182 5b8ebc

Yudt MR, Cidlowski JA. Molecular identification and characterization of a and b forms of the glucocorticoid receptor. *Mol Endocrinol.* (2001) 15:1093– 103. doi:10.1210/mend.15.7.0667

Bamberger CM, Bamberger AM, de Castro M, Chrousos GP. Glucocorticoid receptor beta, a potential endogenous inhibitor of glucocorticoid action in humans. *J Clin Investig.* (1995) 95:2435–41. doi:10.1172/JCI117943

Hernaez R, Solà E, Moreau R, Ginès P. Acute-on-chronic liver failure: an update. *Gut.* (2017) 66:541–53. doi:10.1136/gutjnl-2016-3 12670

Xue R, Zhu Y, Liu H, Meng Q. The clinical parameters for the diagnosis of hepatitis B virus related acute-on-chronic liver failure with sepsis. *Sci Rep.* (2019) 9:2558. doi:10.1038/s41598-019-38866-3

Antisense Tissue Factor Oligodeoxynucleotides Protected Diethyl Nitrosamine/Carbon Tetrachloride-Induced Liver Fibrosis Through Toll Like Receptor4-Tissue Factor-Protease Activated Receptor1 Pathway

Maha M. Shouman[1]*, Rania M. Abdelsalam[2,3], Mahmoud M. Tawfick[4], Sanaa A. Kenawy[2] and Mona M. El-Naa[5]

[1]Department of Pharmacology and Toxicology, Faculty of Pharmacy, Modern Sciences and Arts University (MSA), Giza, Egypt, [2]Department of Pharmacology and Toxicology, Faculty of Pharmacy, Cairo University, Cairo, Egypt, [3]Department of Biology, Faculty of Pharmacy, New Giza University, Giza, Egypt, [4]Department of Microbiology and Immunology, Faculty of Pharmacy (Boys), Al-Azhar University, Cairo, Egypt, [5]Department of Pharmacology and Toxicology, Faculty of Pharmacy, University of Sadat City, Sadat City, Egypt

*Correspondence:
Maha M. Shouman
mamoussa@msa.edu.eg

Tissue factor (TF) is a blood coagulation factor that has several roles in many non-coagulant pathways involved in different pathological conditions such as angiogenesis, inflammation and fibrogenesis. Coagulation and inflammation are crosslinked with liver fibrosis where protease-activated receptor1 (PAR1) and toll-like receptor4 (TLR4) play a key role. Antisense oligodeoxynucleotides are strong modulators of gene expression. In the present study, antisense TF oligodeoxynucleotides (TFAS) was evaluated in treating liver fibrosis via suppression of TF gene expression. Liver fibrosis was induced in rats by a single administration of N-diethyl nitrosamine (DEN, 200 mg/kg; i. p.) followed by carbon tetrachloride (CCl4, 3 ml/kg; s. c.) once weekly for 6 weeks. Following fibrosis induction, liver TF expression was significantly upregulated along with liver enzymes activities and liver histopathological deterioration. Alpha smooth muscle actin (α-SMA) and transforming growth factor-1beta (TGF-1β) expression, tumor necrosis factor-alpha (TNF-α) and hydroxyproline content and collagen deposition were significantly elevated in the liver. Blocking of TF expression by TFAS injection (2.8 mg/kg; s. c.) once weekly for 6 weeks significantly restored liver enzymes activities and improved histopathological features along with decreasing the elevated α-SMA, TGF-1β, TNF-α, hydroxyproline and collagen. Moreover, TFAS decreased the expression of both PAR1 and TLR4 that were induced by liver fibrosis. In conclusion, we reported that blockage of TF expression by TFAS improved inflammatory and fibrotic changes associated with CCl4+DEN intoxication. In addition, we explored the potential crosslink between the TF, PAR1 and TLR4 in liver fibrogenesis. These findings offer a platform on which recovery from liver fibrosis could be mediated through targeting TF expression.

Keywords: TF, PAR1, TLR4, liver fibrosis, inflammation, antisense oligodeoxynucleotides

INTRODUCTION

Liver fibrosis is a response to chronic liver injury induced by diverse causes such as infection, drugs, metabolic disorders, auto-immune diseases and cholestatic liver diseases (Borensztajn et al., 2010). Fibrogenesis is commonly associated with the generation of a chronic inflammation that results in an abnormal wound healing response. Hepatic stellate cells (HSCs) activation is the key pathogenic mechanism for the initiation and progression of liver fibrosis. A complex and tightly regulated cross-talks between HSCs, hepatocytes, Kupffer cells and sinusoidal endothelial cells (SECs) at the level of liver microcirculation are reported during fibrogenesis (Moreira, 2007).

Accumulation of collagen as well as other extracellular matrix (ECM) components in the liver leads to fibrous scar formation, which results in disruption of the liver architecture, hepatocyte loss, deterioration of the normal liver functions and ultimately liver failure (Karsdal et al., 2020). Liver fibrosis is a reversible process, as long as the liver is not at the stage of advanced cirrhosis (Benyon and Iredale, 2000). Given the highly dynamic process of liver fibrosis and the complex and multiple pathways involved in its progress, targeting one pathway that underlies the fibrotic process may not be sufficient to induce its reversal. However, through advances in the understanding of the key events and cellular pathways involved in the pathogenesis of fibrogenesis, the key targets for antifibrotic therapies are likely to be identified (Trautwein et al., 2015).

Recently, the association between chronic liver disease and coagulopathy is well established (Tripodi et al., 2011). Coagulation activity was recorded as a contributor to the pathogenesis of liver toxicity. Furthermore, it was reported that inflammation and coagulation are interrelated for fibrogenesis (Calvaruso et al., 2008).

Tissue factor (TF) is a 47-kDa transmembrane glycoprotein that is normally expressed throughout the body including the liver (Witkowski et al., 2016). TF is the main initiator of the protease coagulation cascade *in vivo*, leading to thrombin generation (Rauch and Nemerson, 2000). It has been reported that under pathological conditions TF expression can be upregulated by many inducers such as cytokines, hypoxia and mechanical injury, thus concentrating TF to the sites of injury (Giesen et al., 1999). TF mediates different pathological signal cascades via a family of G-protein coupled receptors called protease-activated receptors (PARs) (Rao and Pendurthi, 2005).

Four types of PARs have been identified PAR1, PAR2, PAR3 and PAR4. PAR1 receptor was found in the normal liver as well as diseased liver (Rullier et al., 2008; Nault et al., 2016) and has been shown to perform a key role in the pathogenesis of liver fibrosis (Sullivan et al., 2010). PAR1 is expressed by various cells including endothelial cells, fibroblasts, smooth muscle cells and T lymphocytes (Coughlin, 2000). In the liver of patients with cirrhosis and chronic hepatitis, PAR1 was positively stained in fibroblasts in the fibrotic septa in addition to the inflammatory cells infiltrated around newly formed blood vessels and bile ducts (Rullier et al., 2008). PAR1 is primarily activated by thrombin and can be also activated by activated protein C (Riewald et al., 2003), coagulation factor Xa (FXa; Riewald et al., 2001), coagulation

factor VIIa (FVIIa; Camerer et al., 2000) and plasmin (Pendurthi et al., 2002). Thrombin-mediated activation of PAR1 has been reported to contribute to several inflammatory and fibrotic diseases including liver fibrosis (Sullivan et al., 2010).

In the liver, toll-like receptor 4 (TLR4) is found on both Kupffer cells and HSCs (Bai et al., 2013). TLR4 is the main target for lipopolysaccharide (LPS) and is largely involved in the inflammatory reaction associated with liver fibrosis (Beutler, 2004). TLR4 signaling through Kupffer cells leads to the release of proinflammatory cytokines such as TNF-α, IL-1 and IL-6 (Beutler, 2004). Moreover, TLR4 expressed on Kupffer cells is involved in the fibrogenic signaling of HSCs and enhancing their response to transforming growth factor-1β (TGF-1β) thus promoting liver fibrosis (Seki et al., 2007). Interestingly, it has been reported that in patients with hepatitis C infection, specific single-nucleotide polymorphisms of TLR4 affected the rate of fibrosis progression (Huang et al., 2007).

Blocking of specific gene expression has recently gained a growing considerable interest as a tool to decrease the expression of a target protein. DNA encodes RNA, which is then translated into proteins (Chery, 2016). Antisense oligodeoxynucleotides (AS-ODNs) are single-stranded oligodeoxynucleotides that bind to compatible mRNA with a high degree of accuracy, leading to a decline in the target protein level (Bennett and Swayze, 2010). Different types of oligonucleotides antisense sequences, including reverse sequences, antisense sequences containing one or more mismatches and scrambled oligonucleotides have been used as a control of AS-ODNs (Gagnon and Corey, 2019). Over the last years, therapeutic strategies including AS-ODNs that suppress translation of mRNA and other oligonucleotides that interfere with RNA pathway have been substantially improved as a therapy platform at both preclinical and clinical levels (Chi et al., 2005; Kastelein et al., 2006). In 1998, fomivirsen was approved as the first agent that inhibits the translation of mRNA encoding for cytomegalovirus at its early immediate region proteins and permitted for treating cytomegalovirus retinitis (Jabs and Griffiths, 2002). Importantly, by January 2020, 10 oligonucleotide drugs have gained regulatory approval from the FDA (Roberts et al., 2020).

The objective of this work is to study the theory that chemically induced liver fibrosis is TF-dependent and consequently inhibition of TF expression by antisense tissue factor oligodeoxynucleotides (TFAS) could be associated with reduced severity of liver fibrosis. In addition, the study aimed at exploring the TLR4-TF-PAR1 signaling loop as a novel pathway that may be involved in liver fibrosis and the possible role of suppressing TF expression in blocking this loop as a form of cross-talk between coagulation, inflammation and fibrogenesis.

MATERIAL AND METHODS

Experimental Animals

Male Sprague Dawley rats with an average weight of 120–150 gm (5–6 weeks old) were purchased from the Egyptian Organization for Biological Products and Vaccines (Cairo, Egypt). Animals were placed in cages and kept under conventional laboratory conditions throughout the study (room temperature 24–27°C and 55 ± 10% humidity) with alternating 12 h light and dark cycles. Animals were fed normal chow and were permitted water *ad libitum*. They were left in the animal house at Faculty of Pharmacy, Cairo University for acclimatization for one week before the start of the study where rats whose weight exceeded 150 gm were excluded. Male rats are strictly used while female rats are avoided in the experiment to prevent unintended risks. The experimental protocol was approved by the Research Ethics Committee (REC) of Faculty of Pharmacy, Cairo University (PT 1902).

Drugs and Chemicals

N-diethyl nitrosamine (DEN) was purchased from Sigma Chemicals (MO, United States) and dissolved in saline. Carbon tetrachloride (CCl4) was obtained from El Gomhorya Co. (Cairo, Egypt). Tissue factor oligodeoxynucleotides (TF-ODNs) were purchased from Integrated DNA Technologies (San Diego, CA, United States) and dissolved in saline. The sequence of the rat antisense tissue factor oligodeoxynucleotides (TFAS) is 5'-CATGGGGATAGCCAT-3' while the sequence of scrambled control of tissue factor oligodeoxynucleotides (TFSC) is 5'-TGACGCAGAGTCGTA-3'. All chemicals were of the highest purity and analytical grade.

Sample Size Calculation

A total of 40 rats were divided into five groups ($n = 8$) where each group was placed in a cage. The sample size was calculated using G*Power software (GPower 3.1. Ink) where the effect size is 0.77, α level is 0.05 and power (1-β) is 0.95.

Experimental Design

Rats were allocated to cages by simple randomization using a web-based research randomizer and within the same cage, rats received the treatment randomly. The technician was blinded to the group status and the treatment administered to the rats. All the treatments and animals were handled and monitored in the same way. The authors were responsible for treatment preparation, anesthesia and sample collection. The groups were divided as follows:

Control group: healthy rats received saline throughout the experiment, TFAS group: rats treated with TFAS (2.8 mg/kg; s. c.) once a week for six weeks according to Nakamura et al. (2002) and Shimizu et al., (2014).

DEN+CCl4 group: liver fibrosis was induced by injection of a single dose of DEN (200 mg/kg; i. p.) and after one week CCl4 was administered (3 ml/kg; s. c.) once a week for six weeks according to Mansour et al. (2010) with some modification.

TFSC+DEN+CCl4 group: rats intoxicated with DEN and received TFSC (2.8 mg/kg; s. c.) concomitantly with CCl4 for 6 weeks.

TFAS+DEN+CCl4 group: rats intoxicated with DEN and received TFAS (2.8 mg/kg; s. c.) concomitantly with CCl4 for 6 weeks.

Animals were sacrificed following the time frame from starting the experiment till the end of the 7th week.

Sample Collection

Blood samples were collected from the jugular vein and sera were separated. Rats were euthanized using thiopental (85 mg/kg; i. p.; Gonca, 2015). The liver was divided into 2 parts; one part was kept in 10% neutral formalin, whereas the second part was stored in −80°C. The measurements were performed by personnel that were blinded completely to the group status.

Assessment of Liver Functions

Serum liver enzymes activities; alanine aminotransferase (ALT), aspartate aminotransferase (AST) and alkaline phosphatase (ALP) were assessed using colorimetric commercially available assay kits (Biodiagnostic, Giza, Egypt) according to the manufacturer's instructions.

Determination of Liver Content of Tumor Necrosis Factor-alpha

Part of the frozen liver tissue was homogenized in phosphate buffer saline (PBS, pH 7.4) for the assessment of liver TNF-α content using ELISA specific kit (Ray Biotech, United States; ELR-TNFα). The parameter was assessed according to the manufacturer's protocol.

Determination of Liver Hydroxyproline Content

Liver hydroxyproline content was assessed using frozen liver tissue as previously described by Edwards and O'Brien (1980) with slight modifications. Briefly, liver samples were weighed and hydrolyzed in 2.5 ml of 6N HCl at 110°C for 18 h in Teflon coated tubes. The hydrolysate was centrifuged at 3000 rpm for 10 min; the pH of the supernatant was allocated to 7.4 and the absorbance was measured at 558 nm. Total hydroxyproline content was measured against a standard curve established with trans-4-hydroxy-L-proline (Sigma- Aldrich, St Louis, MO, United States).

Analysis of Tissue Factor, Transforming Growth Factor-1beta and Protease-Activated Receptors1 Gene Expression *via* qRT-PCR

Relative quantification of gene expression was performed by extraction of RNA from liver cells using TRIzol plus RNA purification kit (life technologies, Carlsbad, United States) according to the manufacturer's protocol. RNA was reverse transcribed using High Capacity cDNA Reverse Transcription Kit (Applied Biosystems, Foster, CA, United States). Quantification of TGF-1β and PAR1 PCR was carried out using Rotor-Gene Q 5 plex real-time Rotary analyzer (Corbett Life Science, United States). Quantification of TF RNA, TGF-1β RNA and PAR1 RNA was carried out using PCR fluorescence quantitative diagnostic kit, with SYBR Green PCR Master Mix (Applied Biosystems, United States). For quantification of TGF-1β, the primers 5'-TACCATGCCAACTTCTGTCTGGGA-3' (forward primer) and 5'-ATGTTGACAACTGCTCCACCTTG-

3' (reverse primer) were normalized against β-actin 5'-ATCTGG CACCACACCTTC-3' (forward primer) and 5'-AGCCAGGTC CAGACGCA-3' (reverse primer). For quantification of PAR1, primers 5'-CTTGCTGATCGTCGCCC-3' (forward primer) and 5'-TTCACCGTAGCATCTGTCCT-3' (reverse primer) and for quantification of TF, primers 5'-ATGGCTATCCCCATG-3' (forward primer) and 5'-CATGGGGATAGCCAT-3' (reverse primer) were normalized against GADPH 5'-CTGCACCAC CAACTGCTTAC-3' (forward primer) and reverse 5'-CAG AGGTGCCATCCAGAGTT-3' (reverse primer).

Flow Cytometric Analysis of Toll-Like Receptor4

For detection of TLR4 cell surface expression, frozen liver tissue was homogenized then single-cell suspension was washed with staining buffer (PBS containing 1% FBS). Cells were then incubated with biotin-conjugated rat anti-human TLR4 antibody at a concentration of 20 ml/10^6 cells for 30 min on ice. After washing with staining buffer, the cells were mixed with Streptavidin-phycoerythrin and immediately analyzed with a flow cytometer FACScan and CellQuest Software.

Histopathological Examination of Liver With Collagen and Fibrosis Scoring

Liver samples preserved in 10% neutral formalin were washed under tap water; then serial dilutions of alcohol were used for dehydration. Specimens were cleared in xylene and embedded in paraffin. Sections at 4 μm thicknesses were prepared by slide microtome and stained with hematoxylin and eosin (H and E) and Masson's Trichome staining to examine liver histopathological and fibrotic changes. All histopathological examinations were performed by an experienced pathologist who was blinded to the study groups. All methods of tissue sample preparation and staining were carried out as outlined by Drury and Wallington (1983). Qualitative and quantitative scoring of collagen was performed using a full HD microscopic imaging system (Leica Microsystems GmbH, Germany) operated by Leica Application software. The total

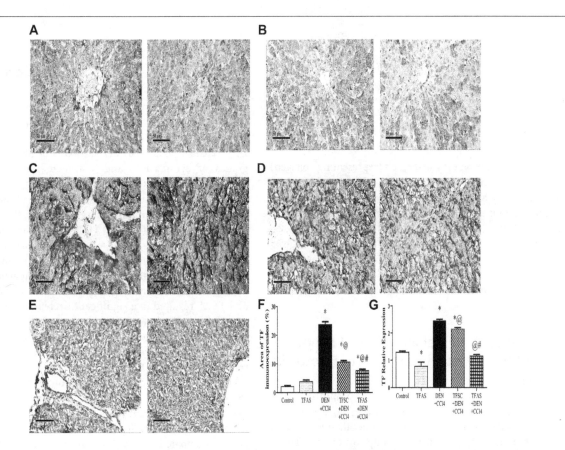

FIGURE 1 | Effect of TF-ODNs on the liver TF expression in DEN+CCl4 intoxicated rats. Immune-stained liver section of TF expression with positive stained grades of cytoplasmic and sub membranous positivity in numerous hepatocytes, (A) control group, (B) TFAS group, (C) DEN+CCl4 group, (D) TFSC+DEN+CCl4 group, (E) TFAS+DEN+CCl4 group and (F) The percentage area of TF immune-expression and (G) qPCR determined TF expression in all study groups. Data are expressed as mean ± SEM (n = 8). (*), (@) and (#) indicate significant difference from Control, DEN+CCl4 and TFSC+DEN+CCl4, respectively at P < 0.05 using one-way ANOVA followed by Tukey-Kramer post-Hoc test. TF: tissue factor; DEN: N-diethyl nitrosamine; CCl4: carbon tetrachloride; TFSC: scrambled tissue factor oligodeoxynucleotides; TFAS: antisense tissue factor oligodeoxynucleotides.

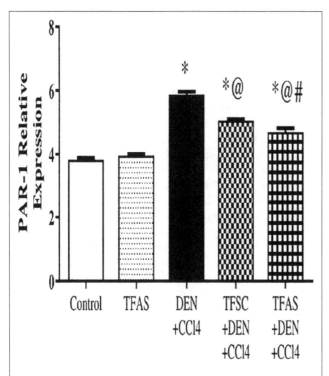

FIGURE 2 | Effect of TF-ODNs on relative expression of PAR1 in liver. Data are expressed as mean ± SEM (n = 8). (*), (@) and (#) indicate significant difference from Control, DEN+CCl4 and TFSC+DEN+CCl4, respectively at *P* < 0.05 using one-way ANOVA followed by Tukey-Kramer post-Hoc test. PAR1: protease activated receptor 1; DEN: N-diethyl nitrosamine; CCl4: carbon tetrachloride; TFSC: scrambled tissue factor oligodeoxynucleotides; TFAS: antisense tissue factor oligodeoxynucleotides.

specimen area and the blue-stained pixels (representing collagen) were segmented. Percent (%) collagen was calculated as the ratio of blue-stained to total specimen pixels. The criteria used for microscopic lesions and fibrosis scoring was listed as follows (Al-Sayed et al., 2019): (−), no lesions were demonstrated; (+), few lesions were demonstrated in one examines section; (++), mild lesions were focally demonstrated in some examined sections; (+++), moderate lesions were diffusely demonstrated in some examined sections; and (++++), severe lesions were diffused in all examined sections.

Immunohistochemical Staining of Alpha Smooth Muscle Actin and Tissue Factor in the Liver

According to the manufacturer's protocol, deparaffinized 4 μm thick tissue sections were treated with 3% H_2O_2 for 20 min, washed, then incubated with anti-alpha smooth muscle actin antibody and anti-tissue factor antibody overnight. Tissue sections were washed with PBS followed by incubation with secondary antibody HRP Envision kit (DAKO) for 20 min and incubated after washing with diaminobenzidine (DAB) for 10 min and then washed finally with PBS and hematoxylin was added for counter staining. Finally, tissue sections were

dehydrated and cleared in xylene. Area percentage of immune-expression levels of α-SMA and TF sections were determined using Leica application module for tissue sections analysis attached to full HD microscopic imaging system (Leica Microsystems GmbH, Germany).

Statistical Analysis

Data analysis was carried out with complete blindness to the study group status. Results were expressed as mean ± SEM. Statistical significance was determined by one-way ANOVA followed by Tukey-Kramer post-Hoc test. P value < 0.05 was considered significant. In addition, correlation and linear regression between TF and the assessed parameters as well as between PAR1 and TLR4 were carried out where slope differences were compared, tested and checked for significance at P< 0.0001. Correlation Coefficient "r" was calculated where the difference in "r" value states that variation of one of the variables will affect the variation in the other one through R^2 calculation. GraphPad Prism 8 for Windows (GraphPad Software, Inc, La Jolla, United States) was used in all analyses.

RESULTS

Effect of Tissue Factor-Oligodeoxynucleotides on the Liver Tissue Factor Expression

Immunohistochemical detection of TF expression in liver sections of control and TFAS groups showed weak basal expression of TF (**Figures 1A,B**). However, liver sections of DEN+CCl4 intoxicated rats showed sharply stained positive grades of cytoplasmic and sub membranous positivity in numerous hepatocytes (**Figure 1C**). The liver sections from DEN+CCl4 intoxicated rats received TFSC showed decreased hepatocellular staining compared to the DEN+CCl4 intoxicated group (**Figure 1D**). Rats that received TFAS showed a profound decrease in TF expression (**Figure 1E**). Area of TF expression showed a significant increase in the DEN+CCl4 intoxicated rats by 943.48% comparing to the basal expression of the control group. Treatment of rats with TFSC and TFAS resulted in a significant decrease in the elevated TF expression by 54.16 and 67.92%, respectively in comparison to untreated intoxicated rats. TFAS treatment significantly decreased TF expression by 30% compared to TFSC treatment (**Figure 1F**).

TF expression was determined by qPCR that showed a significant decrease by 39.78% upon treatment with TFAS alone when compared to the control group. TF expression increased significantly in the DEN+CCl4 intoxicated group by 88.03% compared with control group. Treatment of rats with TFSC and TFAS decreased the elevated TF expression by 12.17 and 52.37%, respectively compared with intoxicated group. Intoxicated rats that were treated with TFAS treatment showed a significant decrease by 45.78% when compared to TFSC treatment (**Figure 1G**).

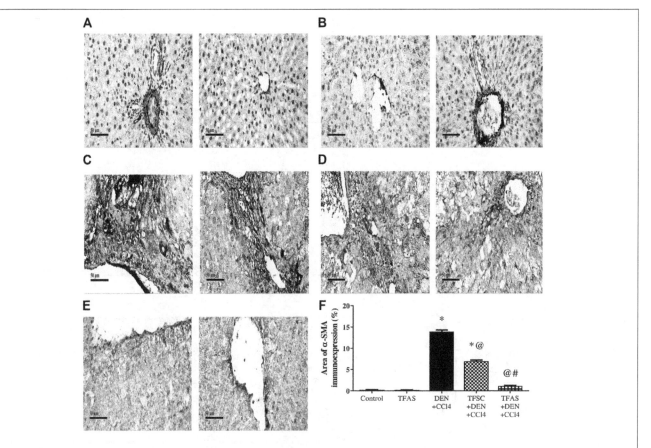

FIGURE 3 | Effect of TF-ODNs on liver α-SMA expression. Immune-stained liver section of α-SMA expression is detected in hepatic stellate cells, fibroblasts and vascular wall, **(A)** control group, **(B)** TFAS group, **(C)** DEN+CCl4 group, **(D)** TFSC+DEN+CCl4 group, **(E)** TFAS+DEN+CCl4 group and **(F)** The percentage of α-SMA expression. Data are expressed as mean ± SEM (n = 8). (*), (@) and (#) indicate significant difference from Control, DEN+CCl4 and TFSC+DEN+CCl4, respectively at $P < 0.05$ using one-way ANOVA followed by Tukey-Kramer post-Hoc test. α-SMA: alpha smooth muscle actin; DEN: N-diethyl nitrosamine; CCl4: carbon tetrachloride; TFSC: scrambled tissue factor oligodeoxynucleotides; TFAS: antisense tissue factor oligodeoxynucleotides.

Effect of Tissue Factor-Oligodeoxynucleotides on Protease-Activated Receptors1 Expression in Liver

PAR1 expression in the livers excised from DEN+CCl4 intoxicated rats was significantly increased by 55.26% compared to the control group. The treatment of intoxicated rats with TFSC and TFAS significantly decreased the elevated level of PAR1 by 13.56 and 20.34%, respectively compared to the DEN+CCl4 group and TFAS treatment manifested a significant decrease in PAR1 expression by 7.84% compared to TFSC (**Figure 2**).

Effect of Tissue Factor-Oligodeoxynucleotides on Liver Alpha-Smooth Muscle Actin Expression

Control and TFAS treated animals showed weak basal expression of α-SMA (**Figures 3A,B**). Rats intoxicated with DEN+CCl4 showed increased α-SMA expression with strongly stained hepatic cells, fibroblasts and vascular wall (**Figure 3C**). DEN+CCl4 intoxicated group treated with

TFSC revealed a decreased area of α-SMA positive cells (**Figure 3D**). In the DEN+CCl4 intoxicated group treated with TFAS, the area of α-SMA expression was nearly similar to that of control animals (**Figure 3E**). Area of α-SMA stained liver cells showed a significant decrease with both TFSC and TFAS treatment when compared to DEN+CCl4 intoxicated animals by 50.71 and 91.43%, respectively. In addition, TFAS treatment showed a significant decrease in α-SMA expression by 82.61% compared to TFSC treatment of intoxicated rats (**Figure 3F**).

Effect of Tissue Factor-Oligodeoxynucleotides on Serum Activities of Alanine aminotransferase, Aspartate aminotransferase and Alkaline Phosphatase

As shown in **Figure 4**, serum activities of ALT (**A**), AST (**B**) and ALP (**C**) are elevated significantly upon DEN+CCl4 intoxication by 18.75, 48.28 and 29.17%, respectively compared to the control group. These elevations were significantly decreased in rats intoxicated with the DEN+CCl4 and treated with TFAS by 7.89, 19.77 and 8.06%, respectively, compared to the untreated

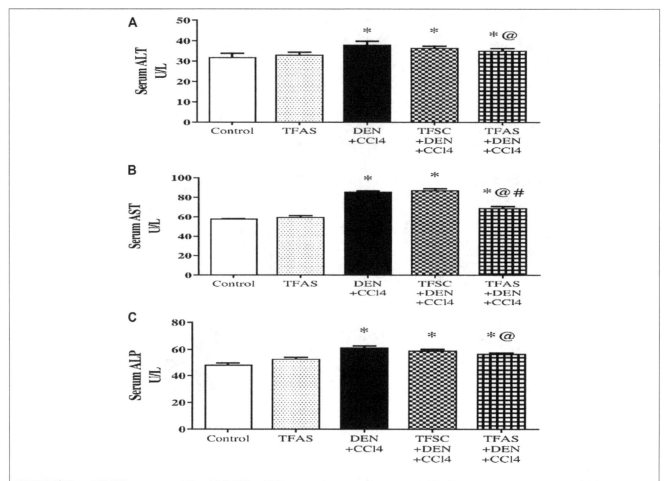

FIGURE 4 | Effect of TF-ODNs on serum activities of ALT, AST and ALP enzymes. Liver enzymes activities of ALT, AST and ALP are presented in figure **(A)**, **(B)** and **(C)**, respectively. Data are expressed as mean ± SEM (n = 8). (*), (@) and (#) indicate significant difference from Control, DEN+CCl4 and TFSC+DEN+CCl4, respectively at P < 0.05 using one-way ANOVA followed by Tukey-Kramer post-Hoc test. ALT: alanine aminotransferase; AST: aspartate aminotransferase; ALP: alkaline phosphatase; DEN: N-diethyl nitrosamine; CCl4: carbon tetrachloride; TFSC: scrambled tissue factor oligodeoxynucleotides; TFAS: antisense tissue factor oligodeoxynucleotides.

intoxicated rats. There was a non-significant difference in serum enzymes activities between the DEN+CCl4 group and that treated with TFSC. On the other hand, serum activity of AST was significantly improved in the intoxicated animals treated TFAS compared to those treated with TFSC.

Effect of Tissue Factor-Oligodeoxynucleotides on Histopathological Features

The control group of rats showed normal histology of the liver (**Figure 5A**) as well as apparent normal features in TFAS-treated rats (**Figure 5B**). However, rats intoxicated with DEN+CCl4 showed a severe loss in hepatic architecture (**Figure 5C**) where degeneration of hepatocytes, area of coagulative hepatocellular necrosis, sinusoidal dilatation, the proliferation of biliary epithelium with periportal infiltration of inflammatory cells in portal areas as well as fibroblastic proliferation and bridging were demonstrated in this group (**Table 1**). These histopathological alterations were moderately reduced in the

group intoxicated and treated with TFAS (**Figure 5E**). In contrast, treatment with TFSC didn't significantly improve the histopathological features (**Figure 5D**).

Effect of Tissue Factor-Oligodeoxynucleotides on Collagen Deposition and Liver Hydroxyproline Content

Control and TFAS-treated normal rats showed uniform collagen distribution (**Figures 6A,B**). Animals intoxicated with DEN+CCl4 showed central vein, portal tract and septal fibrosis that were stained positively for collagen fiber bundles in Masson's Trichome stained liver sections (**Figure 6C**). Treatment with TFSC showed relatively decreased area of collagen accumulation in liver sections (**Figure 6D**) but animals treated with TFAS after intoxication restored collagen distribution nearly to the control rats (**Figure 6E**). The elevated area of collagen deposition in rats intoxicated with DEN+CCl4 was significantly declined with treatment with TFSC and TFAS by 61 and 80%, respectively. In

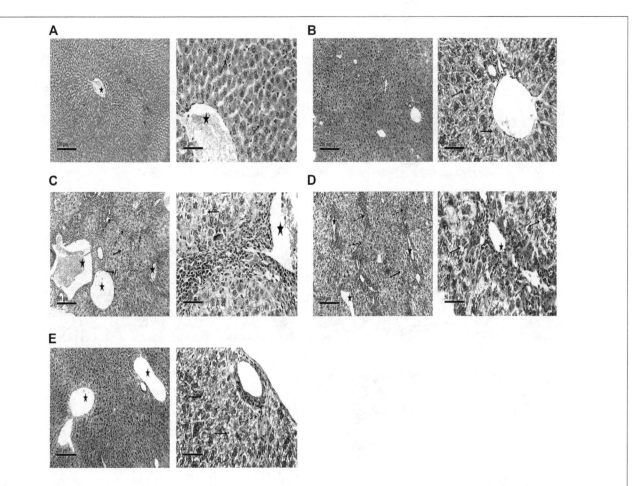

FIGURE 5 | Effect of DEN+CCl4 and TF-ODNs on histopathological features. **(A)** normal histologic structure showing central vein (star) from control group, **(B)** TFAS treated rats showing apparently normal histological features with minimal degenerative changes, **(C)** DEN+CCl4 intoxicated rats showing sever vacuolar degenerative and necrotic hepatocellular changes (black arrow) accompanied with many dilated liver blood vessels (star) and sever periportal inflammatory cells infiltrates (red arrow), **(D)** TFSC treated intoxicated rats showing slight amelioration of abnormal morphological changes with persistence of sever vacuolar degenerative of hepatocytes (arrow), **(E)** TFAS treated intoxicated rats showing moderate amelioration of morphological changes with dilated blood vessels and mild periportal inflammatory cells infiltrates (arrow head); DEN: N-diethyl nitrosamine; CCl4: carbon tetrachloride; TFSC: scrambled tissue factor oligodeoxynucleotides; TFAS: antisense tissue factor oligodeoxynucleotides.

TABLE 1 | Effect of TF-ODNs on liver histopathological and fibrotic changes.

Groups	Degenerative/necrotic changes	Inflammatory cells infiltrates	Fibroblastic proliferation and bridging	Dilated blood vessels
Control	–	–	–	–
TFAS	+	–	–	–
DEN+CCl4	++++	++++	++++	+++
TFSC+DEN+CCl4	++++	+++	+++	+++
TFAS+DEN+CCl4	+++	++	+	+++

– nil: no lesions were demonstrated; +: few lesions were demonstrated in one examined section; ++: mild lesions were focally demonstrated in some examined section; +++: moderate lesions were diffusely demonstrated in some examined section; ++++: severe lesions were diffused in all examined sections.

addition, TFAS showed a more significant decrease by 48.72% compared to rats treated with TFSC (**Figure 6F**). Animals intoxicated with DEN+CCl4 showed a significant increase in liver hydroxyproline content by 42.7% compared to the control group. In contrast to collagen deposition, treatment with TFSC didn't show significant difference in hydroxyproline content, while TFAS showed a significant decrease by 10.68% compared to DEN+CCl4 intoxicated group (**Figure 6G**).

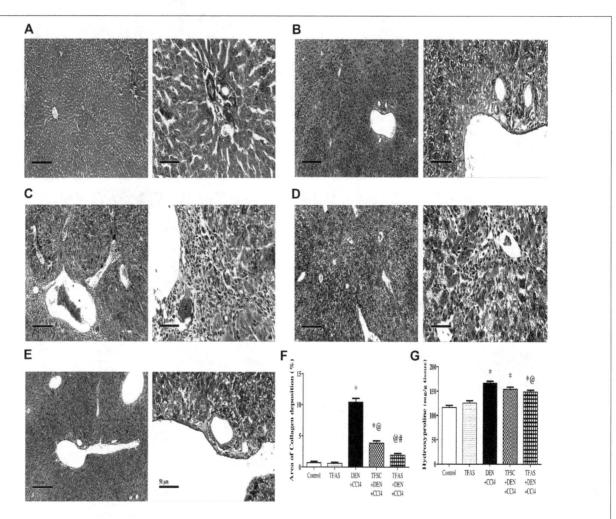

FIGURE 6 | Effect of TF-ODNs on collagen deposition and hydroxyproline content in the liver. **(A)** Masson's Trichome-stained liver section of control group, **(B)** TFAS group, **(C)** DEN+CCl4 group where obvious periportal proliferation of fibroblasts are detected as well as bridging of fibroblasts with abundant formation of collagen fibers, **(D)** TFSC+DEN+CCl4 group and **(E)** TFAS+DEN+CCl4 group showed significant reduction of activated fibroblasts and collagen fibers, **(F)** Percentage area of collagen deposition and **(G)** liver hydroxyproline content in different study groups. Data are expressed as mean ± SEM (n = 8). (*), (@) and (#) indicate significant difference from Control, DEN+CCl4 and TFSC+DEN+CCl4, respectively at $P < 0.05$ using one-way ANOVA followed by Tukey-Kramer post-Hoc test. DEN: N-diethyl nitrosamine; CCl4: carbon tetrachloride; TFSC: scrambled tissue factor oligodeoxynucleotides; TFAS: antisense tissue factor oligodeoxynucleotides.

Effect of Tissue Factor-Oligodeoxynucleotides Effect on Toll-Like Receptor4 Expression in the Liver

Flow cytometric analysis revealed low TLR4 expression on liver cells in the control group as well as TFAS treated normal rats (**Figures 7A,B,F**). Rats intoxicated with DEN+CCl4 showed significant increase in TLR4 expression by 386.67% (**Figures 7C,F**). The intoxicated group treated with TFAS showed a significant reduction in the expression of TLR4 by 47.95% (**Figures 7E,F**). Also, TLR4 expression was significantly decreased in intoxicated group with TFAS treatment by 39.68% compared to TFSC treated one.

Effect of Tissue Factor-Oligodeoxynucleotides on Transforming Growth Factor-1beta Expression and Tumor Necrosis Factor-alpha Content

Induction of liver fibrosis by DEN+CCl4 significantly raised liver TGF-1β expression and TNF-α content by 39.44 and 66.64%, respectively compared to the control group. Treatment with TFAS significantly decreased the elevated levels of liver TGF-1β expression and TNF-α content by 18.18 and 25.43%, respectively. Also, TGF-1β expression and TNF-α content significantly decreased by 12.91 and 18.34%, respectively in TFAS treated intoxicated group compared to the TFSC treatment (**Figure 8A** and **Figure 8B**).

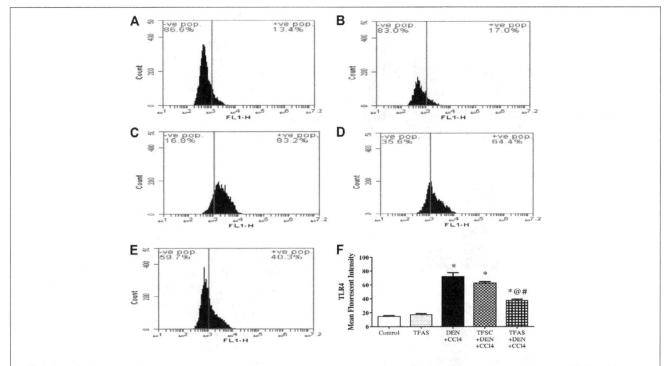

FIGURE 7 | Flow cytometric analysis of the effect of TF-ODNs on TLR4 expression in the liver. Histogram plots of **(A)** Control group, **(B)** TFAS group, **(C)** DEN+CCl4 group, **(D)** TFSC+DEN+CCl4, **(E)** TFAS+DEN+CCl4 and **(F)** Mean fluorescence intensity of TRL4. Data are expressed as mean ± SEM (n = 8). (*), (@) and (#) indicate significant difference from Control, DEN+CCl4 and TFSC+DEN+CCl4, respectively at $P < 0.05$ using one-way ANOVA followed by Tukey-Kramer post-Hoc test. TLR4: toll like receptor 4; DEN: N-diethyl nitrosamine; CCl4: carbon tetrachloride; TFSC: scrambled tissue factor oligodeoxynucleotides; TFAS: antisense tissue factor oligodeoxynucleotides.

Correlation Between Tissue Factor and the Assessed Liver Enzymes Activities, Inflammatory and Fibrotic Markers as Well as Between Protease-Activated Receptors1 and Toll-Like Receptor4 Expression

Figure 9 shows the scatter plot of the positive correlation between TF expression and the assessed parameters; ALT, AST and ALP enzyme activities (**Figure 9A**). There is also a positive correlation between TF expression and the fibrotic markers; α-SMA and PAR1 (**Figure 9B**) as well as collagen and hydroxyproline (**Figure 9C**). A positive correlation was displayed also between TF expression and remodeling and inflammatory markers; TLR4 (**Figure 9D**), TGF-1β (**Figure 9E**) and TNF-α (**Figure 9F**). Also, there is a positive correlation between TLR4 and PAR1 expression (**Figure 9G**) in all study groups.

DISCUSSION

TF is the transmembrane receptor for FVII/VIIa and the TF-FVIIa complex functions as the primary initiator of coagulation *in vivo*. TF is also recognized as a signaling receptor in different pathological conditions such as angiogenesis, tumor, inflammation and fibrogenesis (Lento et al., 2015). In normal liver, TF has been reported to be expressed primarily by hepatocytes (Sullivan et al., 2013) as well as HSCs, SECs and Kupffer cells (Arai et al., 1995).

In accordance with previous studies, liver fibrosis is induced in rats by co-administration of DEN and CCl4 (Uehara et al., 2013; Uehara et al., 2014; Marrone et al., 2016; Sung et al., 2018). Liver sections excised from animals intoxicated with DEN+CCl4 had intense TF staining in hepatocellular cytoplasm. In accordance with these results, overexpression and a profound role of TF have been reported in different models of chemically induced liver injury (Hammad et al., 2011; Abdel-Bakky et al., 2020), including CCl4-induced fibrosis (Duplantier et al., 2004). Furthermore, Knight et al. (2017) reported that mice with deletion of the cytoplasmic TF domain had amelioration of liver fibrosis compared to wild type mice following 8 weeks of CCl4 exposure. Thus, the overexpression of TF observed in this study and the previously reported implementation of TF in the pathogenesis of different models of liver injuries rose the assumption that targeting TF could be of benefit in managing liver fibrosis.

TF-ODNs were reported to inhibit TF production at both transcriptional and translational levels (Yin et al., 2010; Hammad et al., 2013). In addition, TF-ODNs have been reported to be accumulated predominantly in the rat liver following systemic administration (Nakamura et al., 2002; Shimizu et al., 2014). Indeed, in this study, subcutaneous injection of TFAS significantly inhibited the elevated expression of TF in different liver cells. Similarly, Abdel-Bakky et al. (2011);

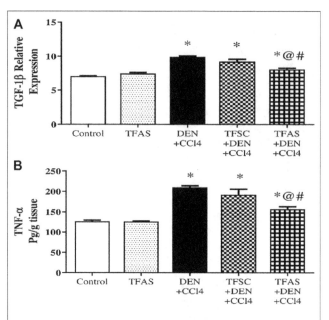

FIGURE 8 | Effect of TF-ODNs on TGF-1β expression and TNF-α content. Data are expressed as mean ± SEM (n = 8). (*), (@) and (#) indicate significant difference from Control, DEN+CCl4 and TFSC+DEN+CCl4, respectively at $P < 0.05$ using one-way ANOVA followed by Tukey-Kramer post-Hoc test. TGF-1β: transforming growth factor beta; TNF-α: tumor necrosis factor alpha; DEN: N-diethyl nitrosamine; CCl4: carbon tetrachloride; TFSC: scrambled tissue factor oligodeoxynucleotides; TFAS: antisense tissue factor oligodeoxynucleotides.

Abdel-Bakky et al. (2015) and Abdel-Bakky et al. (2020) reported significant changes in TF expression pattern in the liver sections excised from mice intoxicated with thioacetamide and CCl4 upon treatment with TFAS.

In this study animals intoxicated with DEN+CCl4 showed significant elevation in the activities of liver enzymes; ALT, AST and ALP along with severe histopathological deterioration of the liver. These observations are consistent with previous findings that animals treated with CCl4 or DEN+CCl4 showed pronounced biochemical and histopathological fibrotic alterations (Poojari et al., 2010; Uehara et al., 2013; Serag et al., 2019; Tripathy et al., 2020). However, treatment with TFAS significantly improved the abnormal activities of liver enzymes and the histopathological inflammatory and fibrotic changes associated with DEN+CCl4 intoxication. The improvement in enzyme activities is positively correlated with TF expression. In agreement with our findings, blockage of TF expression using TFAS improved histopathological and biochemical deteriorations in chemically intoxicated mice (Hammad et al., 2013; Abdel-Bakky et al., 2015 and Abdel-Bakky et al., 2020). Moreover, Luyendyk et al. (2010) demonstrated that liver macrophage and neutrophil aggregation were significantly reduced in mice with low TF expression compared to heterozygous control mice fed diet deficient in methionine and choline.

The distinguished role of HSCs in liver fibrosis was previously documented (Kisseleva and Brenner, 2021). The extent of HSCs activation and proliferation rates is indicated by the expression of characteristic specific receptors such as α-SMA (Jiang and Torok, 2013; Lin et al., 2018) and excessive production of collagen, where the deposition of collagen fibrils in liver connective tissues provides a hallmark of liver fibrosis development (Hernandez-Gea and Friedman, 2011; Bai et al., 2013). The stability of collagen fibrils is maintained by deposition of hydroxyproline amino acid, which is commonly applied as a marker for fibrogenesis and directly correlated with the total collagen and the stage of liver fibrosis (Ding et al., 2017). In the current study, DEN+CCl4-intoxicated rats showed increased α-SMA expression, collagen production and elevation of liver hydroxyproline content. These results indicated a profound activation of HSCs in response to DEN+CCl4 intoxication. Similarly, previous studies showed that α-SMA expression as well as collagen and hydroxyproline content were significantly elevated in response to injection with CCl4 alone or in combination with DEN (Mansour et al., 2010; Abdel-Moneim et al., 2015; Ahmed and Tag, 2017).

In addition to HSCs, activated Kupffer cells and infiltrated macrophages play a pivotal role in liver fibrogenesis. Activated macrophages release TGF-1β which, among growth factors, is the "master" modulator in fibrogenesis and involved in HSCs activation (Nakazato et al., 2010; Meng et al., 2016). Furthermore, they release, among other proinflammatory cytokines, TNF-α which is one of the early events in many types of liver damage and can activate HSCs and modulate innate immune and inflammatory responses (Gupta et al., 2019). In the present study, liver content of both TGF-1β and TNF-α were significantly increased upon administration of DEN+CCl4, the results that are in accordance with that reported by Tork et al. (2016), Elguindy et al. (2016) and Knight et al. (2017).

The role of coagulation proteases in liver fibrosis was recently explored. One of the primary mechanisms whereby coagulation proteases could contribute to liver fibrosis is through direct activation of HSCs. In support of this hypothesis, we found that the expression of TF is positively correlated with HSCs activation markers; α-SMA, collagen and hydroxyproline. Furthermore, these markers were significantly decreased upon TFAS treatment; these findings are consistent with Knight et al., (2017), as the authors suggested that activation of the cytoplasmic domain of TF promoted liver fibrosis by inducing HSCs activation.

Another mechanism that could underlie the pathological role of TF in liver fibrosis is via stimulation of local inflammatory cell activity. Macrophages were reported to express TF which is upregulated during macrophage maturation and fibrogenesis (Knight et al., 2017). In the present study, TFAS significantly reduced the elevated content of TGF-1β and TNF-α; the main products of inflammatory cells accompanied with fibrosis. Furthermore, our study showed a positive correlation between TF and each of TGF-1β and TNF-α. Consequently, we could assume that in addition to inhibition of HSCs, TFAS decrease TGF-1β and TNF-α production with subsequent inhibition of fibrogenesis and inflammation. In the line with our findings, Knight et al. (2017) reported that deletion of the TF cytoplasmic domain significantly lower gene and protein expression of TGF-1β by activated Kupffer cells.

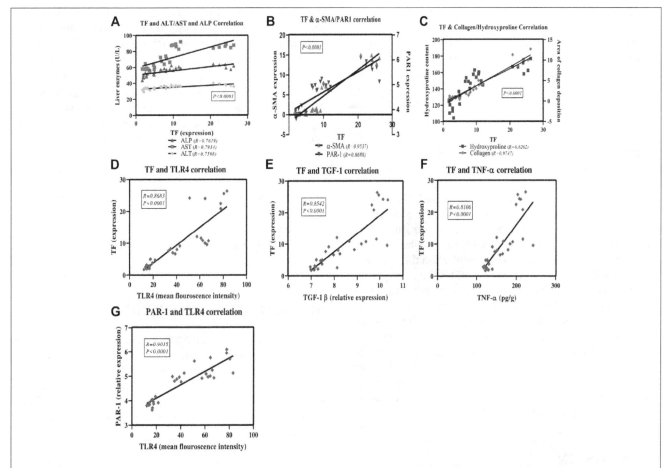

FIGURE 9 | Scatter plots of the correlation between TF and the assessed liver enzymes activities, inflammatory and fibrotic markers as well as between PAR1 and TLR4 expression. The solid lines represent the linear regression and correlation coefficient (r), P is the correlation significance level.

Since inflammation and coagulation are crosslinked with liver fibrosis and given the principal roles of TLR4 and PAR1 in inflammation and coagulation, respectively, we hypothesized that TLR4-TF-PAR1 axis would be a novel pathway involved in the pathogenesis of liver fibrosis and targeting that pathway could underlie the therapeutic benefits of TFAS.

Several studies have explored the role of PARs in liver fibrogenesis (Borensztajn et al., 2010). In chronic liver disease, HSCs express upregulated PAR1 (Fiorucci et al., 2004). Furthermore, it was found that removal of stellate cell-specific PAR1 produced a 35% reduction in the accumulation of liver collagen (Poole et al., 2020) and PAR1 deficient mice appeared to be protected from CCl4-induced liver fibrosis (Rullier et al., 2008; Kallis et al., 2014). In the line with these findings, the current study showed that PAR1 expression was significantly increased in the DEN+CCl4 intoxicated rats.

TLR4 is a main receptor involved in different inflammatory processes (Lucas and Maes, 2013). A crucial role of TLR4 in fibrogenesis was highlighted in experiment where TLR4 mutant mice showed decreased liver fibrosis in response to toxic agents (Seki et al., 2007; El-Kashef and Serrya, 2019). Furthermore, Liang et al. (2016) demonstrated that HSCs activation and proliferation were prohibited through suppression of TLR4 signaling pathway

in DEN-induced liver fibrosis. In accordance with these studies, we reported that liver fibrosis induced by DEN+CCl4 injection was associated with significantly increased expression of TLR4 in the liver tissue.

The contribution of both PAR1 and TLR4 in the beneficial effects of TF blockage was clarified in this study, as rats received TFAS showed a significant reduction in the expression of both PAR1 and TLR4 in liver cells. These findings shed the light on the possibility of crosslinking among the three receptors in controlling liver fibrosis.

Thrombin is produced mainly through cleavage of prothrombin by TF (Mann et al., 2003) and blockage of TF expression resulted in decreased thrombin production (Carraway et al., 2003). Thrombin was reported to produce a dual effect on liver fibrosis via action on PAR1 and through TLR4. Firstly, it was proclaimed that thrombin activates PAR1 on both HSCs and Kupffer cells with subsequent progression of fibrosis (Fiorucci et al., 2004; Rullier et al., 2008). Secondly, thrombin was reported as a critical mediator in LPS-induced liver damage (Rondina et al., 2011) and gut-derived-LPS through TLR4 activation was significantly involved in CCl4-induced liver fibrosis (Seki et al., 2007; Rondina et al., 2011; Wang et al., 2020). Accordingly, blockage of thrombin formation through inhibition of TF could diminish the roles of both PAR1 and TLR4 in the fibrogenic process.

Consequently, based on our findings and the previous studies, we can assume that inhibition of TF expression could censor the downstream production of thrombin with subsequent inhibition of PAR1 and TLR4 mediated fibrogenic and inflammatory process. On the other hand, we can assume that the improvement in the fibrosis observed with TFAS treatment could be reflected in the reduced expression of receptors upregulated under the pathological condition of fibrosis including PAR1 and TLR4.

Notably, the results of this study showed that control oligonucleotides; TFSC resulted in a significant reduction in the expression of TF, PAR1, α-SMA and collagen, although it was significantly less when compared with the effect observed with TFAS. On the other hand, TFSC didn't affect the level of the other assessed parameters compared to DEN+CCl4 group. These results indicate that TFSC may have some specificity towards the TF mRNA binding site and the decreased expression of PAR1, α-SMA and collagen could be the consequences of TFSC-induced inhibition of TF expression. In support of our explanation, it has been reported that various degrees of downregulation of gene expression have been observed with different types of control oligonucleotides that depend on the nature of the used control oligonucleotides, i.e., its base composition, sequence and/or nature of the backbone (Agrawal, 1996).

CONCLUSION

The current study established, for the first time to our knowledge, the potential crosstalk between TF, PAR1 and TLR4 in liver fibrosis. The positive correlation between blockage of TF expression and the downregulation of both PAR1 and TLR4 provides support for the solid crosslink between the receptors. Furthermore, this study reported that blockage of TF expression and gene silencing, using TFAS, reduced liver damage and improved fibrotic changes associated with CCl4+DEN intoxication. These findings offer a platform on which recovery from liver fibrosis could be mediated through targeting TF expression as a key factor in fibrogenesis. Future mechanistic and preclinic studies are recommended to support our findings.

ETHICS STATEMENT

The animal study was reviewed and approved by Research Ethics Committee (REC) of Faculty of Pharmacy, Cairo University, Egypt.

AUTHOR CONTRIBUTIONS

MS, ME-N, MT, RA, and SK contributed to conception and design of the study. MS and ME-N organized the database. ME-N and MS performed the statistical analysis. ME-N and MS wrote the first draft of the manuscript. MS, ME-N, MT, and RA wrote sections of the manuscript. All authors contributed to manuscript revision, read, and approved the submitted version.

REFERENCES

Abdel-Bakky, M. S., Hammad, M. A., Walker, L. A., and Ashfaq, M. K. (2011). Tissue Factor Dependent Liver Injury Causes Release of Retinoid Receptors (RXR-α and RAR-α) as Lipid Droplets. *Biochem. Biophysical Res. Commun.* 410 (1), 146–151. doi:10.1016/j.bbrc.2011.05.127

Abdel-Bakky, M. S., Helal, G. K., El-Sayed, E. M., Alhowail, A. H., Mansour, A. M., Alharbi, K. S., et al. (2020). Silencing of Tissue Factor by Antisense Deoxyoligonucleotide Mitigates Thioacetamide-Induced Liver Injury. *Naunyn-schmiedeberg's Arch. Pharmacol.* 393, 1887–1898. doi:10.1007/s00210-020-01896-0

Abdel-Bakky, M. S., Helal, G. K., El-Sayed, E. M., and Saad, A. S. (2015). Carbon Tetrachloride-Induced Liver Injury in Mice is Tissue Factor Dependent. *Environ. Toxicol. Pharmacol.* 39 (3), 1199–1205. doi:10.1016/j.etap.2015.02.012

Abdel-Moneim, A. M., Al-Kahtani, M. A., El-Kersh, M. A., and Al-Omair, M. A. (2015). Free Radical-Scavenging, Anti-inflammatory/anti-fibrotic and Hepatoprotective Actions of Taurine and Silymarin against CCl4 Induced Rat Liver Damage. *PLoS ONE* 10 (12), e0144509. doi:10.1371/journal.pone.0144509

Agrawal, S. (1996). Antisense Oligonucleotides: Towards Clinical Trials. *Trends Biotechnology* 14 (10), 376–387. doi:10.1016/0167-7799(96)10053-6

Ahmed, A., Hassanin, A., Hassan, A., Ali, S., and El-Anwar, A. (2017). Therapeutic Effects of Milk Thistle Extract against Renal Toxicity Induced by Diethylnitrosamine and Carbon Tetrachloride in Adult Rats. *J. Vet. Anat.* 10 (1), 107–124. doi:10.21608/jva.2017.37166

Al-Sayed, E., Abdel-Daim, M. M., and Khattab, M. A. (2019). Hepatoprotective Activity of Praecoxin a Isolated from Melaleuca Ericifolia against Carbon Tetrachloride-induced Hepatotoxicity in Mice. Impact on Oxidative Stress, Inflammation, and Apoptosis. *Phytotherapy Res.* 33 (2), 461–470. doi:10.1002/ptr.6242

Arai, M., Mochida, S., Ohno, A., Ogata, I., Obama, H., Maruyama, I., et al. (1995). Blood Coagulation Equilibrium in Rat Liver Microcirculation as Evaluated by Endothelial Cell Thrombomodulin and Macrophage Tissue Factor. *Thromb. Res.* 80 (2), 113–123. doi:10.1016/0049-3848(95)00157-M

Bai, T., Lian, L.-H., Wu, Y.-L., Wan, Y., and Nan, J.-X. (2013). Thymoquinone Attenuates Liver Fibrosis via PI3K and TLR4 Signaling Pathways in Activated Hepatic Stellate Cells. *Int. Immunopharmacol.* 15 (2), 275–281. doi:10.1016/j.intimp.2012.12.020

Bennett, C. F., and Swayze, E. E. (2010). RNA Targeting Therapeutics: Molecular Mechanisms of Antisense Oligonucleotides as a Therapeutic Platform. *Annu. Rev. Pharmacol. Toxicol.* 50, 259–293. doi:10.1146/annurev.pharmtox.010909.105654

Benyon, R. C., and Iredale, J. P. (2000). Is Liver Fibrosis Reversible?. *Gut* 46 (4), 443–446. doi:10.1136/gut.46.4.443

Beutler, B. (2004). Inferences, Questions and Possibilities in Toll-like Receptor Signalling. *Nature* 430 (6996), 257–263. doi:10.1038/nature02761

Borensztajn, K., Von Der Thüsen, J. H., Peppelenbosch, M. P., and Spek, C. A. (2010). The Coagulation Factor Xa/protease Activated Receptor-2 axis in the Progression of Liver Fibrosis: A Multifaceted Paradigm. *J. Cell. Mol. Med.* 14 (1–2), 143–153. doi:10.1111/j.1582-4934.2009.00980.x

Calvaruso, V., Maimone, S., Gatt, A., Tuddenham, E., Thursz, M., Pinzani, M., et al. (2008). Coagulation and Fibrosis in Chronic Liver Disease. *Gut* 57 (12), 1722–1727. doi:10.1136/gut.2008.150748

Camerer, E., Huang, W., Coughlin, S. R., and Majerus, P. W. (2000). Tissue Factor- and Factor X-dependent Activation of Protease-Activated Receptor 2 by Factor VIIa. *Proc. Natl. Acad. Sci.* 97 (10), 5255–5260. doi:10.1073/pnas.97.10.5255

Carraway, M. S., Welty-Wolf, K. E., Miller, D. L., Ortel, T. L., Idell, S., Ghio, A. J., et al. (2003). Blockade of Tissue Factor. *Am. J. Respir. Crit. Care Med.* 167 (9), 1200–1209. doi:10.1164/rccm.200204-287OC

Chery, J. (2016). RNA Therapeutics: RNAi and Antisense Mechanisms and Clinical Applications. *Postdoc J.* 4 (7), 35. doi:10.14304/surya.jpr.v4n7.5

Chi, K. N., Eisenhauer, E., Fazli, L., Jones, E. C., Goldenberg, S. L., Powers, J., et al. (2005). A Phase I Pharmacokinetic and Pharmacodynamic Study of OGX-011, a 2'-Methoxyethyl Antisense Oligonucleotide to Clusterin, in Patients with Localized Prostate Cancer. *J. Natl. Cancer Inst.* 97 (17), 1287–1296. doi:10.1093/jnci/dji252

Coughlin, S. R. (2000). Thrombin Signalling and Protease-Activated Receptors. *Nature* 407 (6801), 258–264. doi:10.1038/35025229

Ding, Y.-F., Wu, Z.-H., Wei, Y.-J., Shu, L., and Peng, Y.-R. (2017). Hepatic Inflammation-Fibrosis-Cancer axis in the Rat Hepatocellular Carcinoma Induced by Diethylnitrosamine. *J. Cancer Res. Clin. Oncol.* 143 (5), 821–834. doi:10.1007/s00432-017-2364-z

Drury, R. A. B., and Wallington, E. A. (1983). *Carleton's Histological Technique.* 5th edn. New York: Churchill Livingstone. doi:10.4095/315163

Duplantier, J. G., Dubuisson, L., Senant, N., Freyburger, G., Laurendeau, I., Herbert, J. M., et al. (2004). A Role for Thrombin in Liver Fibrosis. *Gut* 53 (11), 1682–1687. doi:10.1136/gut.2003.032136

Edwards, C. A., and O'Brien, W. D. (1980). Modified Assay for Determination of Hydroxyproline in a Tissue Hydrolyzate. *Clinica Chim. Acta* 104 (2), 161–167. doi:10.1016/0009-8981(80)90192-8

El-Kashef, D. H., and Serrya, M. S. (2019). Sitagliptin Ameliorates Thioacetamide-Induced Acute Liver Injury via Modulating TLR4/NF-KB Signaling Pathway in Mice. *Life Sci.* 228, 266–273. doi:10.1016/j.lfs.2019.05.019

Elguindy, N. M., Yacout, G. A., El Azab, E. F., and Maghraby, H. K. (2016). Chemoprotective Effect of Elettaria Cardamomum against Chemically Induced Hepatocellular Carcinoma in Rats by Inhibiting NF-Kb, Oxidative Stress, and Activity of Ornithine Decarboxylase. *South Afr. J. Bot.* 105, 251–258. doi:10.1016/j.sajb.2016.04.001

Fiorucci, S., Antonelli, E., Distrutti, E., Severino, B., Fiorentina, R., Baldoni, M., et al. (2004). PAR1 Antagonism Protects Against Experimental Liver Fibrosis. Role of Proteinase Receptors in Stellate Cell Activation. *Hepatology* 39 (2), 365–375. doi:10.1002/hep.20054

Gagnon, K. T., and Corey, D. R. (2019). Guidelines for Experiments Using Antisense Oligonucleotides and Double-Stranded RNAs. *Nucleic Acid Ther.* 29 (3), 116–122. doi:10.1089/nat.2018.0772

Giesen, P. L. A., Rauch, U., Bohrmann, B., Kling, D., Roqué, M., Fallon, J. T., et al. (1999). Blood-borne Tissue Factor: Another View of Thrombosis. *Proc. Natl. Acad. Sci.* 96 (5), 2311–2315. doi:10.1073/pnas.96.5.2311

Gonca, E. (2015). Comparison of Thiopental and Ketamine+xylazine Anesthesia Inischemia/reperfusion-Induced Arrhythmias in Rats. *Turk J. Med. Sci.* 45 (6), 1413–1420. doi:10.3906/sag-1403-25

Gupta, G., Khadem, F., and Uzonna, J. E. (2019). Role of Hepatic Stellate Cell (HSC)-derived Cytokines in Hepatic Inflammation and Immunity. *Cytokine* 124, 154542. doi:10.1016/j.cyto.2018.09.004

Hammad, M. A., Abdel-Bakky, M. S., Walker, L. A., and Ashfaq, M. K. (2011). Oxidized Low-Density Lipoprotein and Tissue Factor Are Involved in Monocrotaline/lipopolysaccharide-Induced Hepatotoxicity. *Arch. Toxicol.* 85 (9), 1079–1089. doi:10.1007/s00204-011-0649-6

Hammad, M. A., Abdel-Bakky, M. S., Walker, L. A., and Ashfaq, M. K. (2013). Tissue Factor Antisense Deoxyoligonucleotide Prevents Monocrotaline/LPS Hepatotoxicity in Mice. *J. Appl. Toxicol.* 33 (8), 774–783. doi:10.1002/jat.2728

Hernandez-Gea, V., and Friedman, S. L. (2011). Pathogenesis of Liver Fibrosis. *Annu. Rev. Pathol. Mech. Dis.* 6, 425–456. doi:10.1146/annurev-pathol-011110-130246

Huang, H., Shiffman, M. L., Friedman, S., Venkatesh, R., Bzowej, N., Abar, O. T., et al. (2007). A 7 Gene Signature Identifies the Risk of Developing Cirrhosis in Patients with Chronic Hepatitis C. *Hepatology* 46 (2), 297–306. doi:10.1002/hep.21695

Jabs, D. A., and Griffiths, P. D. (2002). Fomivirsen for the Treatment of Cytomegalovirus retinitis. *Am. J. Ophthalmol.* 133 (4), 552–556. doi:10.1016/s0002-9394(02)01325-9

Jiang, J. X., and Török, N. J. (2013). Liver Injury and the Activation of the Hepatic Myofibroblasts. *Curr. Pathobiol Rep.* 1 (3), 215–223. doi:10.1007/s40139-013-0019-6

Kallis, Y. N., Scotton, C. J., MacKinnon, A. C., Goldin, R. D., Wright, N. A., Iredale, J. P., et al. (2014). Proteinase Activated Receptor 1 Mediated Fibrosis in a Mouse Model of Liver Injury: A Role for Bone Marrow Derived Macrophages. *PLoS ONE* 9 (1), e86241. doi:10.1371/journal.pone.0086241

Karsdal, M. A., Daniels, S. J., Holm Nielsen, S., Bager, C., Rasmussen, D. G. K., Loomba, R., et al. (2020). Collagen Biology and Non-invasive Biomarkers of Liver Fibrosis. *Liver Int.* 40 (4), 736–750. doi:10.1111/liv.14390

Kastelein, J. J. P., Wedel, M. K., Baker, B. F., Su, J., Bradley, J. D., Yu, R. Z., et al. (2006). Potent Reduction of Apolipoprotein B and Low-Density Lipoprotein Cholesterol by Short-Term Administration of an Antisense Inhibitor of Apolipoprotein B. *Circulation* 114 (16), 1729–1735. doi:10.1161/CIRCULATIONAHA.105.606442

Kisseleva, T., and Brenner, D. (2021). Molecular and Cellular Mechanisms of Liver Fibrosis and its Regression. *Nat. Rev. Gastroenterol. Hepatol.* 18 (3), 1–16. doi:10.1038/s41575-020-00372-7

Knight, V., Lourensz, D., Tchongue, J., Correia, J., Tipping, P., and Sievert, W. (2017). Cytoplasmic Domain of Tissue Factor Promotes Liver Fibrosis in Mice. *World J. Gastroenterol.* 23 (31), 5692–5699. doi:10.3748/wjg.v23.i31.5692

Lento, S., Brioschi, M., Barcella, S., Nasim, M. T., Ghilardi, S., Barbieri, S. S., et al. (2015). Proteomics of Tissue Factor Silencing in Cardiomyocytic Cells Reveals a New Role for This Coagulation Factor in Splicing Machinery Control. *J. Proteomics* 119, 75–89. doi:10.1016/j.jprot.2015.01.021

Liang, J., Yang, X., Yu, Y., Li, X., Wu, Y., Shi, R., et al. (2016). Babao Dan Attenuates Hepatic Fibrosis by Inhibiting Hepatic Stellate Cells Activation and Proliferation via TLR4 Signaling Pathway. *Oncotarget* 7 (50), 82554–82566. doi:10.18632/oncotarget.12783

Lin, L., Li, R., Cai, M., Huang, J., Huang, W., Guo, Y., et al. (2018). Andrographolide Ameliorates Liver Fibrosis in Mice: Involvement of TLR4/NF-Kb and TGF-β1/Smad2 Signaling Pathways. *Oxidative Med. Cell. longevity* 2018, 7808656. doi:10.1155/2018/7808656

Lucas, K., and Maes, M. (2013). Role of the Toll like Receptor (TLR) Radical Cycle in Chronic Inflammation: Possible Treatments Targeting the TLR4 Pathway. *Mol. Neurobiol.* 48 (1), 190–204. doi:10.1007/s12035-013-8425-7

Luyendyk, J. P., Sullivan, B. P., Guo, G. L., and Wang, R. (2010). Tissue Factor-Deficiency and Protease Activated Receptor-1-Deficiency Reduce Inflammation Elicited by Diet-Induced Steatohepatitis in Mice. *Am. J. Pathol.* 176 (1), 177–186. doi:10.2353/ajpath.2010.090672

Mann, K. G., Butenas, S., and Brummel, K. (2003). The Dynamics of Thrombin Formation. *Arterioscler. Thromb. Vasc. Biol.* 23 (1), 17–25. doi:10.1161/01.ATV.0000046238.23903.FC

Mansour, M. A., Bekheet, S. A., Al-Rejaie, S. S., Al-Shabanah, O. A., Al-Howiriny, T. A., Al-Rikabi, A. C., et al. (2010). Ginger Ingredients Inhibit the Development of Diethylnitrosoamine Induced Premalignant Phenotype in Rat Chemical Hepatocarcinogenesis Model. *BioFactors* 36 (6), 483–490. doi:10.1002/biof.122

Marrone, A. K., Shpyleva, S., Chappell, G., Tryndyak, V., Uehara, T., Tsuchiya, M., et al. (2016). Differentially Expressed MicroRNAs Provide Mechanistic Insight into Fibrosis-Associated Liver Carcinogenesis in Mice. *Mol. Carcinog.* 55 (5), 808–817. doi:10.1002/mc.22323

Meng, X.-m., Nikolic-Paterson, D. J., and Lan, H. Y. (2016). TGF-β: The Master Regulator of Fibrosis. *Nat. Rev. Nephrol.* 12 (6), 325–338. doi:10.1038/nrneph.2016.48

Moreira, R. K. (2007). Hepatic Stellate Cells and Liver Fibrosis. *Arch. Pathol. Lab. Med.* 131 (11), 1728–1734. doi:10.5858/2007-131-1728-hscalf

Nakamura, K., Kadotani, Y., Ushigome, H., Akioka, K., Okamoto, M., Ohmori, Y., et al. (2002). Antisense Oligonucleotide for Tissue Factor Inhibits Hepatic Ischemic Reperfusion Injury. *Biochem. Biophysical Res. Commun.* 297 (3), 433–441. doi:10.1016/S0006-291X(02)02024-7

Nakazato, K., Takada, H., Iha, M., and Nagamine, T. (2010). Attenuation of N-Nitrosodiethylamine-Induced Liver Fibrosis by High-Molecular-Weight Fucoidan Derived fromCladosiphon Okamuranus. *J. Gastroenterol. Hepatol. (Australia)* 25 (10), 1692–1701. doi:10.1111/j.1440-1746.2009.06187.x

Nault, R., Fader, K. A., Kopec, A. K., Harkema, J. R., Zacharewski, T. R., and Luyendyk, J. P. (2016). From the Cover: Coagulation-Driven Hepatic Fibrosis Requires Protease Activated Receptor-1 (PAR-1) in a Mouse Model of TCDD-Elicited Steatohepatitis. *Toxicol. Sci.* 154 (2), 381–391. doi:10.1093/toxsci/kfw175

Pendurthi, U. R., Ngyuen, M., Andrade-Gordon, P., Petersen, L. C., and Rao, L. V. M. (2002). Plasmin InducesCyr61Gene Expression in Fibroblasts via Protease-Activated Receptor-1 and P44/42 Mitogen-Activated Protein Kinase-dependent Signaling Pathway. *Arterioscler. Thromb. Vasc. Biol.* 22 (9), 1421–1426. doi:10.1161/01.ATV.0000030200.59331.3F

Poojari, R., Gupta, S., Maru, G., Khade, B., and Bhagwat, S. (2010). Chemopreventive and Hepatoprotective Effects of Embelin on N-Nitrosodiethylamine and Carbon Tetrachloride Induced Preneoplasia and Toxicity in Rat Liver. *Asian Pac. J. Cancer Prev.* 11 (4), 1015–1020. doi:10.1016/j.fitote.2005.04.014

Poole, L. G., Pant, A., Cline-Fedewa, H. M., Williams, K. J., Copple, B. L., Palumbo, J. S., et al. (2020). Liver Fibrosis Is Driven by Protease-activated Receptor-1 Expressed by Hepatic Stellate Cells in Experimental Chronic Liver Injury. *Res. Pract. Thromb. Haemost.* 4 (5), 906–917. doi:10.1002/rth2.12403

Rao, L. V. M., and Pendurthi, U. R. (2005). Tissue Factor-Factor VIIa Signaling. *Arterioscler. Thromb. Vasc. Biol.* 25 (1), 47–56. doi:10.1161/01.ATV.0000151624.45775.13

Rauch, U., and Nemerson, Y. (2000). Tissue Factor, the Blood, and the Arterial Wall. *Trends Cardiovascular Medicine* 10 (4), 139–143. doi:10.1016/s1050-1738(00)00049-9

Riewald, M., Kravchenko, V. V., Petrovan, R. J., O'Brien, P. J., Brass, L. F., Ulevitch, R. J., et al. (2001). Gene Induction by Coagulation Factor Xa Is Mediated by Activation of Protease-Activated Receptor 1. *J. Am. Soc. Hematol.* 97 (10), 3109–3116. doi:10.1182/blood.v97.10.3109

Riewald, M., Petrovan, R. J., Donner, A., and Ruf, W. (2003). Activated Protein C Signals through the Thrombin Receptor PAR1 in Endothelial Cells. *J. Endotoxin Res.* 9 (5), 317–321. doi:10.1179/096805103225002584

Roberts, T. C., Langer, R., and Wood, M. J. A. (2020). Advances in Oligonucleotide Drug Delivery. *Nat. Rev. Drug Discov.* 19 (10), 673–694. doi:10.1038/s41573-020-0075-7

Rondina, M. T., Schwertz, H., Harris, E. S., Kraemer, B. F., Campbell, R. A., Mackman, N., et al. (2011). The Septic Milieu Triggers Expression of Spliced Tissue Factor mRNA in Human Platelets. *J. Thromb. Haemost.* 9 (4), 748–758. doi:10.1111/j.1538-7836.2011.04208.x

Rullier, A., Gillibert-Duplantier, J., Costet, P., Cubel, G., Haurie, V., Petibois, C., et al. (2008). Protease-activated Receptor 1 Knockout Reduces Experimentally Induced Liver Fibrosis. *Am. J. Physiol. Gas-Trointest Liver Physiol.* 294 (1), 226–235. doi:10.1152/ajpgi.00444.2007.-Thrombin

Seki, E., De Minicis, S., Österreicher, C. H., Kluwe, J., Osawa, Y., Brenner, D. A., et al. (2007). TLR4 Enhances TGF-β Signaling and Hepatic Fibrosis. *Nat. Med.* 13 (11), 1324–1332. doi:10.1038/nm1663

Serag, H. M., Komy, M. M. El., and Ahmed, H. S. (2019). Assessment the Role of Bisphenol A on Chemotherapeutic Efficacy of Cisplatin against Hepatocellular Carcinoma in Male Rats. *Egypt. J. Hosp. Med.* 74 (2), 352–363. doi:10.12816/EJHM.2019.23057

Shimizu, R., Kitade, M., Kobayashi, T., Hori, S.-I., and Watanabe, A. (2014). Pharmacokinetic-pharmacodynamic Modeling for Reduction of Hepatic Apolipoprotein B mRNA and Plasma Total Cholesterol after Administration of Antisense Oligonucleotide in Mice. *J. Pharmacokinet. Pharmacodyn* 42 (1), 67–77. doi:10.1007/s10928-014-9398-5

Sullivan, B. P., Kopec, A. K., Joshi, N., Cline, H., Brown, J. A., Bishop, S. C., et al. (2013). Hepatocyte Tissue Factor Activates the Coagulation Cascade in Mice. *Blood* 121 (10), 1868–1874. doi:10.1182/blood10.1182/blood-2012-09-455436

Sullivan, B. P., Weinreb, P. H., Violette, S. M., and Luyendyk, J. P. (2010). The Coagulation System Contributes to αVβ6 Integrin Expression and Liver Fibrosis Induced by Cholestasis. *Am. J. Pathol.* 177 (6), 2837–2849. doi:10.2353/ajpath.2010.100425

Sung, Y.-C., Liu, Y.-C., Chao, P.-H., Chang, C.-C., Jin, P.-R., Lin, T.-T., et al. (2018). Combined Delivery of Sorafenib and a MEK Inhibitor Using CXCR4-Targeted Nanoparticles Reduces Hepatic Fibrosis and Prevents Tumor Development. *Theranostics* 8 (4), 894–905. doi:10.7150/thno.21168

Tork, O. M., Khaleel, E. F., and Abdelmaqsoud, O. M. (2016). Altered Cell to Cell Communication, Autophagy and Mitochondrial Dysfunction in a Model of Hepatocellular Carcinoma: Potential Protective Effects of Curcumin and Stem Cell Therapy. *Asian Pac. J. Cancer Prev.* 16 (18), 8271–8279. doi:10.7314/APJCP.2015.16.18.8271

Trautwein, C., Friedman, S. L., Schuppan, D., and Pinzani, M. (2015). Hepatic Fibrosis: Concept to Treatment. *J. Hepatol.* 62 (1), S15–S24. doi:10.1016/j.jhep.2015.02.039

Tripathy, A., Thakurela, S., Sahu, M. K., Uthansingh, K., Singh, A., Narayan, J., et al. (2020). Fatty Changes Associated with N-Nitrosodiethylamine (DEN) Induced Hepatocellular Carcinoma: a Role of Sonic Hedgehog Signaling Pathway. *Genes Cancer* 11 (1-2), 66. doi:10.18632/genesandcancer.203

Tripodi, A., Mannucci, P. M., and Bonomi Hemophilia, B. (2011). The Coagulopathy of Chronic Liver Disease. *N. Engl. J. Med.* 365 (2), 147–156. doi:10.1056/nejmra1011170

Uehara, T., Ainslie, G. R., Kutanzi, K., Pogribny, I. P., Muskhelishvili, L., Izawa, T., et al. (2013). Molecular Mechanisms of Fibrosis-Associated Promotion of Liver Carcinogenesis. *Toxicol. Sci.* 132 (1), 53–63. doi:10.1093/toxsci/kfs342

Uehara, T., Pogribny, I. P., and Rusyn, I. (2014). The DEN and CCl 4 -Induced Mouse Model of Fibrosis and Inflammation-Associated Hepatocellular Carcinoma. *Curr. Protoc. Pharmacol.* 66 (1), 14–30. doi:10.1002/0471141755.ph1430s66

Wang, K., Yang, X., Wu, Z., Wang, H., Li, Q., Mei, H., et al. (2020). Dendrobium Officinale Polysaccharide Protected CCl4-Induced Liver Fibrosis through Intestinal Homeostasis and the LPS-TLR4-NF-Kb Signaling Pathway. *Front. Pharmacol.* 11, 240. doi:10.3389/fphar.2020.00240

Witkowski, M., Landmesser, U., and Rauch, U. (2016). Tissue Factor as a Link between Inflammation and Coagulation. *Trends Cardiovasc. Med.* 26 (4), 297–303. doi:10.1016/j.tcm.2015.12.001

Yin, J., Luo, X., Yu, W., Liao, J., Shen, Y., and Zhang, Z. (2010). Antisense Oligodeoxynucleotide against Tissue Factor Inhibits Human Umbilical Vein Endothelial Cells Injury Induced by Anoxia-Reoxygenation. *Cell Physiol. Biochem.* 25 (4–5), 477–490. doi:10.1159/000303053

Development and Validation of an Interleukin-6 Nomogram to Predict Primary Non-response to Infliximab in Crohn's Disease Patients

Yueying Chen[1], Hanyang Li[1], Qi Feng[2] and Jun Shen[1]*

[1]Division of Gastroenterology and Hepatology, Key Laboratory of Gastroenterology and Hepatology, Ministry of Health, Inflammatory Bowel Disease Research Center, Renji Hospital, School of Medicine, Shanghai Jiao Tong University, Shanghai Institute of Digestive Disease, Shanghai, China, [2]Department of Radiology, Renji Hospital, School of Medicine, Shanghai Jiao Tong University, Shanghai, China

*Correspondence:
Jun Shen
shenjun_renji@163.com

Background: The primary non-response (PNR) rate of infliximab (IFX) varies from 20 to 46% for the treatment of Crohn's disease (CD). Detected PNR reduces the improper use of specific treatments. To date, there is hardly any knowledge regarding early markers of PNR. The aim of this study was to evaluate the role of Interleukin-6 (IL-6) as an early predictor of PNR of IFX for the treatment of CD.

Methods: We enrolled 322 bio-naïve patients diagnosed with CD from January 2016 to May 2020. Primary response was determined at week 14. Multivariable logistic regression was used to construct prediction models. Area under the curve (AUC), calibration and decision curve analyses (DCA) were assessed in the validation cohort. GEO data were analyzed to identify potential mechanisms of *IL-6* in IFX therapy for CD.

Results: PNR occurred in 31.06% (100 of 322) patients who were assessable at week 14. IL-6 levels significantly decreased after IFX therapy ($p < 0.001$). The validation model containing IL-6 presented enhanced discrimination with an AUC of 0.908 and high calibration. Decision curve analysis (DCA) indicated that the model added extra predictive value. GEO data confirmed the IL-6 levels were increased in the PNR group and IL-6-related differentially expressed genes (DEGs) were enriched in the inflammatory response.

Conclusions: We concluded that IL-6 may be used as a predictive factor to assess the risk of PNR to IFX therapy.

Keywords: interleukin-6, primary non-response, crohn's disease, infliximab, bioinfomatics

INTRODUCTION

Crohn's disease (CD) is a chronic inflammatory disease with a relapsing history. The incidence and prevalence of CD have both increased worldwide and this disease has gradually become a more severe socioeconomic burden (Ng et al., 2013). Recently, the treatment of CD entered a new era. Anti-tumor necrosis factor (anti-TNF) therapy has been the first-line therapy for treating CD according to ECCO guidelines (Torres et al., 2020). Infliximab (IFX) is the most widely used anti-TNF agent that promotes mucosal healing and changes the natural history of the disease (Singh et al.,

2018). However, there are still 20–46% of CD patients that show primary non-response (PNR) to IFX (Roda et al., 2016; Yokoyama et al., 2016). Leapfrogging IFX in PNR patients to other medications such as anti-IL-12/23 monoclonal antibodies or anti-leucocyte adhesion molecules avoid ineffective processes of IFX and saves medical resources. Therefore, developing a model to predict PNR to IFX in CD patients will help doctors make better decisions for CD patients.

Previous studies have proposed several factors to predict the efficacy of IFX in CD, including age, BMI, previous surgery history (Billiet et al., 2015), disease behavior (Sprakes et al., 2012), disease duration (Matsuoka et al., 2018), and pro-inflammatory biomarkers (Billiet et al., 2017). Despite evidence, a clinical prediction model is still lacking to assess the possibility of PNR prior to IFX administration based on clinical and biochemical markers. As a chronic inflammatory disease, the regulation of cytokines is associated with the pathogenesis and progression of CD (Chen and Sundrud, 2016). IL-6 is a proinflammatory factor that can exacerbate inflammation by promoting the survival of T cells and the secretion of other cytokines (Hunter and Jones, 2015). IL-6 levels were shown to be elevated in CD patients compared to healthy individuals (Engel et al., 2015). A randomized trial showed that an anti-IL-6 antibody promoted a clinical response and clinical remission in CD patients (Danese et al., 2019). Furthermore, IL-6 served as a predictor of PNR to anti-TNF treatment in CD and patients failing anti-TNF therapy showed increased expression of IL-6 and persistent IL-6 pathway activity (Leal et al., 2015; Soendergaard et al., 2018). A prospective, multicenter study confirmed the predictive roles of IL-6 in patients treated with anti-TNF therapy (Bertani et al., 2020a). Additionally, the single nucleotide polymorphisms of IL-6 may be a promising tool for identifying CD patient response to IFX therapy (Salvador-Martín et al., 2019).

To promote individualized treatment in CD patients, it is crucial to identify predictors to estimate PNR to IFX. Different IL-6 levels present before treatment may contribute to the contrasting response to IFX therapy. Detecting PNR reduces inaccurate treatments while a predictive model determining PNR to IFX in bio-naive CD is lacking. Therefore, we aimed to identify the predictive value of IL-6 in IFX therapy and to construct a model predicting PNR in bio-naive CD patients based on clinical information and IL-6 levels.

METHODS

Patients and Samples
A retrospective and single-center study was performed for CD cases in the Division of Gastroenterology and Hepatology, Renji hospital. Patients enrolled in this study from January 2016 to June 2019 and from July 2019 to May 2020 were assigned to the training and the validation cohorts, respectively. CD was diagnosed based on the ECCO consensus (Maaser et al., 2019). Bio-naïve patients were included and induced with

5 mg/kg of IFX (Janssen Pharmaceutical Ltd, United States). Baseline characteristics were collected prior to treatment.

Levels of biochemical indicators, including IL-6, albumin, hemoglobin, platelets, erythrocyte sedimentation rate (ESR) and CRP were obtained from previous blood analysis, and blood samples were collected for each participant before and after IFX therapy. The Westergren method and nephelometry were used to measure CRP and ESR levels. Enzyme Linked Immunosorbent Assay (ELISA) was used to detect IL-6 levels using a DPC IMMULITE 1000 system of Siemens, and the average CV value about 8.33%. The Clinical Laboratory Department (Renji Hospital, School of Medicine, Shanghai Jiao Tong University, China) performed an analysis of each sample in duplicate. This study was approved by the IRB of Shanghai Jiaotong University School of Medicine, Renji Hospital Ethics Committee (KY2020–115).

Outcomes and Definitions
Our study defined the primary outcome as the proportion of response to IFX, which was determined when achieving clinical response or remission at week 14 (after three IFX injections and before the fourth) using an MDT (multi-disciplinary team) of experienced experts combined with endoscopic and radiological examinations (Hanauer et al., 2002; Wong and Cross, 2017). PNR was defined as: 1) failure to achieve clinical response or clinical remission, clinical response and clinical remission have been defined as a decrease in Harvey Bradshaw indices (HBI) ≥ 2, and total HBI ≤ 4, respectively (Sprakes et al., 2012). 2) need for treatment modification (discontinuation, escalation or surgery) (Roda et al., 2016; Bar-Yoseph et al., 2018; Beltrán et al., 2019).

Statistical Analysis
Results for continuous variables were represented as mean (SDs) or median (interquartile ranges [IQRs]). Categorical variables were shown as proportions. Univariate logistic regression was applied to analyze the relationships between different factors and PNR to IFX therapy. A Chi-square test was used to compare categorical variables. The t test or Mann-Whitney U test were used to compare continuous variables.

Multivariable regression models with forward stepwise likelihood ratio algorithms were used to develop models predicting the response to infliximab 5 mg/kg through 14 weeks. Akaike information criterion (AIC) was performed to assessed the goodness of fit of two models. Discrimination of the prediction models was evaluated by receiver operating characteristics (ROC) analysis and presented as area under the curve (AUC). Odds ratios (OR) having 95% confidence intervals (CI) of final predictors were calculated. Calibration curves were used to assess the calibration of nomograms by comparing the predicted and observed probabilities. The clinical effectiveness of the models was assessed using decision curve analysis (DCA). Integrated Discrimination Improvement (IDI) was a reclassification measures showed the difference in discrimination slopes of two models, and was used to assess the improvement of risk differences between cases and non-cases (Pencina et al., 2008;

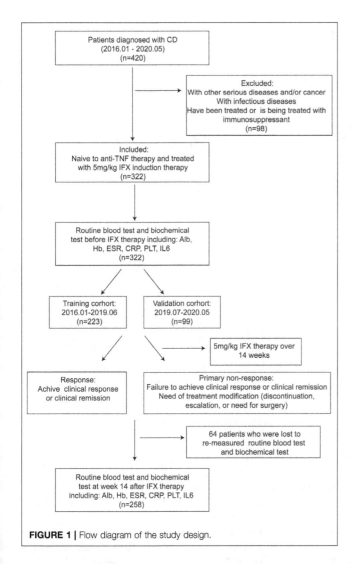

FIGURE 1 | Flow diagram of the study design.

Steyerberg et al., 2010; Kerr et al., 2011). All statistical analyses were performed using SPSS 25.0 and R 3.6.3 with a statistical significance of $p < 0.05$.

Bioinformatic Analysis
Data Source
A gene expression microarray dataset (GSE111761) of Schmitt's study from the GEO database was selected (Schmitt et al., 2019). GSE111761 contained three samples from anti-TNF non-responders and three from responders. The patients were diagnosed as CD and defined as responders or non-responders when they had ongoing anti-TNF therapy for over 3 months. The GSE111761 dataset was available on the GPL13497 platform (Agilent-026652 Whole Human Genome Microarray 4 × 44K v2).

Identification of Differentially Expressed Genes (DEGs)
R software (version 3.6.3) and the limma package in Bioconductor were used to detect DEGs in GSE111761 (Ritchie et al., 2015). DEGs were identified using selection criteria of an adjusted p value < 0.05 and $|logFC| > 1.0$.

TABLE 1 | Multivariate regression analyses of the model 1 and model 2.

Variables	B	Or (95% CI)	P	s.e
(a) Multivariate regression analysis including BMI, behavior, and CRP				
BMI	−0.217	0.805 (0.731–0.908)	0.000	0.061
Behavior	1.281	3.602 (1.881–6.895)	0.000	0.331
CRP	0.025	1.025 (1.009–1.041)	0.002	0.008
(b) Multivariate regression analysis including BMI, behavior, CRP, and IL-6				
BMI	−0.212	0.809 (0.716–0.914)	0.001	0.062
Behavior	1.252	3.499 (1.809–6.766)	0.000	0.336
CRP	0.024	1.024 (1.008–1.041)	0.003	0.008
IL-6	0.237	1.267 (1.041–1.541)	0.018	0.100

BMI, Body Mass Index; CRP, C-reactive protein; IL6, interleukin-6; CI, confidence interval; OR, odds ratio; s.e., standard error.

Enrichment Analysis
Gene Set Enrichment Analysis (GSEA) was performed using the ClusterProfile package in Bioconductor with a statistical significance of $p < 0.05$ (Yu et al., 2012).

Protein-Protein Interaction (PPI) Network Construction
PPI network reveals the specific and unspecific interactions of proteins, and promotes to identify therapeutic target (Petta et al.,

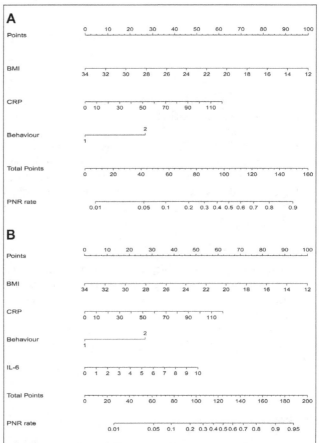

FIGURE 2 | Nomograms for model 1 and model 2 were developed in the training cohort **(A)** Nomogram one for model 1, with BMI, behavior, and CRP. BMI, Body Mass Index; CRP, C-reactive protein **(B)** Nomogram two for model 2, with BMI, behavior, CRP, and IL6. IL6, interleukin-6.

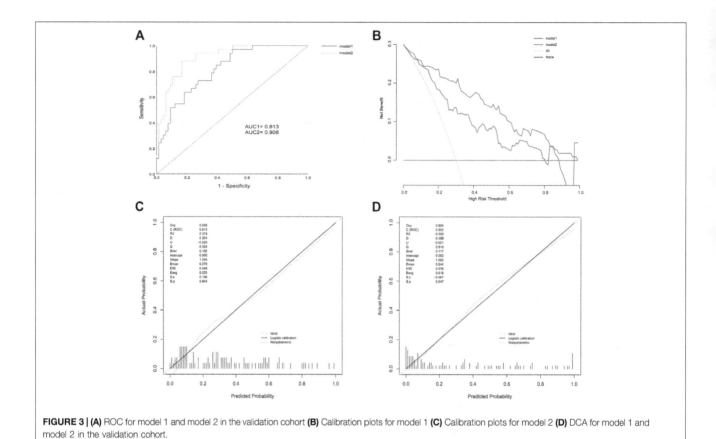

FIGURE 3 | (A) ROC for model 1 and model 2 in the validation cohort **(B)** Calibration plots for model 1 **(C)** Calibration plots for model 2 **(D)** DCA for model 1 and model 2 in the validation cohort.

2016; Maurel et al., 2019). STRING (version 11.0), a freely accessible database that collects, scores and integrates data, was used to predict functional relationships between proteins (Szklarczyk et al., 2019). A PPI network of genes with a score > 0.4 in STRING was constructed using Cytoscape software (version 3.7.2) (Smoot et al., 2011). The degree of protein nodes was calculated using the Cytoscape plugin CytoHubba to identify hub genes (Chin et al., 2014). Hub genes were selected with a score ≥ 4.5 based on the EPC algorithm.

Construction of Regulatory Network

The network of genes and their corresponding miRNAs and lncRNAs was constructed using starbase, a publicly available database mainly focusing on miRNA-target interactions (Li et al., 2014). Transcription factors (TFs) were downloaded from TRRUST (http://www.grnpedia.org/trrust/), a public database for predicting TFs of various genes through DNA sequences (Farre et al., 2003). These tools were combined to construct a multi-factor regulation network.

RESULTS

Baseline Characteristics and Univariate Analyses

From a total of 322 active CD patients receiving 5 mg/kg IFX induction therapy, 223 and 99 were assigned to training and

validation groups, respectively (**Figure 1**). Disease behavior was merged into two categories, including nonstricturing and nonpenetrating (B1) into one category, and stricturing and/or penetrating (B2/B3) subtypes into another category. The baseline characteristics are shown in **Supplementary Table S1**. The incidence of PNR in the training cohort was 30.0% (n = 67), while the incidence in the validation cohort was 33.3% (n = 33). Baseline characteristics of patients were similar between the two cohorts. Univariate regressions showed that BMI ($p <$ 0.001), disease behavior ($p <$ 0.001), CRP levels ($p =$ 0.001), and IL-6 levels before IFX therapy ($p =$ 0.002) were strongly associated with PNR to IFX treatment (**Supplementary Table S2**).

IL-6 levels were measured in 258 of the studied 322 patients before initiation and at week 14 before the fourth IFX injection. IL-6 levels were found to significantly decrease after IFX therapy ($p <$ 0.001) and were obviously different between PNR and response groups ($p =$ 0.001) (**Supplementary Figure S1**).

Development of Prediction Models and Nomogram Construction

Results of multiple logistic regression suggested BMI, disease behavior, CRP levels and IL-6 levels before IFX therapy were determined as predicting factors. To identify the true predictive effects of IL-6, we built a model contained IL-6 and the other one did

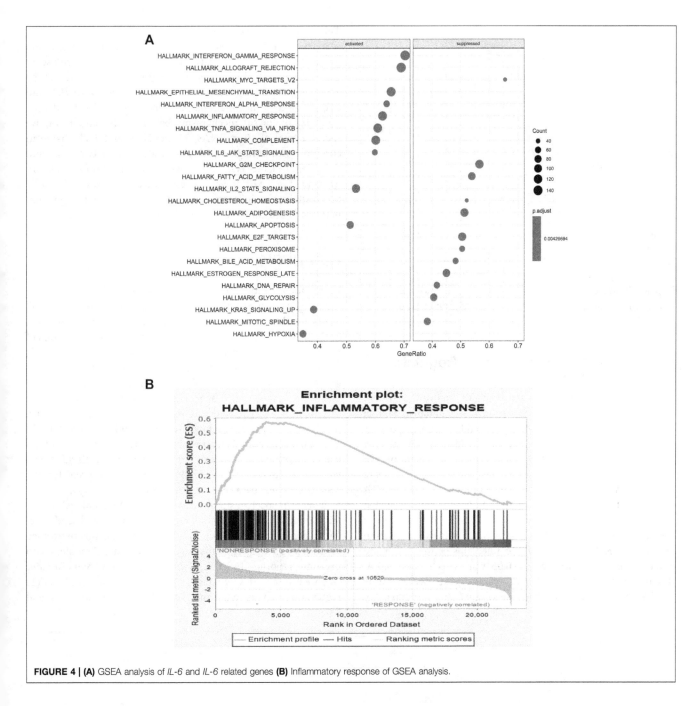

FIGURE 4 | (A) GSEA analysis of *IL-6* and *IL-6* related genes **(B)** Inflammatory response of GSEA analysis.

not. The diagnostic equations of models were: logitP = 1.162–0.217* BMI +1.281 * behavior +0.025 * CRP, and logitP = 0.144–0.212* BMI +1.252 * behavior +0.024 * CRP +0.237* IL-6, respectively. The results of multivariate regression analyses are shown in **Table 1**. These two models are presented as nomograms, which containing these independent predictors to calculate the risk of PNR based on the total points **(Figure 2)**.

Validation of Prediction Models

Efficacies of the two models were compared to the validation cohort. AIC was 111.3 and 99.1 of model1 and model2, respectively. ROC analysis indicated and the AUC of BMI,

behavior, CRP, and IL-6 were 0.652 (95% CI: 0.540–0.764), 0.674 (95% CI: 0.563–0.785), 0.744 (95% CI: 0.646–0.842), and 0.787 (95% CI: 0.698–0.877) respectively. An AUC of 0.813 (95% CI: 0.729–0.897) in model 1 and 0.908 (95% CI: 0.851–0.966) in model 2 **(Figure 3)**. The *p* value = 0.005 of DeLong's test showed that an AUC of model 2 was significantly better than model 1. Calibration plots showed that the average differences (E aver) were 2.5 and 1.8% in model 1 and 2, and no significant differences ($P_1 = 0.844$, $P_2 = 0.947$) between the predicted and the calibrated probabilities. DCA showed that if the risk thresholds were between 12 and 85%, model 2 added more clinical net benefit compared to model 1. To explore additional benefits conferred by

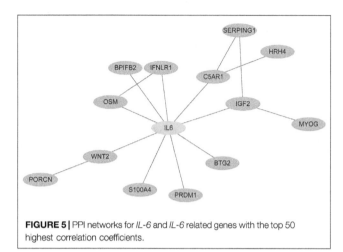

FIGURE 5 | PPI networks for *IL-6* and *IL-6* related genes with the top 50 highest correlation coefficients.

IL-6 levels, we compared IDI between models and found this improvement index was improved upon addition of IL-6 (IDI = 19%; 95% CI, 0.10–0.28; $p < 0.000$).

Identification of Pathway and Regulatory Network of IL-6

To identify potential pathways and regulatory network of IL-6 in IFX therapy of CD, the GSE111761 dataset contained lamina propria mononuclear cells from three anti-TNF non-responders and three responders were included to identify DEGs. The samples were obtained from the patients with anti-TNF therapy for over 3 months and the Simple Endoscopic Score for Crohn's disease (SES-CD) <5. There were 2,228 DEGs including 1,384 upregulated genes and 844 downregulated genes and IL-6 expression levels were significantly elevated in PNR patients (**Supplementary Figure S2**). Spearman correlation was performed to investigate the connections between *IL-6* and other DEGs. Genes with a $p < 0.05$ were selected for GSEA. Results indicated that *IL-6* and relative genes were mainly involved in inflammatory response (**Figure 4**; **Supplementary**

Table S3). We selected *IL-6* related genes with the top 50 highest correlation coefficients to create PPIs, and identified five hub genes, including *IL-6, IGF2, C5AR1, IFNLR1* and *OSM* with score ≥ 4.5 based on the EPC algorithm (**Figure 5**). We found that the expression of Oncostatin M (*OSM*) coordinated with *IL-6* and also belonged to the inflammatory response in GSEA. To identify potential biological mechanisms between *IL-6* and *OSM*, we found a total of 10 miRNAs, 25 lncRNAs, and 1 TF shared in common with both *IL-6* and *OSM*. Data of these two genes and their miRNAs, lncRNAs and TF were integrated into a regulatory network (**Figure 6**). It was suggested that *IL-6* and *OSM* may be involved in the inflammatory response through a regulation network based on common lncRNAs, miRNAs and TF.

DISCUSSION

Even though anti-TNF agents have shown to be effective in inducing clinical response and mucosal healing, there are still a considerable proportion of patients who do not respond (Ding et al., 2016). Previous studies have identified several predictors of PNR to IFX in CD, such as BMI, fecal calprotectin (Pavlidis et al., 2016), proinflammatory biomarkers (Billiet et al., 2017), and genetic markers (Barber et al., 2016). These studies have also established prediction models based on these factors. IL-6 is a proinflammatory cytokine and expression levels alter after IFX therapy. It is considered a good predictor of IFX response (Suzuki et al., 2015; Salvador-Martín et al., 2019). However, there are few prediction models for PNR to IFX treatment in CD. In this study, we showed that IL-6 levels before IFX therapy predicted the response to IFX treatment and alter after IFX therapy.

This retrospective study included 322 CD patients who were naive to anti-TNF therapy and both their clinical and serological data were collected. Logarithmic transformation was performed for IL-6 levels to decrease the undulation of data. Consistent with previous reports, IL-6 levels were significantly reduced after 14 weeks of IFX therapy. Univariate and multivariate regression analyses found that BMI, disease behavior, CRP and

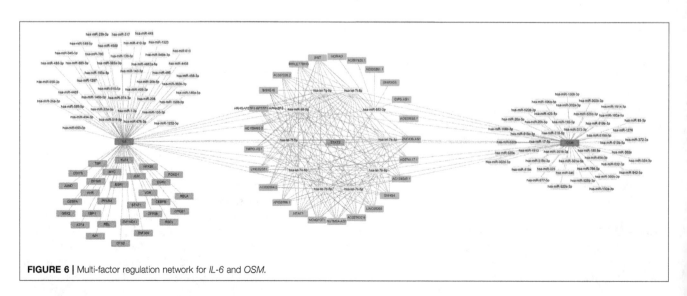

FIGURE 6 | Multi-factor regulation network for *IL-6* and *OSM*.

IL-6 levels before IFX therapy independently predicted the response to IFX treatment. To explore the predictive ability of IL-6, we established two prediction models, one containing BMI, disease behavior and CRP levels, and the other including BMI, disease behavior, CRP levels, and IL-6 levels. Results of AIC and ROC in the validation cohort, indicated that the goodness of fit and discrimination of model containing IL-6 was better than the model not including IL-6. And the AUC of the model incorporating IL-6 was higher than that in single factors, including BMI, disease behavior and CRP levels. The calibration curve and DCA curve demonstrated a greater consistency and clinical validity in the model containing IL-6. IDI analysis showed that incorporation of IL-6 with BMI, behavior, and CRP significantly improved the discriminatory accuracy for PNR with IDI of 19% ($p < 0.000$). Furthermore, the improvement of IDI for discriminating PNR to IFX therapy is consistent with previous studies, such as Leal et al. (Leal et al., 2015), which revealed the predictive effect of IL-6 on risk of PNR to anti-TNF therapy in CD patients. Therefore, we suggested that IL-6 played a central role in assessing the possibility of PNR to IFX therapy.

Furthermore, we analyzed GEO data to verify the predictive power of IL-6. It was found that expression of *IL-6* significantly increased in non-responders compared with responders to IFX therapy. GSEA of *IL-6* and its relative genes with high correlation coefficients showed that these genes mainly were enriched in the inflammatory response. Through the construction of PPI networks, we found that *OSM* directly connected to *IL-6* and its expression was consistent with *IL-6* in the inflammatory response. *OSM* regulates the production of proinflammatory cytokines such as IL-6 through the JAK-STAT pathway (Hermanns, 2015). Studies demonstrated that *OSM* induced intestinal inflammation, while mechanisms remained unclear (Thomas, 2017). Furthermore, *OSM* has been considered a novel biomarker to predict the efficacy of anti-TNF therapy. One study showed that *OSM* was enriched in CD mucosa and complete mucosal healing was more likely to occur in patients with low *OSM* expression levels. Notably, the expression of *OSM* was strongly correlated with PNR to IFX (West et al., 2017). Another clinical study suggested that *OSM* was an appreciable biomarker in predicting the possibility of mucosal healing compared with fecal calprotectin, which indicated *OSM* may be a predictive indicator for IFX therapy (Bertani et al., 2020b). To explore the common mechanisms of *IL-6* and *OSM* in IFX treatment, we found that they both shared 10

miRNAs, 25 lncRNAs and 1 TF, which provides potential targets and pathways research diving into deeper mechanistic studies.

Although this study developed a new prediction model based on clinical and serological data, it faced several limitations. First, as a retrospective study, we defined PNR through chart review rather than prospectively collected disease activity indices. To ensure homogeneousness of the study, all CD patients were evaluated by the same physician group over the duration of IFX treatment. Second, IL-6 levels were detected in peripheral blood rather than mucosal tissue. As a result, findings represented the state of the peripheral immune system instead of the inflamed mucosa. Furthermore, external validation is required to confirm the validity of these results in clinical practice.

CONCLUSION

This study found IL-6 levels altered after IFX therapy and added IL-6 to enhance the predictive value of PNR to IFX therapy in CD bio-naïve patients. A novel prediction model was developed, including IL-6 levels combined with BMI, disease behavior and CRP levels. With this model, clinicians can estimate the risk of PNR to IFX therapy and select the optimal treatment for individual patients. Furthermore, this study also constructed a multi-factor regulation network of *IL-6* and its relative gene *OSM*, providing stronger direction for exploring the predictive and therapeutic targets of IFX treatment in CD. Further investigation is needed to determine the association between IL-6 from either peripheral or inflamed mucosal and anti-TNF treatment responses.

ETHICS STATEMENT

This study was approved by the IRB of Shanghai Jiaotong University School of Medicine, Renji Hospital Ethics Committee (KY2020-115).

AUTHOR CONTRIBUTIONS

YC and HL, collected the papers and analyzed data, analyzed the conclusions, drafted the manuscript; QF reviewed the data and conclusions; JS presented the idea of this paper, supported the funding, analyzed the conclusions, drafted and revised the manuscript.

REFERENCES

Bar-Yoseph, H., Levhar, N., Selinger, L., Manor, U., Yavzori, M., Picard, O., et al. (2018). Early drug and anti-infliximab antibody levels for prediction of primary nonresponse to infliximab therapy. *Aliment. Pharmacol. Ther.* 47 (2), 212–218. doi:10.1111/apt.14410

Barber, G. E., Yajnik, V., Khalili, H., Giallourakis, C., Garber, J., Xavier, R., et al.

(2016). Genetic markers predict primary non-response and durable response to anti-TNF biologic therapies in crohn's disease. *Am. J. Gastroenterol.* 111 (12), 1816–1822. doi:10.1038/ajg.2016.408

Beltrán, B., Iborra, M., Sáez-González, E., Marqués-Miñana, M. R., Moret, I., Cerrillo, E., et al. (2019). Fecal calprotectin pretreatment and induction infliximab levels for prediction of primary nonresponse to infliximab therapy in crohn's disease. *Dig. Dis.* 37 (2), 108–115. doi:10.1159/000492626

Bertani, L., Caviglia, G. P., Antonioli, L., Pellicano, R., Fagoonee, S., Astegiano, M., et al. (2020a). Serum interleukin-6 and -8 as predictors of response to vedolizumab in inflammatory bowel diseases. *J. Clin. Med.* 9 (5). doi:10.3390/jcm9051323

Bertani, L., Fornai, M., Fornili, M., Antonioli, L., Benvenuti, L., Tapete, G., et al. (2020b). Serum oncostatin M at baseline predicts mucosal healing in Crohn's disease patients treated with infliximab. *Aliment. Pharmacol. Ther.* 52 (2), 284–291. doi:10.1111/apt.15870

Billiet, T., Cleynen, I., Ballet, V., Claes, K., Princen, F., Singh, S., et al. (2017). Evolution of cytokines and inflammatory biomarkers during infliximab induction therapy and the impact of inflammatory burden on primary response in patients with Crohn's disease. *Scand. J. Gastroenterol.* 52 (10), 1086–1092. doi:10.1080/00365521.2017.1339825

Billiet, T., Papamichael, K., de Bruyn, M., Verstockt, B., Cleynen, I., Princen, F., et al. (2015). A matrix-based model predicts primary response to infliximab in crohn's disease. *Eccojc* 9 (12), 1120–1126. doi:10.1093/ecco-jcc/jjv156

Chen, M. L., and Sundrud, M. S. (2016). Cytokine networks and T-cell subsets in inflammatory bowel diseases. *Inflamm. Bowel Dis.* 22 (5), 1157–1167. doi:10.1097/mib.0000000000000714

Chin, C.-H., Chen, S.-H., Wu, H.-H., Ho, C.-W., Ko, M.-T., and Lin, C.-Y. (2014). cytoHubba: identifying hub objects and sub-networks from complex interactome. *BMC Syst. Biol.* 8 (Suppl. 4), S11. doi:10.1186/1752-0509-8-s4-s11

Danese, S., Vermeire, S., Hellstern, P., Panaccione, R., Rogler, G., Fraser, G., et al. (2019). Randomised trial and open-label extension study of an anti-interleukin-6 antibody in Crohn's disease (ANDANTE I and II). *Gut* 68 (1), 40–48. doi:10.1136/gutjnl-2017-314562

Ding, N. S., Hart, A., and De Cruz, P. (2016). Systematic review: predicting and optimising response to anti-TNF therapy in Crohn's disease - algorithm for practical management. *Aliment. Pharmacol. Ther.* 43 (1), 30–51. doi:10.1111/apt.13445

Engel, T., Ben-Horin, S., and Beer-Gabel, M. (2015). Autonomic dysfunction correlates with clinical and inflammatory activity in patients with crohn's disease. *Inflamm. Bowel Dis.* 21 (10), 2320–2326. doi:10.1097/MIB.0000000000000508

Farre, D., Roset, R., Huerta, M., Adsuara, J. E., Rosello, L., Alba, M. M., et al. (2003). Identification of patterns in biological sequences at the ALGGEN server: PROMO and MALGEN. *Nucleic Acids Res.* 31 (13), 3651–3653. doi:10.1093/nar/gkg605

Hanauer, S. B., Feagan, B. G., Lichtenstein, G. R., Mayer, L. F., Schreiber, S., Colombel, J. F., et al. (2002). Maintenance infliximab for Crohn's disease: the ACCENT I randomised trial. *The Lancet* 359 (9317), 1541–1549. doi:10.1016/s0140-6736(02)08512-4

Hermanns, H. M. (2015). Oncostatin M and interleukin-31: cytokines, receptors, signal transduction and physiology. *Cytokine Growth Factor. Rev.* 26 (5), 545–558. doi:10.1016/j.cytogfr.2015.07.006

Hunter, C. A., and Jones, S. A. (2015). IL-6 as a keystone cytokine in health and disease. *Nat. Immunol.* 16 (5), 448–457. doi:10.1038/ni.3153

Kerr, K. F., McClelland, R. L., Brown, E. R., and Lumley, T. (2011). Evaluating the incremental value of new biomarkers with integrated discrimination improvement. *Am. J. Epidemiol.* 174 (3), 364–374. doi:10.1093/aje/kwr086

Leal, R. F., Planell, N., Kajekar, R., Lozano, J. J., Ordás, I., Dotti, I., et al. (2015). Identification of inflammatory mediators in patients with Crohn's disease unresponsive to anti-TNFα therapy. *Gut* 64 (2), 233–242. doi:10.1136/gutjnl-2013-306518

Li, J.-H., Liu, S., Zhou, H., Qu, L.-H., and Yang, J.-H. (2014). starBase v2.0: decoding miRNA-ceRNA, miRNA-ncRNA and protein-RNA interaction networks from large-scale CLIP-Seq data. *Nucl. Acids Res.* 42, D92–D97. doi:10.1093/nar/gkt1248

Maaser, C., Sturm, A., Vavricka, S. R., Kucharzik, T., Fiorino, G., Annese, V., et al. (2019). ECCO-ESGAR Guideline for Diagnostic Assessment in IBD Part 1: initial diagnosis, monitoring of known IBD, detection of complications. *J. Crohn's colitis* 13 (2), 144–164K. doi:10.1093/ecco-jcc/jjy113

Matsuoka, K., Hamada, S., Shimizu, M., Nanki, K., Mizuno, S., Kiyohara, H., et al. (2018). Factors predicting the therapeutic response to infliximab during maintenance therapy in Japanese patients with Crohn's disease. *PloS one* 13 (10), e0204632. doi:10.1371/journal.pone.0204632

Maurel, M., Obacz, J., Avril, T., Ding, Y. P., Papadodima, O., Treton, X., et al. (2019). Control of anterior GRadient 2 (AGR2) dimerization links endoplasmic reticulum proteostasis to inflammation. *EMBO Mol. Med.* 11 (6). doi:10.15252/emmm.201810120

Ng, S. C., Tang, W., Ching, J. Y., Wong, M., Chow, C. M., Hui, A. J., et al. (2013). Incidence and phenotype of inflammatory bowel disease based on results from the Asia-pacific Crohn's and colitis epidemiology study. *Gastroenterology* 145 (1), 158–165. doi:10.1053/j.gastro.2013.04.007

Pavlidis, P., Gulati, S., Dubois, P., Chung-Faye, G., Sherwood, R., Bjarnason, I., et al. (2016). Early change in faecal calprotectin predicts primary non-response to anti-TNFα therapy in Crohn's disease. *Scand. J. Gastroenterol.* 51 (12), 1447–1452. doi:10.1080/00365521.2016.1205128

Pencina, M. J., D' Agostino, R. B., D' Agostino, Vasan, R. S., Jr., and Vasan, R. S. (2008). Evaluating the added predictive ability of a new marker: from area under the ROC curve to reclassification and beyond. *Statist. Med.* 27 (2), 157–172. discussion 207-12. doi:10.1002/sim.2929

Petta, I., Lievens, S., Libert, C., Tavernier, J., and De Bosscher, K. (2016). Modulation of protein-protein interactions for the development of novel therapeutics. *Mol. Ther.* 24 (4), 707–718. doi:10.1038/mt.2015.214

Ritchie, M. E., Phipson, B., Wu, D., Hu, Y., Law, C. W., Shi, W., et al. (2015). Limma powers differential expression analyses for RNA-sequencing and microarray studies. *Nucleic Acids Res.* 43 (7), e47. doi:10.1093/nar/gkv007

Roda, G., Jharap, B., Neeraj, N., and Colombel, J.-F. (2016). Loss of response to anti-TNFs: definition, epidemiology, and management. *Clin. translational Gastroenterol.* 7, e135. doi:10.1038/ctg.2015.63

Salvador-Martín, S., López-Cauce, B., Nuñez, O., Laserna-Mendieta, E. J., García, M. I., Lobato, E., et al. (2019). Genetic predictors of long-term response and trough levels of infliximab in crohn's disease. *Pharmacol. Res.* 149, 104478. doi:10.1016/j.phrs.2019.104478

Schmitt, H., Billmeier, U., Dieterich, W., Rath, T., Sonnewald, S., Reid, S., et al. (2019). Expansion of IL-23 receptor bearing TNFR2+ T cells is associated with molecular resistance to anti-TNF therapy in Crohn's disease. *Gut* 68 (5), 814–828. doi:10.1136/gutjnl-2017-315671

Singh, S., Fumery, M., Sandborn, W. J., and Murad, M. H. (2018). Systematic review and network meta-analysis: first- and second-line biologic therapies for moderate-severe Crohn's disease. *Aliment. Pharmacol. Ther.* 48 (4), 394–409. doi:10.1111/apt.14852

Smoot, M. E., Ono, K., Ruscheinski, J., Wang, P.-L., and Ideker, T. (2011). Cytoscape 2.8: new features for data integration and network visualization. *Bioinformatics* 27 (3), 431–432. doi:10.1093/bioinformatics/btq675

Soendergaard, C., Seidelin, J. B., Steenholdt, C., and Nielsen, O. H. (2018). Putative biomarkers of vedolizumab resistance and underlying inflammatory pathways involved in IBD. *BMJ open Gastroenterol.* 5 (1), e000208. doi:10.1136/bmjgast-2018-000208

Sprakes, M. B., Ford, A. C., Warren, L., Greer, D., and Hamlin, J. (2012). Efficacy, tolerability, and predictors of response to infliximab therapy for Crohn's disease: a large single centre experience. *J. Crohn's Colitis* 6 (2), 143–153. doi:10.1016/j.crohns.2011.07.011

Steyerberg, E. W., Vickers, A. J., Cook, N. R., Gerds, T., Gonen, M., Obuchowski, N., et al. (2010). Assessing the performance of prediction models. *Epidemiology (Cambridge, Mass)* 21 (1), 128–138. doi:10.1097/ede.0b013e3181c30fb2

Suzuki, Y., Matsui, T., Ito, H., Ashida, T., Nakamura, S., Motoya, S., et al. (2015). Circulating interleukin 6 and albumin, and infliximab levels are good predictors of recovering efficacy after dose escalation infliximab therapy in patients with loss of response to treatment for Crohn's disease. *Inflamm. Bowel Dis.* 21 (9), 2114–2122. doi:10.1097/mib.0000000000000475

Szklarczyk, D., Gable, A. L., Lyon, D., Junge, A., Wyder, S., Huerta-Cepas, J., et al. (2019). STRING v11: protein-protein association networks with increased coverage, supporting functional discovery in genome-wide experimental datasets. *Nucleic Acids Res.* 47 (D1), D607–D613. doi:10.1093/nar/gky1131

Thomas, H. (2017). Oncostatin M promotes inflammation in IBD. *Nat. Rev. Gastroenterol. Hepatol.* 14 (5), 261. doi:10.1038/nrgastro.2017.47

Torres, J., Bonovas, S., Doherty, G., Kucharzik, T., Gisbert, J. P., Raine, T., et al. (2020). ECCO guidelines on therapeutics in crohn's disease: medical treatment. *J. Crohn's colitis* 14 (1), 4–22. doi:10.1093/ecco-jcc/jjz180

West, N. R., Hegazy, A. N., Hegazy, A. N., Owens, B. M. J., Bullers, S. J., Linggi, B., et al. (2017). Oncostatin M drives intestinal inflammation and predicts response to tumor necrosis factor-neutralizing therapy in patients with inflammatory bowel disease. *Nat. Med.* 23 (5), 579–589. doi:10.1038/nm.4307

Wong, U., and Cross, R. K. (2017). Primary and secondary nonresponse to infliximab: mechanisms and countermeasures. *Expert Opin. Drug Metab. Toxicol.* 13 (10), 1039–1046. doi:10.1080/17425255.2017.1377180

Development and Validation of an Interleukin-6 Nomogram to Predict Primary Non-response to Infliximab...

141

Yokoyama, K., Yamazaki, K., Katafuchi, M., and Ferchichi, S. (2016). A retrospective claims database study on drug utilization in Japanese patients with crohn's disease treated with adalimumab or infliximab. *Adv. Ther.* 33 (11), 1947–1963. doi:10.1007/s12325-016-0406-6

Yu, G., Wang, L.-G., Han, Y., and He, Q.-Y. (2012). clusterProfiler: an R package for comparing biological themes among gene clusters. *OMICS: A J. Integr. Biol.* 16 (5), 284–287. doi:10.1089/omi.2011.0118

13

NLRP6 Plays an Important Role in Early Hepatic Immunopathology Caused by *Schistosoma mansoni* Infection

Rodrigo C. O. Sanches[1†], Cláudia Souza[1†], Fabio Vitarelli Marinho[1], Fábio Silva Mambelli[2], Suellen B. Morais[1], Erika S. Guimarães[1] and Sergio Costa Oliveira[1,3]*

[1] *Departamento de Bioquímica e Imunologia, Instituto de Ciências Biológicas, Universidade Federal de Minas Gerais, Belo Horizonte, Brazil,* [2] *Departamento de Genética, Ecologia e Evolução, Instituto de Ciências Biológicas, Universidade Federal de Minas Gerais, Belo Horizonte, Brazil,* [3] *Instituto Nacional de Ciência e Tecnologia em Doenças Tropicais (INCT-DT), CNPq MCT, Salvador, Brazil*

*Correspondence:
Sergio Costa Oliveira
scozeus1@gmail.com

[†] *These authors have contributed equally to this work*

Schistosomiasis is a debilitating parasitic disease that affects more than 200 million people worldwide and causes approximately 280,000 deaths per year. Inside the definitive host, eggs released by *Schistosoma mansoni* lodge in the intestine and especially in the liver where they induce a granulomatous inflammatory process, which can lead to fibrosis. The molecular mechanisms initiating or promoting hepatic granuloma formation remain poorly understood. Inflammasome activation has been described as an important pathway to induce pathology mediated by NLRP3 receptor. Recently, other components of the inflammasome pathway, such as NLRP6, have been related to liver diseases and fibrotic processes. Nevertheless, the contribution of these components in schistosomiasis-associated pathology is still unknown. In the present study, using dendritic cells, we demonstrated that NLRP6 sensor is important for IL-1β production and caspase-1 activation in response to soluble egg antigens (SEA). Furthermore, the lack of NLRP6 has been shown to significantly reduce periovular inflammation, collagen deposition in hepatic granulomas and mRNA levels of α-SMA and IL-13. Livers of $Nlrp6^{-/-}$ mice showed reduced levels of CXCL1/KC, CCL2, CCL3, IL-5, and IL-10 as well as Myeloperoxidase (MPO) and Eosinophilic Peroxidase (EPO) enzymatic activity. Consistently, the frequency of macrophage and neutrophil populations were lower in the liver of NLRP6 knockout mice, after 6 weeks of infection. Finally, it was further demonstrated that the onset of hepatic granuloma and collagen deposition were also compromised in $Caspase-1^{-/-}$, $IL-1R^{-/-}$ and $Gsdmd^{-/-}$ mice. Our findings suggest that the NLRP6 inflammasome is an important component for schistosomiasis-associated pathology.

Keywords: *Schistosoma mansoni*, immunopathology, inflammasome, NLRP6, fibrosis

INTRODUCTION

Schistosomiasis is a debilitating parasitic disease which affects 78 countries worldwide. This disease leads to approximately 200,000 deaths annually and severely compromises the life quality from those affected. Among causative species, *Schistosoma haematobium, Schistosoma japonicum,* and *Schistosoma mansoni* stand out as those of major importance to human health (1–3). Infection occurs through the direct contact of the host with the parasite's larval form. After parasite penetration and sexual development, egg laying begins. The release of eggs in the feces and its hatching in the environment closes the parasite's life cycle (4). However, a significant amount of these eggs is trapped in some of the host's organs, such as liver and intestine, where they induce a granulomatous inflammatory reaction (5, 6). Hepatic granulomatous inflammation arises from the egg-secreted antigens, which perform hepatotoxic and immunological activities capable of recruiting immune cells to the organ and forming periovular granuloma. The composition of the granuloma includes macrophages, eosinophils, neutrophils, T and B lymphocytes and especially fibroblasts, responsible for the fibrotic characteristic of the structure (7, 8).

Although the process of hepatic granuloma formation is extensively studied, all cellular events and key participants have not been fully established yet. The role of intracellular immune receptors in granuloma formation, for instance, was first described in a seminal study conducted by Ritter and colleagues (9). However, a better understanding of cytosolic sensors during *S. mansoni* infection is required. These intracellular receptors are those responsible for activating the inflammasome pathway. This pathway induces the formation of an intracellular protein complex typically consisting of Nucleotide-binding oligomerization domain (NOD), leucine-rich repeat (LRR)-containing protein (NLR) family members, an adapter molecule known as ASC, and the cysteine protease caspase-1 as an effector molecule. Activation of this pathway leads to cleavage of immature forms of IL-1β and IL-18 into their mature forms. It might also induce cell death by pyroptosis. The inflammasome activation takes place in both immune and non-immune cells and is essentially triggered by pathogen-associated molecular patterns (PAMPs) and Danger-associated molecular patterns (DAMP) (10, 11).

It is known that the inflammasome pathway plays an important role during chronic liver diseases (12). Besides fighting pathogens such as bacteria (13) and viruses (14), inflammasome also participates in aggravating sterile liver inflammations such as Alcoholic Liver Disease (ALD) (15) and Non-alcoholic Steatohepatitis (NASH) (16). NLRP3 is the most widely studied receptor in this context since it is activated by several types of insults (17). On the other hand, the participation of other NLR family receptors in hepatic pathological processes, such as NLRP6, is still elusive.

The inflammasome pathway plays an essential role in schistosomiasis-associated liver pathology. It has been demonstrated that NLRP3 is critical for granuloma formation and hepatic stellate cells (HSCs) activation (18) in *S. japonicum* infections. Regarding *S. mansoni* infection this same sensor has

been shown to be involved in the adaptive immune response and also granuloma formation (9). Recent studies have reported that NLRP3 and NLRP6 expression are simultaneously modulated in some processes, including those occurring in the liver (19, 20). Additionally, the role of NLRP6 in fibrotic diseases has already been described (21, 22). Thus, we decided to investigate whether the NLRP6 sensor plays a role in the course of *S. mansoni* infection and liver pathology. In this study, we demonstrate that lack of NLRP6 modulates the formation of hepatic granuloma, influencing local chemokine and cytokine production as well as macrophage and neutrophil recruitment into the liver. Also, this receptor is important for promoting collagen deposition.

MATERIALS AND METHODS

Ethics Statement
This study was carried out in accordance with Brazilian laws #6638 and #9605 in Animal Experiments. The protocol was approved by the Committee on Ethics of Animal Experiments of the Universidade Federal de Minas Gerais (UFMG) (Permit Number: #367/2017).

Mice and Parasite
Wild-type C57BL/6 mice were purchased from the Universidade Federal de Minas Gerais (UFMG). $Nlrp3^{-/-}$, $Nlrp6^{-/-}$, $Casp-1^{-/-}$, $IL-1R^{-/-}$, and $Gsdmd^{-/-}$ were described previously (23–26). The animals were maintained at UFMG and used at 6–10 week of age. *Schistosoma mansoni* (LE strain) cercariae at Fundação Oswaldo Cruz – Centro de Pesquisas René Rachou (CPqRR-Brazil) were routinely obtained from infected *Biomphalaria glabrata* snails exposed to light, inducing the shedding of parasites.

Eggs, SEA, and SWAP
Eggs were obtained from 50-day-infected Swiss mice livers. Briefly, the liver was blender processed in cold saline (2% NaCl) for 2 min. Next, the material was decanted into a glass goblet for 35 min at low temperature. Part of the decanting supernatant was discarded and the remaining solution was washed with cold saline. Decantation-washing was repeated until reaching a translucent solution. Eggs were recovered by filtration. For the preparation of Soluble Egg Antigens (SEA), eggs were disrupted for 40 min at low temperature in PBS and then the homogenate was centrifuged at $100,000 \times g$ for 1 h at 4°C. The resulting supernatant was frozen at −80°C. Soluble adult worm antigen (SWAP) was obtained by mechanical maceration of worms in cold PBS. After centrifugation ($13,000 \times g$ – 7 min), the supernatant was collected and stored at −80°C. The protein concentration of SEA and SWAP was determined using BCA™ protein assay kit (Thermo Fisher Scientific, Waltham, MA, United States).

BMDC Generation and Activation
To obtain bone marrow-derived dendritic cells (BMDCs), bone marrow cells were cultured in RPMI with 10% FBS, 100 U/mL penicillin, 100 µg/mL streptomycin and 20 ng/mL murine

recombinant GM-CSF (Peprotech, Riberão Preto, Brazil). Petri dishes containing 1×10^7 cells were incubated at 37°C in 5% CO_2. At day 3 of incubation, 5 mL of fresh complete medium with GM-CSF was added, and 5 mL of medium was replaced with fresh supplemented medium containing GM-CSF on days 5 and 7. At day 10, non-adherent cells were harvested and seeded in 24-well plates (5×10^5 cells/well). Stimulation of BMDCs was performed by priming cells with 1 μg/ml of Pam_3Cys (Sigma-Aldrich, St. Louis, MO, United States) for 5 h and then stimulating with 50 μg/mL of SEA for 17 and 24 h. As positive control for inflammasome activation, cells were primed with 1 μg/ml of Pam_3Cys (5 h) or 1 μg/ml of LPS (4 h) and stimulated with ATP (5 mM) (50 min) or Nigericin (20 μM) (50 min). Culture supernatants were collected and cells were lysed with M-PER Mammalian Protein Extraction Reagent (Thermo Fisher Scientific) supplemented with 1:100 protease inhibitor mixture (Sigma-Aldrich).

Western Blotting

Cell lysates and supernatants from DCs culture were subjected to SDS-PAGE analysis and western blotting. The proteins were resolved on a 15% SDS-PAGE gel, and transferred to nitrocellulose membranes (Amersham Biosciences, Uppsala, Sweden). Membranes were blocked for 1 h in TBS (0.1% Tween-20; 5% non-fat dry milk) and incubated with primary antibodies at 4°C, overnight. Primary antibody used was mouse monoclonal against the p20 subunit of caspase-1 (Adipogen, San Diego, CA, United States). Monoclonal antibody against β-actin (Cell Signaling Technology, Danvers, MA, United States) was used as a loading control blot (1:1,000). The membranes were washed three times for 10 min in TBS with 0.1% Tween 20. Next, membranes were incubated for 1 h at room temperature with the suitable HRP-conjugated secondary antibody (1:1,000). Immunoreactive bands were visualized using Luminol chemiluminescent HRP substrate (Millipore).

Splenocyte Culture

Spleen cells were obtained from macerated spleens of individual C57BL/6 and $Nlrp6^{-/-}$ mice after 6 weeks of infection with S. mansoni cercariae (n = 5/group). Cells were washed with PBS and the erythrocytes were lysed with a hemolytic solution (155 mM NH4Cl, 10 mM KHCO3, pH 7.2). Cells were adjusted to 1×10^6/well in complete RPMI medium (10% fetal bovine serum, 100 U/mL penicillin and 100 μg/mL streptomycin). Spleen cells were cultured in 96-well plates with medium and stimulated with SWAP (200 μg/mL), SEA (20 μg/mL), Eggs (50/well) or concanavalin A (ConA) (5 μg/mL). Culture supernatants were collected after 24 h for IL-5 and after 72 h for IFN-γ, IL-10, and IL-13 measurements by ELISA.

Liver Processing

Right lobe of liver from 6-week-infected C57BL/6 and $Nlrp6^{-/-}$ mice was collected and 1 mL of cytokine extraction solution (0.4 M NaCl, 0.05% Tween 20, 0.5% BSA, 0.1 mM PMSF, 0.1 mM benzethoniumchloride, 10 mM EDTA and 20 KI aprotinin) was

added to each 100 mg of tissue. Ultra-Turrax homogenizer-dispenser was used to homogenize solutions containing the organs. Next, the samples were centrifuged at 10,000 × g for 10 min at 4°C. Non-parenchymal cells from left lobe were used for flow cytometry analysis. Tissue was removed without perfusion, cut into small pieces, incubated in RPMI medium containing 30 μg/ml of Liberase TM (Roche) and 20 U/mL of DNAse I (GE) for 40 min, and passed through a 70 μm pore-size cell strainer. After centrifugation, the cells were resuspended in PBS containing 2% fetal bovine serum (FBS) and 5 mM EDTA. Low-speed centrifugation (50 × g – 5 min) was used to remove parenchymal cells. Erythrocytes were lysed with a hemolytic solution (155 mM NH4Cl, 10 mM KHCO3, pH 7.2). The remaining non-parenchymal cells were resuspended in RPMI culture medium.

Cytokine Measurements

Cytokine/Chemokine production was evaluated using the Duoset ELISA kit (R&D Diagnostic, Minneapolis, MN, United States) according to the manufacturer's instructions.

EPO and MPO Activity Assays

Eosinophilic Peroxidase and Myeloperoxidase assays were performed as described by Cançado et al. (27). Right lobe of the liver was homogenized, red blood cells subjected to hypotonic lysis and the remaining liver cells subjected to detergent lysis and freeze-thaw cycles. The enzymatic assay was performed using the suitable substrates and the result was measured on a microplate reader at the appropriate wavelength (492 nm for EPO and 450 nm for MPO). The result was expressed in absorbance units.

Flow Cytometry Analysis

Spleen and non-parenchymal liver cells were stained for CD11b, CD11c, Ly6G, F4/80, CD3, and CD4. Briefly, cells were incubated for 20 min with anti-mouse CD16/32 (BD Biosciences) in FACS buffer (PBS, 1% FBS, 1 mM NaN3) and were stained for surface markers for 20 min using: APC-Cy7-conjugated anti-mouse CD11b (1:200, M1/70; BD Biosciences), FITC-conjugated anti-mouse CD11c (1:100, HL3; BD Biosciences), PE-conjugated anti-mouse Ly6G (1:200, 1A8; BD Biosciences), biotinylated anti-mouse F4/80 (1:200, BM8; BD Biosciences), PE-Cy7-conjugated anti-mouse CD3 (1:100, BD Biosciences) and APC-conjugated anti-mouse CD4 (1:200, BD Biosciences). The appropriate isotype controls were used. Next, cells were washed and incubated for 20 min at 4°C in the dark with PerCP-Cy5.5 conjugated streptavidin (1:200 BD Biosciences). Lastly, cells were washed and resuspended in PBS. Attune Flow Cytometer (Applied Biosystems, Waltham, MA, United States) was used for collecting approximately 100,000 events and data were analyzed using FlowJo software (Tree Star, Ashland, OR, United States).

In order to evaluate macrophage polarization, non-parenchymal liver cells were stained as described above using APC-Cy7-conjugated anti-mouse CD11b (1:200, M1/70; BD Biosciences), biotinylated anti-mouse F4/80 (1:200, BM8; BD Biosciences), BB700-conjugated anti-mouse CD197 (1:200, 4B12

BD Biosciences), FITC-conjugated anti-mouse CD80 (1:200, 16-10A1, BD Biosciences), PE-conjugated anti-mouse CD163 (1:200, TNKUPJ, eBioscience) and APC-conjugated anti-mouse CD206 (1:200, MR5D3, BD Biosciences).

Quantitative Real-Time PCR

Liver middle lobe of 6-week-infected C57BL/6 and $Nlrp6^{-/-}$ mice was used for RNA extraction. The tissue was homogenized in TRIzol (Invitrogen) and total RNA was isolated in accordance with the manufacturer's instructions. Reverse transcription of total RNA was performed and quantitative real-time RT-PCR was conducted in a final volume of 20 μL containing SYBR Green PCR Master Mix (Applied Biosystems, Foster City, CA, United States), oligo-dT cDNA as the PCR template and 2.5 μM of primers. The PCR reaction was performed with QuantStudio3 real-time PCR instrument (Applied Biosystems). Primers were used to amplify a specific fragment (100–120 bp) corresponding to specific gene targets as follows: *18S* Forward (5'-CGTTCC ACCAACTAAGAACG-3') and *18S* Reverse (5'-CTCAACACGG GAAACCTCAC-3'; α-*SMA* Forward (5'-GTCCCAGACATCAG GGAGTAA-3') and α-*SMA* Reverse (5'-TCGGATACTTCA GCGTCAG-3'); *IL-13* Forward (5'-CCTGGCTCTTGCTTGCC-3') and *IL-13* Reverse (5'-GGTCTTGTGTGATGTTGCTCA-3'); *IL-1β* Forward (5'-TGACCTGGGCTGTCCAGATG-3') and *IL-1β* Reverse (5'-CTGTCCATTGAGGTGGAGAG-3'); *Casp-1* Forward (5'-GGAAGCAATTTATCAACTCAGTG-3') and *Casp-1* Reverse (5'-GCCTTGTCCATAGCAGTAATG-3').

Mice Infection and Parasite Burden

Six-to-eight-week-old wild-type and knockout mice were anesthetized with 5% ketamine, 2% xylazine and 0.9% NaCl and then infected with 100 cercariae (LE strain) through exposure of percutaneous abdominal skin, for 1 h. After 6 weeks of infection, mice were euthanized and perfused from the portal veins, the recovered worms were counted and the mean difference between groups of mice was evaluated.

Pathological Parameters

Number of eggs was obtained from liver median lobe. The tissue was weighed and digested in an aqueous solution of KOH (5%) for 16 h at 37°C. After, eggs were washed in saline and centrifuged twice at 270 × g for 10 min and counted using a light microscope. The number of calculated eggs was corrected by considering the mass of the tissue, resulting in number of eggs per gram of liver. The left lobe was fixed with 10% buffered formaldehyde in PBS. Histological sections were performed using microtome at 6 μm and stained on a slide with Hematoxylin-Eosin (HE) and Masson blue. For measurement of granuloma size and collagen deposition, a JVC TK-1270/RBG camera, attached to the microscope (10 × objective lens), was used to obtain the images. Analysis were carried out using ImageJ software (U.S. National Institutes of Health, Bethesda, MD, United States)[1]. Granuloma size was measured, in μm², for all granulomas found in liver sections.

---

[1] http://rsbweb.nih.gov/ij/index.html

Statistical Analysis

The statistical tests were performed using Student's *t-test*, one-way and two-way ANOVA followed by Bonferroni adjustments for comparison between groups. *P*-values obtained were considered significant if they were <0.05. Statistical analysis was performed using GraphPad Prism 6 (La Jolla, CA, United States).

RESULTS

IL-1β Production and Caspase-1 Activation Are Partially Dependent on NLRP6 in SEA/Eggs-Stimulated Dendritic Cells

During *S. mansoni* infection, hepatic dendritic cells (DCs) are the main cells responsible for promoting the shift from Th1 to Th2 immune profile, which is triggered by egg antigens (28). Ritter and colleagues (2010) reported that SEA induces inflammasome activation in DCs and described the involvement of NLRP3 (9). Thus, given the relevance of these cells, we decided to use bone marrow-derived dendritic cells (BMDCs) in order to investigate whether the NLRP6 sensor is involved in IL-1β secretion in response to different parasite antigens. Using Pam₃Cys (P₃Cys) as the first signal, we observed that eggs and their soluble antigens (SEA) induce high levels of IL-1β and this production was partially influenced by NLRP6 (**Figure 1A**). In contrast, IL-1β production induced by soluble adult worm antigens (SWAP) was much lower compared to SEA (**Figure 1A**). Additionally, TNF-α levels were not altered comparing both WT and NLRP6 knockout (KO) mice (**Figure 1B**). Since SEA was sufficient to induce IL-1β production, we used this stimulus to evaluate the role of NLRP6 in caspase-1 (casp-1) activation. **Figures 1C,D** demonstrate that SEA induces activation of casp-1 in WT DCs and this process was clearly inhibited in $Nlrp6^{-/-}$ DCs.

NLRP6 Influences Granuloma Formation and Collagen Deposition in the Liver

Since the liver is one of the main entrapment tissues for parasite's eggs and once the participation of NLRP6 in the egg and SEA-induced immune response has been observed, we wondered if this sensor could play any role in liver pathology. First, we observed that in livers of 4- and 6-week infected animals the levels of *IL-1β* and *caspase-1* mRNA did not significantly change between $Nlrp6^{-/-}$ and WT mice (**Supplementary Figure S1**). Initially, we observed that the number of eggs per gram of tissue was not altered between WT and knockout mice (**Figure 2A**). Consistently, the worm burden recovery was the same comparing both groups (**Supplementary Figure S2**). On the other hand, NLRP6 has been shown to influence the periovular inflammatory response, contributing significantly to granuloma formation (**Figure 2B**). In addition, collagen deposition within the granulomatous structure was reduced in $Nlrp6^{-/-}$ mice when compared to WT (**Figures 2B,C,H**). We also evaluated levels of cytokines and fibrotic markers within the tissue, such as the cytokines IL-5, IL-10, IL-13, and the protein Alpha-smooth muscle actin (α-SMA). IL-5 and IL-10 cytokines

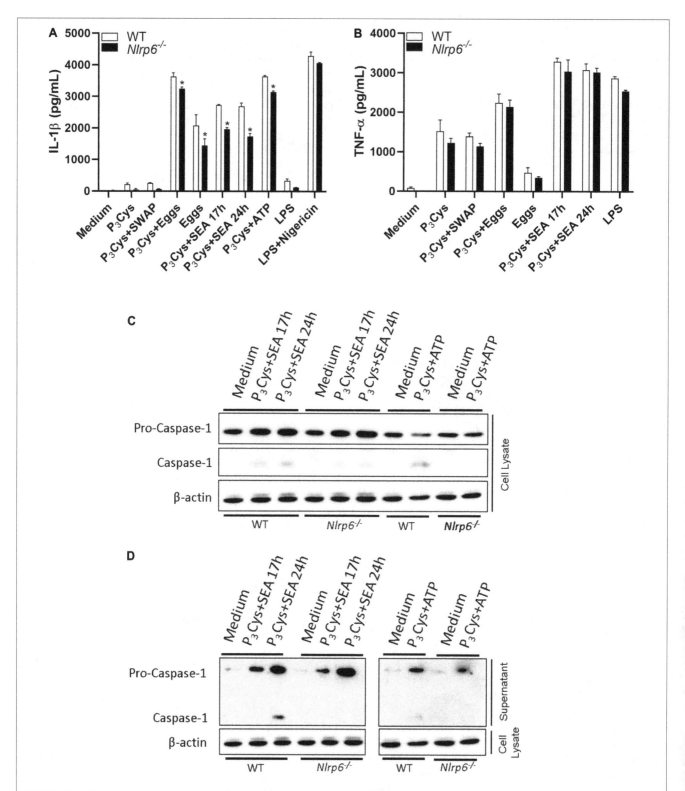

FIGURE 1 | NLRP6 regulates IL-1β production and Casp-1 activation induced by SEA. WT or *Nlrp6⁻/⁻* deficient BMDCs were primed with P₃Cys (1 μg/ml – 5 h) and stimulated with SEA (50 μg/mL – 17 h, 24 h), Eggs (100 eggs/well – 24 h), SWAP (200 μg/mL – 24 h) or ATP (5 mM – 50 min). For nigericin control (20 μM), cells were primed with LPS (1 μg/ml – 4 h) and stimulate for 50 min. **(A)** IL-1β and **(B)** TNF-α were measured by ELISA. Casp-1 activation was analyzed by western blot in **(C)** cell lysate and **(D)** supernatant using antibody against p20 subunit. An asterisk denotes statistically significant differences between NLRP6 versus WT animals (*p* < 0.05).

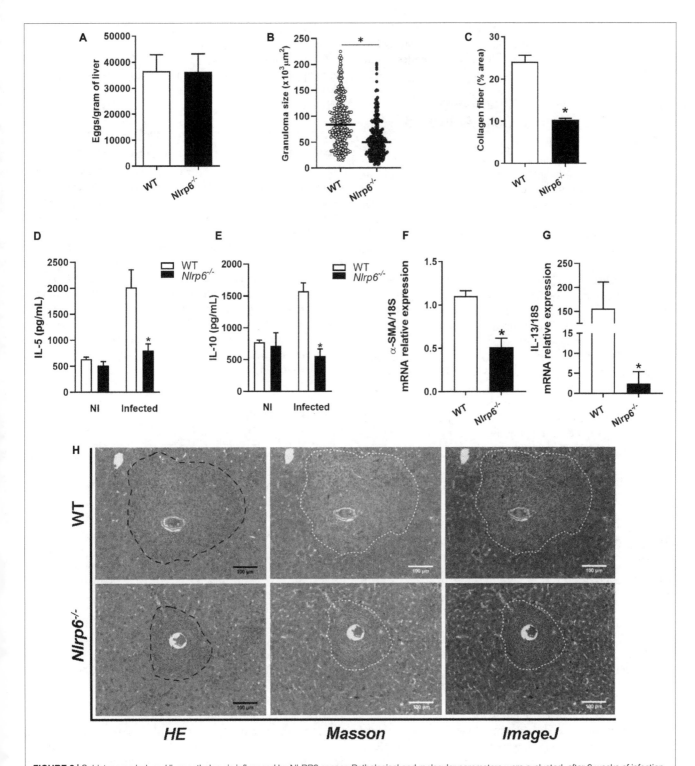

FIGURE 2 | *Schistosoma*-induced liver pathology is influenced by NLRP6 sensor. Pathological and molecular parameters were evaluated, after 6 weeks of infection in WT and *Nlrp6*−/− mice. **(A)** Number of eggs per gram of liver, **(B)** Granuloma size (μm^2) and **(C)** Collagen deposition. **(D)** IL-5 and **(E)** IL-10 cytokine levels were detected. **(F)** α-SMA and **(G)** IL-13 transcripts were also measured. **(H)** Representative images of granulomas detected in hematoxylin-eosin, masson blue and the output from ImageJ software, respectively. An asterisk denotes statistically significant differences between NLRP6 versus WT animals ($p < 0.05$). The bar represents 100 μm. NI stands for Non-infected mice.

levels, as well as, α-SMA and IL-13 mRNA measurements were reduced in $Nlrp6^{-/-}$ group when compared to WT (**Figures 2D–G**). These data demonstrate that NLRP6 contributes to the pathology caused by *S. mansoni*.

NLRP6 Influences IL-10 and IFN-γ Production by Spleen Cells Activated With Egg Antigens

After determining the impact of NLRP6 on inflammasome activation and granuloma formation in response to egg antigens, we decided to investigate the frequency of dendritic cells and CD4$^+$ T lymphocytes in spleen cells derived from *S. mansoni* infected mice. Cells were obtained following the gate strategy described in **Supplementary Figure S3**. We observed that 6-week-infected $Nlrp6^{-/-}$ and WT mice presented no significant difference regarding CD11b$^+$CD11c$^+$ (dendritic cells) and CD3$^+$CD4$^+$ (CD4$^+$ lymphocytes) cell populations (**Figures 3A,B**). Interestingly, when spleen cells were stimulated with eggs or SEA, the cytokine production was altered. Both antigens induced increased levels of IL-10 and IFN-γ in splenocyte culture supernatants from $Nlrp6^{-/-}$ compared to WT mice (**Figures 3E,F**). Additionally, NLRP6 appears to have no effect on IL-5 and IL-13 production (**Figures 3C,D**). Curiously, when $Nlrp6^{-/-}$ and WT spleen cells from *S. mansoni* infected mice were stimulated with SWAP, no significant difference on IFN-γ, IL-10, IL-5, and IL-13 levels was observed (**Supplementary Figure S4**). These data emphasize the relevance of NLRP6 during egg antigen response regulating IL-10 and IFN-γ production. Furthermore, enhanced IL-10 production in $Nlrp6^{-/-}$ may be related to reduced granuloma formation and fibrosis.

NLRP6 Mediates Innate Immune Cells Recruitment in *Schistosoma*-Infected Liver

Since lack of NLRP6 has been shown to modulate hepatic granuloma formation, we decided to investigate how this sensor influences liver pathology. Initially, we evaluated the level of chemokines (CCL2, CCL3, CCL11, and CXCL1) in livers of *Schistosoma*-infected mice. These chemokines have already been described as related to granuloma formation. In *Schistosoma*-infected $Nlrp6^{-/-}$ mice only the production of CCL11 was not reduced in comparison to WT mice (**Figure 4D**). CCL2, CXCL1, and CCL3 were diminished in $Nlrp6^{-/-}$ mice compared to WT animals (**Figures 4A–C**). Additionally, we observed that the enzymes MPO and EPO were also reduced in $Nlrp6^{-/-}$ mice when compared to WT (**Figures 4E,F**). Our next step was to evaluate which non-parenchymal cell populations could be altered in *Schistosoma*-infected $Nlrp6^{-/-}$ mice. Cells were obtained following the gate strategy described in **Supplementary Figure S5**. Neutrophils and macrophages were the major cell populations reduced in $Nlrp6^{-/-}$ mice when compared to WT (**Figures 4G,H**). The frequency of dendritic cells and CD4$^+$ T lymphocytes remained unaltered in either mouse groups (**Figures 4I,J**). We also found that the lack of NLRP6 does not affect macrophage polarization, even though

there is a strong tendency of reduction in anti-inflammatory macrophages (CD206$^+$CD163$^+$) in $Nlrp6^{-/-}$ compared to WT mice (**Supplementary Figure S6**). Therefore, the NLRP6 sensor possibly induces the formation of hepatic granuloma by favoring chemokine production and the recruitment of immune cells to the liver.

Inflammasome Pathway Is Broadly Relevant to Granuloma Formation

The NLR family receptors perform their functions depending on tissue and cell type, as already demonstrated for NLRP3 and NLRP6 (29, 30). For this reason, we decided to evaluate whether other inflammasome pathway-related molecules, such as Casp-1, GSDMD, and IL-1R, played a role in the formation of hepatic granuloma. Similarly to what we observed here for $Nlrp6^{-/-}$ mice, a significant reduction in periovular inflammatory response in $Casp-1^{-/-}$, $Gsdmd^{-/-}$, and $IL-1R^{-/-}$ mice was observed. In addition, a reduction in collagen deposition was observed in the granulomas of $Casp-1^{-/-}$, $Gsdmd^{-/-}$, and $IL-1R^{-/-}$ mice when compared to WT (**Figures 5B–D**). This was accompanied by no alteration in the number of eggs in the tissue (**Figure 5A**), and worm burden recovery (**Supplementary Figure S2**) when compared to WT mice.

DISCUSSION

The role of the inflammasome pathway in the pathogenesis of chronic liver diseases has been investigated in the last few years (31, 32). Hepatic injuries from different sources are capable of leading to inflammasome activation, as described for drug-induced damage (33), ischemia-reperfusion (34), alcoholic and non-alcoholic fatty liver disease (15, 16), and viral hepatitis (14). Inflammasome triggers or amplify liver diseases by releasing pro-inflammatory cytokines such as IL-1β, IL-1α, IL-18, and also through other inflammatory mediators such as High Mobility Group Box 1 (HMGB1) (35). Release of such cytokines and DAMPs occur, in part, due to Gasdermin-D cleavage and subsequent pyroptosis of the cell (36). The fibrotic process resulting from chronic liver diseases has also involved the inflammasome pathway. IL-1β and danger signals induce Hepatic Stellate Cells (HSC) to transdifferentiate and perform extracellular matrix remodeling function. In addition, HSCs can internalize pre-formed inflammasome complexes released by other pyroptosis dying cells (37–39).

The participation of the NLRP3 receptor in chronic liver diseases such as non-alcoholic fatty liver disease (NAFLD) is well described (16, 17). On the other hand, the role of the NLRP6 sensor in these liver pathologies is still elusive. Recently, Xiao and colleagues (2018) reported that in the NAFLD model induced by methionine-choline deficient (MCD) diet, NLRP3 and NLRP6 expression is highly detected in the liver. After *Lycium barbarum* polysaccharides (LBP) treatment, NAFLD condition improves and the expression of both NLR receptors decreases (20). Besides, a previous study with NAFLD obese patients demonstrates that when hepatic portal fibrosis is present, the expression of *NLRP6* mRNA in adipose tissues is higher compared to cases when

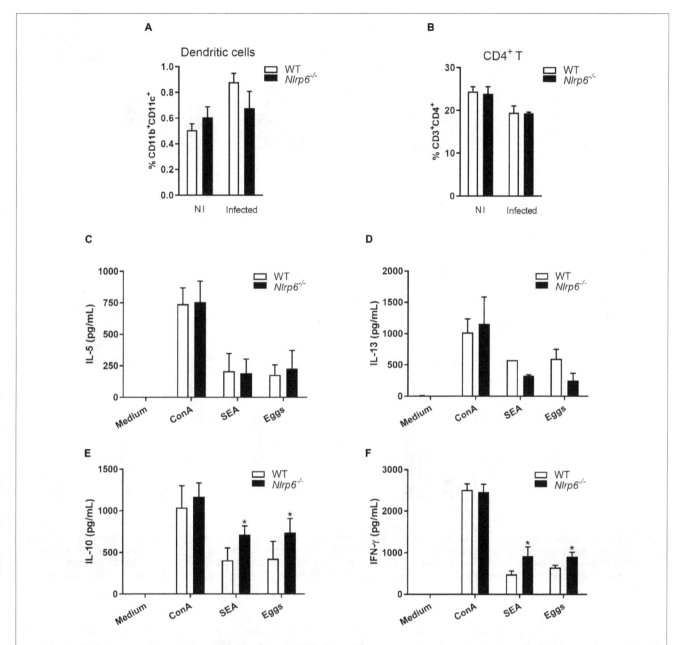

FIGURE 3 | Cytokine profile induced by SEA/Eggs in *Nlrp6⁻ᐟ⁻* mice. Six-weeks post infection the percentage of **(A)** dendritic cells (CD11b⁺CD11c⁺) and **(B)** CD4⁺ T lymphocytes (CD3⁺CD4⁺) in spleens from non-infected (NI) and infected animals were analyzed by flow cytometry. Spleen cells of infected mice were restimulated with ConA (5 μg/mL), SEA (20 μg/mL) or Eggs (50/well). Cytokine levels were measured by ELISA in cell supernatants from antigen restimulated cells, **(C)** IL-5, **(D)** IL-13, **(E)** IL-10 and **(F)** IFN-γ. An asterisk denotes statistically significant differences between NLRP6 versus WT animals (*p* < 0.05).

hepatic portal fibrosis is not observed (21). These findings suggest that NLRP6 might play important role in chronic liver disease and fibrosis. All those findings intrigued us to evaluate the role of this sensor in *S. mansoni* infection.

Schistosoma mansoni and *S. japonicum* infections are sources of injury and are able to induce chronic liver disease. The long survival period of *Schistosoma* worms within the human host implies recurrent inflammation and wound-healing cycles in the liver, triggered by egg antigens which can result in fibrosis, portal hypertension and hepatosplenomegaly (4, 8). Among

non-parenchymal liver cells, DCs stand out as key cells during this pathological process. Broadly responsive to egg antigens, DCs are essential for promoting systemic shift in the immune response profile (from Th1 to Th2), which is crucial for host survival upon infection (28, 40). In addition, the first report of inflammasome pathway activation by *S. mansoni* antigens involved dendritic cells responding to SEA. For these reasons, we initially decided to evaluate the role of NLRP6 in DCs. Our findings suggest that NLRP6 is important for the formation of the inflammasome complex, since it influences IL-1β secretion

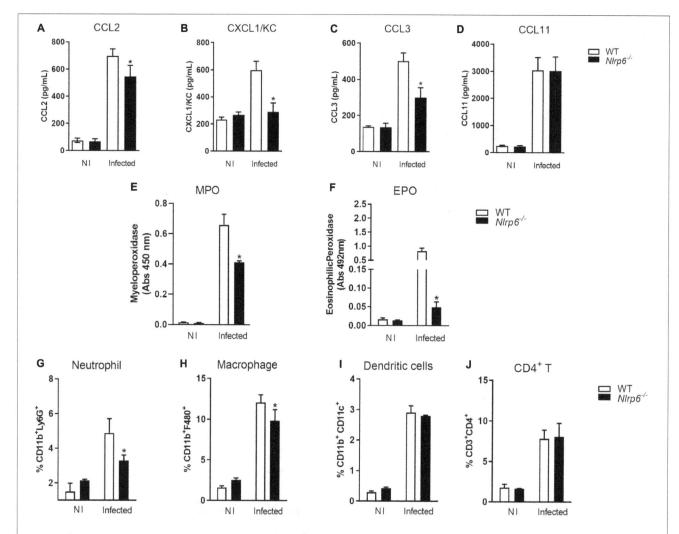

FIGURE 4 | NLRP6 regulates chemokine production and immune cell recruitment into the liver. After 6 weeks of infection, the liver was used to measure chemokine levels, MPO and EPO activities and the frequency of immune cells. Levels of **(A)** CCL2, **(B)** CXCL1 **(C)** CCL3 and **(D)** CCL11 were measured by ELISA. **(E,F)** MPO and EPO activities were also detected. The percentage of **(G)** CD11b⁺Ly6G⁺, **(H)** CD11b⁺F4/80, **(I)** CD11b⁺CD11c⁺ and **(J)** CD3⁺CD4⁺ T lymphocyte populations were measured by flow cytometry. An asterisk denotes statistically significant differences between NLRP6 versus WT animals ($p < 0.05$). NI stands for Non-infected mice.

and caspase-1 activation in response to SEA. Previous studies demonstrate that NLRP6 structurally has the ability to form the inflammasome complex and does so in response to gram-positive bacteria cell wall components, activating both caspase-1 and caspase-11 in the same complex (41, 42).

The activation of intracellular receptors was not expected to occur in response to multicellular parasites such as S. mansoni. Surprisingly, Ritter and colleagues (2010) demonstrated that SEA triggers NLRP3 inflammasome pathway in DCs (9). Following this seminal study, NLRP3 inflammasome role has been investigated, especially in S. japonicum infection. In this context, NLRP3 has been shown to be pivotal for inducing hepatic granuloma formation and collagen deposition in the granulomatous structure (18, 43). In this study, we confirmed that NLRP3 is pivotal for hepatic granuloma formation, but we did not find any alteration in collagen deposition in Nlrp3⁻/⁻ mice when compared to WT (**Supplementary Figure S7**).

This observation may be related to the early time point infection of our model (6 weeks), which also could explain the distribution of collagen throughout the granuloma structure and not only peripherally, as typically observed in later granulomas. Surprisingly, we have demonstrated for the first time that NLRP6 also plays an important role in S. mansoni-induced pathology. We found that this sensor influences the formation of hepatic granuloma, altering local chemokine (CCL2, CCL3, and CXCL1) and cytokine (IL-5, IL-10, and IL-13) production, macrophage and neutrophil recruitment into the liver, and also is important for promoting collagen deposition. In Schistosoma egg-induced pathology, chemokine production is essential to modulate granuloma formation (44, 45). CCL3-deficient mice, for instance, showed size reduced granuloma, lower fibrosis and lower EPO activity in the liver (46). Although classically responsible for neutrophil recruitment, CXCL1 also impacts on the recruitment of HSCs, which are responsible for collagen

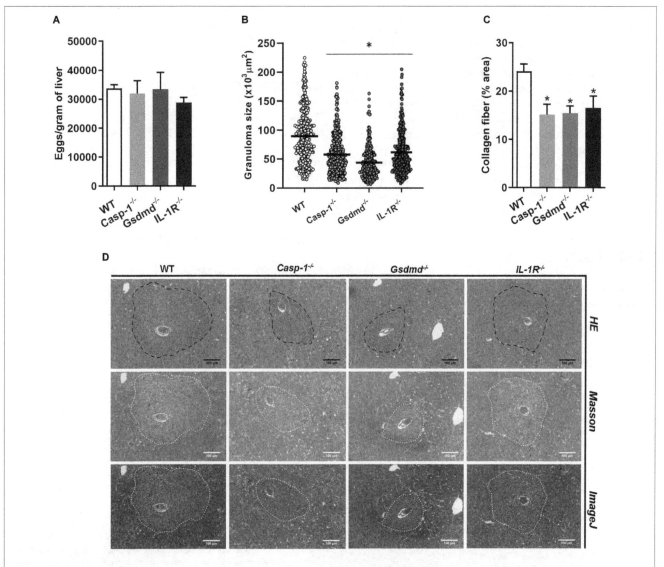

FIGURE 5 | Inflammasome activation influences granuloma formation and collagen deposition. Pathological parameters were analyzed for other inflammasome components such as Casp-1, GSDMD and IL-1R in mouse livers. **(A)** Number of eggs per gram of liver, **(B)** Granuloma size and **(C)** collagen deposition were measured in WT and Casp-1, GSDMD and IL-1R deficient animals. **(D)** Representative images of granulomas detected in hematoxylin and eosin, masson blue and the output from ImageJ software, respectively. An asterisk denotes statistically significant differences between deficient mice versus WT animals ($p < 0.05$). The bar represents 100 μm.

deposition in the granuloma structure (47). Following injury, hepatic resident cells produce CCL2, important for monocyte and macrophage recruitment (48).

NLRP6 is known as an atypical sensor with wide functional capability, performing activities integrated and/or independent on the inflammasome complex (30). Our findings demonstrate that Casp-1 activation and IL-1β production, in response to SEA, can be regulated by NLRP6. Therefore, our findings suggest that the role of this receptor in hepatic granuloma formation is due to the inflammasome activation, since $Nlrp3^{-/-}$ mice have demonstrated a similar phenotype. It is clear that the inflammasome pathway is important for Schistosoma-induced liver pathology, once we have observed granuloma reduction and lower collagen deposition in $Casp\text{-}1^{-/-}$, $Gsdmd^{-/-}$, and

$IL\text{-}1R^{-/-}$ mice when compared to WT. Previous liver disease studies support our observations for $Casp\text{-}1^{-/-}$ and $IL\text{-}1R^{-/-}$ mice. In a high fat diet-induced NASH model, deficient Casp-1 animals showed improvement in hepatic steatosis, inflammation and fibrogenesis (49). Similarly, IL-1R signaling has been shown to be critical for the progression of steatohepatitis and hepatic fibrosis in hypercholesterolemic mice (50). The role of Gasdermin- D and pyroptosis has also been described in chronic liver diseases (51, 52). During human NAFLD/NASH, GSDMD and its N-terminal peptide (GSDMD-N) are upregulated, besides MCD-fed $Gsdmd^{-/-}$ mice showed decreased severity of steatosis and inflammation comparing to WT (52). During Schistosoma infection, Liu and colleagues (2019) demonstrated that S. japonicum induces expression of the GSDMD-N in the liver, and that this expression is modulated by NLRP3 sensor (53). In addition, it has been reported that SEA from *S. japonicum* eggs induces pyroptosis in HSCs (54). However, no *in vivo* mouse study has been reported correlating GSDMD deficiency and granuloma formation and fibrosis induced by *S. mansoni* infection as demonstrated here.

In summary, the data presented here demonstrate that lack of NLRP6 modulates activation of the inflammasome pathway in response to *S. mansoni* egg antigens. In addition, NLRP6 and the inflammasome components are important in liver pathology induced by *S. mansoni* infection. Taken together, these data reinforce the relevance of understanding the inflammasome signaling pathway, given its potential to influence the severe pathological conditions induced by this disease.

ETHICS STATEMENT

The animal study was reviewed and approved by the Committee on Ethics of Animal Experiments of the Federal University of Minas Gerais (Permit Number: #367/2017) and carried out in accordance with Brazilian laws #6638 and #9605 in Animal Experiments.

AUTHOR CONTRIBUTIONS

RS and SO designed the project and experiments, and wrote the manuscript. RS, CS, FVM, FSM, EG, and SM carried out most of the experiments. RS carried out statistical analysis and prepared the figures. SO submitted this manuscript. All authors reviewed the manuscript.

ACKNOWLEDGMENTS

We thank Dr. Cristina T. Fonseca from Fundação Oswaldo Cruz – Centro de Pesquisas René Rachou (CPqRR-Brazil) for providing *S. mansoni* cercariae to carry out the experiments.

REFERENCES

Hotez PJ, Alvarado M, Basáñez M-G, Bolliger I, Bourne R, Boussinesq M, et al. The global burden of disease study 2010: interpretation and implications for the neglected tropical diseases. *PLoS Negl Trop Dis*. (2014) 8:e2865. doi: 10.1371/journal.pntd.0002865

Steinmann P, Keiser J, Bos R, Tanner M, Utzinger J. Schistosomiasis and water resources development: systematic review, meta-analysis, and estimates of people at risk. *Lancet Infect Dis*. (2006) 6:411–25. doi: 10.1016/S1473-3099(06)70521-7

Utzinger J, Raso G, Brooker S, De Savigny D, Tanner M, Ørnbjerg N, et al. Schistosomiasis and neglected tropical diseases: towards integrated and sustainable control and a word of caution. *Parasitology*. (2009) 136:1859–74. doi: 10.1017/S0031182009991600

Colley DG, Bustinduy AL, Secor WE, King CH. Human schistosomiasis. *Lancet*. (2014) 383:2253–64. doi: 10.1016/S0140-6736(13)61949-2

Hams E, Aviello G, Fallon PG. The *Schistosoma* granuloma: friend or foe? *Front Immunol*. (2013) 4:89. doi: 10.3389/fimmu.2013.00089

Moore DV, Sandground JH. The relative egg producing capacity of *Schistosoma Mansoni* and *Schistosoma Japonicum* 1, 2. *Am J Trop Med Hyg*. (1956) 5:831–40. doi: 10.4269/ajtmh.1956.5.831

Almadi MA, Aljebreen AM, Sanai FM, Marcus V, AlMeghaiseeb ES, Ghosh S. New insights into gastrointestinal and hepatic granulomatous disorders. *Nat Rev Gastroenterol Hepatol*. (2011) 8:455. doi: 10.1038/nrgastro.2011.115

Wilson MS, Mentink-Kane MM, Pesce JT, Ramalingam TR, Thompson R, Wynn TA. Immunopathology of schistosomiasis. *Immunol Cell Biol*. (2007) 85:148–54. doi: 10.1038/sj.icb.7100014

Ritter M, Gross O, Kays S, Ruland J, Nimmerjahn F, Saijo S, et al. *Schistosoma mansoni* triggers Dectin-2, which activates the Nlrp3 inflammasome and alters adaptive immune responses. *Proc Natl Acad Sci USA*. (2010) 107:20459–64. doi: 10.1073/pnas.1010337107

Broz P, Dixit VM. Inflammasomes: mechanism of assembly, regulation and signalling. *Nat Rev Immunol*. (2016) 16:407. doi: 10.1038/nri. 2016.58

Martinon F, Burns K, Tschopp J. The inflammasome: a molecular platform triggering activation of inflammatory caspases and processing of proIL-β. *Mol Cell*. (2002) 10:417–26. doi: 10.1016/s1097-2765(02)00599-3

Luan J, Ju D. Inflammasome: a double-edged sword in liver diseases. *Front Immunol*. (2018) 9:2201. doi: 10.3389/fimmu.2018.02201

Maltez VI, Tubbs AL, Cook KD, Aachoui Y, Falcone EL, Holland SM, et al. Inflammasomes coordinate pyroptosis and natural killer cell cytotoxicity to clear infection by a ubiquitous environmental bacterium. *Immunity*. (2015) 43:987–97. doi: 10.1016/j.immuni.2015.10.010

Zalinger ZB, Elliott R, Weiss SR. Role of the inflammasome-related cytokines Il-1 and Il-18 during infection with murine coronavirus. *J Neurovirol*. (2017) 23:845–54. doi: 10.1007/s13365-017-0574-4

Petrasek J, Bala S, Csak T, Lippai D, Kodys K, Menashy V, et al. IL-1 receptor antagonist ameliorates inflammasome-dependent alcoholic steatohepatitis in mice. *J Clin Invest*. (2012) 122:3476–89. doi: 10.1172/JCI60777

Wree A, McGeough MD, Peña CA, Schlattjan M, Li H, Inzaugarat ME, et al. NLRP3 inflammasome activation is required for fibrosis development in NAFLD. *J Mol Med (Berl)*. (2014) 92:1069–82. doi: 10.1007/s00109-014-1170- 1

Wu X, Dong L, Lin X, Li J. Relevance of the NLRP3 inflammasome in the pathogenesis of chronic liver disease. *Front Immunol*. (2017) 8:1728. doi: 10.3389/fimmu.2017.01728

Lu Y-Q, Zhong S, Meng N, Fan Y-P, Tang W-X. NLRP3 inflammasome activation results in liver inflammation and fibrosis in mice infected with *Schistosoma japonicum* in a Syk-dependent manner. *Sci Rep*. (2017) 7:8120. doi: 10.1038/s41598-017-08689-1

Chen H, Li Y, Gu J, Yin L, Bian F, Su L, et al. TLR4-MyD88 pathway promotes the imbalanced activation of NLRP3/NLRP6 via caspase-8 stimulation after lkali burn injury. *Exp Eye Res*. (2018) 176:59–68. doi: 10.1016/j.exer.2018.07. 001

Xiao J, Wang F, Liong EC, So K-F, Tipoe GL. *Lycium barbarum polysaccharides* improve hepatic injury through NFkappa-B and NLRP3/6 pathways in a methionine choline deficient diet steatohepatitis mouse model. *Int J Biol Macromol*. (2018) 120:1480–9. doi: 10.1016/j.ijbiomac.2018.09.151

Mehta R, Neupane A, Wang L, Goodman Z, Baranova A, Younossi ZM. Expression of NALPs in adipose and the fibrotic progression of non-alcoholic fatty liver disease in obese subjects. *BMC Gastroenterol*. (2014) 14:208. doi: 10.1186/s12876-014-0208-8

Zhu Y, Ni T, Deng W, Lin J, Zheng L, Zhang C, et al. Effects of NLRP6 on the proliferation and activation of human hepatic stellate cells. *Exp Cell Res*. (2018) 370:383–8. doi: 10.1016/j.yexcr.2018.06.040

Kayagaki N, Stowe IB, Lee BL, O'Rourke K, Anderson K, Warming S, et al.

Caspase-11 cleaves gasdermin D for non-canonical inflammasome signalling. *Nature*. (2015) 526:666. doi: 10.1038/nature15541

Lara-Tejero M, Sutterwala FS, Ogura Y, Grant EP, Bertin J, Coyle AJ, et al. Role of the caspase-1 inflammasome in *Salmonella typhimurium* pathogenesis. *J Exp Med*. (2006) 203:1407–12. doi: 10.1084/jem.20060206

Mayer-Barber KD, Barber DL, Shenderov K, White SD, Wilson MS, Cheever A, et al. Cutting edge: caspase-1 independent IL-1β production is critical for host resistance to *Mycobacterium tuberculosis* and does not require TLR signaling in vivo. *J Immunol*. (2010) 184:3326–30. doi: 10.4049/jimmunol.09 04189

Vandanmagsar B, Youm Y-H, Ravussin A, Galgani JE, Stadler K, Mynatt RL, et al. The NLRP3 inflammasome instigates obesity-induced inflammation and insulin resistance. *Nat Med*. (2011) 17:179. doi: 10.1038/nm.2279

Cançado GGL, Fiuza JA, de Paiva NCN, de Carvalho Dhom Lemos L, Ricci ND, Gazzinelli-Guimaraes PH, et al. Hookworm products ameliorate dextran sodium sulfate-induced colitis in BALB/c mice. *Inflamm Bowel Dis*. (2011) 17:2275–86. doi: 10.1002/ibd.21629

Kaisar MM, Ritter M, del Fresno C, Jónasdóttir HS, van der Ham AJ, Pelgrom LR, et al. Dectin-1/2–induced autocrine PGE2 signaling licenses dendritic cells to prime Th2 responses. *PLoS Biol*. (2018) 16:e2005504. doi: 10.1371/journal.pbio.2005504

Bruchard M, Rebé C, Derangère V, Togbé D, Ryffel B, Boidot R, et al. The receptor NLRP3 is a transcriptional regulator of T H 2 differentiation. *Nat Immunol*. (2015) 16:859. doi: 10.1038/ni.3202

Levy M, Shapiro H, Thaiss CA, Elinav E. NLRP6: a multifaceted innate immune sensor. *Trends Immunol*. (2017) 38:248–60. doi: 10.1016/j.it.2017.01. 001

Alegre F, Pelegrin P, Feldstein AE. Inflammasomes in liver fibrosis. *Semin Liver Dis*. (2017) 37:119–27. doi: 10.1055/s-0037-1601350

Szabo G, Csak T. Inflammasomes in liver diseases. *J Hepatol*. (2012) 57:642–54. doi: 10.1016/j.jhep.2012.03.035

Chen C-J, Kono H, Golenbock D, Reed G, Akira S, Rock KL. Identification of a key pathway required for the sterile inflammatory response triggered by dying cells. *Nat Med*. (2007) 13:851. doi: 10.1038/nm1603

Zhu P, Duan L, Chen J, Xiong A, Xu Q, Zhang H, et al. Gene silencing of NALP3 protects against liver ischemia–reperfusion injury in mice. *Hum Gene Ther*. (2010) 22:853–64. doi: 10.1089/hum.2010.145

Yang D, Postnikov YV, Li Y, Tewary P, de la Rosa G, Wei F, et al. High- mobility group nucleosome-binding protein 1 acts as an alarmin and is critical for lipopolysaccharide-induced immune responses. *J Exp Med*. (2012) 209:157–71. doi: 10.1084/jem.20101354

Miao EA, Rajan JV, Aderem A. Caspase−1−induced pyroptotic cell death. *Immunol Rev*. (2011) 243:206–14. doi: 10.1111/j.1600-065X.2011.01044.x

Franklin BS, Bossaller L, De Nardo D, Ratter JM, Stutz A, Engels G, et al. The adaptor ASC has extracellular and 'prionoid' activities that propagate inflammation. *Nat Immunol*. (2014) 15:727. doi: 10.1038/ni.2913

Reiter FP, Wimmer R, Wottke L, Artmann R, Nagel JM, Carranza MO, et al. Role of interleukin-1 and its antagonism of hepatic stellate cell proliferation and liver fibrosis in the Abcb4-/-mouse model. *World J Hepatol*. (2016) 8:401. doi: 10.4254/wjh.v8.i8.401

Tang N, Zhang Y-P, Ying W, Yao X-X. Interleukin-1β upregulates matrix metalloproteinase-13 gene expression via c-Jun N-terminal kinase and p38 MAPK pathways in rat hepatic stellate cells. *Mol Med Rep*. (2013) 8:1861–5. doi: 10.3892/mmr.2013.1719

Brunet LR, Finkelman FD, Cheever AW, Kopf MA, Pearce EJ. IL-4 protects against TNF-alpha-mediated cachexia and death during acute schistosomiasis. *J Immunol*. (1997) 159:777–85.

Hara H, Seregin SS, Yang D, Fukase K, Chamaillard M, Alnemri ES, et al. The NLRP6 inflammasome recognizes lipoteichoic acid and regulates gram-positive pathogen infection. *Cell*. (2018) 175:1651–1664.e14. doi: 10.1016/j.cell.2018.09.047

Shen C, Lu A, Xie WJ, Ruan J, Negro R, Egelman EH, et al. Molecular mechanism for NLRP6 inflammasome assembly and activation. *Proc Natl Acad Sci USA*. (2019) 116:2052–7. doi: 10.1073/pnas.1817221116

Meng N, Xia M, Lu YQ, Wang M, Boini KM, Li PL, et al. Activation of NLRP3 inflammasomes in mouse hepatic stellate cells during *Schistosoma J.* infection. *Oncotarget*. (2016) 7:39316–31. doi: 10.18632/oncotarget.10044

Burke ML, McManus DP, Ramm GA, Duke M, Li Y, Jones MK, et al. Temporal expression of chemokines dictates the hepatic inflammatory infiltrate in a murine model of schistosomiasis. *PLoS Negl Trop Dis*. (2010) 4:e598. doi: 10.1371/journal.pntd.0000598

Chuah C, Jones MK, Burke ML, McManus DP, Gobert GN. Cellular and chemokine-mediated regulation in schistosome-induced hepatic pathology. *Trends Parasitol*. (2014) 30:141–50. doi: 10.1016/j.pt.2013.12.009

Souza AL, Roffê E, Pinho V, Souza DG, Silva AF, Russo RC, et al. Potential role of the chemokine macrophage inflammatory protein 1α in human and experimental schistosomiasis. *Infect Immun*. (2005) 73:2515–23. doi: 10.1128/IAI.73.4.2515-2523.2005

Saiman Y, Friedman SL. The role of chemokines in acute liver injury. *Front Physiol*. (2012) 3:213. doi: 10.3389/fphys.2012.00213

Warmington KS, Boring L, Ruth JH, Sonstein J, Hogaboam CM, Curtis JL, et al. Effect of CC chemokine receptor 2 (CCR2) knockout on type-2 (schistosomal antigen-elicited) pulmonary granuloma formation: analysis of cellular recruitment and cytokine responses. *Am J Pathol*. (1999) 154:1407–16. doi: 10.1016/S0002-9440(10)65394-1

Dixon LJ, Flask CA, Papouchado BG, Feldstein AE, Nagy LE. Caspase-1 as a central regulator of high fat diet-induced non-alcoholic steatohepatitis. *PLoS One*. (2013) 8:e56100. doi: 10.1371/journal.pone.0056100

Kamari Y, Shaish A, Vax E, Shemesh S, Kandel-Kfir M, Arbel Y, et al. Lack of interleukin-1α or interleukin-1β inhibits transformation of steatosis to steatohepatitis and liver fibrosis in hypercholesterolemic mice. *J Hepatol*. (2011) 55:1086–94. doi: 10.1016/j.jhep.2011.01.048

Guo H, Xie M, Zhou C, Zheng M. The relevance of pyroptosis in the pathogenesis of liver diseases. *Life Sci*. (2019) 223:69–73. doi: 10.1016/j.lfs. 2019.02.060

Xu B, Jiang M, Chu Y, Wang W, Chen D, Li X, et al. Gasdermin D plays a key role as a pyroptosis executor of non-alcoholic steatohepatitis in humans and mice. *J Hepatol*. (2018) 68:773–82. doi: 10.1016/j.jhep.2017.11.040

Liu X, Zhang Y-R, Cai C, Ni X-Q, Zhu Q, Ren J-L, et al. Taurine alleviates *Schistosoma*-induced liver injury by inhibiting the TXNIP/NLRP3 inflammasome signal pathway and pyroptosis. *Infect Immun*. (2019) 87:12. doi: 10.1128/IAI.00732-19

Kong D-L, Kong F-Y, Liu X-Y, Yan C, Cui J, Tang R-X, et al. Soluble egg antigen of *Schistosoma japonicum* induces pyroptosis in hepatic stellate cells by modulating ROS production. *Parasit Vectors*. (2019) 12:1–12. doi: 10.1186/s13071-019-3729-8

14

Hepatoprotective Effect and Molecular Mechanisms of Hengshun Aromatic Vinegar on Non-Alcoholic Fatty Liver Disease

Shenghu Zhu[1†], Linshu Guan[2†], Xuemei Tan[2], Guoquan Li[1], Changjie Sun[2], Meng Gao[2], Bao Zhang[1]* and Lina Xu[2,3]*

[1]Jiangsu Hengshun Vinegar Industry Co., Ltd., Zhenjiang, China, [2]College of Pharmacy, Dalian Medical University, Dalian, China, [3]Key Laboratory for Basic and Applied Research on Pharmacodynamic Substances of Traditional Chinese Medicine of Liaoning Province, Dalian Medical University, Dalian, China

*Correspondence:
Bao Zhang
zhangbao_nng@163.com
Lina Xu
xulina627@163.com

†These authors have contributed equally to this work and share first authorship

Aromatic vinegar with abundant bioactive components can be used as a food additive to assist the treatment of various diseases. However, its effect on non-alcoholic fatty liver disease (NAFLD) is still unknown. The purpose of this study was to investigate the mechanism of Hengshun aromatic vinegar in preventing NAFLD in vivo and in vitro. Aromatic vinegar treatment was applied to rats fed with a high-fat diet (HFD) and HepG2 cells challenged with palmitic acid (PA). Our results showed that aromatic vinegar markedly improved cell viabilities and attenuated cell damage in vitro. The levels of TC, TG, FFA, AST, ALT, and malondialdehyde (MDA) in HFD-induced rats were significantly decreased by aromatic vinegar. Mechanism investigation revealed that aromatic vinegar markedly up-regulated the level of silent information regulator of transcription 1 (Sirt1), and thereby inhibited inflammation of the pathway through down-regulating the expressions of high mobility group box 1, toll-likereceptor-4, nuclear transcription factor-κB, tumor necrosis factor receptor-associated factor-6, and inflammatory factors. Aromatic vinegar simultaneously increased the expression of farnesoid X receptor and suppressed expressions of lipogenesis related proteins, including fatty acid synthase, acetyl-CoA carboxylase-1, sterol regulatory element binding transcription factor 1, and stearoyl-CoA desaturase-1. These results were further validated by knockdown of Sirt1 using siRNAs silencing in vitro. In conclusion, Hengshun aromatic vinegar showed protective effects against NAFLD by enhancing the activity of SIRT1 and thereby inhibiting lipogenesis and inflammation pathways, which is expected to become a new assistant strategy for NAFLD therapy in the future.

Keywords: non-alcoholic fatty liver disease, aromatic vinegar, inflammation, lipid metabolism, silent information regulator of transcription 1

INTRODUCTION

Non-alcoholic fatty liver disease (NAFLD) is a clinicopathological syndrome characterized by excessive fatty deposition of hepatocytes, excluding alcohol and other well-defined liver damage factors. It is strongly associated with dyslipidemia, obesity, hypertension, and insulin resistance (Dowman et al., 2011). NAFLD encompasses a series of pathological changes ranging from simple hepatic lipid accumulation (steatosis) to non-alcoholic steatohepatitis (NASH) accompanied by inflammation and varying degrees of fibrosis (Soares e Silva et al., 2015). What is more serious is that NAFLD may even develop into eventual cirrhosis, hepatocellular carcinoma, and death related to liver disease (Farrell and Larter, 2006). In 2016, the global prevalence of NAFLD was about 25%, with the highest rates in South America and the Middle East and the lowest in Africa (Younossi et al., 2016). Statistics showed an upward trend in global morbidity, with an estimated increase of 3.6 million cases per year. It is estimated that the overall prevalence of NAFLD among adults will reach 33.5% by 2030 (Estes et al., 2018). Therefore, NAFLD has become an increasingly serious public health problem due to its rising incidence whether in developed or semi-developed countries.

Due to the occult nature of the disease, the specific pathogenesis of NAFLD is still unclear, and it is believed that NAFLD is affected by a variety of factors. At present, the "two-hit" hypothesis on the pathogenesis of NAFLD has been widely summarized and provides a profound theoretical basis for a series of subsequent studies (Basaranoglu et al., 2013). In the development of NAFLD, the "first hit" refers primarily to the abnormal accumulation of triglyceride (TG) in hepatocytes which has been confirmed to be associated with excessive lipid intake and insulin resistance (IR) (Bugianesi et al., 2010). Based on the first attack, the accumulation of lipids in hepatocytes destroys the oxidative capacity of mitochondria, leading to an increase in the number of reactive oxygen species involved in the re-reaction. Under the combined action of multiple cytokines, such mitochondrial oxidative stress ultimately leads to the "second hit" of NAFLD. It may trigger inflammation, fibrosis, and even hepatocytes apoptosis, ultimately causing end-stage liver disease (Rolo et al., 2012; Xia et al., 2019). Accordingly, we conclude that targeting the regulation of blood lipids and inflammatory responses will play an important role in the treatment of NAFLD.

At present, there is no effective treatment method for NAFLD, and commonly accepted treatment strategies mainly include weight loss, dietary changes, and physical exercise. With the widespread prevalence of NAFLD, people pay more and more attention to dietary changes as a preventive measure and therapeutic strategy for the disease. Studies have shown that Patchouli alcohol, a kind of medicinal food in Asian countries, has a protective effect against NAFLD by altering the metabolism (Wu et al., 2019). Other studies have indicated that tomato juice intake reduces triglycerides and cholesterol levels in the liver and serum, as well as the degree of hepatic steatosis (García-Alonso et al., 2017). Therefore, consumption of tomato juice or its extracts can improve the metabolic patterns of NAFLD induced by a high-fat diet (HFD). In addition, spinach can alleviate HFD-induced obesity, through increasing the number of Lactobacillus counts, lowering fasting blood glucose and total LDL-cholesterol, and preventing excessive cholesterol accumulation in the liver (Elvira-Torales et al., 2019).

Vinegar is a kind of fermented acidic liquid food, which is used as a condiment in cuisine. Previous studies have indicated that vinegar supplementation has a positive effect on the prevention of cardiovascular diseases, ulcerative colitis (UC), the recurrence of kidney stones, and that it can regulate blood glucose and blood pressure (Jing et al., 2015; Shen et al., 2016; Zhu et al., 2019). Moreover, dietary vinegar plays a certain role in reducing body weight, visceral and subcutaneous fat, and regulating lipid metabolism, it also has functional properties including antibacterial effects, antioxidation, control of blood glucose, anticancer properties and so on (Kondo et al., 2009; Budak et al., 2014; Chen et al., 2016). A recent study demonstrated that synthetic acetic acid vinegar and Nipa vinegar had weight loss and anti-inflammatory effects on mice maintaining a HFD (Beh et al., 2017). However, the effect and molecular mechanism of aromatic vinegar on NAFLD remains unclear. Therefore, we conducted the following studies to investigate the hypolipidemic and hepatoprotective effects of Hengshun aromatic vinegar on NAFLD rats induced by a HFD and HepG2 cells induced by palmitic acid (PA) and elucidate the underlying molecular mechanism.

MATERIALS AND METHODS

Chemicals and Materials

Hengshun aromatic vinegar was obtained from Jiangsu Hengshun Vinegar Industry Co., Ltd. (Zhenjiang, China). Dulbecco's Modified Eagle's medium (DMEM) and fetal bovine serum (FBS) were purchased from Gibco (California, United States). Oil Red O staining kit, 3-(4,5-Dimethylthiazol-2-yl)-2,5-diphenyltetrazolium bromide (MTT), PA, and simvastatin were supplied by Solarbio Science and Technology Co., Ltd. (Beijing, China). Total cholesterol (TC), TG, alanine aminotransferase (ALT), aspartate amino-transferase (AST), free fatty acids (FFA), and malondialdehyde (MDA) detection kits were obtained from Nanjing Jiancheng Institute of Biotechnology (Nanjing, China). The tissue protein extraction kit was purchased from KEYGEN Biotech (Nanjing, China). Enhanced bicinchoninic acid (BCA) protein assay kit was purchased from Beyotime Institute of Biotechnology (Jiangsu, China). TransZolTM, TransScript All-in-One First-Strand cDNA Synthesis SuperMix for qPCR, TransStart Top Green qPCR SuperMix, protein marker, EasySee Western blot kit were purchased from TransGen Biotech (Beijing, China). silent information regulator of transcription 1 (Sirt1) SiRNA (Sequences, sense: 5'-GGAGAUGAUCAAGAGGCAATT-3', antisense: 5'-UUGCCUCUUGAUCAUCUCCTT-3') was designed and obtained from GenePharma Co., Ltd. (Shanghai, China). Lipofectamine2000 reagent was purchased from Thermo Fisher Scientific (Waltham, America).

Cell Culture

HepG2 cells were purchased from the Shanghai Institute of Biochemistry and Cell Biology (Shanghai, China) and cultured in DMEM medium supplemented with 10% FBS in a humidified environment containing 5% CO_2 and 95% O_2 at 37°C.

Cytotoxicity of Aromatic Vinegar

HepG2 cells were seeded into 96-well plates at a density of 5×10^4 cells/well overnight, and treated with various concentrations of aromatic vinegar (0.125, 0.25, 0.5, 1, 1.5, 2, 3, and 4%) for 12, 24 and 36 h, respectively, and then the toxicity of the compound was assayed through the MTT method. A total of 10 μl MTT solution (5 mg/ml) was added to each well and incubated for 4 h, and then the formazan crystals were dissolved by 150 μl of DMSO. The absorbance of the specimen was quantified at 490 nm by a microplate reader (Thermo Fisher Scientific, MA, United States), and cell viabilities were calculated.

Palmitic Acid Induced Injury in HepG2 Cells

A series of working dilutions of PA were prepared in a serum-free DMEM medium. HepG2 cells were seeded into 96-well plates at a density of 5×10^4 cells/well overnight, and then treated with various concentrations (0.1, 0.2, 0.3, 0.4, 0.5, 0.6, 0.8 and 1.0 mmol/L) of PA for 12, 24 and 36 h. Cell viabilities were detected using the MTT method as described above and a suitable concentration of PA (0.3 mmol/L) was optimized.

HepG2 cells (5×10^4 cells/well) were seeded into 96-well plates and incubated overnight. The cells in treatment groups were pretreated with aromatic vinegar at concentrations of 0.5, 1, and 1.5% for 24 h, and then treated with 0.3 mmol/L of PA for 24 h. Cells in the control group were cultured in serum-free DMEM medium under normal conditions for 48 h, and those for the model group were treated with 0.3 mmol/l of PA for 24 h. Finally, the viability of cell was determined with the MTT method as described above.

Animals and Treatment

Seventy male Sprague-Dawley (SD) rats, weighing 180–220 g, were obtained from Liaoning Changsheng Biotechnology (SYXK (Liao) 2018-0007). The rats were kept under the controlled condition with constant temperature (23 ± 2°C), relative humidity (55% ± 5%), a 12 h light/dark cycle, and free access to water and food.

After 1 week of acclimatization, the rats were randomly divided into seven groups (n = 10), including the control group, the aromatic vinegar control group, the model group, the aromatic vinegar-treated groups (2.50, 1.25, 0.83 ml/kg aromatic vinegar), and the positive control group (4 mg/kg simvastatin). Normal saline was intragastrically administrated to the rats in the control and model group, and Hengshun aromatic vinegar and simvastatin were given to the treated animals once daily for 9 weeks. During this period, rats in the control and aromatic vinegar control group were fed a normal chow diet, while rats in other groups were fed a (HFD, consisting of 10% fat, 20% sucrose, 2.5% cholesterol, 1% cholate, 1% egg, 30% bean sprout and 35.5% chow diet) (Qin et al., 2018; Tang et al., 2018). Finally, the animals were sacrificed after an overnight fast, and serum samples were extracted from blood samples, centrifuged (3,500 rpm, 4°C) for 10 min and stored at −20°C until detection. The liver tissues were rapidly collected and stored at −80°C for other assays.

Biochemical Assay

The levels of AST, ALT, TC, TG, and FFA in serum, and MDA in the liver tissue were determined using the detection kits based on the manufacturer's instructions.

H&E and Oil Red O Staining

In vivo experiments, liver tissues were fixed in 10% polyoxymethylene solution, processed by standard histological procedures, and ultimately embedded in paraffin wax. Then, the tissues were sectioned into 5-μm slices, which were stained with H&E. To evaluate lipid droplets in the liver, the frozen liver sections were stained with Oil Red O. In vitro experiments, HepG2 cells were treated with vinegar for 24 h and then the PA model was established for 24 h. After washing with PBS for 3 times, the cells were fixed with 10% paraformaldehyde solution for 30 min, and then stained with Oil Red O for 30 min finally washed with 60% isopropanol and PBS in sequence. Eventually, images of the stained sections and cells were obtained using a light microscope (NIKON, Tokyo, Japan).

Immunofluorescence Assay

The paraffin sections of the liver were dewaxed twice with xylene for 15 min each time and rehydrated with different concentrations of alcohol (100, 90, 80, 70, and 60%) for 5 min. We then treated them with citrate buffer (pH = 6.0) in boiling water for 15 min for thermal repair. The deparaffinized liver tissue sections were incubated with rabbit anti-Sirt1, anti-farnesoid X receptor (FXR), or anti-high mobility group box 1 (HMGB1) (1:70, dilution) antibodies in a humidified box at 4°C overnight. After washing with PBS three times, the sections were incubated with a fluorescein-labeled secondary antibody for 1 h at 37°C. Eventually, the immunostained samples were imaged by fluorescence microscopy (Olympus, Tokyo, Japan).

Real-Time PCR Assay

Total RNA samples were obtained from HepG2 cells and liver tissues using RNAiso Plus reagent following the manufacturer's protocol. After purity determination, cDNA was synthesized using a PrimeScript® RT reagent Kit with a TC-512 PCR system (TECHNE, United Kingdom). The levels of mRNA were performed by using real-time PCR with SYBR® PremixEx Taq TM II (Tli RNaseH Plus) in an ABI 7500 Real Time PCR System (Applied Biosystems, United States). The forward (F) and reverse (R) primers for the tested genes are listed in **Table 1**. Among the data from each sample, the Ct value of the target genes was normalized to that of GAPDH. The relative quantification of mRNAs was calculated using the $2^{-\triangle\triangle Ct}$ method.

Western Blotting Assay

Total protein samples from the liver tissues of rats and cells were extracted using a protein extraction kit and the protein content was determined by BCA Kit. Then, the proteins were loaded onto the SDS-PAGE gel (8–12%), separated electrophoretically, and transferred to PVDF membranes (Millipore, Massachusetts, United States). After being blocked with 5% dried skim milk for 3 h, the membranes were incubated with appropriate primary antibodies overnight at 4°C. The blots were then incubated with the goat anti-rabbit IgG-horseradish peroxidase-conjugated secondary antibody for 3 h. Protein expressions were detected by the enhanced chemiluminescence (ECL) method and the images were obtained by Bio-Spectrum Gel Imaging System (UVP, Upland, CA, United States). The intensity values of the

TABLE 1 | The primer sequences used for real-time PCR assay.

Genes	Forward primer (5'-3')	Reverse primer (5'-3')
Rats GAPDH	GGCACAGTCAAGGCTGAGAATG	ATGGTGGTGAAGACGCCAGTA
IL-1β	CCCTGAACTCAACTGTGAAATAGCA	CCCAAGTCAAGGGCTTGGAA
IL-6	ATTGTATGAACAGCGATGATGCAC	CCAGGTAGAAACGGAACTCCAGA
TNF-α	TCAGTTCCATGGCCCAGAC	GTTGTCTTTGAGATCCATGCCATT
Human GAPDH	GCACCGTCAAGGCTGAGAAC	TGGTGAAGACGCCAGTGGA
IL-1β	CTGAGCACCTTCTTTCCCTTCA	TGGACCAGACATCACCAAGCT
IL-6	TGGCTGAAAAAGATGGATGCT	TCTGCACAGCTCTGGCTTGT
TNF-α	TGTAGCCCATGTTGTAGCAAACC	GAGGACCTGGGAGTAGATGAGGTA

TNF-α, tumor necrosis factor-α; IL-1β, interleukin-1β; IL-6, interleukin-6.

relative protein levels were normalized with GAPDH as an internal control.

Silent Information Regulator of Transcription 1 siRNA Treatment

HepG2 cells were cultured for approximately 24 h to 70–80% confluence in six-well plates. The cells were then transfected with Sirt1-targeted siRNA or empty vector plasmid (negative control, NC) using lipofectamine2000 reagent according to the manufacturer's protocol. After transfection for 6 h, the medium was replaced with a complete medium. When the cells reached the appropriate density, they were exposed to aromatic vinegar (1.5%) for 24 h and treated with PA (0.3 mmol/l) for an additional 24 h. Then, the cells were collected for further experiments.

Statistical Analysis

All data were expressed as the mean ± SD. Statistical analysis was performed using GraphPad Prism 5.0 software (San Diego, CA, United States). Significant differences among multiple groups were analyzed by a one-way ANOVA test followed by the Newman-Keuls test when comparing multiple independent groups. An unpaired t-test was carried out in the comparison two different groups. The results were considered to be statistically significant at $p < 0.05$. The data and statistical analysis were in accordance with standard recommendations for pharmacological experiment design and analysis.

RESULTS

Aromatic Vinegar Attenuates Palmitic Acid-Induced Damage in HepG2 Cells

The results indicate that when the concentration of aromatic vinegar was higher than 1.5%, aromatic vinegar induced cell damage in HepG2 cells (**Figure 1A**). When the concentration of aromatic vinegar was less than 1.5%, the viability of HepG2 cells has no significant difference compared with the control group, indicating that aromatic vinegar was safe for HepG2 cells under the treatment conditions. Therefore, aromatic vinegar at

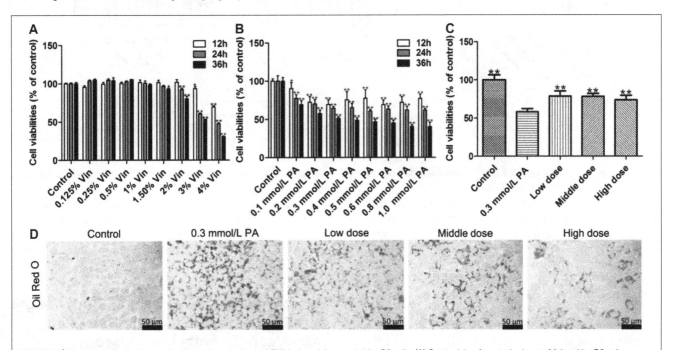

FIGURE 1 | Protective effects of aromatic vinegar on palmitic acid (PA)-induced damage in HepG2 cells. **(A)** Cytotoxicity of aromatic vinegar (Vin) on HepG2 cells; **(B)** Effects of PA on cell viability; **(C)** Effects of aromatic vinegar attenuated on PA-induced cell damage; **(D)** Effects of aromatic vinegar on Oil Red O staining in HepG2 cells (×400 magnification; Scale bar = 50 µm). Values are expressed as the mean ± SD (n = 5). *p < 0.05, **p < 0.01 compared with model groups.

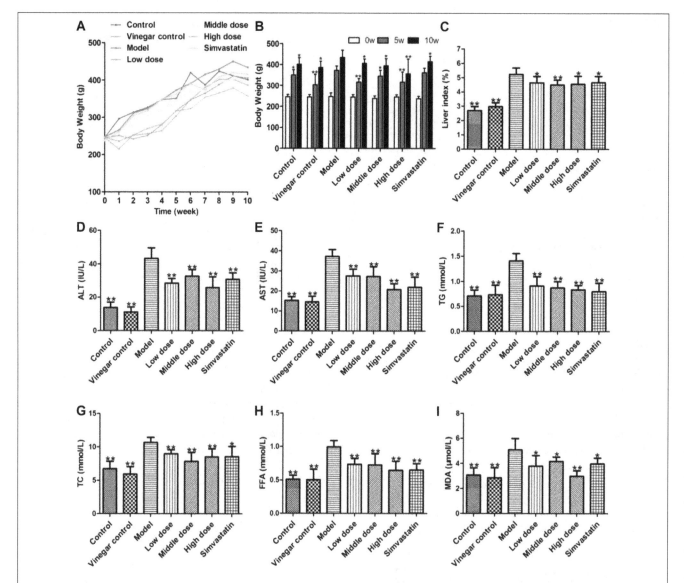

FIGURE 2 | Effects of aromatic vinegar on biochemical indexes of rats. **(A,B)** Effect of aromatic vinegar on body weight **(C)** Effects of aromatic vinegar on the ratio of liver to body weight (%); **(D–I)** Effects of aromatic vinegar on the levels of alanine transaminase (ALT), aspartate transaminase (AST), TG, total cholesterol (TC), and free fatty acid (FFA) in serum and malondialdehyde (MDA) in liver tissue. Values are expressed as the mean ± SD (n = 8). *$p < 0.05$, **$p < 0.01$ compared with model groups.

concentrations of 0.5, 1, and 1.5% for 24 h were selected to protect HepG2 cells against PA-induced injury.

According to the results, the suitable concentration and treatment time of PA *in vitro* experiments were optimized. As shown in **Figure 1B**, compared with control groups, the viability rates of HepG2 cells were significantly decreased by 0.1–1.0 mmol/L PA treatment, which was decreased to 64.31% by 0.3 mmol/L of PA treatment for 24 h. Therefore, HepG2 cells were treated with 0.3 mmol/L PA for 24 h to establish the injury model.

In treatment groups, HepG2 cells were pretreated with aromatic vinegar at the concentrations of 0.5, 1, and 1.5% for 24 h, and then treated with 0.3 mmol/L of PA for 24 h. Subsequently, the results showed that aromatic vinegar pretreatment can significantly reverse the PA-induced cell

damage and has an obvious protective effect on cells in a dose-dependent manner (**Figure 1C**).

As shown in **Figure 1D**, Oil Red O staining indicated that a large number of lipid droplet accumulations were observed in HepG2 cells after PA modeling, while aromatic vinegar treatment groups improved PA-induced lipid droplet accumulation compared with the model group.

Effects of Aromatic Vinegar on Body Weight and Biochemical Indexes in Rats With Non-Alcoholic Fatty Liver Disease

The body weights of each group of rats were measured weekly. As shown in **Figures 2A,B**, the body weight of rats increased in each group after 10 weeks of feeding, while it was significantly

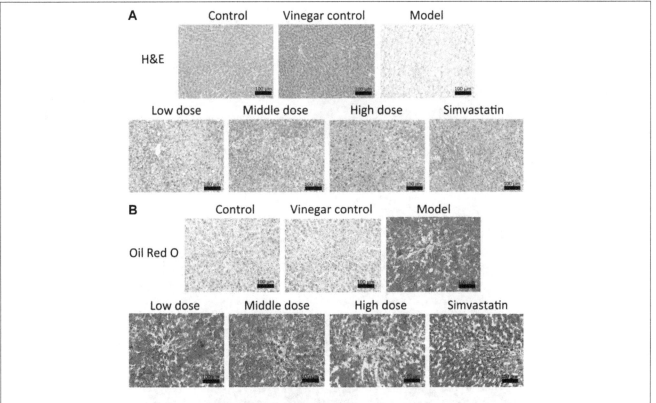

FIGURE 3 | Effects of aromatic vinegar against non-alcoholic fatty liver disease in rats based on staining. **(A)** Effects of aromatic vinegar on HE staining images of liver tissues in rats (×200 magnification); **(B)** Effects of aromatic vinegar on Oil Red O staining images of liver tissues in rats (×200 magnification). Scale bar = 100 μm. Values are expressed as the mean ± SD. *p < 0.05, **p < 0.01 compared with model groups.

improved in the aromatic vinegar and simvastatin administration groups compared with that of the model group. Similarly, the ratios of liver to body weight in aromatic vinegar groups and the simvastatin group were dramatically decreased compared with the model group (**Figure 2C**).

AST and ALT are specific aminotransferases in the liver, and their levels increase when the liver is damaged. As shown in **Figures 2D,E**, the levels of serum ALT and AST were significantly increased in the model group, while aromatic vinegar and simvastatin could markedly reduce these levels. Therefore, we concluded that feeding a HFD can cause liver damage in rats, while aromatic vinegar or simvastatin treatment can ameliorate liver damage. Similar results were shown in **Figures 2F,G,H**, the TG, TC, and FFA levels significantly increased in rats fed a HFD compared with the control group, while those were significantly reduced in aromatic vinegar groups. Moreover, as shown in **Figure 2I**, aromatic vinegar significantly reduced the MDA level in liver tissue compared with the model group. These data indicated that aromatic vinegar can ameliorate obesity and dyslipidaemia induced by a HFD, and significantly alleviate NAFLD via suppressing oxidative stress.

Effect of Aromatic Vinegar on Liver Pathology

H&E staining showed that livers had an intact lobular architecture with a clear central vein and radiation line, and

the cell cord is arranged neatly in the control group and vinegar control group. A large number of fat vacuoles and inflammatory cell infiltration appeared in the liver tissues of the model group, while aromatic vinegar and simvastatin administration significantly improved this condition (**Figure 3A**). In addition, compared with the control group, lipid droplets increased significantly in the HFD induced model, while administration groups significantly improved lipid accumulation in a dose-dependent way (**Figure 3B**). Oil Red O staining further showed that aromatic vinegar could inhibit excessive lipid accumulation in the liver. These data indicated that aromatic vinegar had a good effect on protecting the liver and reducing lipid.

Aromatic Vinegar Activates Silent Information Regulator of Transcription 1 Pathway to Regulate Hepatic Lipid Synthesis and Inflammation *In Vitro* and *In Vivo*

As shown in **Figures 4A,B**, the expression levels of SIRT1, FXR and HMGB1 in HepG2 cells and the liver tissues of rats were assessed by western blotting assay. The results indicated that the expression levels of SIRT1 and FXR were significantly down-regulated, and the level of HMGB1 was markedly up-regulated compared with control groups in vitro and in vivo. However,

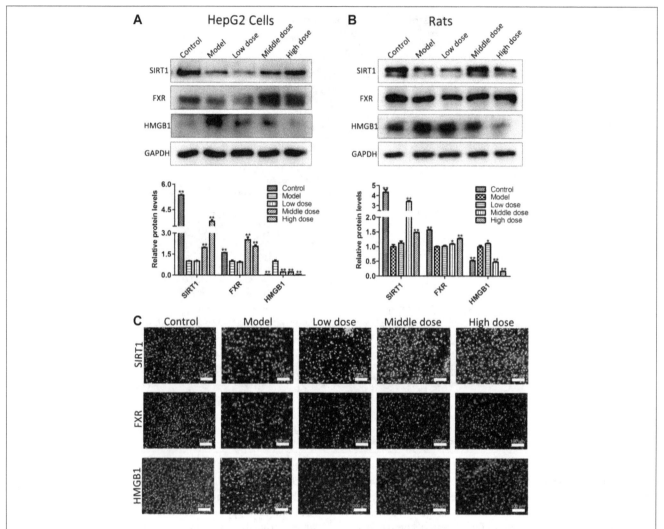

FIGURE 4 | Aromatic vinegar activates the silent information regulator of transcription 1 pathway *in vitro* and *in vivo*. **(A)** Effects of aromatic vinegar on the expression levels of SIRT1, farnesoid X receptor (FXR) and high mobility group box 1 (HMGB1) *in vitro*; **(B)** Effects of aromatic vinegar on the expression levels of SIRT1, FXR and HMGB1 *in vivo*; **(C)** Effects of aromatic vinegar on SIRT1, FXR and HMGB1 levels based on immunofluorescence staining *in vivo* (×200 magnification). Scale bar = 100 μm. Values are expressed as the mean ± SD (n = 3). *$p < 0.05$, **$p < 0.01$ compared with model groups.

compared with model groups, aromatic vinegar significantly increased the expression levels of SIRT1 and FXR, and decreased the levels of HMGB1.

As shown in **Figure 4C**, the results indicate that the levels of SIRT1 and FXR-positive cells were substantially increased, and HMGB1-positive areas were obviously decreased in liver tissues by aromatic vinegar compared with the control groups based on immunofluorescence assays. These results indicated that aromatic vinegar activated the SIRT1 pathway, and then affected the expression levels of FXR and HMGB1.

Aromatic Vinegar Ameliorates Lipid Metabolism *In Vitro* and *In Vivo*

The results in **Figure 5** show that aromatic vinegar markedly down-regulated the expression levels of proteins and genes associated with lipogenesis compared with the model groups

in vitro and *in vivo*, including sterol regulatory element binding transcription factor 1 (SREBP1), fatty acid synthase (FASN), acetyl-CoA carboxylase-1 (ACC1) and stearoyl-CoA desaturase-1 (SCD1). The data indicated that aromatic vinegar could play an anti-NAFLD role by regulating lipid metabolism related proteins.

Aromatic Vinegar Attenuates Inflammation *In Vitro* and *In Vivo*

As shown in **Figures 6A,B**, compared with control groups, the protein levels of toll-like receptor-4 (TLR4), nuclear transcription factor-κB (NF-κB) and tumor necrosis factor receptor-associated factor-6 (TRAF6) were all significantly increased, while the expression of which was significantly reversed by administrating aromatic vinegar *in vitro* and *in vivo*. As shown in **Figures 6C,D**, *in vitro* and *in vivo*, increased mRNA

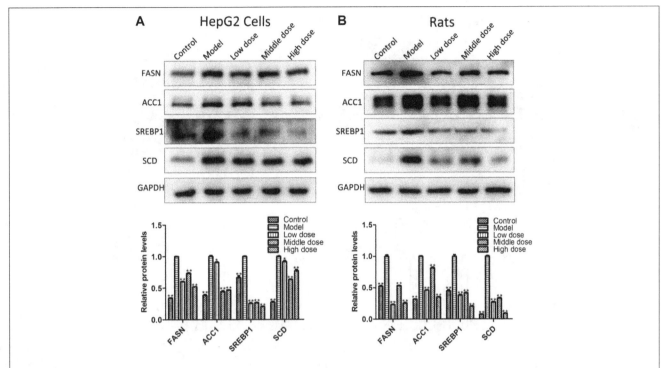

FIGURE 5 | Effect of aromatic vinegar on the levels of some proteins related to lipid metabolism. **(A)** Effects of aromatic vinegar on the protein levels of fatty acid synthase (FASN), acetyl-CoA carboxylase-1 (ACC1), sterol regulatory element binding transcription factor 1 (SREBP1) and stearoyl-CoA desaturase-1 (SCD) *in vitro*; **(B)** Effects of aromatic vinegar on the protein levels of FASN, ACC1, SREBP1 and SCD *in vivo*. Values are expressed as the mean ± SD (n = 3). *$p < 0.05$, **$p < 0.01$ compared with model groups.

levels of tumor necrosis factor-α (TNF-α), interleukin-1β (IL-1β) and interleukin-6 (IL-6) were observed in the model groups, which were markedly decreased by aromatic vinegar. These results indicated that aromatic vinegar delayed NAFLD through ameliorating inflammation.

Effect of Aromatic Vinegar on Lipid Metabolism and Inflammation After Transfecting Silent Information Regulator of Transcription 1 SiRNA *In Vitro*

To further determine the effect of aromatic vinegar on SIRT1 pathway, HepG2 cells were transfected with SIRT1 siRNA and pretreated with aromatic vinegar for 24 h before other tests. As shown in **Figure 7A**, transfecting SIRT1 siRNA aggravated PA-induced injury compared with the group transfected with negtive control siRNA. In addition, the protein levels of SIRT1 and FXR were markedly increased, and HMGB1 was markedly decreased in aromatic vinegar-treated groups after transfection. Obviously, SIRT1 siRNA reduced the protective effect of aromatic vinegar on PA-induced injury. What's more, SIRT1 siRNA blocked the effects of aromatic vinegar on the mRNA levels of IL-1β, IL-6 and TNF-α (**Figure 7B**). Based on the Oil Red O staining shown in **Figure 7C**, aromatic vinegar treatment groups obviously improved PA-induced lipid droplet accumulation with or without SIRT1 siRNA. These results further strongly demonstrated that the regulatory effect of aromatic vinegar on lipid metabolism and inflammation was achieved through

regulation of the SIRT1/FXR and SIRT1/HMGB1 signal pathways.

DISCUSSION

NAFLD is a type of acquired metabolic stress liver injury, which is closely related to insulin resistance and genetic susceptibility (Cheung and Sanyal, 2010). With the epidemic trend of obesity caused by unhealthy diet, the prevalence of NAFLD are rising worldwide, and NAFLD has become the main cause of chronic liver disease in developed countries (Safari and Gérard, 2019; Stefan et al., 2019). NAFLD is a major global health issue that deserves close attention. The pathogenesis of NAFLD is a complex process, in which the occurrence of hepatic lipotoxicity may further lead to mitochondrial dysfunction, thereby activating inflammatory responses (Zhang et al., 2018). The liver provides a central store for excessive lipid accumulation (Chung et al., 2017). NAFLD is characterized primarily by fatty deposition of hepatocytes, which accounts for more than 5% of the liver weight (Gong et al., 2017). As is known to all, Hengshun aromatic vinegar is one of the most famous traditional fermented vinegars in China, and is generally produced from glutinous rice, wheat bran, and rice hulls through a unique solid layered fermentation process (Xu et al., 2011a). It has the characteristics of "color, fragrance, acid, alcohol, thick," and has a strong taste that is sour and not astringent, fragrant and slightly sweet, colory and strong taste. Although there is no

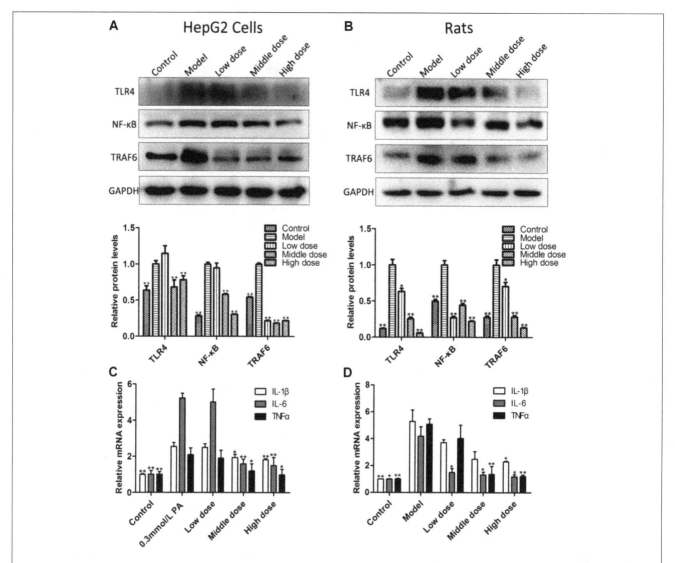

FIGURE 6 | Effect of aromatic vinegar on the levels of some proteins related to inflammation and inflammatory mediators. **(A)** Effects of aromatic vinegar on the protein levels of toll-likereceptor-4 (TLR4), nuclear transcription factor-κB (NF-κB) and tumor necrosis factor receptor-associated factor-6 (TRAF6) *in vitro*; **(B)** Effects of aromatic vinegar on the protein levels of TLR4, NF-κB and TRAF6 *in vivo*; **(C)** Effects of aromatic vinegar on the mRNA levels of tumor necrosis factor-α (TNF-α), interleukin-1β (IL-1β) and interleukin-6 (IL-6) *in vitro*; **(D)** Effects of aromatic vinegar on the mRNA levels of TNF-α, IL-1β and IL-6 *in vivo*. Values are expressed as the mean ± SD (n = 3). *$p < 0.05$, **$p < 0.01$ compared with model groups.

accurate formulation for aromatic vinegar, it has a hundred years of mature, reliable production technology and quality control. What's more, Chinese literature has found that Hengshun aromatic vinegar contains 88.09% water and volatile matter and 11.91% solid matter (w/v), and is rich in organic acids, sugar, protein, amino acids and other aromatic ingredients, which largely affect its taste characteristics and organoleptic quality (Zhao et al., 2018). The effective components in it are relatively abundant and stable through the fingerprint analysis and amino acid analysis. During the brewing process, aromatic vinegar produces many bioactive compounds, such as organic acids, amino acids and phenolic compounds, which play important roles in antioxidant activities (Zhang et al., 2019). In addition, polyphenols, flavonoids, and melanoidins were found in

Hengshun aromatic vinegar, which play crucial roles in diseases prevention and contribute benefits to human health (Zhao et al., 2018; Duan et al., 2019). Studies have also showed that the alkylpyrazine named ligustrazine was found as a bioactive compound in Hengshun aromatic vinegar, which has the health effects such as reducing blood pressure, promoting blood circulation and removing stasis, improving coronary heart disease, thrombolytic therapy and liver protection (Xu et al., 2011b; Chen et al., 2019). In the present study, PA-induced HepG2 cells and HFD-induced SD rats were used as NAFLD models *in vitro* and *in vivo* to investigate the pharmacodynamic actions and molecular mechanism of Hengshun aromatic vinegar. Aromatic vinegar showed significant effects against NAFLD due to the evidences with

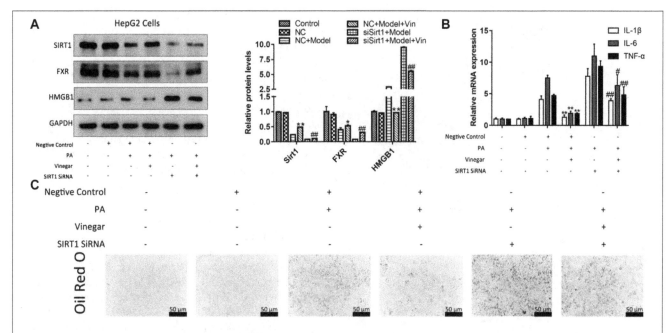

FIGURE 7 | Effffect of aromatic vinegar on silent information regulator of transcription 1 (SIRT1)/FXR and SIRT1/high mobility group box 1 (HMGB1) pathway in HepG2 cells transfected with SIRT1 siRNA. **(A)** The protein levels of SIRT1, FXR and HMGB1; **(B)** The mRNA levels of interleukin-1β (IL-1β), interleukin-6 (IL-6) and TNF-α; **(C)** Oil Red O staining (×400 magnification; Scale bar = 50 μm). Values are expressed as the mean ± SD (n = 3). *$p < 0.05$, **$p < 0.01$ compared with model group transfected with negtive control siRNA (NC + Model); #$p < 0.05$, #$p < 0.01$ compared with model group transfected with SIRT1 siRNA (siSirt1 + Model).

the decreased levels of AST, ALT, TC, TG, FFA and MDA, and the alleviation of histopathological changes.

SIRT1, a nonamide adenine dinucleotide (NAD⁺)-dependent protein deacetylase, acts as an important modulator of metabolic pathways and plays a critical role in the pathophysiology of many metabolic diseases. It's a member of silent information regulator 2 family, which are a group of proteins with either histone deacetylase or mono-ADP-ribosyltransferase activity (Colak et al., 2011). In recent years, studies have shown that SIRT1 with an extensive spectrum of biological functions plays an important role in the regulation related to metabolism, cell survival and apoptosis (Silva and Wahlestedt, 2010). In addition, it has been found that the pathophysiological mechanism of NAFLD may be affected by the activation of SIRT1 (Colak et al., 2014). Studies have shown that dioscin regulated lipid metabolism through SIRT1/AMPK signal pathway and significantly prevented NAFLD (Yao et al., 2018). Similarly, it has also been reported that celastrol ameliorated NAFLD by SIRT1 pathway, which had an important role in improving liver metabolic injury induced by HFD (Zhang et al., 2016). In this study, we did find the result that the expression of SIRT1 was down-regulated in model group, which was consistent with SIRT1 expression in other studies. Moreover, our SIRT1 siRNA experimental results proved that the main target of aromatic vinegar was SIRT1. It attenuated NAFLD by activating the SIRT1 pathway to regulate liver lipid metabolism and inflammation *in vitro* and *in vivo*.

As a key regulator of hepatic metabolic homeostasis, hepatic SIRT1 acts as an endogenous activator of its downstream protein FXR in hepatocytes (Yang et al., 2017). FXR, a member of the nuclear receptor super family of ligand-activated transcription factors, has recently been demonstrated to play a key role in the molecular mechanism of regulating lipid glucose homeostasis (Nie et al., 2017). At the same time, FXR is the primary nuclear receptor for bile acids and plays an important role in bile acid homeostasis (Yang et al., 2017). In addition, FXR is a crucial target protein downstream of SIRT1, which plays a connecting role after being regulated by SIRT1. Generally speaking, hepatic FXR regulates lipid homeostasis through a variety of mechanisms, including reducing fatty acid synthesis, decreasing fatty acid uptake, and increasing β-oxidation (Cave et al., 2016). Celastrol has a protective effect on cholestatic liver injury by regulating SIRT1/FXR pathway (Zhao et al., 2019). Other research revealed that imperatorin exerts the protective effect against hepatotoxicity induced by excessive acetaminophen similarly by stimulating the SIRT1/FXR pathway (Gao et al., 2020). Moreover, studies have showed that NAFLD may be mitigated through the regulation of SIRT1/FXR signaling pathway (Han et al., 2019). Through the activation of FXR, a major adipogenic regulator called SREBP1 will be regulated and further reduced the protein levels of FASN, ACC1 and SCD in its downstream which are related to lipogenesis (Dong et al., 2019). Consistent with other research results, we found that FXR regulated by SIRT1 activates downstream protein SREBP1, which affects the protein levels of FASN, ACC1 and SCD, thereby reducing adipogenesis (**Figure 8**). Our results indicated that aromatic vinegar could alleviate NAFLD by reducing lipogenesis through SIRT1/FXR signaling pathway. What's more, the SIRT1 siRNA experimental results also confirmed this conclusion.

It has been confirmed that SIRT1 not only regulates FXR, but also activates HMGB1, a key inflammatory mediator in the inflammatory

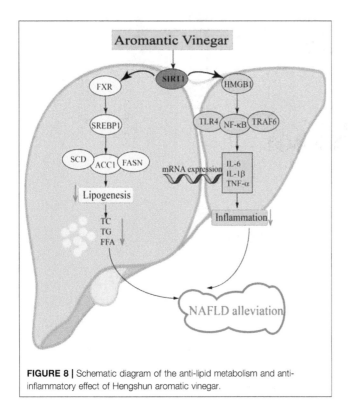

FIGURE 8 | Schematic diagram of the anti-lipid metabolism and anti-inflammatory effect of Hengshun aromatic vinegar.

signaling pathway (Qi et al., 2017). Recent study has demonstrated that SIRT1 is a key factor in the negative regulation of HMGB1, whose release is regulated by SIRT1 acetylation mediated direct interaction (Hwang et al., 2015). It has been reported that SIRT1 induces HMGB1 expression, thereby modulating ovarian cancer behaviors (Jiang et al., 2018). Le K et al. have demonstrated that resveratrol plays a neuroprotective role in neonatal hypoxic-ischemic brain injury by activating SIRT1 to inhibit HMGB1 signaling (Le et al., 2019). Moreover, The SIRT1/HMGB1 pathway has been proved to be an important target for inhibiting of NAFLD inflammation (Zeng et al., 2015). HMGB1, ubiquitously and highly expressed in hepatocytes, is a critical chromosomal non-histone protein that can regulate DNA structure. As we all know, it plays a pivotal role in the initiation and maintenance inflammation responses, which is a key process that takes place in ordinary liver diseases such as NAFLD (Khambu et al., 2019). The inflammation responses during NAFLD may be the result of stress, damage and cell death of hepatocytes caused by lipid, and such lipotoxicity further leads to the release of HMGB1 (Ibrahim et al., 2018). The downstream inflammation-related proteins such as TLR4, TRAF6 and NF-κB are activated due to the release of HMGB1 (Li et al., 2011; Lan et al., 2017). Researches have shown that liver inflammation is caused by pro-inflammatory cytokines and chemokines generated by adipocytes, lipid-laden hepatocytes and hepatic macrophages (Manne et al., 2018). NF-κB, activated by HMGB1, acts as a major transcriptional regulator regulating inflammation and cell death during the development of NAFLD (Jiang et al., 2019). After NF-κB activation, it is transferred from the cytoplasm to the nucleus, releasing a great deal of inflammatory factors. The alteration of NF-κB activity can affect the expression of hepatic pro-inflammatory

cytokines, such as IL-1β, IL-6 and TNF-α, and the excessive production of which may lead to inflammatory reaction (Gäbele et al., 2009). In the present study, we obtained the following results that SIRT1 induced the release of HMGB1, which regulated the downstream inflammation-related proteins TLR4, TRAF6, and NF-κB. After activation, NF-κB released a large number of inflammatory factors including IL-1β, IL-6, and TNF-α (**Figure 8**). These results supported the view that aromatic vinegar played a critical role in relieving NAFLD by regulating inflammation through SIRT1/HMGB1 signaling pathway. In addition, the experimental results of SIRT1 siRNA also confirmed this conclusion.

There are some shortages in the current study. The anti-NAFLD effects of aromatic vinegar were evaluated only in cell and rats model, which needs to be further evaluated in clinical studies. It has been reported in Chinese journal that Hengshun aromatic vinegar concentrate, extract and its different molecular weight components could inhibit the oxidative modification of human low density lipoprotein. It provids the possibility for the clinical application of aromatic vinegar in treating NAFLD combined with our findings in this study. As flavoring, aromatic vinegar is difficult to be developed into a medicine for the treatment of diseases. Previous studies have suggested that osteoporosis was alleviated in rats by consumption of aromatic vinegar alone or in combination with calcium salt (Yu et al., 2020). Consequently, it will be a direction in the future that aromatic vinegar could be developed as a clinical adjunctive therapy to alleviate NAFLD and further studies could investigate the combination effect of Hengshun aromatic vinegar with other medicines.

CONCLUSION

Our study demonstrated that Hengshun aromatic vinegar showed valid effects against NAFLD via regulating lipid metabolism and inflammation by targeting SIRT1. This study provided new evidence for the recommendation that Hengshun aromatic vinegar can be used as an adjuvant strategy for the therapy and health care of NAFLD.

ETHICS STATEMENT

The animal study was reviewed and approved by Animal Research Committee of Dalian Medical University.

AUTHOR CONTRIBUTIONS

Data curation, LX; Funding acquisition, GL; Methodology, SZ and LG; Project administration and resources, BZ; Software, MG; Validation, LG, XT, and CS; Writing – original draft, LG and LX; Writing – review and editing, LX. SZ and LG contributed same work to this paper and they are the co-first authors.

REFERENCES

Basaranoglu, M., Basaranoglu, G., and Sentürk, H. (2013). From fatty liver to fibrosis: a tale of "second hit". World J. Gastroenterol 19, 1158–1165. doi:10.3748/wjg.v19.i8.1158

Beh, B. K., Mohamad, N. E., Yeap, S. K., Ky, H., Boo, S. Y., Chua, J. Y. H., et al. (2017). Anti-obesity and anti-inflammatory effects of synthetic acetic acid vinegar and Nipa vinegar on high-fat-diet-induced obese mice. Sci. Rep. 7, 6664. doi:10.1038/s41598-017-06235-7

Budak, N. H., Aykin, E., Seydim, A. C., Greene, A. K., and Guzel-Seydim, Z. B. (2014). Functional properties of vinegar. J. Food Sci. 79, R757–R764. doi:10.1111/1750-3841.12434

Bugianesi, E., Moscatiello, S., Ciaravella, M. F., and Marchesini, G. (2010). Insulin resistance in nonalcoholic fatty liver disease. Curr. Pharm. Des. 16, 1941–1951. doi:10.2174/138161210791208875

Cave, M. C., Clair, H. B., Hardesty, J. E., Falkner, K. C., Feng, W., Clark, B. J., et al. (2016). Nuclear receptors and nonalcoholic fatty liver disease. Biochim. Biophys. Acta 1859, 1083–1099. doi:10.1016/j.bbagrm.2016.03.002

Chen, B., Ma, Y., Xue, X., Wei, J., Hu, G., and Lin, Y. (2019). Tetramethylpyrazine reduces inflammation in the livers of mice fed a high fat diet. Mol. Med. Rep. 19, 2561–2568. doi:10.3892/mmr.2019.9928

Chen, H., Chen, T., Giudici, P., and Chen, F. (2016). Vinegar functions on health: Constituents, sources, and formation mechanisms. Compr. Rev. Food Sci. Food Saf. 15, 1124–1138. doi:10.1111/1541-4337.12228

Cheung, O. and Sanyal, A. J. (2010). Recent advances in nonalcoholic fatty liver disease. Curr. Opin. Gastroenterol. 26, 202–208. doi:10.1097/MOG.0b013e328337b0c4

Chung, K. W., Kim, K. M., Choi, Y. J., An, H. J., Lee, B., Kim, D. H., et al. (2017). The critical role played by endotoxin-induced liver autophagy in the maintenance of lipid metabolism during sepsis. Autophagy 13, 1113–1129. doi:10.1080/15548627.2017.1319040

Colak, Y., Ozturk, O., Senates, E., Tuncer, I., Yorulmaz, E., Adali, G., et al. (2011). SIRT1 as a potential therapeutic target for treatment of nonalcoholic fatty liver disease. Med. Sci. Mon. Int. Med. J. Exp. Clin. Res. 17, HY5. doi:10.12659/msm.881749

Colak, Y., Yesil, A., Mutlu, H. H., Caklili, O. T., Ulasoglu, C., Senates, E., et al. (2014). A potential treatment of non-alcoholic fatty liver disease with SIRT1 activators. J. Gastrointestin. Liver Dis. 23, 311–319. doi:10.15403/jgld.2014.1121.233.yck

Dong, R., Yang, X., Wang, C., Liu, K., Liu, Z., Ma, X., et al. (2019). Yangonin protects against non-alcoholic fatty liver disease through farnesoid X receptor. Phytomedicine 53, 134–142. doi:10.1016/j.phymed.2018.09.006

Dowman, J. K., Armstrong, M. J., Tomlinson, J. W., and Newsome, P. N. (2011). Current therapeutic strategies in non-alcoholic fatty liver disease. Diabetes Obes. Metabol. 13, 692–702. doi:10.1111/j.1463-1326.2011.01403.x

Duan, W., Xia, T., Zhang, B., Li, S., Zhang, C., Zhao, C., et al. (2019). Changes of physicochemical, bioactive compounds and antioxidant capacity during the brewing process of zhenjiang aromatic vinegar. Molecules 24, 3935. doi:10.3390/molecules24213935

Elvira-Torales, L. I., Periago, M. J., González-Barrio, R., Hidalgo, N., Navarro-González, I., Gómez-Gallego, C., et al. (2019). Spinach consumption ameliorates the gut microbiota and dislipaemia in rats with diet-induced non-alcoholic fatty liver disease (NAFLD). Food Funct. 10, 2148–2160. doi:10.1039/c8fo01630e

Estes, C., Razavi, H., Loomba, R., Younossi, Z., and Sanyal, A. J. (2018). Modeling the epidemic of nonalcoholic fatty liver disease demonstrates an exponential increase in burden of disease. Hepatology 67, 123–133. doi:10.1002/hep.29466

Farrell, G. C. and Larter, C. Z. (2006). Nonalcoholic fatty liver disease: from steatosis to cirrhosis. Hepatology 43, S99–S112. doi:10.1002/hep.20973

Gäbele, E., Froh, M., Arteel, G. E., Uesugi, T., Hellerbrand, C., Schölmerich, J., et al. (2009). TNFα is required for cholestasis-induced liver fibrosis in the mouse. Biochem. Biophys. Res. Commun. 378, 348–353. doi:10.1016/j.bbrc.2008.10.155

Gao, Z., Zhang, J., Wei, L., Yang, X., Zhang, Y., Cheng, B., et al. (2020). The protective effects of imperatorin on acetaminophen overdose-induced Acute liver injury. Oxidat. Med. Cell Longev. 2020, 1. doi:10.1155/2020/8026838

García-Alonso, F. J., González-Barrio, R., Martín-Pozuelo, G., Hidalgo, N., Navarro-González, I., Masuero, D., et al. (2017). A study of the prebiotic-like effects of tomato juice consumption in rats with diet-induced non-alcoholic fatty liver disease (NAFLD). Food Funct. 8, 3542–3552. doi:10.1039/c7fo00393e

Gong, Z., Tas, E., Yakar, S., and Muzumdar, R. (2017). Hepatic lipid metabolism and non-alcoholic fatty liver disease in aging. Mol. Cell. Endocrinol. 455, 115–130. doi:10.1016/j.mce.2016.12.022

Han, X., Cui, Z.-Y., Song, J., Piao, H.-Q., Lian, L.-H., Hou, L.-S., et al. (2019). Acanthoic acid modulates lipogenesis in nonalcoholic fatty liver disease via FXR/LXRs-dependent manner. Chem. Biol. Interact. 311, 108794. doi:10.1016/j.cbi.2019.108794

Hwang, J. S., Choi, H. S., Ham, S. A., Yoo, T., Lee, W. J., Paek, K. S., et al. (2015). Deacetylation-mediated interaction of SIRT1-HMGB1 improves survival in a mouse model of endotoxemia. Sci. Rep. 5, 15971. doi:10.1038/srep15971

Ibrahim, S. H., Hirsova, P., and Gores, G. J. (2018). Non-alcoholic steatohepatitis pathogenesis: sublethal hepatocyte injury as a driver of liver inflammation. Gut 67, 963–972. doi:10.1136/gutjnl-2017-315691

Jiang, J., Yan, L., Shi, Z., Wang, L., Shan, L., and Efferth, T. (2019). Hepatoprotective and anti-inflammatory effects of total flavonoids of Qu Zhi Ke (peel of Citrus changshan-huyou) on non-alcoholic fatty liver disease in rats via modulation of NF-κB and MAPKs. Phytomedicine 64, 153082. doi:10.1016/j.phymed.2019.153082

Jiang, W., Jiang, P., Yang, R., and Liu, D. F. (2018). Functional role of SIRT1-induced HMGB1 expression and acetylation in migration, invasion and angiogenesis of ovarian cancer. Eur. Rev. Med. Pharmacol. Sci. 22, 4431–4439. doi:10.26355/eurrev_201807_15494

Jing, L., Yanyan, Z., and Junfeng, F. (2015). Acetic acid in aged vinegar affects molecular targets for thrombus disease management. Food Funct. 6, 2845–2853. doi:10.1039/c5fo00327j

Khambu, B., Yan, S., Huda, N., and Yin, X.-M. (2019). Role of high-mobility group box-1 in liver pathogenesis. Int. J. Mol. Sci. 20, 5314. doi:10.3390/ijms20215314

Kondo, T., Kishi, M., Fushimi, T., Ugajin, S., and Kaga, T. (2009). Vinegar intake reduces body weight, body fat mass, and serum triglyceride levels in obese Japanese subjects. Biosci. Biotechnol. Biochem. 73, 1837–1843. doi:10.1271/bbb.90231

Lan, K.-C., Chao, S.-C., Wu, H.-Y., Chiang, C.-L., Wang, C.-C., Liu, S.-H., et al. (2017). Salidroside ameliorates sepsis-induced acute lung injury and mortality via downregulating NF-κB and HMGB1 pathways through the upregulation of SIRT1. Sci. Rep. 7, 12026. doi:10.1038/s41598-017-12285-8

Le, K., Chibaatar Daliv, E., Wu, S., Qian, F., Ali, A. I., Yu, D., et al. (2019). SIRT1-regulated HMGB1 release is partially involved in TLR4 signal transduction: a possible anti-neuroinflammatory mechanism of resveratrol in neonatal hypoxic-ischemic brain injury. Int. Immunopharm. 75, 105779. doi:10.1016/j.intimp.2019.105779

Li, L., Chen, L., Hu, L., Liu, Y., Sun, H.-Y., Tang, J., et al. (2011). Nuclear factor high-mobility group box1 mediating the activation of toll-like receptor 4 signaling in hepatocytes in the early stage of nonalcoholic fatty liver disease in mice. Hepatology 54, 1620–1630. doi:10.1002/hep.24552

Manne, V., Handa, P., and Kowdley, K. V. (2018). Pathophysiology of nonalcoholic fatty liver disease/nonalcoholic steatohepatitis. Clin. Liver Dis. 22, 23–37. doi:10.1016/j.cld.2017.08.007

Nie, H., Song, C., Wang, D., Cui, S., Ren, T., Cao, Z., et al. (2017). MicroRNA-194 inhibition improves dietary-induced non-alcoholic fatty liver disease in mice through targeting on FXR. Biochim. Biophys. Acta 1863, 3087–3094. doi:10.1016/j.bbadis.2017.09.020

Qi, Z., Zhang, Y., Qi, S., Ling, L., Gui, L., Yan, L., et al. (2017). Salidroside inhibits HMGB1 acetylation and release through upregulation of SirT1 during inflammation. Oxidat. Med. Cell Longev. 2017, 1. doi:10.1155/2017/9821543

Qin, G., Ma, J., Huang, Q., Yin, H., Han, J., Li, M., et al.. (2018). Isoquercetin improves hepatic lipid accumulation by activating AMPK pathway and suppressing TGF-β signaling on an HFD-induced nonalcoholic fatty liver disease rat model. Int. J. Mol. Sci. 19, 4126. doi:10.3390/ijms19124126

Rolo, A. P., Teodoro, J. S., and Palmeira, C. M. (2012). Role of oxidative stress in the pathogenesis of nonalcoholic steatohepatitis. Free Radic. Biol. Med. 52, 59–69. doi:10.1016/j.freeradbiomed.2011.10.003

Safari, Z. and Gérard, P. (2019). The links between the gut microbiome and non-alcoholic fatty liver disease (NAFLD). Cell. Mol. Life Sci. 76, 1541–1558. doi:10.1007/s00018-019-03011-w

Shen, F., Feng, J., Wang, X., Qi, Z., Shi, X., An, Y., et al. (2016). Vinegar treatment prevents the development of murine experimental colitis via inhibition of inflammation and apoptosis. *J. Agric. Food Chem.* 64, 1111–1121. doi:10.1021/acs.jafc.5b05415

Silva, J. P. and Wahlestedt, C. (2010). Role of Sirtuin 1 in metabolic regulation. *Drug Discov. Today* 15, 781–791. doi:10.1016/j.drudis.2010.07.001

Soares e Silva, A. K., de Oliveira Cipriano Torres, D., dos Santos Gomes, F. O., dos Santos Silva, B., Lima Ribeiro, E., Costa Oliveira, A., et al. (2015). LPSF/GQ-02 inhibits the development of hepatic steatosis and inflammation in a mouse model of non-alcoholic fatty liver disease (NAFLD). *PLoS One* 10, e0123787. doi:10.1371/journal.pone.0123787

Stefan, N., Häring, H.-U., and Cusi, K. (2019). Non-alcoholic fatty liver disease: causes, diagnosis, cardiometabolic consequences, and treatment strategies. *Lancet Diabetes Endocrinol.* 7, 313–324. doi:10.1016/S2213-8587(18)30154-2

Tang, W., Yao, X., Xia, F., Yang, M., Chen, Z., Zhou, B., et al. (2018). Modulation of the gut microbiota in rats by hugan qingzhi tablets during the treatment of high-fat-diet-induced nonalcoholic fatty liver disease. *Oxidat. Med. Cell Longev.* 2018, 1. doi:10.1155/2018/7261619

Wu, X., Xu, N., Li, M., Huang, Q., Wu, J., Gan, Y., et al. (2019). Protective effect of patchouli alcohol against high-fat diet induced hepatic steatosis by alleviating endoplasmic reticulum stress and regulating VLDL metabolism in rats. *Front. Pharmacol.* 10, 1134. doi:10.3389/fphar.2019.01134

Xia, H., Zhu, X., Zhang, X., Jiang, H., Li, B., Wang, Z., et al. (2019). Alpha-naphthoflavone attenuates non-alcoholic fatty liver disease in oleic acid-treated HepG2 hepatocytes and in high fat diet-fed mice. *Biomed. Pharmacother.* 118, 109287. doi:10.1016/j.biopha.2019.109287

Xu, W., Huang, Z., Zhang, X., Li, Q., Lu, Z., Shi, J., et al. (2011a). Monitoring the microbial community during solid-state acetic acid fermentation of Zhenjiang aromatic vinegar. *Food Microbiol.* 28, 1175–1181. doi:10.1016/j.fm.2011.03.011

Xu, W., Xu, Q., Chen, J., Lu, Z., Xia, R., Li, G., et al. (2011b). Ligustrazine formation in Zhenjiang aromatic vinegar: changes during fermentation and storing process. *J. Sci. Food Agric.* 91, 1612–1617. doi:10.1002/jsfa.4356

Yang, J., Sun, L., Wang, L., Hassan, H. M., Wang, X., Hylemon, P. B., et al. (2017). Activation of SIRT1/FXR signaling pathway attenuates triptolide-induced hepatotoxicity in rats. *Front. Pharmacol.* 8, 260. doi:10.3389/fphar.2017.00260

Yao, H., Tao, X., Xu, L., Qi, Y., Yin, L., Han, X., et al. (2018). Dioscin alleviates non-alcoholic fatty liver disease through adjusting lipid metabolism via SIRT1/AMPK signaling pathway. *Pharmacol. Res.* 131, 51–60. doi:10.1016/j.phrs.2018.03.017

Younossi, Z. M., Koenig, A. B., Abdelatif, D., Fazel, Y., Henry, L., and Wymer, M. (2016). Global epidemiology of nonalcoholic fatty liver disease-meta-analytic assessment of prevalence, incidence, and outcomes. *Hepatology* 64, 73–84. doi:10.1002/hep.28431

Yu, Y., Zhang, Z., Zhang, B., Zeng, Y., Li, X., Ji, H., et al. (2020). Implication of vinegar alone or in combination with caltrate in a rat osteoporosis model induced by a low calcium diet and retinoic acid. *Chin. Tradit. Med. J.* 3, 1–8.

Zeng, W., Shan, W., Gao, L., Gao, D., Hu, Y., Wang, G., et al. (2015). Inhibition of HMGB1 release via salvianolic acid B-mediated SIRT1 up-regulation protects rats against non-alcoholic fatty liver disease. *Sci. Rep.* 5, 16013. doi:10.1038/srep16013

Zhang, B., Xia, T., Duan, W., Zhang, Z., Li, Y., Fang, B., et al. (2019). Effects of organic acids, amino acids and phenolic compounds on antioxidant characteristic of Zhenjiang aromatic vinegar. *Molecules* 24, 3799. doi:10.3390/molecules24203799

Zhang, X., Ji, X., Wang, Q., and Li, J. Z. (2018). New insight into inter-organ crosstalk contributing to the pathogenesis of non-alcoholic fatty liver disease (NAFLD). *Protein Cell* 9, 164–177. doi:10.1007/s13238-017-0436-0

Zhang, Y., Geng, C., Liu, X., Li, M., Gao, M., Liu, X., et al. (2017). Celastrol ameliorates liver metabolic damage caused by a high-fat diet through SIRT1. *Mol. Metabol.* 6, 138–147. doi:10.1016/j.molmet.2016.11.002

Zhao, C., Xia, T., Du, P., Duan, W., Zhang, B., Zhang, J., et al. (2018). Chemical composition and antioxidant characteristic of traditional and industrial Zhenjiang aromatic vinegars during the aging process. *Molecules* 23, 2949. doi:10.3390/molecules23112949

Zhao, Q., Liu, F., Cheng, Y., Xiao, X.-R., Hu, D.-D., Tang, Y.-M., et al. (2019). Celastrol protects from cholestatic liver injury through modulation of SIRT1-

FXR signaling. *Mol. Cell. Proteomics* 18, 520–533. doi:10.1074/mcp.RA118.000817

Zhu, W., Liu, Y., Lan, Y., Li, X., Luo, L., Duan, X., et al. (2019). Dietary vinegar prevents kidney stone recurrence via epigenetic regulations. *EBioMedicine* 45, 231–250. doi:10.1016/j.ebiom.2019.06.004

15

Perforin Acts as an Immune Regulator to Prevent the Progression of NAFLD

Qian Wang [1,2*†], Dehai Li [1,2†], Jing Zhu [1,2†], Mingyue Zhang [1,2], Hua Zhang [1,2], Guangchao Cao [1,2], Leqing Zhu [1,2], Qiping Shi [3], Jianlei Hao [1,2], Qiong Wen [1,2], Zonghua Liu [1,2], Hengwen Yang [1,2*] and Zhinan Yin [1,2*]

[1] Zhuhai Precision Medical Center, Zhuhai People's Hospital (Zhuhai Hospital Affiliated with Jinan University), Jinan University, Zhuhai, China, [2] The Biomedical Translational Research Institute, Faculty of Medical Science, Jinan University, Guangzhou, China, [3] The First Affiliated Hospital of Jinan University, Guangzhou, China

*Correspondence:
Qian Wang
wangqian@jnu.edu.cn
Hengwen Yang
hengwenyang@jnu.edu.cn
Zhinan Yin
zhinan.yin@yale.edu

[†] These authors share first authorship

Non-alcoholic fatty liver disease (NAFLD) is one of the main causes of cirrhosis and major risk factors for hepatocellular carcinoma and liver-related death. Despite substantial clinical and basic research, the pathogenesis of obesity-related NAFLD remains poorly understood. In this study, we show that perforin can act as an immune regulator to prevent the progression of NAFLD. Aged perforin-deficient (Prf$^{-/-}$) mice have increased lipid accumulation in the liver compared to WT mice. With high-fat diet (HFD) challenge, Prf$^{-/-}$ mice have increased liver weight, more severe liver damage, and increased liver inflammation when compared with WT controls. Mechanistic studies revealed that perforin specifically regulates intrinsic IFN-γ production in CD4 T cells, not CD8 T cells. We found that CD4 T cell depletion reduces liver injury and ameliorates the inflammation and metabolic morbidities in Prf$^{-/-}$ mice. Furthermore, improved liver characteristics in HFD Prf$^{-/-}$ and IFN-γR$^{-/-}$ double knockout mice confirmed that IFN-γ is a key factor for mediating perforin regulation of NAFLD progression. Overall, our findings reveal the important regulatory role perforin plays in the progression of obesity-related NAFLD and highlight novel strategies for treating NAFLD.

Keywords: perforin, NAFLD, CD4 T cells, IFN-γ, inflammation

INTRODUCTION

Non-alcoholic fatty liver disease (NAFLD) pathogenesis is tightly linked to obesity and therefore is an emerging healthcare problem worldwide (1, 2). NAFLD, along with related inflammation, progressive subtype non-alcoholic steatohepatitis (NASH), fibrosis, and ultimately hepatocellular carcinoma, is becoming one of the leading causes of liver-related morbidity and mortality worldwide (3–5). The pathogenesis of NAFLD remains incompletely understood. It is appreciated that multiple concurrent intrahepatic and extrahepatic events contribute to development and progression of NAFLD, including cell senescence, insulin resistance, and immune system dysfunction (6, 7). Cellular senescence refers to the irreversible arrest of cell growth that occurs when cells are exposed to various stresses (8–10). Recent experimental evidence suggests that hepatocyte senescence is linked to the fibrosis that develops as NAFLD progresses; hepatocyte expression of p21, the universal cell cycle inhibitor, is positively correlated with fibrosis stage in liver sections from 70 NAFLD patients (11). Dysregulated lipid metabolism plays a key role in initiation and progression of hepatic steatosis and is frequently associated with inflammation of the liver (12, 13). Elevated inflammation promotes the development of insulin resistance, which in turn further promotes ectopic fat accumulation in the liver, thus forming a vicious cycle (14, 15). Inflammation and fibrogenesis are regulated by complex immunologic pathways that may present possible new therapeutic targets in the liver for NAFLD (7).

Perforin, which is primarily released by CD8$^+$ T cells and natural killer (NK) cells, helps eliminate infected or dangerous cells and induce apoptosis (16, 17). Following degranulation, pores formed by perforin enable granzyme entry into cells and subsequent caspase activation. Perforin-mediated cytotoxicity is also involved in the homeostatic regulation of CD4 and CD8 T cells *in vivo* (18, 19). Recent reports revealed that perforin-mediated exocytosis (but not death-receptor-mediated apoptosis) is essential for immune surveillance of senescent cells, and disruption of this pathway as a result of disease or inflammation can lead to the accumulation of senescent cells in the liver (20). Interestingly, a recent study showed that mice on a high-fat diet (HFD) lacking perforin developed more severe obesity, glucose tolerance, and insulin resistance and had higher triglyceride levels in the liver when compared with wild-type (WT) controls (21). However, the precise role of perforin in the context of HFD-induced NAFLD has not been systematically researched yet.

We show that perforin acts as an important immune regulator to prevent NAFLD progression. Aged Prf$^{-/-}$ mice had more severe liver injury and lipid accumulation than did WT control mice. In the condition of HFD-induced NAFLD, we also found that Prf$^{-/-}$ mice developed more severe hepatic steatosis with more macrophage and IFN-γ, producing CD4$^+$ T cell infiltration of the liver. Depletion of CD4$^+$ T cells in Prf$^{-/-}$ mice almost completely rescued the observed phenotypes, suggesting an important regulatory role for CD4$^+$ T cells. Moreover, when IFN-γ receptor signaling is ablated by using perforin and IFN-γ receptor double knockout mice, both liver injury and lipid accumulation were dramatically diminished, indicating that IFN-γ signaling plays a pivotal role in mediating NAFLD pathogenesis.

Overall, our studies reveal that perforin acts as an important immune regulator for NAFLD progression. This finding expands our understanding of inflammation in regulating NAFLD and may have therapeutic implications for NAFLD in the future.

MATERIALS AND METHODS

Mice

Prf$^{-/-}$ and IFN-γR$^{-/-}$ mice were purchased from the Jackson Laboratory. C57BL/6J mice were purchased from Guangdong Medical Laboratory Animal Center (Guangzhou, China). All mice were males and received either a normal control diet (SFD) or HFD (60 kcal % fat; Research Diets) beginning at an age of 6–8 weeks old. All mice were maintained under specified pathogen-free conditions at Jinan University (Guangzhou, China). Animal procedures were approved by and performed in accordance with the Jinan University's Institutional Laboratory Animal Care and Use Committee guidelines.

Isolation of Liver Mononuclear Cells

The protocol used for isolating murine liver mononuclear cells (MNCs) was as described previously (22). Liver tissue was obtained from mice, and the tissue was dissociated to procure MNCs. To obtain liver MNCs, murine livers were pressed through a 200-gauge stainless steel mesh and suspended in either RPMI-1640 medium or PBS. The cells were then centrifuged at 50 g for 1 min. The cell suspension was collected and centrifuged again at 974 g for 10 min. The cell pellet containing MNCs was then resuspended in 40% Percoll (GE Healthcare, Uppsala, Sweden), after which the cell suspension was overlaid on 70% Percoll and centrifuged at 1,260 g for 30 min. The resulting cell pellets were collected from the interphase following two additional washings in PBS or RPMI-1640 medium.

Serum Biochemistry

Mice were fasted overnight. Then, whole blood was collected, and serum alanine aminotransferase (ALT) and cholesterol levels were determined using an automatic biochemistry analyzer (7600-020, Hitachi, Japan).

Cytokine Detection With ELISA

Mice were fasted overnight, and 0.1 g of liver tissue was harvested from the mice in 1 ml of PBS. Liver tissue was then homogenized by hand and centrifuged at 3,000 rpm for 10 min, after which the supernatant was carefully collected. All steps were performed at 4°C. IL-6, IFN-γ, and TNF-α levels in liver supernatants were determined using a commercially available mouse enzyme-linked immunosorbent assay (ELISA) kit (eBioscience, San Diego, CA, USA) according to the manufacturer's instructions.

Flow Cytometry Analysis

Non-parenchymal cells were transferred to a new well and treated with 1:1000 GolgiPlug, 1 ng/ml ionomycin, and 50 ng/ml PMA for 4–6 h. Intracellular and cell surface staining was performed as described in the fixation/permeabilization kit (554714; BD) protocol. Cells were stained with the surface markers PEcy7-anti-mouse CD3, PE-anti-mouse NK1.1, FITC-anti-mouse CD4, and PerCPCY5.5-anti-mouse CD8 for 15 min at 4°C. Cells were stained for cytokines with BV421 anti–mouse IFN-γ and APC-IL-17A for 30 min at 4°C, washed with PBS, and analyzed using FACS verse flow cytometry (BD). Data were analyzed using FlowJo (TreeStar).

CD4$^+$ T Cell Depletion

To deplete CD4$^+$ T cells, 200-μg doses of anti-CD4 monoclonal antibody (clone: GK1.5; Sungene Biotech) per mouse were intraperitoneally injected weekly during HFD challenge. Sterile-filtered PBS was used as a control.

Histological Examination

Liver tissue was harvested and fixed in 4% (w/v) paraformaldehyde, and 4 mm-thick sections that had been affinized and rehydrated were stained with hematoxylin and eosin (H&E). Hepatic lipid content was determined using frozen sections embedded in Tissue-Tek O.C.T. compound and stained with Oil Red O (Sigma-Aldrich, St. Louis, MO, USA). Images were acquired on a Leica DM3000 microscope.

Immunofluorescence

Liver tissue was harvested, fixed in 4% (w/v) paraformaldehyde, and cut in 4 mm-thick sections. Liver sections were then perfused with 30 ml of 4% paraformaldehyde for fixation. Sections were then incubated with the following dilutions of mouse-specific primary antibodies: 1:200 anti-F4/80 (ab16911, Abcam) and 1:200 iNOS antibody (GTX74171, Gentex). For visualization, 1:200 fluorescent Alexa Fluor 594 and FITC 488 secondary antibodies (Invitrogen Vector) were used for both individual staining and co-staining at room temperature for 2 h. After washing, tissue sections were fixed with Vectashield containing DAPI for visualization. A laser cofocal microscopy (TCS SP8, Leica) was used to capture images and conduct further analysis. For the microscopy images displaying M1 (iNOS+ F4/80+) or total macrophages (F4/80+), 4 slides per mouse liver tissue were prepared and 4 fields were captured from each slide. The quantification of M1 or total macrophages was conducted in these 16 fields and designated as one biological independent sample, and the percentage of M1 in total macrophages was calculated and shown.

Tissue Triglyceride Quantification

The protocol for quantifying hepatic triglyceride (TG) levels was carried out as described previously (23). Briefly, 20–30 mg of liver tissue was homogenized in 500 μl of PBS and mixed with chloroform/methanol 2:1 (vol/vol). The organic phase was transferred, air-dried overnight, and resuspended in 1% Triton X-100 in absolute ethanol. The concentration of TGs was then quantified using a serum triglyceride determination kit (Sigma, Triglyceride Reagent T2449 and Free Glycerol Reagent F6428).

RNA Extraction and Quantitative Real-Time PCR

Total liver RNA was isolated using TRIzol Reagent (DP424, Tiangen, China). cDNA synthesis was performed using a Prime Script RT Reagent Kit (Takara, Shiga, Japan). Levels of mRNA expression were quantified by real-time PCR (RT-PCR). RT-PCR was performed using TB Green (Takara). Primer sequences are shown in the **Table 1**.

Statistical Analysis

Data are presented as the mean ± SEM. Statistical significance between two groups was evaluated using a two-tailed unpaired Student's t-test. Values of $P < 0.05$ were considered to be statistically significant. The data shown in each panel of these figures were collected from a single experiment; each experiment was repeated for at least three times and showed consistent results. Moreover, the statistical analysis was conducted on each single experiment.

RESULTS

Perforin Deficiency Accelerates Liver Injury and Enhances Lipid Accumulation in 14 Month-Old Mice

NAFLD is common in the elderly, in whom it carries a more substantial burden of hepatic (non-alcoholic steatohepatitis,

TABLE 1 | Primers for real-time RT-PCR.

Hprt forward	5'-CGTCGTGATTAGCGATGATGAAC-3'
Hprt reverse	5'-TCACTAATGACACAAACGTGATTC-3'
Fabp4 forward	5'-GACGACAGGAAGGTGAAGAG-3'
Fabp4 reverse	5'-ACATTCCACCACCAGCTTGT-3'
Cebpα forward	5'-AAGAACAGCAACGAGTACCGG-3'
Cebpα reverse	5'-CATTGTCACTGGTCAGCTCCA-3'
SREBP-1C forward	5'-GATCAAAGAGGAGCCAGTGC-3'
SREBP-1C reverse	5'-TAGATGGTGGCTGCTGAGTG-3'
PPARγ forward	5'-GCCCTTTGGTGACTTTATGG-3'
PPARγ reverse	5'-CAGCAGGTTGTCTTGGATGT-3'
PPARα forward	5'-TCGGACTCGGTCTTCTTGAT-3'
PPARα reverse	5'-TCTTCCCAAAGCTCCTTCAA-3'
Cox-1 forward	5'-CTCACAGTGCGGTCCAAC-3'
Cox-1 reverse	5'-CCAGCACCTGGTACTTAA-3'
AOX forward	5'-TCGGGCAAGTGAGGCGCATT-3'
AOX reverse	5'-AGCAACAGCATTGGGGCGGA-3'
Cpt1α forward	5'-CCCAAGTATCCACAGGGTCA-3'
Cpt1α reverse	5'-TTTGAATCGGCTCCTAATGG-3'
Lipe forward	5'-GTGGAGGCACATTTAGTTCT-3'
Lipe reverse	5'-GTGACCTGTTTGTTTGTTCT-3'
Lpl forward	5-TAGATGAGGCCAACCTGTCC-3'
Lpl reverse	5-CTGCGTAGTCGGGGTACATT-3'
CD36 forward	5'-AGATGACGTGGCAAAGAACAG-3'
CD36 reverse	5'-CCTTGGCTAGATAACGAACTCTG-3'
Scd1 forward	5'-TTCTTGCGATACACTCTGGTGC-3'
Scd1 reverse	5'-CGGGATTGAATGTTCTTGTCGT-3'
Cidea forward	5'-TGACATTCATGGGATTGCAGAC-3'
Cidea reverse	5'-GGCCAGTTGTGATGACTAAGAC-3'
Chrebpβ forward	5'-TCTGCAGATCGCGTGGAG-3'
Chrebpβ reverse	5'-CTTGTCCCGGCATAGCAAC-3'
Fasn forward	5'-CCTTGGCTAGATAACGAACTCTG−3'
Fasn reverse	5'-ATCCATAGAGCCCAGCCTTCCATC−3'

cirrhosis, and hepatocellular carcinoma) and extra-hepatic manifestations and complications (cardiovascular disease, extrahepatic neoplasms) than in younger age groups (24). Aged Prf$^{-/-}$ mice have been reported to have accumulation of senescent cells and development of chronic systemic and local inflammation in the liver (25, 26). We hypothesized that aged Prf$^{-/-}$ mice might also have more severe hepatic morbidities since inflammation correlates with liver dysfunction. To test this hypothesis, we first determined liver weights and liver injury (ALT) levels in aged WT and Prf$^{-/-}$ mice at 14 months of age. As expected, the aged Prf$^{-/-}$ mice showed significantly increased liver weight (**Figure 1A**), elevated liver damage, and increased lipid accumulation as shown by levels of ALT that trended as increased and significantly increased liver TG levels (**Figure 1B**). Furthermore, liver histological analysis revealed more severe hepatic steatosis and significantly increased accumulation of lipid in aged Prf$^{-/-}$ mice compared with WT mice (**Figure 1C**). These results indicated that the perforin deficiency aggravates liver injury and steatosis in aged mice.

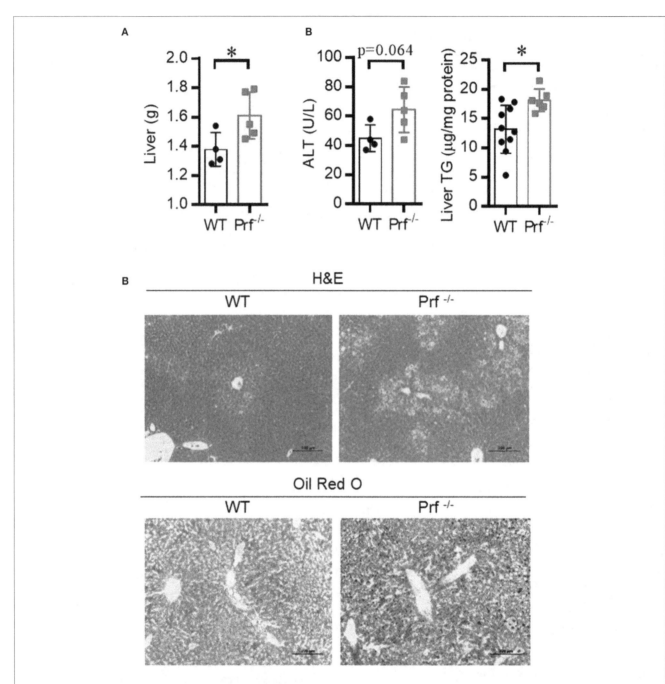

FIGURE 1 | Perforin deficiency accelerates liver injury and enhances lipid accumulation in 14 month-old mice. **(A)** Liver weight was determined for WT and Prf$^{-/-}$ mice on a normal chow diet (n = 4–5). **(B)** Serum levels of ALT (left, n = 4–5) and liver TG content (right, n = 6–10) were measured. **(C)** Representative images of liver sections stained with H&E and Oil red O in WT and Prf$^{-/-}$ mice at the age of 14 months. ALT, alanine aminotransferase; WT, wild-type; TG, triglyceride. The data shown in each panel of the figures were collected from a single experiment, and each experiment was repeated for at least three times and rendered consistent results. Means ± SEM, *p < 0.05.

Perforin Deficiency Aggravates HFD-Induced Liver Injury and Steatohepatitis

The role of perforin in NAFLD was then investigated using an HFD-induced NAFLD model. Prf$^{-/-}$ and WT mice at 6–8 weeks of age were fed on SFD or HFD for 10 weeks to induce NAFLD.

As expected, HFD challenge was associated with elevated body weight and ALT activation in WT mice (**Figures 2A,B**). The increase in body weight in response to HFD challenge was comparable between WT and Prf$^{-/-}$ mice; however, Prf$^{-/-}$ mice had significantly enlarged livers (**Figure 2A**). Additionally, the Prf$^{-/-}$ mice had more severe liver damage as indicated

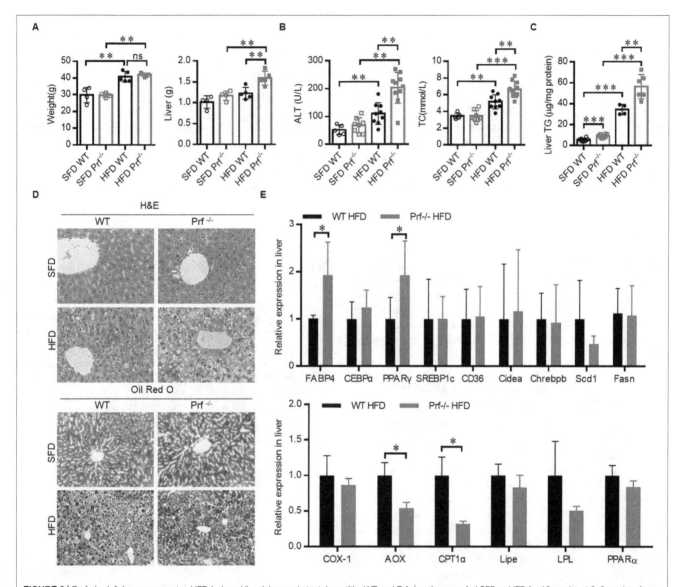

FIGURE 2 | Perforin deficiency aggravates HFD-induced liver injury and steatohepatitis. WT and Prf$^{-/-}$ mice were fed SFD or HFD for 10 weeks at 6–8 weeks of age. **(A)** Body weight (left panel) and liver weights (right panel) ($n = 4$–5), **(B)** measurements of serum ALT (left panel) and cholesterol levels (right panel) ($n = 5$–10), and **(C)** measurements of liver TG content ($n = 4$–8). **(D)** Representative images of liver sections stained with H&E and Oil red O. **(E)** Expression levels of lipogenic genes (top) and fatty acid oxidation genes (bottom) in the liver, relative to Hprt expression levels ($n = 4$–9). The data shown in each panel of the figures were collected from a single experiment, and each experiment was repeated for at least three times and rendered consistent results. Means ± SEM, *$p < 0.05$; **$p < 0.01$, ***$p < 0.001$.

by higher ALT levels. The livers of HFD Prf$^{-/-}$ mice exhibited significantly increased lipid accumulation (**Figure 2C**). Histological analysis of livers indicated that HFD Prf$^{-/-}$ mice had more severe hepatic steatosis and lipid accumulation when compared with WT controls (**Figure 2D**). Moreover, RT-PCR analysis of liver samples from HFD mice showed that the expression levels of genes involved in lipid production such as fatty acid binding protein 4 (Fabp4) and peroxisome proliferator-activated receptor gamma (PPARγ) were significantly increased, whereas expression levels of lipid catabolism-related genes such as carnitine palmitoyl transferase 1 (CPT-1α) and aldehyde oxidase (AOX-1) were significantly decreased in HFD Prf$^{-/-}$ mice (**Figure 2E**). These results indicated that

perforin deficiency with HFD challenge aggravated liver injury and steatohepatitis.

Perforin Deficiency Promotes an Inflammatory Response in the Liver After HFD Challenge

Pro-inflammatory T cells promote M1 macrophage activation and intensively contribute to HFD-induced NAFLD (27). To explore the mechanism that drives more severe NAFLD in Prf$^{-/-}$ mice, we analyzed the composition of the immune cell infiltrate in the liver by flow cytometry. Perforin deficiency did not alter the infiltration of CD4, CD8, NK, NK1.1+ T cells, or total macrophages in the liver (**Figures 3A–C**). However, the cell number of CD11c+ macrophages was significantly increased (**Figure 3D**). We next evaluated inflammatory cytokine production by these immune cell subsets. Interestingly, we observed that IFN-γ production from CD4 T, but not CD8 T cells, NK cells, or NK1.1+ T cells, was significant increased, while IL-17 was barely detectable and largely unaffected in all subsets (**Figures 3E–H**). We characterized the cell number in each category and found no significant difference of CD4 T cells, CD8 T cells, and NK and NK1.1+T cells. The cell numbers of CD11c+ macrophages (M1) and IFN-γ+CD4 T cells were significantly increased in perforin KO liver, which equivalent as the percentage analysis (**Figure 3I**).

We also determined the levels of pro-inflammatory cytokines secreted by the liver in HFD-challenged Prf$^{-/-}$ and WT mice. As expected, Prf$^{-/-}$ livers produced more IL-6, TNF-α, and IFN-γ compared with livers from WT controls (**Figure 4A**). Immunofluorescence analysis showed that perforin deficiency robustly promoted the enrichment of M1 macrophage in the liver, which was consistent with the previous percentage and cell number analysis (**Figure 4B**). These findings suggest that upon HFD challenge, the IFN-γ level and M1 macrophage-mediated inflammation are enhanced in Prf$^{-/-}$ mice.

Perforin Regulates Fatty Liver Disease Through CD4 T Cells in the Liver

To determine whether increased IFN-γ production from CD4 T cells in Prf$^{-/-}$ mice was associated with the exacerbated liver phenotypes that develop after HFD challenge, we depleted CD4 T cells in Prf$^{-/-}$ mice and then fed the mice with HFD. As expected, CD4 T cell depletion predisposed Prf$^{-/-}$ mice to decreased liver weights, lipid accumulation, and diminished liver damage (**Figures 5A–C**). Notably, levels of the pro-inflammatory cytokine TNF-α, as well as macrophage accumulation, were also significantly decreased following CD4 T cell depletion in Prf$^{-/-}$ mice; so was the IFN-γ level, though CD4 T cells are not the only cells producing IFN-γ (**Figures 5D,E**). Furthermore, the mRNA expression levels of genes involved in lipogenesis such as Fabp4, CEBPα, PPARγ, SREBP1c, Chrebpβ, and Scd1 were decreased following CD4 T cell depletion in Prf$^{-/-}$ mice, whereas lipolysis-related genes such as AOX1, CPT1α, and LPL were unchanged following CD4 T cell depletion in Prf$^{-/-}$ mice (**Figure 5F**). These findings indicate that CD4 T cells play a critical role in perforin-mediated regulation of NAFLD progression.

Hepatic Steatosis in Prf$^{-/-}$ Mice Is Dependent on IFN-γ-Mediated Inflammation

Since the level of IFN-γ was significantly increased in the livers of Prf$^{-/-}$ mice, we next explored whether CD4 T cells contribute to exacerbated NAFLD in these mice via IFN-γ activity. Therefore, we crossed Prf$^{-/-}$ mice with IFN-γ receptor-deficient mice to get double knockout mice (IFN-γR$^{-/-}$ and Prf$^{-/-}$). Following HFD challenge, IFN-γR$^{-/-}$ and Prf$^{-/-}$ mice gained similar amounts of body weight but had significantly decreased liver weights when compared to Prf$^{-/-}$ mice (**Figures 6A,B**). Notably,

IFN-γR$^{-/-}$ and Prf$^{-/-}$ mice showed significantly rescued NAFLD symptoms, including diminished hepatic steatosis, cellular ballooning, and lipid accumulation (**Figure 6C**). We also found that IFN-γR$^{-/-}$ & Prf$^{-/-}$ mice had reduced serum ALT, cholesterol, and liver TG levels, as well as diminished pro-inflammatory cytokine production, while the level of IFN-γ was no significantly changed after IFN-γ receptor deficiency (**Figure 6D**). Moreover, the cell number of pro-inflammatory (F4/80$^+$iNOS$^+$) macrophage in the livers of IFN-γR$^{-/-}$Prf$^{-/-}$ mice was also dramatically decreased when compared to Prf$^{-/-}$ mice (**Figure 6E**). Taken together, these findings strongly support an important role for elevated IFN-γ in promoting NAFLD progression in the context of perforin deficiency, given that ablation of IFN-γ signaling had a protective effect on the liver in an NAFLD mouse model.

CD4 T Cells Demonstrate Intrinsically Elevated IFN-γ Production in Prf$^{-/-}$ Mice

To define the functional properties of CD4 T cells from Prf$^{-/-}$ mice, total spleen lymphocytes from WT and Prf$^{-/-}$ mice were stimulated *in vitro* with anti CD3/anti-CD28 in the presence of Golgi-Stop. CD4 but not CD8 T cells from Prf$^{-/-}$ mice showed increased levels of IFN-γ production upon CD3/CD28 stimulation (**Figures 7A,B**). To further study whether elevated IFN-γ production by CD4 T cells in Prf$^{-/-}$ mice was an intrinsic property of these mice, naïve CD4 T cells were sorted from WT and Prf$^{-/-}$ spleens and directly differentiated into Th1 cells. Interestingly, naïve CD4 T cells from Prf$^{-/-}$ mice showed an elevated ability to differentiate into Th1 cells (**Figure 7C**). These findings support the conclusion that CD4 T cells undergo an intrinsic functional change in Prf$^{-/-}$ mice.

DISCUSSION

HFD-induced NAFLD is a well-established mouse model for studying the pathophysiological mechanisms of human fatty liver disease. NAFLD is a prevalent liver disease worldwide that can have severe complications such as liver fibrosis and even development of hepatocellular carcinoma, for which there are no effective therapeutic approaches (28). Numerous factors such as leptin, TNF-α, and IL-6 are involved in the initiation and progression of hepatic steatosis and related metabolic dysfunction (29–31). However, the precise role of perforin, a cytotoxic factor released by T cells, has not been precisely studied in the context of HFD-induced NAFLD. Here we described an important protective role for perforin in regulating NAFLD progression. We found that perforin regulates intrinsic IFN-γ production in CD4 T cells, which influences pro-inflammatory macrophage accumulation to affect the progression of NAFLD.

One major finding of this study is the discovery of the protective role perforin plays in regulating NAFLD progression. Perforin is a ~67-kDa pore-forming protein that is stored in the secretory vesicles (granules) of CTLs and NK cells (32). Perforin is known to have potent and extensive functions in mediating targeted killing together with various other factors

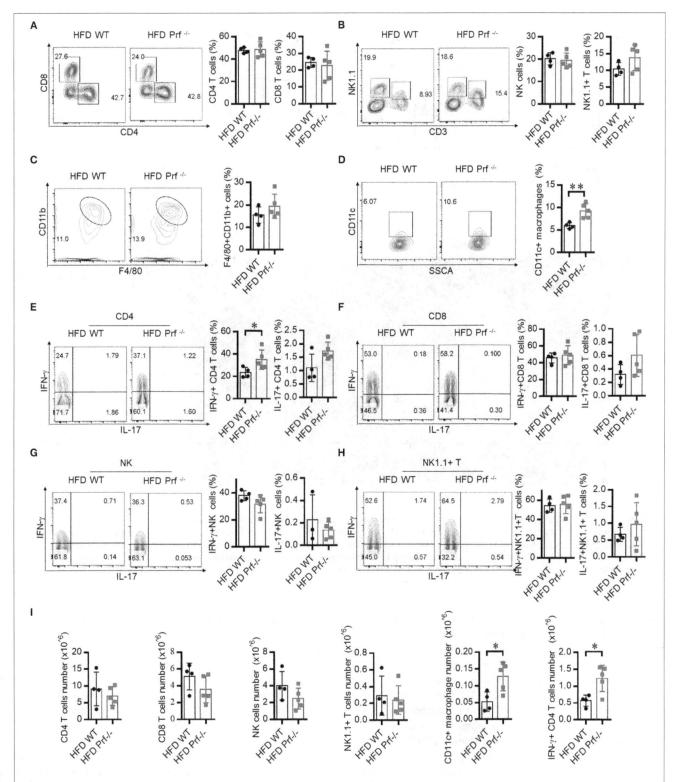

FIGURE 3 | Perforin deficiency drives inflammatory reactions in liver after HFD challenge. WT and Prf$^{-/-}$ mice were fed HFD for 10 weeks. Flow cytometry analysis of the representative histogram (left) and frequency (right) of liver CD4 T cells, CD8 T cells **(A)**, NK cells, NK1.1+ T cells **(B)**, macrophages **(C)**, and CD11c+ macrophages **(D)** and intracellular staining in the liver for IFN-γ and IL-17 in CD4 T cells **(E)**, CD8 T cells **(F)**, NK cells **(G)**, and NK1.1+ T cells **(H)**. **(I)** The total number of CD4 T cells, CD8 T cells, NK cells, and NK1.1+ T cells, CD11c+ macrophages and IFN-γ+CD4 T cells. $n = 4$–5 mice per group. The data shown in each panel of the figures were collected from a single experiment, and each experiment was repeated for at least three times and rendered consistent results. Means ± SEM; *$p < 0.05$.

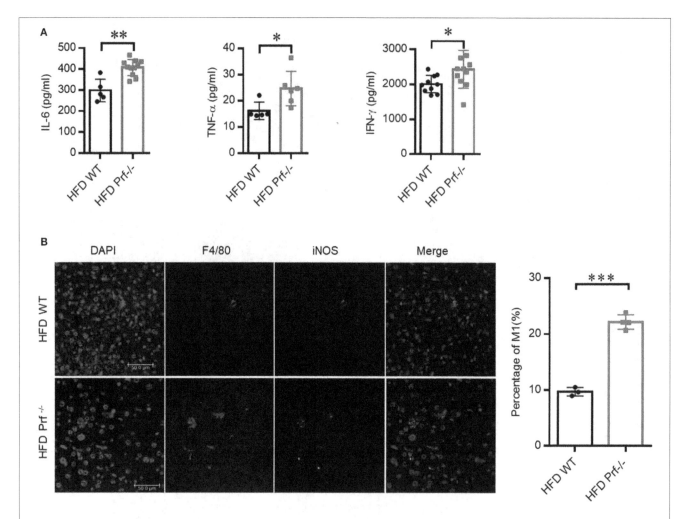

FIGURE 4 | Perforin deficiency drives the accumulation of M1 macrophages and releases of pro-inflammatory cytokines in the liver with HFD challenge. WT and Prf$^{-/-}$ mice were fed HFD for 10 weeks. **(A)** IL-6 (left panel, $n = 5$–11), TNF-α (middle panel, $n = 5$–6), and IFN-γ (right panel, $n = 10$–11) levels in liver supernatants. **(B)** Representative immunofluorescence images from liver with DAPI (blue), F4/80 (red), iNOS (green), and co-localization (merged image) (left) and the percentage of M1/M (refers to iNOS+F4/80+cells/F4/80+ cells) was calculated (right). The data shown in each panel of the figures were collected from a single experiment, and each experiment was repeated for at least three times and rendered consistent results. Means ± SEM, *$p < 0.05$; **$p < 0.01$; ***$p < 0.001$.

secreted by immune cells (19). Previous studies have shown that perforin-deficient mice are sensitive to obesity-induced insulin resistance as a result of restricted T cell expansion and activation in adipose tissue. Perforin has also been reported to play critical roles in promoting inflammation-mediated diseases, including type 1 diabetes (33), cerebral malaria (34), and viral myocarditis (35). A recent study revealed that perforin expressed in CD8 T cells regulates innate and adaptive immunity in the liver and exerts a protective effect in MCD (methionine/choline-deficient diet) diet-induced NASH models (36). Interestingly, MCD diet-induced non-obese NAFLD displays characteristics distinct from those of obesity-induced NAFLD. The precise role of perforin in liver metabolic disorders such as obesity-induced fatty liver disease has not been systematically researched yet. Using 14 month-old Prf$^{-/-}$ mice fed either normal chow or HFD, we demonstrated that perforin played a critical protective role in obesity-induced NAFLD.

In our mouse experiments, we chose male mice fed on HFD (60% fat) for 10 weeks to induce NAFLD and found that Prf$^{-/-}$ mice had more liver weight and liver TG accumulation in hepatocytes. These data are seemingly in contrast to a recent paper published by Cuff et al. which showed that after 24 weeks of obesogenic diet [22.6% fat, 23.0% protein, and 40.2% carbohydrate (w/w) supplement with sweetened condensed milk (Nestle) *ad libitum*], there was no difference in hepatomegaly and liver weight between the wild-type and perforin knockout female mice; otherwise, the fibrosis was significantly lower, and perforin KO mice suffer from less severe NAFLD mediated by NK cells (37). These conflicting findings may be due to the different diets, gender, and feeding time. In Cuff et al.'s paper, they chose 24 weeks as the timepoint so that they could compare the development of fibrosis, which is not usually pronounced at 10 weeks in NAFLD. Several reports indicated that free access to condensed milk induced an increase in serum AST activity

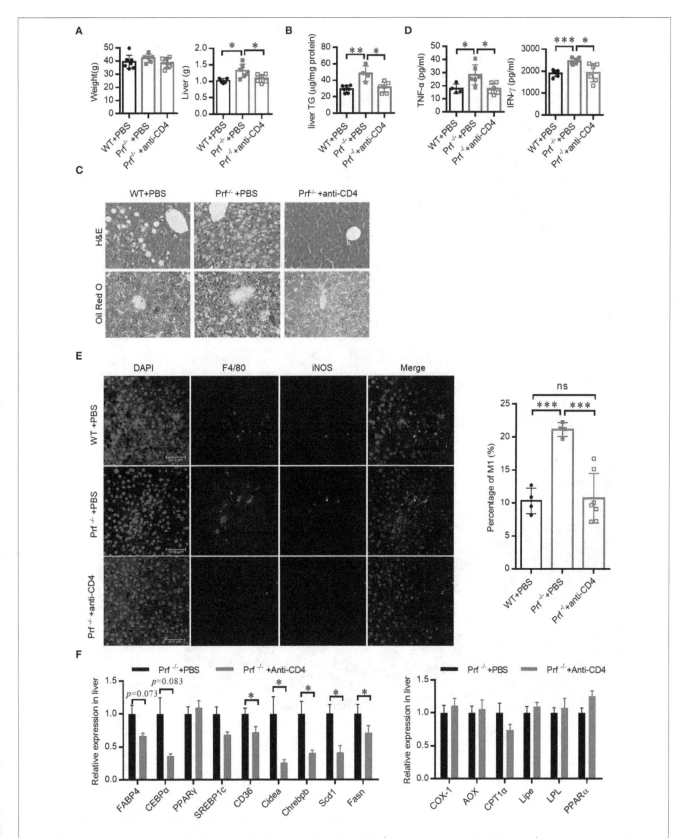

FIGURE 5 | Perforin regulates fatty liver disease through CD4 T cells in the liver. WT and Prf$^{-/-}$ mice were injected with PBS, or Prf$^{-/-}$ mice were injected with an anti-CD4 antibody weekly during 10 weeks of HFD challenge. **(A)** Body and liver weight were measured (n = 6–8). **(B)** Measurements of liver TG content (n = 4–7). **(C)**
(Continued)

FIGURE 5 | Representative images of liver sections stained with H&E (top) and Oil red O (bottom). **(D)** Serum TNF-α and IFN-γ levels were determined (n = 4–6). **(E)** Representative immunofluorescence images from liver with DAPI (blue), F4/80 (red), iNOS (green), and co-localization (merged image) (left) and the percentage of M1/M (refers to iNOS+F4/80+cells/F4/80+ cells) was calculated (right). **(F)** Expression levels of lipogenic genes (left) and fatty acid oxidation genes (right) in the liver relative to Hprt expression levels (n = 6–11). The data shown in each panel of the figures were collected from a single experiment, and each experiment was repeated for at least three times and rendered consistent results. Means ± SEM, *p < 0.05; **p < 0.01, ***p < 0.001.

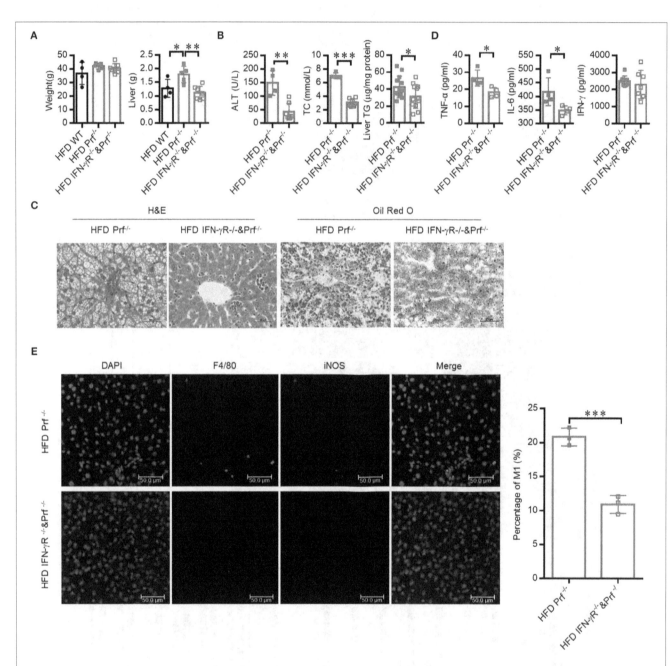

FIGURE 6 | Hepatic steatosis in Prf$^{-/-}$ mice is dependent on IFN-γ mediated inflammation. Prf$^{-/-}$ and IFN-γR$^{-/-}$ and Prf$^{-/-}$ mice were fed HFD for 10 weeks. **(A)** Body and liver weight were measured (n = 4–7). **(B)** Serum levels of ALT (left panel, n = 4–7), cholesterol (middle panel, n = 4–7), and liver TG (right panel) were measured (n = 12–13). **(C)** Representative images of liver sections stained with H&E (left) and Oil red O (right). **(D)** TNF-α, IL-6, and IFN-γ levels were detected in liver culture supernatants (n = 4). **(E)** Representative immunohistochemistry of DAPI (blue), F4/80 (red), iNOS (green), and co-localization (merged image) in liver, and the percentage of M1/M (refers to iNOS+F4/80+cells/ F4/80+ cells) was calculated (right). The data shown in each panel of the figures were collected from a single experiment, and each experiment was repeated for at least three times and rendered consistent results. Means ± SEM, *p < 0.05; **p < 0.01, ***p < 0.001.

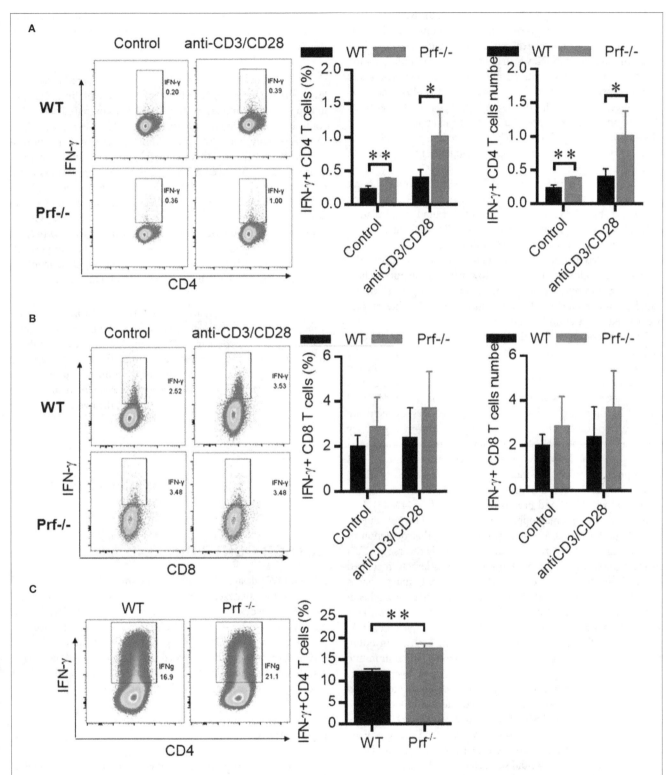

FIGURE 7 | CD4 T cells in Prf⁻/⁻ mice have an intrinsically elevated ability of IFN-γ production. CD4 T cells **(A)** and CD8 T cells **(B)** from WT and Prf⁻/⁻ mouse spleens were cultured in media supplemented with GolgiStop in the presence or absence of plate-bound anti-CD3 plus anti-CD28 for 4–6 h and then stained for intracellular IFN-γ (left, percentage; right, cell number, n = 5–6). **(C)** Naive CD4+ T cells were sorted from the spleen of WT or KO mice and differentiated to Th1 cells for 3 days. The IFN-γ production in these cells was detected by flow cytometry. Representative FACS plots and total cell number of IFN-γ+CD4+T cells were shown. The data shown in each panel of the figures were collected from a single experiment, and each experiment was repeated for at least three times and rendered consistent results. Means ± SEM, *p < 0.05; **p < 0.01.

and type I collagen deposition in the liver (38). NAFLD refers to a spectrum of liver diseases, including non-alcoholic fatty liver, which is characterized by steatosis with no or minor inflammation, and NASH, which is associated with inflammation and ballooning with or without fibrosis, and it may progress to liver cirrhosis and hepatocellular carcinoma (39, 40). The livers from mice fed a high-fat diet lacked fibrosis and showed mild steatosis and focal hepatocellular necrosis and apoptosis (41, 42). These contradictory findings suggest that perforin might have different actions at different stages during the pathogenesis of NAFLD and NASH.

Compared with WT controls, SFD-fed $Prf^{-/-}$ mice showed increased liver TG levels at an early age (**Figure 2C**), which suggests that perforin may regulate early liver lipid accumulation independent of diet. After 10 weeks of HFD challenge, $Prf^{-/-}$ mice had more IFN-γ-producing CD4 T cells in the liver. Further studies revealed that $Prf^{-/-}$ mice had intrinsically increased IFN-γ-producing ability in CD4 T cells. However, it is still unclear how perforin, a cytotoxic factor that helps mediate target cell death, could stimulate CD4 T cells to produce IFN-γ. Further studies are needed to better understand this phenomenon.

The promotion of hepatic steatosis resulting from perforin deficiency was associated with a strong increase in hepatic macrophage accumulation and inflammation as evaluated by the expression of TNF-α, IL-6, and iNOS. Traditionally, macrophages are divided into pro-inflammatory (M1) and wound-healing (M2) classes. M1 macrophages, which are induced by IFN-γ and LPS and express pro-inflammatory cytokines such as TNF-α, IL-6, and IL-1β, are implicated in the pathogenesis of chronic liver inflammation. M2 macrophages, which are induced by IL-4, IL-10, and IL-13 and produce IL-10, TGF-β, PDGF, and EGF, have anti-inflammatory effects and promote wound healing (43–45). It is well established that macrophages play an important role during NAFLD pathogenesis. Previous studies found that depletion of macrophages with clodronate could significantly reverse NAFLD in mice (3, 46). Liver immune homeostasis is largely regulated within the hepatic sinusoid, where resident macrophages (Kupffer cells) are located as part of the liver reticuloendothelial system (also known as the mononuclear phagocyte system). This system forms a highly active, dynamic, and complex network, constituting the primary line of defense against invading microorganisms along with the involvement of other immune cells such as neutrophils. In different stages of liver disease, resident Kupffer cells and freshly recruited monocyte-derived macrophages play a key role in the regulation of inflammation, fibrogenesis, and fibrolysis (47). In our study, $Prf^{-/-}$ mice had more macrophages, especially M1-type macrophage accumulation in liver after HFD challenge when compared with WT controls. However, we did not determine the mechanism of M1-type macrophage accumulation in the liver in this study. Is the increased accumulation due to the proliferation of resident Kupffer cells, or recruitment from peripheral circulatory systems, or the polarization of monocytes? We speculated that the increase in M1-type macrophage accumulation in the liver might be the result of monocyte polarization, since liver injury and lipid accumulation were almost non-existent in IFN-γR$^{-/-}$ &Prf$^{-/-}$ mice with decreased M1-type macrophage accumulation in

the liver when compared with $Prf^{-/-}$ mice. Further studies are necessary to better understand the mechanism behind this observation.

Depletion of CD4 T cells in $Prf^{-/-}$ mice rendered these mice less sensitive to NAFLD, with similar levels of liver TG and macrophage accumulation detected when compared with WT controls. This finding highlights the indispensable role of CD4 T cells, especially Th1 cells, in NAFLD progression. In clinical studies, it was reported that the peripheral CD4 compartment in obese children displayed a Th1-prone phenotype, and pediatric patients with NASH also showed increased expression of IFN-γ in the liver. Dysregulated lipid metabolism in NAFLD was reported to cause a selective loss of intrahepatic CD4+ lymphocytes, leading to accelerated hepatocarcinogenesis (48). In this study, we demonstrated that the protective effect of perforin in HFD-induced NAFLD was almost completely dependent on Th1 cells, which is consistent with the existing literature.

In conclusion, we demonstrated that perforin acts as an important immune regulator in NAFLD progression through regulating INF-γ-producing CD4 T cells to decrease macrophage accumulation in the liver. Based on these findings, therapeutic strategies targeting perforin might be a promising approach for the development of novel strategies to prevent or treat hepatic steatosis and related metabolic disorders in the liver.

ETHICS STATEMENT

The animal study was reviewed and approved by Laboratory Animal Ethics Committee Jinan University.

AUTHOR CONTRIBUTIONS

DL and QWa designed the project, performed experiments, and collected and analyzed the data. QWa wrote the manuscript. JZ and MZ worked on the mouse model. GC and JH helped modify and revise the article. QWe, HZ, and ZL maintained and genotyped the mice. LZ and QS performed RT-PCR. ZY, HY, and QWa supervised and coordinated the work, designed the overall research study, and helped write the manuscript. All authors have read, discussed, and approved the final manuscript.

FUNDING

This work was supported by the National Natural Science Foundation of China (the Key Program, 31830021), and the State Bureau of Foreign Experts Affairs (111 project, B16021) to ZY and HY. This work was also supported by the Science and Technology Department of the Guangdong Province of China (2018B030312008) to HY, the National Natural Science Foundation of China (grant 31800721 to QWa), the China Postdoctoral Fund (grant 2018M633278 to QWa), the National Natural Science Foundation of China (81630025, 31970830 to

JH), the Traditional Chinese Medicine Bureau of Guangdong Province (2018071 to JH), the Guangzhou Municipal Science and Technology Bureau (201904010090 to JH) and the Health Commission of Guangdong Province (A2019520 to JH).

ACKNOWLEDGMENTS

We thank Tucker Sarah for helping us correct typos and grammar errors and polish the text.

REFERENCES

Vernon G, Baranova A, Younossi ZM. Systematic review: the epidemiology and natural history of non-alcoholic fatty liver disease and non- alcoholic steatohepatitis in adults. *Aliment Pharm Ther.* (2011) 34:274–85. doi: 10.1111/j.1365-2036.2011.04724.x

Temple JL, Cordero P, Li J, Nguyen V, Oben JA. A guide to non-alcoholic fatty liver disease in childhood and adolescence. *Int J Mol Sci.* (2016) 17:947. doi: 10.3390/ijms17060947

Kazankov K, Jorgensen SMD, Thomsen KL, Moller HJ, Vilstrup H, George J, et al. The role of macrophages in nonalcoholic fatty liver disease and nonalcoholic steatohepatitis. *Nat Rev Gastroenterol Hepatol.* (2019) 16:145– 59. doi: 10.1038/s41575-018-0082-x

Cha JY, Kim DH, Chun KH. The role of hepatic macrophages in nonalcoholic fatty liver disease and nonalcoholic steatohepatitis. *Lab Anim Res.* (2018) 34:133–39. doi: 10.5625/lar.2018.34.4.133

Osayande AS, Kale N. Nonalcoholic fatty liver disease: identifying patients at risk of inflammation or fibrosis. *Am Family Phys.* (2017) 95:796–97.

Hardy T, Oakley F, Anstee QM, Day CP. Nonalcoholic fatty liver disease: pathogenesis and disease spectrum. *Annu Rev Pathol Mech.* (2016) 11:451– 96. doi: 10.1146/annurev-pathol-012615-044224

Koyama Y, Brenner DA. Liver inflammation and fibrosis. *J Clin Invest.* (2017) 127:55–64. doi: 10.1172/JCI88881

Campisi J. Aging, cellular senescence, and cancer. *Annu Rev Physiol.* (2013) 75:685–705. doi: 10.1146/annurev-physiol-030212-183653

Provinciali M, Cardelli M, Marchegiani F, Pierpaoli E. Impact of cellular senescence in aging and cancer. *Curr Pharm Des.* (2013) 19:1699– 709. doi: 10.2174/1381612811319090017

Herranz N, Gil J, Mechanisms and functions of cellular senescence. *J Clin Invest.* (2018) 128:1238–46. doi: 10.1172/JCI95148

Aravinthan A, Scarpini C, Tachtatzis P, Verma S, Penrhyn-Lowe S, Harvey R, et al. Hepatocyte senescence predicts progression in non-alcohol-related fatty liver disease. *J Hepatol.* (2013) 58:549–56. doi: 10.1016/j.jhep.2012. 10.031

Tacke F. Targeting hepatic macrophages to treat liver diseases. *J Hepatol.* (2017) 66:1300–12. doi: 10.1016/j.jhep.2017.02.026

Cai DS, Yuan MS, Frantz DF, Melendez PA, Hansen L, Lee J, et al. Local and systemic insulin resistance resulting from hepatic activation of IKK-beta and NF-kappaB. *Nat Med.* (2005) 11:183–90. doi: 10.1038/nm1166

Glass CK, Olefsky JM. Inflammation and lipid signaling in the etiology of insulin resistance. *Cell Metab.* (2012) 15:635– 45. doi: 10.1016/j.cmet.2012.04.001

Seki E, Schwabe RF. Hepatic inflammation and fibrosis: functional links and key pathways. *Hepatology.* (2015) 61:1066–79. doi: 10.1002/hep.27332

Badovinac VP, Tvinnereim AR, Harty JT. Regulation of antigen-specific CD8(+) T cell homeostasis by perforin and interferon-gamma. *Science.* (2000) 290:1354–7. doi: 10.1126/science.290.5495.1354

Bolitho P, Voskoboinik I, Trapani JA, Smyth MJ. Apoptosis induced by the lymphocyte effector molecule perforin. *Curr Opin Immunol.* (2007) 19:339– 47. doi: 10.1016/j.coi.2007.04.007

Voskoboinik I, Smyth MJ, Trapani JA. Perforin-mediated target- cell death and immune homeostasis. *Nat Rev Immunol.* (2006) 6:940–52. doi: 10.1038/nri1983

Voskoboinik I, Whisstock JC, Trapani JA. Perforin and granzymes: function, dysfunction and human pathology. *Nat Rev Immunol.* (2015) 15:388– 400. doi: 10.1038/nri3839

Spicer BA, Conroy PJ, Law RHP, Voskoboinik I, Whisstock JC. Perforin-A key (shaped) weapon in the immunological arsenal. *Semin Cell Dev Biol.* (2017) 72:117–23. doi: 10.1016/j.semcdb.2017.07.033

Revelo XS, Tsai S, Lei H, Luck H, Ghazarian M, Tsui H, et al. Perforin is a novel immune regulator of obesity-related insulin resistance. *Diabetes.* (2015) 64:90–103. doi: 10.2337/db13-1524

Zhang S, Liang R, Luo W, Liu C, Wu X, Gao Y, et al. High susceptibility to liver injury in IL-27 p28 conditional knockout mice involves intrinsic interferon-gamma dysregulation of CD4+ T cells. *Hepatology.* (2013) 57:1620–31. doi: 10.1002/hep.26166

Shan B, Wang X, Wu Y, Xu C, Xia Z, Dai J, et al. The metabolic ER stress sensor IRE1alpha suppresses alternative activation of macrophages and impairs energy expenditure in obesity. *Nat Immunol.* (2017) 18:519– 29. doi: 10.1038/ni.3709

Bertolotti M, Lonardo A, Mussi C, Baldelli E, Pellegrini E, Ballestri S, et al. Nonalcoholic fatty liver disease and aging: epidemiology to management. *World J Gastroenterol.* (2014) 20:14185–204. doi: 10.3748/wjg.v20.i39.14185

Ovadya Y, Landsberger T, Leins H, Vadai E, Gal H, Biran A, et al. Impaired immune surveillance accelerates accumulation of senescent cells and aging. *Nat Commun.* (2018) 9:5435. doi: 10.1038/s41467-018-07825-3

Sagiv A, Biran A, Yon M, Simon J, Lowe SW, Krizhanovsky V. Granule exocytosis mediates immune surveillance of senescent cells. *Oncogene.* (2013) 32:1971–7. doi: 10.1038/onc.2012.206

Alisi A, Carpino G, Oliveira FL, Panera N, Nobili V, Gaudio E. The role of tissue macrophage-mediated inflammation on NAFLD pathogenesis and its clinical implications. *Mediat Inflamm.* (2017) 2017:8162421. doi: 10.1155/2017/8162421

Friedman SL, Neuschwander-Tetri BA, Rinella M, Sanyal AJ. Mechanisms of NAFLD development and therapeutic strategies. *Nat Med.* (2018) 24:908– 22. doi: 10.1038/s41591-018-0104-9

Stojsavljevic S, Gomercic Palcic M, Virovic Jukic L, Smircic Duvnjak L, Duvnjak M. Adipokines and proinflammatory cytokines, the key mediators in the pathogenesis of nonalcoholic fatty liver disease. *World J Gastroenterol.* (2014) 20:18070–91. doi: 10.3748/wjg.v20.i48.18070

Angulo P, Alba LM, Petrovic LM, Adams LA, Lindor KD, Jensen MD. Leptin, insulin resistance, and liver fibrosis in human nonalcoholic fatty liver disease. *J Hepatol.* (2004) 41:943–9. doi: 10.1016/j.jhep.2004.08.020

Canbakan B, Tahan V, Balci H, Hatemi I, Erer B, Ozbay G, et al. Leptin in nonalcoholic fatty liver disease. *Ann Hepatol.* (2008) 7:249– 54. doi: 10.1016/S1665-2681(19)31856-3

Walch M, Latinovic-Golic S, Velic A, Sundstrom H, Dumrese C, Wagner CA, et al. Perforin enhances the granulysin-induced lysis of Listeria innocua in human dendritic cells. *BMC Immunol.* (2007) 8:14. doi: 10.1186/1471-2172-8-14

Kagi D, Odermatt B, Ohashi PS, Zinkernagel RM, Hengartner H. Development of insulitis without diabetes in transgenic mice lacking perforin-dependent cytotoxicity. *J Exp Med.* (1996) 183:2143–52. doi: 10.1084/jem.183.5.2143

Nitcheu J, Bonduelle O, Combadiere C, Tefit M, Seilhean D, Mazier D, et al. Perforin-dependent brain-infiltrating cytotoxic CD8+ T lymphocytes mediate experimental cerebral malaria pathogenesis. *J Immunol.* (2003) 170:2221–8. doi: 10.4049/jimmunol.170.4.2221

Koike H, Kanda T, Sumino H, Yokoyama T, Arai M, Motooka M, et al. Reduction of viral myocarditis in mice lacking perforin. *Res Commun Mol Pathol Pharmacol.* (2001) 110:229–37.

Wang T, Sun G, Wang Y, Li S, Zhao X, Zhang C, et al. The immunoregulatory effects of CD8 T-cell-derived perforin on diet-induced nonalcoholic steatohepatitis. *FASEB J.* (2019) 33:8490–503. doi: 10.1096/fj.201802534RR

Cuff AO, Sillito F, Dertschnig S, Hall A, Luong TV, Chakraverty R, et al. The obese liver environment mediates conversion of NK cells to a less cytotoxic ILC1-like phenotype. *Front Immunol.* (2019) 10:2180. doi: 10.3389/fimmu.2019.02180

Brown GT, Kleiner DE. Histopathology of nonalcoholic fatty liver disease and nonalcoholic steatohepatitis. *Metab Clin Exp.* (2016) 65:1080. doi: 10.1016/j.metabol.2015.11.008

Karagozian R, Derdak Z, Baffy G. Obesity-associated mechanisms of hepatocarcinogenesis. *Metab Clin Exp.* (2014) 63:607– 17. doi:

10.1016/j.metabol.2014.01.011

Starley BQ, Calcagno CJ, Harrison SA. Nonalcoholic fatty liver disease and hepatocellular carcinoma: a weighty connection. *Hepatology.* (2010) 51, 1820– 32. doi: 10.1002/hep.23594

Hebbard L, George J. Animal models of nonalcoholic fatty liver disease. *Nat Rev Gastro Hepat.* (2011) 8:34–44. doi: 10.1038/nrgastro.2010.191

Masi LN, Martins AR, Crisma AR, do Amaral CL, Davanso MR, Serdan TDA, et al. Combination of a high-fat diet with sweetened condensed milk exacerbates inflammation and insulin resistance induced by each separately in mice. *Sci Rep.* (2017) 7:3937. doi: 10.1038/s41598-017-04308-1

Murray PJ. Macrophage polarization. *Ann Rev Physiol.* (2017) 79:541– 66. doi: 10.1146/annurev-physiol-022516-034339

Saradna A, Do DC, Kumar S, Fu QL, Gao P. Macrophage polarization and allergic asthma. *Transl Res.* (2018) 191:1–14. doi: 10.1016/j.trsl.2017.09.002

Sica A, Erreni M, Allavena P, Porta C. Macrophage polarization in pathology. *CMLS.* (2015) 72:4111–26. doi: 10.1007/s00018-015-1995-y

Sica A, Invernizzi P, Mantovani A. Macrophage plasticity and polarization in liver homeostasis and pathology. *Hepatology.* (2014) 59:2034–42. doi: 10.1002/hep.26754

Freitas-Lopes MA, Mafra K, David BA, Carvalho-Gontijo R, Menezes GB. Differential location and distribution of hepatic immune cells. *Cells.* (2017) 6:E48. doi: 10.3390/cells6040048

Ma C, Kesarwala AH, Eggert T, Medina-Echeverz J, Kleiner DE, Jin P, et al. NAFLD causes selective CD4(+) T lymphocyte loss and promotes hepatocarcinogenesis. *Nature.* (2016) 531:253–7. doi: 10.1038/nature16969

16

Role of Kupffer Cells in Driving Hepatic Inflammation and Fibrosis in HIV Infection

Lumin Zhang and Meena B. Bansal*

Divison of Liver Diseases, Icahn School of Medicine at Mount Sinai, New York, NY, United States

Correspondence:
Meena B. Bansal
meena.bansal@mssm.edu

While the interactions between HIV and various liver cell populations have been explored, the relevance of these interactions when patients are well-controlled on ART is less clear. Therefore, we focus this perspective on HIV-related alterations that may drive hepatic inflammation and fibrosis in aviremic patients, with a focus on Kupffer cells and Hepatic Stellate Cells. Persistent CD4+ T cell depletion in the gut resulting in increased gut permeability has been postulated to play a role in systemic immune activation in HIV patients. The liver, with its unique location, remains the gatekeeper between the gut and the systemic circulation. The resident liver macrophage, Kupffer cell, is responsible for clearing and responding to these products. We propose that changes in Kupffer cell biology, in the context of HIV infection, creates a mileu that drives hepatic inflammation and fibrosis in response to microbial translocation. Targeting these pathways may be helpful in improving liver-related outcomes in HIV patients.

Keywords: liver fibrosis, HIV - human immunodeficiency virus, hepatic stellate cell (HSCs), Kupffer cells, microbial translocation

INTRODUCTION

End-stage liver disease is a major cause of non-AIDS related mortality in HIV+ patients even with effective anti-retroviral therapy, accounting for almost 15% of deaths (1–7). As a result of shared routes of transmission, HCV and HBV are the most common liver diseases in HIV-infected patients, although other chronic liver diseases are emerging (8, 9). Most data, therefore, regarding fibrosis progression rates is derived from those with coinfection. These patients have a higher relative risk (RR) of cirrhosis, increased development of decompensated cirrhosis and accelerated fibrosis progression rates compared with those who are only infected with HCV or HBV (10, 11). Furthermore, rapid fibrosis correlates with reduced CD4+ T cell counts and detectable plasma HIV levels. HIV patients are also more susceptible to other liver diseases, which synergize to accelerative liver fibrosis. Alcohol consumption is associated with increased relative risk of fibrosis progression in HIV mono-infected patients (12) while NASH is emerging as a major cause of liver disease, with half of mono-infected patients with unexplained liver enzyme elevations having NASH (13). While many may have an unrecognized chronic liver injury, a higher frequency of liver fibrosis was demonstrated in HIV-1–monoinfected patients (range 11–40.9%) compared with uninfected patients even without coinfection of hepatitis viruses and alcohol abuse, suggesting a correlation between HIV-1 infection and advanced liver fibrosis (14–19). Therefore, persistent HIV-1 infection and viral associated liver immune dysfunction may independently contribute to the progression of liver diseases (20). Lastly, in those on ART, drug-induced liver injury and increased rates of NASH due to both medications and metabolic derangements common in HIV are being observed. While hepatic stellate cells are the downstream effector of liver fibrosis, this perspective focuses on the role Kupffer cells play in promoting a mileu conducive to fibrosis progression in patients with HIV infection, particularly in aviremic patients.

THE LIVER AS THE GATEKEEPER

Shortly after HIV infection, a severe CD4+ T cell depletion in the gut-associated lymphoid tissues leads to a disruption of the intestinal barrier, consequently promoting translocation of microbial products into the portal circulation. The liver, which derives the majority of its blood flow from the portal circulation, is uniquely positioned to protect the systemic circulation from gut-derived products. In particular, the resident hepatic macrophage, the Kupffer cell, located within the hepatic sinusoid is charged with clearing translocated bacterial products in an immunotolerant manner. However, when products provoke a pro-inflammatory response by Kupffer cells, a cascade of intrahepatic inflammatory respones is initiated with numerous secreted cytokines, such as IL-1β, TNF-α, and IL-6, serving as major drivers in the progression of liver injury and fibrosis.

KUPFFER CELLS AT THE NEXUS OF LIVER INFLAMMATORY RESPONSES

Kupffer cells (KCs) are the largest population of resident tissue macrophages in the liver. They reside within the hepatic sinusoid in close proximity to hepatic stellate cells, liver sinusoidal endothelia cells, and intrahepatic lymphocytes. Both the low flow state of the portal circulation and the uniquely fenestrated endothelium create a conducive environment for interaction of KCs with neighboring cells and circulating cells of the immune system. Physiologically, KCs are the first line of defense to eliminate macromolecules, immune complexes, senescent cells, virally-infected cells, and translocated microbial products from the gut to avoid liver injury and systemic immune responses (21). Given the dynamic nature of cell surface receptor expression on macrophage populations and some controversy regarding their origins, CD163 or CD68, CD14 and CD16 are often used to identify human KCs. However, murine KCs display phenotypic patterns characterized by F4/80+, MHCII, and CD11b^{Int} expression. A detailed discussion of markers for various macrophage subpopulations within the liver is beyond the scope of this perspective and discussed elsewhere (22). The focus of this perspective is on the role of CD68+human KCs in promoting liver inflammation and fibrosis in patients with HIV.

The importance of KCs in liver injury and inflammation have been established with depletion studies wherein GdCl$_3$ was associated with AST reduction and inflammation in an alcohol model of liver injury (23). Crosstalk between KCs and HSCs is also evidenced by KC depletion as mRNA levels of TGF-β, α-SMA and collagen I are significantly decreased (24). Although GdCl3 is not specific to KCs, and thus interpretation is complex, GdCl3 treatment dramatically decreased cytokines predominantly produced by KCs, TNF-α, IL-6, and IL-1β, in

response to LPS stimulation in murine livers (25, 26). Similarly, liposome/clodronate can suppress pro-inflammatory responses through the depletion of KCs (27).

In homeostasis, KCs are central to intrahepatic immune tolerance through an antigen-mediated induction of functional arrest of CD4 cells and regulatory T cells. However, in an inflamed microenvironment this delicate equilibrium is disrupted resulting in immune dysfunction and tolerance break (28). Indeed, knockout of TREM-1 (Triggering receptor expressed on myeloid cells), which is highly expressed on KCs in liver fibrosis, reduced liver fibrosis through the inhibition of TNF-α and IL-6 responses in a number of chronic injury models (29). Similarly, knock down of Jun N-terminal kinase ½ (JNK-1/2) from KCs reversed liver fibrosis in a choline-deficient L-aminoacid-defined (CDAA) model, with a decline in inflammatory responses, including TNF-α, IL6, IL-1β, and TGF-β (30).

While KCs display M1-like features in acute liver injury, with protracted chronic inflammation, due to exhaustion of M1-like macrophages and immune cells, M2-like macrophages emerge and secrete protective cytokines upon chronic cytotoxic stimulation such as IL-4, IL-10, and TGF-β (31, 32). IL-10, an anti-inflammatory cytokine, down-regulates macrophage effector functions and differentiation of neighboring cells to maintain immune microenvironment homeostasis. For example, administration of IL-10 decreased TNF-α produced from LPS-treated KCs (33). While very complex, the manipulation of KC mediated immune responses or approaches to limit their stimulation may be exploited therapeutically.

MICROBIAL TRANSLOCATION AND KUPFFER CELLS

The impact of translocated microbial products on KCs is well-established. pretreatment with 2.5% dextran sulphate sodium (DSS) causes increased intestinal permeability and promotes translocation of microbial products into the portal blood in mice. The resulting amplified TLR4 mediated inflammatory responses in KCs resulted in significant livery injury (34). Using a liver slice model, LPS stimulation increased IL-1β and TNF-α production compared to the control (35). Consistently, in mouse models, LPS administration rapidly induces the release of inflammatory cytokines in the liver with a higher IL-6 production obtained from LPS stimulated KCs than splenic and alveolar macrophages (36).

THE ROLE OF TLR4 SIGNALING IN INFLAMMATORY RESPONSES OF KUPFFER CELLS

TLR4, as one member of Toll-like receptors, belongs to the pattern recognition receptor (PRR) family. After stimulation by TLR4 ligands, for example lipopolysaccharides, TLR4 is activated through conformational changes and interaction with TIR-domain-containing adapter proteins via hydrophilic interactions. Intracellular TLR4 signaling is mediated by two classical pathways: the TIRAP–MyD88-NF-κB pathway and the TRIF–TRAM-interferon regulatory factor-3 (IRF3)-NF-κB pathway. TLR4 signaling participates in the initiation of pro-inflammatory response, especially TRIF mediated TNF-α and synthesis of chemokines and have been reveiwed in detail elswhere (37).

In addition to TNF-α, TLR4 signaling also contributes to the transmission of two priming signals for the IL-1β pathway through the NLRP3 inflammasome. IL-1β is a crucial proinflammatory cytokine in response to microbial infection. IL-1β from LPS-treated KCs can produce a deleterious effect on hepatocytes and promote the secretion of VLDL apo B and lipid (38). IL-1β was also found to inhibit IFN-α induced STAT1 activation in hepatocytes, attenuating the innate immune response to viral infection in hepatocytes (39). In general, NLRP3 mediated-cleavage of caspase 1 is the critical step to promote the maturation of IL-1β. The formation of the NLRP3 inflammasome is initiated by ATP or microbial stimulation (40). Blockage of NLRP3 activation in KCs decreased IL-1β response to Ischemia/Reperfusion induced liver injury and improved survival (41, 42). Administration of MCC950, a small molecule selective inhibitor of NLRP3, suppressed LPS primed IL-1β response in NPC cells, subsequently, decreasing liver injury (43). Given the important role of TLR4 signaling in KCs, the modulation of this pathway in the context of HIV infection and persistent microbial translocation is critical.

MODULATION OF INFLAMMATORY RESPONSES BY HIV-1 INFECTION IN KCS

In addition to CD4, both CCR5 and CXCR4, HIV-1 co-receptors, are detected on human KCs isolated from non-HIV-1 individuals, suggesting that KCs are permissive for HIV-1 infection. HIV-1 infection of KCs in viremic patients has been shown by *in situ* hybridization for HIV-1 RNA and PCR for proviral DNA on FACS-purifed KCs from livers of patients with Acquired Immunodeficiency Sydnrome (AIDs) (44–46). Moreover, retrieval of HIV-1 from KCs derived from patients either not on ART (47) or on ART for short durations has been shown and supported by studies in SIV$_{DH12R}$-infected macaques (48, 49). Recently it has been shown that KCs derived from patients on long term ART, while containing evidence of HIV-1 transcripts, do not secrete replication competent virus (50). While macrophages are known to be able to transmit infectious virus to susceptible CD4+ cells via cell-cell contact (51, 52), the ability of KCs in patients on long-term ART to do so has not yet been explored though warrants investigation.

We have shown that Kupffer cells are highly permissive for HIV-1 infection *in vitro* with robust and sustained viral replication (53). HIV-1$_{BaL}$, a laboratory adapted CCR5-tropic HIV, infection rendered KCs more sensitive to LPS treatment through an increase in CD14 and TLR4 expression on the cell surface, resulting in increased secretion of TNF-α and IL-6, which was blocked by a small molecule TLR4 inhibitor. Interestingly, despite AZT and ritonavir abrogated viral replication, KCs maintained their sensitivity to the pro-inflammatory response to LPS. These findings suggest that even in patients on

ART, KC biology may be impacted and promote a mileu supporting hepatic inflammation and fibrosis in response to microbial translocation. While no change in IFNα or IFNβ expression in HIV-1 infected KCs was observed, IL-1β mRNA and both intracellular and secreted IL-1β was increased by HIV-1$_{BaL}$ infection. Similar to the IL-6 and TNF-α response, this HIV-related sensitization was found to be TLR4-dependent and further determined to be via the NLRP3-caspase 1 pathway. Immunostaining on liver tissue derived from aviremic HIV+ patients demonstrated an increased expression of IL-1β compared to normal liver with a high degree of colocalization in CD68+ macrophages (54). These studies show that TLR4 mediated NLRP3 activation is critical for the inflammatory responses to microbial products in KCs. Importantly, liver injury and resulting damage-associated molecular patterns (DAMPS) also activate TLR4 signals in KCs and thus may play a role in other forms of liver injury in HIV patients such as drug-induced liver injury. Interestingly, it has also been shown that CCR5 and TLR may co-cluster on monocyte-derived macrophages (MDMs) as secretion of CCL2 and CXCL8 in response to either R5 gp120, recombinant envelope protein from CCR5-tropic HIV-1, or LPS can be blocked by either a CCR5 inhibitor or TLR4 blocking. These results suggest another mechanism for synergistic effects of HIV and LPS on macrophage biology and should be specifically examined in human KCs (55).

INFLAMMATORY RESPONSES TO HIV-1 INFECTION IN OTHER LIVER IMMUNE CELLS

While beyond the scope of this perspective, HIV-1 infection impacts a number of other cells critical to the inflammatory response in the liver. In line with circulating CD4+ T cells, HIV infection leads to a depletion of CD4+ T cell in the liver with relative reversal of CD4/CD8 ratio typically seen. Viral infection also makes IL2+ CD4+ T cells dysfunctional and attenuates hepatic immune response to microbial infection (56–58). CD4+ T cells from HIV mono-infected patients exhibit a low regulatory effect on Natural killer (NK). Co-cultured with NK cells, CD4+ T cells from HIV-1+ individuals greatly reduced anti-fibrotic effect of NK cells on HSCs (59). Therefore, reduction in CD4+ T cells influences progression of liver fibrosis in HIV+ patients (10, 60) while increased relative CD8+T cells correlates with a higher fibrosis scores in HIV-1 infected patients (61).

NK cells, which account for up to 30–50% human liver lymphocytes, play an important role in clearing virally infected cells trough NK cell antibody dependent cell cytotoxicity (ADCC). The activation and NK cellular numbers are spontaneously increased early in response to HIV-1 infection but with chronic infection exhaustion results in NK dysfunction with persistent viremia (62).

While the role of DCs in HIV-1 infection and progression and ability to transmit infectious virus to CD4 cells by cell-cell contact has been shown, HIV interaction with DCs in the liver is less studied. TLR7 is constitutively expressed by human pDCs. The delivery of HIV-1 viral nucleic acids in early endosome of pDCs can be blocked by TLR7 inhibitor (63), suggesting that TLR7 is involved in the antigen presentation by pDCs. In addition, mDC express TLR4 and the frequency of mDCs, especially CXCL16-producing mDCs has been shown to be associated with the level of microbial products in the liver of HIV+ patients (64).

INTERACTIONS BETWEEN HIV AND HEPATOCYTES AND IMPLICATIONS FOR HEPATIC INFLAMMATION AND FIBROSIS

In vitro studies have shown that the envelope protein, HIV gp 120, which binds either CXCR4 (X4) or CCR5 (R5) on its target cell can promote hepatocyte apoptosis (65) and along with the HCV glycoprotein E2 promote the secretion of the pro-inflammatory cytokine IL-8 (66, 67). It has been known that Kupffer cells play a primary role in the clearance of apoptotic hepatocytes/cellular debris within the liver and thus play a key role in sterile inflammation and repair (68). More recently, Ganesan et. al demonstrated that ethanol exposure promotes HIV accumulation within hepatocytes, ultimately leading to increased oxidative stress and apoptosis. These apoptotic hepatocytes then stimulate inflammasome activation in KCs and pro-fibrogenic genes in hepatic stellate cells (69). Moreover, hepatic stellate cells can also engulf apoptotic hepatocytes resulting in NAPDH oxidation, stellate cell activation, and fibrogenesis (70). Therefore, effects on HIV on hepatocytes can promote both KC and HSC activation, synergistically driving hepatic inflammation and fibrosis.

DIRECT INTERACTIONS BETWEEN HIV AND HUMAN STELLATE CELLS

HSCs express both HIV CCR5 and CXCR4 co-receptors. We have shown that HIV and its envelope protein gp120 promote HSC activation, collagen I production, and CCL2 secretion through interactions with CXCR4 (71) and others have shown that the envelope protein on HIV that preferentially uses CCR5 for cellular entry (R5 gp120) promotes HSC chemotaxis and CCL2 secretion (72). While HIV can infect HSCs *in vitro*, infection *in vivo* has not been established. Similar to what has recently been shown for KCs, *in vitro* infected HSCs do not secrete replication competent virus though, like DCs, may be able to transmit virus by cell-cell contact (71, 73, 74). Similar to what has been shown on MDMs, CCR5 and TLR4 seem to co-cluster on HSCs and result in increased CCL2 and CXCL8 in response to gp120 and LPS, with effects of ligands blocked by inhibiting either receptor alone (55). As CCL2 is an important chemokine for attracting circulating monocytes into the liver, this may be important for propagating hepatic inflammation. R5 gp120 also promotes IL-6 secretion from HSCs through Jun-NF-kB activation (75). These studies suggest that HIV promotes inflammation and fibrosis by interacting with CXCR4 and CCR5 via gp120 and synergizes with TLR4 signals. While the

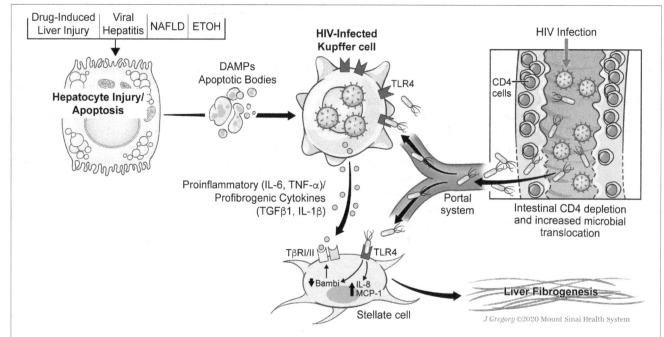

FIGURE 1 | Role of HIV and associated microbial translocation in driving hepatic inflammation and fibrosis through kupffer cell and stellate cell interactions. HIV infection causes early CD4 gut depletion which promotes increased microbial translocation and the delivery of pathogen-associated molecular patterns to the liver (PAMPs). At the same time, patients with HIV have multiple secondary chronic liver injuries (NAFLD, DILI, HCV, HBV, Alcohol) which promote direct injury to hepatocytes and give rise to damage-associated molecular patterns (DAMPs) or endogenous TLR ligands. HIV infected KCs are sensitized to effects of both the translocated microbial products as well as DAMPs. These signals converge on the HIV-infected KCs resulting in the secretion of a number of pro-inflammatory (IL-6, TNF-α) and pro-fibrogenic cytokines (IL-1β and TGFβ1). Additionally, TLR ligands have pro-inflammatory effects on HSCs and sensitize them to KC-derived TGFβ1. Used with permission from @Mount Sinai Health System.

latter is important in viremic patients, relevance for those on ART are not clear. For those on ART, the impact of HIV on microbial translocation and KC biology may be more important.

INTERPLAY BETWEEN KUPFFER CELLS AND HEPATIC STELLATE CELLS

While the ultimate effector cell in liver fibrosis is the hepatic stellate cell, the signals generated by KCs are critically important in promoting the activation of HSCs and then perpetuating the activated state. TLR4 activation on HSCs results in downregulation of the TGFβ1 pseudoreceptor, BAMBI, which sensitizes HSCs to the pro-fibrogenic effects of TGFβ1 (76), much of which is derived by KCs. Therefore, in the context of HIV-1 and associated microbial translocation, the effects on both KCs and HSCs are compounded and drive hepatic inflammation and fibrosis (**Figure 1**). Overall association between microbial translocation and liver fibrosis progression has been shown in a variety of liver diseases and thus HIV simply compounds this effect.

CONCLUSION

As patients with HIV live longer, liver disease will continue to emerge as a leading cause of morbidity and mortality.

Understanding how HIV may set the stage for hepatic injury, inflammation and fibrosis may lead to novel therapeutic strategies. While treatment of underlying diseases, ranging from viral hepatitis to NASH or alcohol, remains the most imporant strategy, the alterations unique to this population need to be kept in mind. With this perspective, HIV related alterations in KC biology and microbial translocation may be at the nexus of creating a milue conducive to hepatic fibrosis. Targeting either the KC response to TLR4 ligands, PAMPs or DAMPS, decreasing the burden of microbial products from reaching the portal circulation, or blocking downstream pro-inflammatory or pro-fibrogenic effects on stellate cells are important to consider. Much will be learned from current treatments undergoing investigation for non-HIV related liver fibrosis that may be additionally leveraged for this special population.

AUTHOR CONTRIBUTIONS

LZ and MB wrote and reviewed this manuscript.

REFERENCES

Lifson AR, Group ICODW, Belloso WH, Carey C, Davey RT, Duprez D, et al. Determination of the underlying cause of death in three multicenter international HIV clinical trials. *HIV Clin Trials.* (2008) 9:177–85. doi: 10.1310/hct0903-177

Data Collection on Adverse Events of Anti-HIV drugs (D:A:D) Study Group, Smith C, Sabin CA, Lundgren JD, Thiebaut R, Weber R, et al. Factors associated with specific causes of death amongst HIV- positive individuals in the D:A:D Study. *AIDS.* (2010) 24:1537–48. doi:10.1097/QAD.0b013e32833a0918

Price JC, Thio CL. Liver disease in the HIV-infected individual. *Clin Gastroenterol Hepatol.* (2010) 8:1002–12. doi:10.1016/j.cgh.2010.08.024

Leone S, Gregis G, Quinzan G, Velenti D, Cologni G, Soavi L, et al. Causes of death and risk factors among HIV-infected persons in the HAART era: analysis of a large urban cohort. *Infection.* (2011) 39:13–20. doi:10.1007/s15010-010-0079-z

Puoti M, Moioli MC, Travi G, Rossotti R. The burden of liver disease in human immunodeficiency virus-infected patients. *Semin Liver Dis.* (2012) 32:103–13. doi:10.1055/s-0032-1316473

Weber R, Ruppik M, Rickenbach M, Spoerri A, Furrer H, Battegay M, et al. Decreasing mortality and changing patterns of causes of death in the Swiss HIV Cohort Study. *HIV Med.* (2013) 14:195–207. doi:10.1111/j.1468-1293.2012.01051.x

Salmon-Ceron D, Rosenthal E, Lewden C, Bouteloup V, May T, Burty C, et al. Emerging role of hepatocellular carcinoma among liver-related causes of deaths in HIV-infected patients: the French national Mortalite 2005 study. *J Hepatol.* (2009) 50:736–45. doi:10.1016/j.jhep.2008.11.018

Vallet-Pichard A, Mallet V, Pol S. Nonalcoholic fatty liver disease and HIV infection. *Semin Liver Dis.* (2012). 32:158–66. doi:10.1055/s-0032-1316471

Stabinski L, Reynolds SJ, Ocama P, Laeyendecker O, Ndyanabo A, Kiggundu V. et al. High prevalence of liver fibrosis associated with HIV infection: a study in rural Rakai, Uganda. *Antivir Ther.* (2011) 16:405–11. doi: 10.3851/IMP1783

Benhamou Y, Bochet M, Di Martino V, Charlotte F, Azria F, Coutellier A, et al. Liver fibrosis progression in human immunodeficiency virus and hepatitis C virus

coinfected patients. *The Multivirc Group Hepatol.* (1999) 30:1054–8. doi: 10.1002/hep.510300409

Macías J, Berenguer J, Japón MA, Girón JA, Rivero A, López-Cortés LF, et al., Fast fibrosis progression between repeated liver biopsies in patients coinfected with human immunodeficiency virus/hepatitis C virus. *Hepatology.* (2009) 50:1056–63. doi: 10.1002/hep.23136

Chaudhry AA, Sulkowski MS, Chander G, Moore RD. Hazardous drinking is associated with an elevated aspartate aminotransferase to platelet ratio index in an urban HIV-infected clinical cohort. *HIV Med.* (2009) 10:133–42. doi: 10.1111/j.1468-1293.2008.00662.x

Joshi D, O'grady J, Dieterich D, Gazzard B, Agarwal K. Increasing burden of liver disease in patients with HIV infection. *Lancet.* (2011) 377:1198–209. doi: 10.1016/S0140-6736(10)62001-6

Dallapiazza M, Amorosa VK, Localio R, Kostman JR, Lo Re V III. Prevalence and risk factors for significant liver fibrosis among HIV-monoinfected patients. *BMC Infect Dis.* (2010). 10:116. doi: 10.1186/1471-2334-10-116

Merchante N, Perez-Camacho I, Mira JA, Rivero A, Macias J, Camacho A, et al. Prevalence and risk factors for abnormal liver stiffness in HIV-infected patients without viral hepatitis coinfection: role of didanosine. *Antivir Ther.* (2010) 15:753–63. doi: 10.3851/IMP1612

Han SH, Kim SU, Kim CO, Jeong SJ, Park JY, Choi JY, et al. Abnormal liver stiffness assessed using transient elastography (Fibroscan(R)) in HIV-infected patients without HBV/HCV coinfection receiving combined antiretroviral treatment. *PLoS ONE.* (2013) 8:e52720. doi: 10.1371/journal.pone.0052720

Tahiri M, Sodqi M, Lahdami FE, Marih L, Lamdini H, Hliwa W, et al. Risk factors for liver fibrosis among human immunodeficiency virus monoinfected patients using the FIB4 index in Morocco. *World J Hepatol.* (2013) 5:584–8. doi:10.4254/wjh.v5.i10.584

Rockstroh JK, Mohr R, Behrens G, Spengler U. Liver fibrosis in HIV: which role does HIV itself, long-term drug toxicities and metabolic changes play? *Curr Opin HIV AIDS.* (2014) 9:365–70. doi: 10.1097/COH.0000000000000064

Anadol E, Lust K, Boesecke C, Schwarze-Zander C, Mohr R, Wasmuth JC, et al. Exposure to previous cART is associated with significant liver fibrosis and cirrhosis in human immunodeficiency virus-infected patients. *PLoS ONE.* (2018) 13:e0191118. doi: 10.1371/journal.pone.0191118

Lamers SL, Rose R, Maidji E, Agsalda-Garcia M, Nolan DJ, Fogel GB, et al. HIV

DNA is frequently present within pathologic tissues evaluated at autopsy from combined antiretroviral therapy-treated patients with undetectable viral loads. *J Virol.* (2016) 90:8968–83. doi: 10.1128/JVI.00674-16

Shi J, Fujieda H, Kokubo Y, Wake K. Apoptosis of neutrophils and their elimination by Kupffer cells in rat liver. *Hepatology.* (1996) 24:1256–63. doi: 10.1002/hep.510240545

Guillot A, Tacke F. Liver macrophages: old dogmas and new insights. *Hepatol Commun.* (2019) 3:730–43. doi: 10.1002/hep4.1356

Adachi Y, Bradford BU, Gao W, Bojes HK, Thurman RG. Inactivation of Kupffer cells prevents early alcohol-induced liver injury. *Hepatology.* (1994) 20:453–60. doi: 10.1002/hep.1840200227

Canbay A, Feldstein AE, Higuchi H, Werneburg N, Grambihler A, Bronk SF, et al. Kupffer cell engulfment of apoptotic bodies stimulates death ligand and cytokine expression. *Hepatology.* (2003) 38:1188–98. doi: 10.1053/jhep.2003.50472

Rizzardini M, Zappone M, Villa P, Gnocchi P, Sironi M, Diomede L, et al. Kupffer cell depletion partially prevents hepatic heme oxygenase 1 messenger RNA accumulation in systemic inflammation in mice: role of interleukin 1beta. *Hepatology.* (1998) 27:703–10. doi: 10.1002/hep.510270311

Tomiyama K, Ikeda A, Ueki S, Nakao A, Stolz DB, Koike Y, et al. Inhibition of Kupffer cell-mediated early proinflammatory response with carbon monoxide in transplant-induced hepatic ischemia/reperfusion injury in rats. *Hepatology.* (2008) 48:1608–20. doi: 10.1002/hep.22482

Ju C, Reilly TP, Bourdi M, Radonovich MF, Brady JN, George JW, et al. Protective role of Kupffer cells in acetaminophen-induced hepatic injury in mice. *Chem Res Toxicol.* (2002) 15:1504–13. doi: 10.1021/tx0255976

Heymann F, Peusquens J, Ludwig-Portugall I, Kohlhepp M, Ergen C, Niemietz P, et al. Liver inflammation abrogates immunological tolerance induced by Kupffer cells. *Hepatology.* (2015) 62:279–91. doi: 10.1002/hep.27793

Nguyen-Lefebvre AT, Ajith A, Portik-Dobos V, Horuzsko DD, Arbab AS, Dzutsev A, et al. The innate immune receptor TREM-1 promotes liver injury and fibrosis. *J Clin Invest.* (2018) 128:4870–83. doi: 10.1172/JCI98156

Kodama Y, Kisseleva T, Iwaisako K, Miura K, Taura K, De Minicis S, et al. c-Jun N-terminal kinase-1 from hematopoietic cells mediates progression from hepatic steatosis to steatohepatitis and fibrosis in mice. *Gastroenterology.* (2009) 137:1467–77 e1465. doi: 10.1053/j.gastro.2009.06.045

Mantovani A, Sica A. Macrophages, innate immunity and cancer: balance, tolerance, and diversity. *Curr Opin Immunol.* (2010) 22:231–7. doi: 10.1016/j.coi.2010.01.009

Coussens LM, Zitvogel L, Palucka AK. Neutralizing tumor-promoting chronic inflammation: a magic bullet? *Science.* (2013) 339:286–91. doi: 10.1126/science.1232227

Wan J, Benkdane M, Teixeira-Clerc F, Bonnafous S, Louvet A, Lafdil F, et al. M2 Kupffer cells promote M1 Kupffer cell apoptosis: a protective mechanism against alcoholic and nonalcoholic fatty liver disease. *Hepatology.* (2014) 59:130–42. doi: 10.1002/hep.26607

El Kasmi KC, Anderson AL, Devereaux MW, Fillon SA, Harris JK, Lovell MA, et al. Toll-like receptor 4-dependent Kupffer cell activation and liver injury in a novel mouse model of parenteral nutrition and intestinal injury. *Hepatology.* (2012) 55:1518–28. doi: 10.1002/hep.25500

Olinga P, Merema MT, De Jager MH, Derks F, Melgert BN, Moshage H, et al. Rat liver slices as a tool to study LPS-induced inflammatory response in the liver. *J Hepatol.* (2001) 35:187–94. doi: 10.1016/S0168-8278(01)00103-9

Ogle CK, Wu JZ, Mao X, Szczur K, Alexander JW, Ogle JD. Heterogeneity of Kupffer cells and splenic, alveolar, and peritoneal macrophages for the production of TNF, IL-1, and IL-6. *Inflammation.* (1994) 18:511–23. doi: 10.1007/BF01560698

Vaure C, Liu Y. A comparative review of toll-like receptor 4 expression and functionality in different animal species. *Front Immunol.* (2014) 5:316. doi: 10.3389/fimmu.2014.00316

Bartolome N, Arteta B, Martinez MJ, Chico Y, Ochoa B. Kupffer cell products and interleukin 1beta directly promote VLDL secretion and apoB mRNA up-regulation in rodent hepatocytes. *Innate Immun.* (2008) 14:255–66. doi: 10.1177/1753425908094718

Tian Z, Shen X, Feng H, Gao B. IL-1 beta attenuates IFN-alpha beta- induced antiviral activity and STAT1 activation in the liver: involvement of proteasome-dependent pathway. *J Immunol.* (2000) 165:3959–65. doi: 10.4049/jimmunol.165.7.3959

He Y, Hara H, Nunez G. Mechanism and regulation of NLRP3 inflammasome activation. *Trends Biochem Sci.* (2016) 41:1012–21. doi: 10.1016/j.tibs.2016.09.002

Huang H, Chen HW, Evankovich J, Yan W, Rosborough BR, Nace GW, et al. Histones activate the NLRP3 inflammasome in Kupffer cells during sterile inflammatory liver injury. *J Immunol.* (2013) 191:2665–79. doi: 10.4049/jimmunol.1202733

Xu Y, Yao J, Zou C, Zhang H, Zhang S, Liu J, et al. Asiatic acid protects against hepatic ischemia/reperfusion injury by inactivation of Kupffer cells via PPARgamma/NLRP3 inflammasome signaling pathway. *Oncotarget.* (2017) 8:86339–55. doi: 10.18632/oncotarget.21151

Mridha AR, Wree A, Robertson A, a,B, Yeh MM, Johnson CD, et al. NLRP3 inflammasome blockade reduces liver inflammation and fibrosis in experimental NASH in mice. *J Hepatol.* (2017) 66:1037–46. doi: 10.1016/j.jhep.2017.01.022

Housset C, Lamas E, Brechot C. Detection of HIV1 RNA and p24 antigen in HIV1-infected human liver. *Res Virol.* (1990) 141:153–9. doi:10.1016/0923-2516(90)90017-D

Hoda SA, White JE, Gerber MA. Immunohistochemical studies of human immunodeficiency virus-1 in liver tissues of patients with AIDS. *Mod Pathol.* (1991) 4:578–81.

Schmitt MP, Steffan AM, Gendrault JL, Jaeck D, Royer C, Schweitzer C, et al. Multiplication of human immunodeficiency virus in primary cultures of human Kupffer cells–possible role of liver macrophage infection in the physiopathology of AIDS. *Res Virol.* (1990) 141:143–52. doi:10.1016/0923-2516(90)90016-C

Schweitzer C, Keller F, Schmitt MP, Jaeck D, Adloff M, Schmitt C, et al. Morphine stimulates HIV replication in primary cultures of human Kupffer cells. *Res Virol.* (1991) 142:189–95. doi: 10.1016/0923-2516(91)90056-9

Persidsky Y, Steffan AM, Gendrault JL, Hurtrel B, Berger S, Royer C, et al. Permissiveness of Kupffer cells for simian immunodeficiency virus (SIV) and morphological changes in the liver of rhesus monkeys at different periods of SIV infection. *Hepatology.* (1995) 21:1215–25. doi: 10.1002/hep.1840210502

Igarashi T, Brown CR, Endo Y, Buckler-White A, Plishka R, Bischofberger N, et al. Macrophage are the principal reservoir and sustain high virus loads in rhesus macaques after the depletion of CD4+ T cells by a highly pathogenic simian immunodeficiency virus/HIV type 1 chimera (SHIV): implications for HIV-1 infections of humans. *Proc Natl Acad Sci USA.* (2001) 98:658–63. doi: 10.1073/pnas.98.2.658

Kandathil AJ, Sugawara S, Goyal A, Durand CM, Quinn J, Sachithanandham J, et al. No recovery of replication-competent HIV-1 from human liver macrophages. *J Clin Invest.* (2018) 128:4501–9. doi: 10.1172/JCI121678

Poli G. Cell-to-cell vs. cell-free HIV-1 transmission from macrophages to CD4+ T lymphocytes: lessons from the virology textbook. *AIDS.* (2013) 27:2307–8. doi: 10.1097/QAD.0b013e328363619a

Bracq L, Xie M, Benichou S, Bouchet J. Mechanisms for Cell- to-Cell Transmission of HIV-1. *Front Immunol.* (2018) 9:260. doi: 10.3389/fimmu.2018.00260

Mosoian A, Zhang L, Hong F, Cunyat F, Rahman A, Bhalla R, et al. Frontline Science: HIV infection of Kupffer cells results in an amplified proinflammatory response to LPS. *J Leukoc Biol.* (2017) 101:1083–90. doi: 10.1189/jlb.3HI0516-242R

Zhang L, Mosoian A, Schwartz ME, Florman SS, Gunasekaran G, Schiano T, et al. HIV infection modulates IL-1beta response to LPS stimulation through a TLR4-NLRP3 pathway in human liver macrophages. *J Leukoc Biol.* (2019) 105:783–95. doi: 10.1002/JLB.4A1018-381R

Del Corno M, Cappon A, Donninelli G, Varano B, Marra F, Gessani S. HIV-1 gp120 signaling through TLR4 modulates innate immune activation in human macrophages and the biology of hepatic stellate cells. *J Leukoc Biol.* (2016) 100:599–606. doi: 10.1189/jlb.4A1215-534R

Ostrowski SR, Gerstoft J, Pedersen BK, Ullum H. Impaired production of cytokines is an independent predictor of mortality in HIV-1-infected patients. *AIDS.* (2003) 17:521–30. doi: 10.1097/00002030-200303070-00007

Sun Z, Denton PW, Estes JD, Othieno FA, Wei BL, Wege AK, et al. Intrarectal transmission, systemic infection, and CD4+ T cell depletion in humanized mice infected with HIV-1. *J Exp Med.* (2007) 204:705–14. doi: 10.1084/jem.20062411

Erikstrup C, Kronborg G, Lohse N, Ostrowski SR, Gerstoft J, Ullum H. T-cell dysfunction in HIV-1-infected patients with impaired recovery of CD4 cells despite suppression of viral replication. *J Acquir Immune Defic Syndr.* (2010) 53:303–10. doi:10.1097/QAI.0b013e3181ca3f7c

Glassner A, Eisenhardt M, Kokordelis P, Kramer B, Wolter F, Nischalke HD, et al. Impaired CD4(+) T cell stimulation of NK cell anti-fibrotic activity may contribute to accelerated liver fibrosis progression in HIV/HCV patients. *J Hepatol.* (2013) 59:427–33. doi: 10.1016/j.jhep.2013.04.029

Brau N, Salvatore M, Rios-Bedoya CF, Fernandez-Carbia A, Paronetto F, Rodriguez-Orengo JF, et al. Slower fibrosis progression in HIV/HCV- coinfected patients with successful HIV suppression using antiretroviral therapy. *J Hepatol.* (2006) 44:47–55. doi: 10.1016/j.jhep.2005.07.006

Kooij KW, Wit FW, Van Zoest RA, Schouten J, Kootstra NA, Van Vugt M, et al. Liver fibrosis in HIV-infected individuals on long- term antiretroviral therapy: associated with immune activation, immunodeficiency and prior use of didanosine. *AIDS.* (2016) 30:1771–80. doi:10.1097/QAD.0000000000001119

Lucar O, Reeves RK, Jost S. A Natural Impact: NK Cells at the Intersection of Cancer and HIV Disease. *Front Immunol.* (2019) 10:1850. doi: 10.3389/fimmu.2019.01850

Beignon AS, Mckenna K, Skoberne M, Manches O, Dasilva I, Kavanagh DG, et al. Endocytosis of HIV-1 activates plasmacytoid dendritic cells via Toll-like receptor-viral RNA interactions. *J Clin Invest.* (2005) 115:3265–75. doi: 10.1172/JCI26032

Evans TI, Li H, Schafer JL, Klatt NR, Hao XP, Traslavina RP, et al. SIV-induced translocation of bacterial products in the liver mobilizes myeloid dendritic and natural killer cells associated with liver damage. *J Infect Dis.* (2016) 213:361–9. doi: 10.1093/infdis/jiv404

Vlahakis S, Villasis-Keever A, Gomez T, Al E. Human immunodeficiency virus-induced apoptosis of human hepatocytes via CXCR4. *J Infect Dis.* (2003) 188:1455–60. doi: 10.1086/379738

Balasubramanian S, Ganju R, Groopman J. Hepatitis C virus and HIV envelope proteins collaboratively mediate interleukin-8 secretion through activation of p38 MAP kinase and SHP2 in hepatocytes. *J Biol Chem.* (2003) 278:35755–66. doi: 10.1074/jbc.M302889200

Munshi N, Balasbramanian A, Koziel M, Ganju R, Groopman J. Hepatitis C and human immunodeficiency virus envelope proteins cooperatively induce hepatocytic apoptosis via an innocent bystander mechanism. *J Infect Dis.* (2003) 188:1192–204. doi: 10.1086/378643

Yang L, Seki E. Toll-like receptors in liver fibrosis: cellular crosstalk and mechanisms. *Front Physiol.* (2012) 3:138. doi: 10.3389/fphys.2012.00138

Ganesan M, New-Aaron M, Dagur RS, Makarov E, Wang W, Kharbanda KK, et al. Alcohol metabolism potentiates HIV-induced hepatotoxicity: contribution to end-stage liver disease. *Biomolecules.* (2019) 9:20851. doi: 10.3390/biom9120851

Zhan SS, Jiang JX, Wu J, Halsted C, Friedman SL, Zern MA, et al. Phagocytosis of apoptotic bodies by hepatic stellate cells induces NADPH oxidase and is associated with liver fibrosis *in vivo*. *Hepatology.* (2006) 43:435–43. doi: 10.1002/hep.21093

Hong F, Saiman Y, Si C, Mosoian A, Bansal MB. X4 Human immunodeficiency virus type 1 gp120 promotes human hepatic stellate cell activation and collagen I expression through interactions with CXCR4. *PLoS ONE.* (2012) 7:e33659. doi: 10.1371/journal.pone.0033659

Bruno R, Galastri S, Sacchi P, Cima S, Caligiuri A, Defranco R, et al. gp120 modulates the biology of human hepatic stellate cells: a link between HIV infection and liver fibrogenesis. *Gut.* (2010) 59:513–20. doi: 10.1136/gut.2008.163287

Tuyama AC, Hong F, Saiman Y, Wang C, Ozkok D, Mosoian A, et al. Human immunodeficiency virus (HIV)-1 infects human hepatic stellate cells and promotes collagen I and monocyte chemoattractant protein-1 expression: implications for the pathogenesis of HIV/hepatitis C virus-induced liver fibrosis. *Hepatology.* (2010) 52:612–22. doi: 10.1002/hep.23679

Salloum S, Holmes JA, Jindal R, Bale SS, Brisac C, Alatrakchi N, et al. Exposure to human immunodeficiency virus/hepatitis C virus in hepatic and stellate cell lines reveals cooperative profibrotic transcriptional activation between viruses and cell types. *Hepatology.* (2016) 64:1951–68. doi: 10.1002/hep.28766

Gupta D, Rani M, Khan N, Jameel S. HIV-1 infected peripheral blood mononuclear cells modulate the fibrogenic activity of hepatic stellate cells through secreted TGF-beta and JNK signaling. *PLoS ONE.* (2014) 9:e91569. doi:10.1371/journal.pone.0091569

Seki E, De Minicis S, Osterreicher CH, Kluwe J, Osawa Y, Brenner DA, et al. TLR4 enhances TGF-beta signaling and hepatic fibrosis. *Nat Med.* (2007) 13:1324–32. doi: 10.1038/nm1663

17

Carveol a Naturally-Derived Potent and Emerging Nrf2 Activator Protects Against Acetaminophen-Induced Hepatotoxicity

Zaif Ur Rahman[1,2], Lina Tariq Al Kury[3], Abdullah Alattar[4], Zhen Tan[1], Reem Alshaman[4], Imran Malik[5], Haroon Badshah[2], Zia Uddin[6], Atif Ali Khan Khalil[7], Naveed Muhammad[2], Saifullah Khan[8], Amjad Ali[9], Fawad Ali Shah[5]*, Jing Bo Li[1]* and Shupeng Li[10]*

[1]Shenzhen University Clinical Research Center for Neurological Diseases, Health Management Center, Shenzhen University General Hospital, Shenzhen University Clinical Medical Academy, Shenzhen University, Shenzhen, China, [2]Department of Pharmacy, Abdul Wali Khan University, Khyber Pakhtunkhwa, Pakistan, [3]College of Natural and Health Sciences, Zayed University, Abu Dhabi, United Arab Emirates, [4]Department of Pharmacology and Toxicology, Faculty of Pharmacy, University of Tabuk, Tabuk, Saudi Arabia, [5]Riphah Institute of Pharmaceutical Sciences, Riphah International University, Islamabad, Pakistan, [6]Department of Pharmacy, COMSATS University Islamabad, Abbottabad Campus, Abbottabad, Pakistan, [7]Department of Biological Sciences, National University of Medical Sciences, Rawalpindi, Pakistan, [8]Department of Microbiology and Biotechnology, Abasyn University Peshawar, Khyber Pakhtunkhwa, Pakistan, [9]Department of Botany, University of Malakand, Khyber Pakhtunkhwa, Pakistan, [10]State Key Laboratory of Oncogenomics, School of Chemical Biology and Biotechnology, Shenzhen Graduate School, Peking University, Shenzhen, China

*Correspondence:
Fawad Ali Shah
fawad.shah@riphah.edu
Shupeng Li
lisp@pkusz.edu.cn
Jing Bo Li
lijb_003@163.com

Acetaminophen (N-acetyl p-aminophenol or APAP) is used worldwide for its antipyretic and anti-inflammatory potential. However, APAP overdose sometimes causes severe liver damage. In this study, we elucidated the protective effects of carveol in liver injury, using molecular and *in silico* approaches. Male BALB/c mice were divided into two experimental cohorts, to identify the best dose and to further assess the role of carveol in the nuclear factor E2-related factor; nuclear factor erythroid 2; p45-related factor 2 (Nrf2) pathway. The results demonstrated that carveol significantly modulated the detrimental effects of APAP by boosting endogenous antioxidant mechanisms, such as nuclear translocation of Nrf2 gene, a master regulator of the downstream antioxidant machinery. Furthermore, an inhibitor of Nrf2, called all-trans retinoic acid (ATRA), was used, which exaggerated APAP toxicity, in addition to abrogating the protective effects of carveol; this effect was accompanied by overexpression of inflammatory mediators and liver = 2ltoxicity biomarkers. To further support our notion, we performed virtual docking of carveol with Nrf2-keap1 target, and the resultant drug-protein interactions validated the *in vivo* findings. Together, our findings suggest that carveol could activate the endogenous master antioxidant Nrf2, which further regulates the expression of downstream antioxidants, eventually ameliorating the APAP-induced inflammation and oxidative stress.

Keywords: acetaminophen, carveol, hepatotoxicity, anti-inflammatory, Nrf2 pathway

INTRODUCTION

Liver diseases are associated with an increased number of disability cases, and approximately 50 million liver-associated morbidity and mortality reports are documented each year (Gorrell, 2005). Because of the persistent and continuous involvement of the liver in metabolic processes, the accumulation of free radicals overwhelms the natural defense system, making the liver one of the

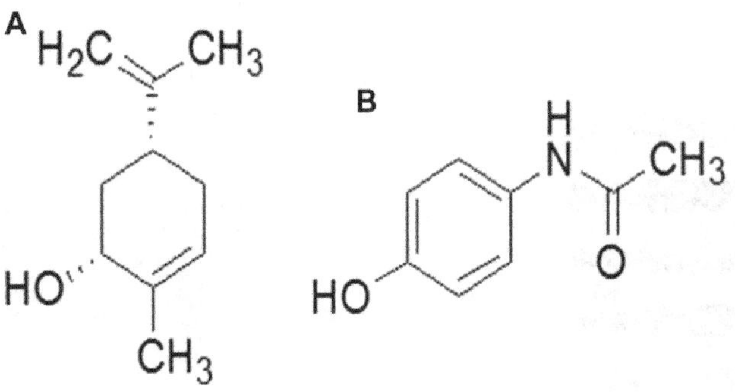

Figure 1 | Chemical structure of **(A)** carveol and **(B)** paracetamol.

most vulnerable organ. These free radicals are the prominent cause of oxidative stress-induced thiol depletion and lipid peroxidation, which subsequently trigger toxic cascading events and eventually lead to various hepatic pathologies, such as cirrhosis and acute or chronic hepatitis (Abo-Haded et al., 2017).

Paracetamol (acetaminophen, N-acetyl p-aminophenol, or APAP) is a non-prescription drug with both analgesic and antipyretic activities, and this drug is included in several preparations, either as a single moiety or in combination (Ghaffar and Tadvi, 2014). It has a large therapeutic window and is generally safe; however, when abused in large doses, it leads to severe hepatic necrosis and hepatic failure (Al-Fartosi et al., 2011). Currently, paracetamol is considered the chief causative agent of acute liver failure due to accidental overdose, which requires a liver transplant in some extreme cases (Gopal et al., 2011; Du et al., 2016). At a high dose, APAP is metabolized to glucuronic acid or sulfate conjugates (Sharma et al., 2016) and is transformed into the pro-reactive cytotoxic intermediate N-acetyl-phenzoquinoneimine (NAPQI), which is responsible for oxidative stress and intracellular glutathione (GSH) depletion (Shah et al., 2014; Hellerbrand et al., 2017; Zai et al., 2018). The covalent binding of NAPQI to mitochondria initiates cascading pathological processes, such as free radical formation and peroxynitrite accumulation, further supplemented by the release of pro-inflammatory cytokines and mediators, all of which collectively exacerbate acute and chronic liver necrosis (Dalaklioglu et al., 2013; Hennig et al., 2018). Various hepatoprotective strategies have been evaluated to protect the liver from toxins. The current clinical practice recommends silymarin as a hepatoprotective supplement to cope with various liver insults, including APAP and methotrexate (MTX) (Crowell et al., 1992). The transcription factor Nrf2 is an integral part of the host cellular defense mechanism against oxidative stress and electrophilic insult. Nrf2 binds to antioxidant response elements (ARE) at the promoter site, which in turn encodes several antioxidant/phase-II detoxifying enzymes and other relevant stress-responding factors (Thompson Coon and Ernst, 2002). Previous studies have revealed the involvement of Nrf2-ARE signaling in attenuating inflammation in several pathologies, such as stroke, and other disorders (Ma and He, 2012; Ning et al., 2018). Hence, dysregulation of Nrf2 signaling results in increased

susceptibility to oxidative stress and inflammatory damage. Previous studies have demonstrated that Nrf2 plays a critical role in the regulation of inflammation and oxidative stress, which are linked to the pathophysiologies of several diseases. Therefore, Nrf2 can be considered a potential pharmacological target to be investigated against various insults, including APAP.

Natural drug moieties are an attractive source of new drugs, owing to their rich antioxidant potential. Several natural drugs have hepatoprotective potential against a variety of mediators, including free radicals and inflammatory factors (James et al., 2003; Lee et al., 2006). Carveol, a monoterpene phenol, is isolated from the essential oils extracted from the plant family *Lamiaceae* or *Labiatae*, which includes the genera *Thymbra*, *Origanum*, *Corydothymus*, *Satureja*, and *Thymus* (**Figure 1**) (Pastore et al., 2003). It has long been used in traditional Chinese medicine as an antispasmodic, a carminative, and an astringent (Aleksunes et al., 2008) and has been evaluated in the treatment of indigestion and dyspepsia (Guo and White, 2016). Carveol has been demonstrated to have antioxidative, antihyperlipidemic, and anti-inflammatory activities, and ameliorate liver toxicity in a mouse model of carbon tetrachloride (Patterson et al., 2013). However, to date, the potential hepatoprotective effects of carveol against APAP have not been evaluated. Taking into consideration the pharmacological value of essential oils extracted from plant sources and the significance of new drug discovery, the current study sought to investigate whether carveol mitigates APAP-induced detrimental effects. If so, the potential underlying molecular and cellular mechanisms should be further delineated to explain the effects of carveol on hepatocellular protection. This will not only expand the understanding of the molecular cascading mechanism of cell death but will also provide some clues to unveil the therapeutic potential of carveol.

MATERIALS AND METHODS

Chemicals and Reagents

The pharmaceutical drugs (silymarin and N-acetyl para aminophenol (paracetamol CAS: 103-90-2, C8H9NO2: APAP) of HPLC grade (99%) were supplied by a local pharmaceutical manufacturer and used as raw material. All the antibodies were procured from Santa Cruz Biotechnology, United States, or Abcam, United Kingdom. Phosphate-buffered saline (PBS) tablets were used for all morphological analyses or fresh buffers were prepared for each use. The details and corresponding catalog numbers of the primary antibodies are HO-1 (SC-13691), TRX (SC-20146), Nrf2 (SC-722), COX-2 (SC-514489), p-JNK (SC-6254), TNF-α (SC-52B83), and p-NFκB (SC-271908). Other immunohistochemistry-related consumables, such as AB and C Elite kit (two vials-SC-2018) and 3,3-diaminobenzidine (DAB) (SC-216567), were also provided by Santa Cruz Biotechnology, United States. The biotin secondary antibody (ab-6789) and DPX mounting media were purchased from Abcam United Kingdom. The p-NFκB enzyme-linked immunosorbent assay (ELISA) kit (Cat # SU-B28069) and Nrf2 kit (cat. no. SU-B30429) were purchased

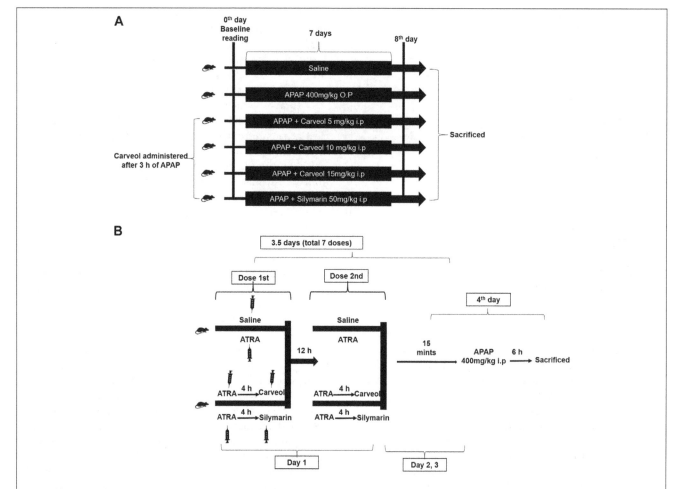

Figure 2 | Experimental design 1 **(A)**. Carveol, APAP, and silymarin were prepared in 0.9% NaCl, while ATRA was prepared in a mixture of 2% dimethyl sulfoxide and 0.9% NaCl (*n* = 10/group). Baseline reading was recorded at the beginning (0th day of the experiment), and mean weight and food intake were monitored during the entire experiment **(B)** Diagrammatic illustration of *in vivo* study for the Nrf2 signaling pathway. The treatment protocol was continued for 3.5 days. In all these groups, a single loading dose of paracetamol was injected (400 mg/kg, i. p.) 15 min after the last dose of ATRA or carveol or silymarin, except in the saline group. Serum samples and liver tissues were collected after 6 h of the last dose.

from Shanghai Yuchun Biotechnology, China. HO-1 (cat. No. E-EL-R0488), and TNF-α (E-EL-R0019) ELISA kits were purchased from Elabscience.

Animals and Drug Treatment

Male BLAB/c mice, weighing 30–35 g and 8–10 weeks old, were housed (three per cage) at the facility of the Riphah Institute of Pharmaceutical Sciences (RIPS), under-documented protocols (temperature: 22 ± 1 °C; humidity: 50 ± 10%). Strict laboratory protocols were followed during all experimental procedures. The animals were kept for some days at the facility before the experimental procedures, and the body weights were constantly checked every day throughout the study. Furthermore, we strictly followed the approved protocols and guidelines of the institutional research ethical committee (REC) of the Riphah Institute of Pharmaceutical Sciences (RIPS), Islamabad (Approval ID: Ref. No. REC/RIPS/2018-19/A202), which are similar to the ARRIVE guidelines, with some minor exemptions. We adopted the human endpoint criteria for

euthanizing the mice if they displayed a severe sign of distress or suffering. The mice were subjected to the following experimental protocols. Two separate cohorts of animals were used for the experiments as follows:

Experimental Cohort 1

The mice treatment protocol is indicated in **Figure 2A**, and the following groups were employed. 1) Saline group: the mice received saline (0.9% NaCl) injection intraperitoneally (i. p.) for seven consecutive days, 2) APAP group: the mice received a single dose of paracetamol orally/per os (400 mg/kg, p. o.) for 7 days, 3) Three different groups of APAP + carveol: the mice received paracetamol orally for seven consecutive days, followed by a single i. p. injection of different doses of carveol, namely APAP + carveol 5 mg (5 mg/kg, i. p.); APAP + carveol 10 mg (10 mg/kg, i. p.); APAP + carveol 15 mg (15 mg/kg, i. p.), 4) APAP + silymarin group: the mice received paracetamol orally for seven consecutive days, followed by silymarin (50 mg/kg, i.p.). Carveol, APAP, and silymarin were prepared in 0.9% NaCl (*n* = 14 per/group). At the end of the experiment, the mice were anesthetized with xylazine and ketamine (i. p.); blood was collected via cardiac puncture and was processed for biochemical analysis. Samples from the liver were taken and frozen at −50 °C or preserved in 4% paraformaldehyde for ELISA or paraffin sectioning, respectively. Next, 4 μm thin hepatic tissue sections were made with a rotary microtome from the paraffin block, for histological analysis. Overall, three mice died during the experimental procedures, two from APAP and one from the Carveol + APAP groups, which we excluded from the experiment. The saline-treated mice survived throughout the experiments.

Experimental Cohort 2

The mice treatment protocol is indicated in **Figure 2B**, and the following groups were employed with $n = 10$/gp. 1) Saline group: the mice received saline (i. p.), 2) APAP + ATRA group: the mice received seven injections of ATRA (10 mg/kg, i. p.) at 12 h intervals, 3) APAP + ATRA + Carveol group: the mice received carveol 15 mg/kg i.p 4 h after each ATRA dose, and 4) APAP + ATRA + silymarin group: the mice received silymarin 50 mg/kg i.p 4 h after each ATRA dose. For all the groups except saline, APAP 400 mg/kg was administered (i. p.) 15 min after the last dose of ATRA (APAP + ATRA group) or carveol (APAP + ATRA + carveol) or silymarin (APAP + ATRA + silymarin). At the end of the treatment, the mice were sacrificed and samples were collected.

Hematoxylin and Eosin (H and E) Staining

Hematoxylin and eosin staining was performed according to our previous protocols (Ali et al., 2019; Ansari et al., 2019; Ullah et al., 2020). Briefly, the non-coated slides initially underwent a deparaffinization step with xylene, followed by hydration (graded ethanolic series), and finally with water. The slides were incubated in a Coplin jar containing hematoxylin to stain the nucleus. The slides were washed with water and traced for nuclear staining, using a compound microscope. The slides were then dipped in 1% HCl, 1% ammonia water, and rinsed with water. Eosin staining was then performed, the slides were subjected to dehydration, fixed in xylene, and covered with coverslips. Five images per slide were obtained using a light microscope (Olympus, Japan) at the same threshold intensity, and were later analyzed using ImageJ software to quantify the number of distorted, vacuolated, infiltrated, and surviving cells.

Liver Functional Biomarkers

Enzymes, such as AST, ALT, phosphatases, and total bilirubin (TB), were spectroscopically analyzed using an autoanalyzer (Olympus AU-2700) according to the manufacturer's instructions.

Oxidative Enzyme Analysis and Lipid Peroxidation

The non-enzymatic glutathione (GSH) level and the enzymatic glutathione S-transferase (GST) activity were determined as previously described (Ullah et al., 2020). After homogenizing liver tissue samples (cohort 1), the supernatant was collected. For the assay, the stock of 0.2 M sodium phosphate buffer was prepared as $Na_2HPO_4.2H_2O$ and NaH_2PO_4 (pH 8). For sample loading, buffer (153 μL), freshly prepared 1 mmol DTNB (40 μL), and the supernatant (6.6 μL) were sequentially mixed, and after 15 min, the absorbance of this mixture was determined using a spectrophotometer at 412 nm. A mixture of DTNB solution and phosphate buffer served as the control, whereas the buffer was used as a blank. The absorbance was calculated from the values of the absorbance of the control and the sample and expressed as μmol/mg protein. To detect GST activity (Imran et al., 2020), the stock of 0.1 M potassium phosphate buffer was prepared as $KHPO_4$ and KH_2PO_4 (at a 1:2 ratio, pH 6.5). For the assay, 1 mmol GST and 1 mmol CDNB were also prepared; then GST solution, CDNB, potassium buffer, and tissue homogenate were mixed (at a 1:1:27:1 ratio) and the optical density was determined at 340 nm. The phosphate buffer was used as a blank, and the assay mixture without homogenate was used as a control. GST activity was calculated using the extinction coefficient of the product and expressed as nmoles of CDNB conjugated/min/mg protein.

Determination of Lipid Peroxidation (LPO) in Tissue

Oxidative stress augmented the oxidation of macromolecules, such as lipids, which can be quantified by the thiobarbituric acid reactive substance (TBARS) levels. A previously reported protocol was adopted for the LPO assay, with minor changes (Imran et al., 2020). Approximately 40 μL of tissue supernatant was added to a freshly prepared solution of ferric ammonium sulfate and incubated for some time. Next, after the addition of 75 μL of thiobarbituric acid (TBA) to the mixture, the color changed, and the absorbance of the resultant mixture was immediately measured using a microplate reader (at 532 nm). The levels were expressed as nmol Tbras/min/mg protein (Iqbal et al., 2020).

Immunohistochemical Analysis

We used coated slides for immunohistochemical studies as described in a previous study (Rana et al., 2020). The slides were subjected to deparaffinization and hydration protocols as discussed for H and E. To unlock the antigenic epitopes from paraformaldehyde, proteinase K was applied to the tissue, followed by PBS rinsing. After hydration, the slides were not allowed to dry at any stage of the immunohistochemical analysis. Before blocking with normal goat serum the slides were treated with H_2O_2 to eradicate peroxidase activity. The selectivity of serum depends upon the source of the secondary antibody. After blocking for an appropriate time, primary antibodies, such as nuclear factor-κB (p-NFκB), COX2, c-Jun N-terminal kinase (p-JNK), HO-1, TNF-α, and Nrf2 (dilution 1:100, Santa Cruz Biotechnology), were applied overnight in a moistened box in the refrigerator. The following morning, the slides were removed and kept for 1 h at room temperature in a moistened chamber. After rinsing with PBS, the biotinylated secondary antibody (goat anti-mouse and goat anti-rabbit) was applied, followed by the application of ABC reagent (SCBT United States) in a humidified chamber, and the slides were rinsed with PBS and stained with DAB. The slides were then dried, dehydrated in ascending ethanolic series, fixed in xylene, and covered with coverslips. The liver positive cells for all the primary antibodies were quantified using the ImageJ software.

Enzyme-Linked Immunosorbent Assay (ELISA)

p-NFκB, HO-1, Nrf2, and TNF-α levels were quantified using an ELISA kit as per the manufacturer's instructions (for detailed chemicals and reagents). Approximately 50 mg of the tissue sample was homogenized, using PBS (also containing PMSF as a serine inhibitor), at 15,000 RPM, followed by centrifugation and collection of the supernatant. Protein concentration in each homogenate was calculated using the BCA kit (Thermo Fisher), and the resultant protein concentration was added to each well to determine the level of the respective proteins, using an ELISA reader. The resultant picograms of cytokines per milliliter (pg/ml) were then converted pg/mg total protein).

Real-Time Polymerase Chain Reaction (RT-PCR)

Total RNA was extracted from the freshly isolated liver of mice in experimental duplicates using the TRIzol method. 20 μL of M-MuLV reverse transcriptase was used to dilute 1 μg of RNA and used this mix to synthesize cDNA with a cDNA synthesis kit (vivantis cDSK01-050 Sdn. Bhd, Malaysia). To estimate the gene expression of Nrf2 quantitatively, real-time PCR was performed using the 2X HOT SYBR Green qPCR master mix (Solar Bio cat # SR1110) and real-time Mic PCR (BioMolecular System) according to the manufacturer specifications. The sequence of the primers used for amplification was Nrf2 Forward: CCATTT ACGGAGACCCACCGCCTG and Reverse: CTCGTGTGAGAT GAGCCTCTAAGCGG and GAPDH, Forward: AGGTCGGTG TGAACGGATTTG and Reverse: TGTAGACCATGTAGTTGA GGTCA (Wakabayashi et al., 2014). The relative gene expressions of Nrf2 was determined by the $2^{-\Delta\Delta CT}$ method for real-time quantitative PCR.

Bioinformatic Studies

In silico studies were performed as previously described (Shah and Rashid, 2020). Briefly, the 3-dimensional structures of cyclooxygenase (COX2) PDB ID: IPXX, interleukin (IL-1β) PDB ID: 2MIB, PDB ID: 2TNF for TNF-α, PDB ID: 3TTI for JNK, PDB ID: ILE5 for nuclear factor-kB (NFκB), PDB ID: 1DVE for HO-1, and PDB ID: 2LZ1 for Nrf2 were downloaded from the RCSB protein data bank in Discovery Studio (DSV). Docking studies require PDB and mol2 format, for which the 3D structure of the proteins and ligand carveol were downloaded in the respective format. Both protein and ligand were loaded into the PyRx docking software, and drug-receptor interactions were evaluated by binding the energy values (E-value). The E-values further validated the best pose of the ligand in the complex, and by DSV, the best orientation and interaction were

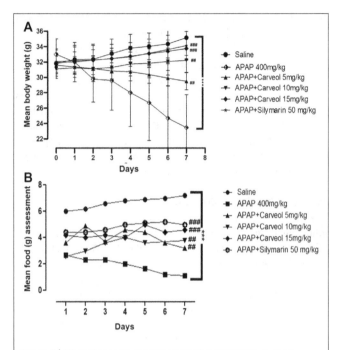

Figure 3 | Effect of carveol treatment on physical parameters, such as body weight and food intake. **(A)** Bodyweight changes **(B)** Mean food intake. The number of animals was 14/group, and the results were analyzed using a repeated two-way ANOVA test. ###$p < 0.001$, ##$p < 0.01$ compared to the APAP group, ***$p < 0.001$, compared to the saline group.

prepared and analyzed. The structure of carveol was collected from online sources.

Statistical Analysis

The symbols *, #, \$, and β were used to indicate a significant difference. * or β indicates differences compared to saline, while # to APAP and \$ represents a significant difference to APAP + ATRA. All the data are expressed as mean ± SEM, and ImageJ software was used to analyze all the histological data (ImageJ 1.30; https://imagej.nih.gov/ij/). Bodyweight and food intake data were analyzed using a repeated two-way ANOVA, and the remaining data were analyzed using one-way ANOVA with Tukey's multiple comparison test as a post-hoc test.

RESULTS

Results of Experimental Design one
Effect of Carveol on Body Weight and Food Intake

Our results showed that APAP induced a dramatic and persistent loss of body weight. However, carveol prevented body weight loss in a dose-dependent manner (**Figure 3A**). Carveol, at 15 mg/kg per day, showed the most significant effect on body weight ($p < 0.001$). Bodyweight reduction could be attributed to decreased food intake, as APAP-treated mice consumed significantly less amount of food; however, carveol ameliorated this effect in a dose-dependent manner, which is comparable to that of silymarin (50 mg/kg) (**Figure 3B**, $p < 0.001$).

TABLE 1 | The protective effect of carveol on liver functional enzymes: APAP augmented the serum level of LFTs and attenuated high-density lipoprotein (HDL) level, while carveol, with respect to APAP, mitigated LFT levels and increased HDL levels.

Treatment	ALT (U/L)	AST (U/L)	TP (g/dl)	TB (mg/dl)	ALP (U/L)	Albumin (g/dl)	LDL (mg/dl)	HDL (mg/dl)
Saline	59 ± 8.71	106 ± 13.89	7.8 ± 0.30	0.33 ± 0.18	98.66 ± 15.53	4.93 ± 0.65	39 ± 5.56	78.66 ± 8.02
APAP 400 mg/kg	194.66 ± 6.02***	276.66 ± 27.02***	3.53 ± 0.40***	2.16 ± 0.30***	220.33 ± 49.44***	2.23 ± 0.30***	102.66 ± 13.05***	37.66 ± 2.51***
APAP + Carveol 5 mg/kg	164.66 ± 10.69	269.33 ± 81.5	5.7 ± 0.45##	1.23 ± .37##	177 ± 11.78	3.5 ± 36	78.66 ± 17.4	41.66 ± 3.05
APAP + Carveol 10 mg/kg	148.33 ± 11.37#	258.66 ± 36.67	5.53 ± 1.19##	1.03 ± .20##	136.66 ± 3.05##	4.23 ± .41#	64 ± 21#	52.66 ± 6.5#
APAP + Carveol 15 mg/kg	95.33 ± 7.37###	172.33 ± 14.7##	6.6 ± 0.55###	0.525 ± 0.03###	122.66 ± 8.50###	4.5 ± 0.36##	65.66 ± 17.67##	64.66 ± 7.76##
APAP + Silymarin 50 mg/kg	81.33 ± 8.50###	138.66 ± 14.22##	6.16 ± 0.40###	0.67 ± 0.29###	130 ± 16.70###	5.93 ± 0.85##	51.33 ± 9.29##	52.33 ± 2.08#

*The data are presented as means ± SEM and were analyzed using one-way ANOVA with n = 7/group. The symbols *** and ### represent p < 0.001 and the symbol ## represents p < 0.01 values of significant differences. The samples were processed from cohort 1.*

TABLE 2 | Effect of carveol on oxidative enzymes.

Treatment	GSH (µmol/mg protein)	GST (nmoles of CDNS conjugated/min/mg protein)	TBARS (nmoles Tbras/min/mg protien)
Saline	74.88 ± 13.78	25.42 ± 1.30	79.32 ± 0.70
APAP 400 mg/kg	6.30 ± 4.97***	1.78 ± 1.50***	215.58 ± 5.82***
APA + Carveol 5 mg/kg	44.4 ± 9.26#	4.67 ± 0.91	192.54 ± 2.80
APA + Carveol 10 mg/kg	54.49 ± 9.98##	8.83 ± 1.62#	167.78 ± 2.164#
APA + Carveol 15 mg/kg	62.29 ± 18.82###	14.2 ± 1.43##	131.74 ± 0.64##
APAP + Silymarin 50 mg/kg	66.68 ± 11.45###	18.20 ± 2.31##	115.83 ± 2.164##

*The symbols *** and ### represent p < 0.001, while the symbol ## or # represents p < 0.01 and p < 0.05, n = 7/group. The data are expressed as mean ± SEM and were analyzed using one-way ANOVA followed by Tukey's multiple comparison test. The samples were processed from cohort 1.*

Carveol Improved the Liver Detriments of APAP

Table 1 shows that APAP significantly disturbed the functional markers ($p < 0.001$), while carveol at different doses normalized the values in the APAP-administered group; carveol at 15 mg exhibited similar effects as those of silymarin.

Carveol Alleviated the Liver Metabolic Deficits Induced by APAP

The liver plays a principal role in the synthesis, storage, secretion, and catabolism of proteins, bilirubin, lipoproteins, and lipids, which represent sensitive markers during liver damage. Our results showed a significant increase in the levels of total protein (TP), albumin, and HDL, accompanied by decreased total bilirubin (TB) and low-density lipoprotein levels (**Table 1**). These results suggest that liver anabolic and catabolic functions were both severely hampered. Moreover, carveol showed a dose-dependent protective effect, which was comparable to the effects of silymarin at a dose of 15 mg/kg. Furthermore, the effect of carveol on HDL levels was more significant ($p < 0.01$) than that of the silymarin-treated group ($p < 0.05$).

Effects of Carveol on Antioxidant Enzymes

Table 2 summarizes the effects of carveol on changes in endogenous enzyme activities, following APAP treatment. APAP stimulated GSH depletion (6.30 ± 4.97), and antioxidant enzyme glutathione-S-transferase (GST) (1.78 ± 1.50) in the hepatic tissue ($p < 0.001$). Treatment with carveol at different doses attenuated the downregulation of GSH (62.29 ± 8.82) and GST (14.2 ± 1.43).

Effect of Carveol on LPO

The LPO content in the liver homogenate of the APAP group was increased to 215.58 ± 5.82, compared to that in the saline group ($p < 0.001$, **Table 2**). Carveol at 15 mg/kg dose significantly ($p < 0.01$, **Table 2**) attenuated this content (131.74 ± 0.64), an effect that could be matched to that of the silymarin group.

Carveol Protected the Liver From APAP-Induced Cellular Damage

The results of H and E staining revealed significant histopathological changes in the APAP-intoxicated animals (**Figure 4**, ###$p < 0.001$). Significant alterations were observed in the APAP group, compared to those in the saline-treated

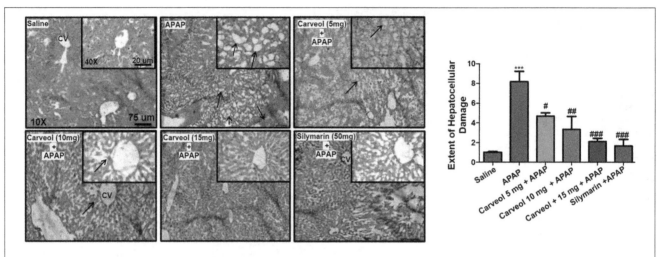

Figure 4 | Carveol restored the morphological integrity of the liver, as shown by histological examination. Liver tissue was stained with H and E (magnification, ×10 scale bar 75 μm and 40× scale bar 20 μm). The data are presented as means ± SEM and were analyzed using one-way ANOVA followed by Tukey's multiple comparison test; n = 7/group. The symbols *** and ### represent significant difference values of $p < 0.001$, and ## or # represent significant difference values of $p < 0.01$ or $p < 0.05$ respectively. The slides were processed from cohort 1.

TABLE 3 | Effect of carveol on histopathological scoring.

Groups	Hepatocytes necrosis	Inflammatory cells infiltration	Fatty degeneration/vacuolization
Saline	—	—	—
APAP 400 mg/kg	+++	+++	+++
APA + Carveol 5 mg/kg	+++	++	++
APA + Carveol 10 mg/kg	+	+	+
APA + Carveol 15 mg/kg	—	—	±
APAP + Silymarin 50 mg/kg	—	—	±

+++ significant, ++ high, + moderate, —nil.

animals. The saline group showed normal hepatic cell shape, and there was no vacuolization or lipid globule. Nevertheless, many aberrant morphological features, such as sinusoidal dilatation, hepatocyte degeneration with loss of lobular architecture/ hepatocyte disarray, pericentral lymphocytic infiltration, moderate steatosis/fatty degeneration, and abundant inflammatory cell infiltration, were observed in the APAP-treated groups (**Table 3**). Carveol treatment significantly reversed these histopathological abnormalities induced by APAP, in a dose-dependent manner, as revealed by the microscopic scores (Carveol histopathological score).

Effect of Carveol on APAP-Mediated Inflammatory Markers

The JNK signaling pathway mediates the stress-induced inflammatory cascade and is implicated in mitochondrial apoptosis, and its activation results in the phosphorylation of numerous transcription factors, such as AP-1, p53, Bax, and Bim. Furthermore, JNK can trigger other mediators, such as TNF-α, p-NFκB, and COX-2 (Ali A et al., 2020). To reveal the possible involvement of JNK and TNF-α, immunohistochemical staining was performed, and the results showed higher

expression of these mediators in the APAP-administered group ($p < 0.001$) (**Figures 5A,B**), whereas carveol dose at 15 mg significantly reduced their hyperexpression ($p < 0.01$, **Figure 5A**, $p < 0.001$, **Figure 5B**). Moreover, COX-2 and p-NFκB expression were also evaluated, and the results showed that both were highly expressed in the APAP group ($p < 0.001$, **Figures 5C,D**). Carveol attenuated the expression of p-NFκB and TNF-α in a dose-dependent manner.

Effect of Carveol on the Nrf2 Signaling Pathway

To examine the possible effect of carveol on the Nrf2 signaling pathway, the expression of Nrf2, HO-1, and TRX was determined via immunohistochemistry (**Figure 6**). APAP activated the expression of Nrf2 (**Figure 6A**) and TRX ($p < 0.05$, **Figure 6C**) due to oxidative stress, and carveol, at 15 mg/kg, further expressed these antioxidative proteins to counteract oxidative stress ($p < 0.001$, **Figure 6A**, $p < 0.01$, **Figure 6C**). HO-1 and thioredoxin TRX exhibit similar characteristics, as both are antioxidants and eradicate reactive oxygen species, thereby protecting the cell from inflammation and apoptosis (Shah et al., 2018; Li and Liu, 2019). The effect of carveol on the thioredoxin protein level was evaluated in different

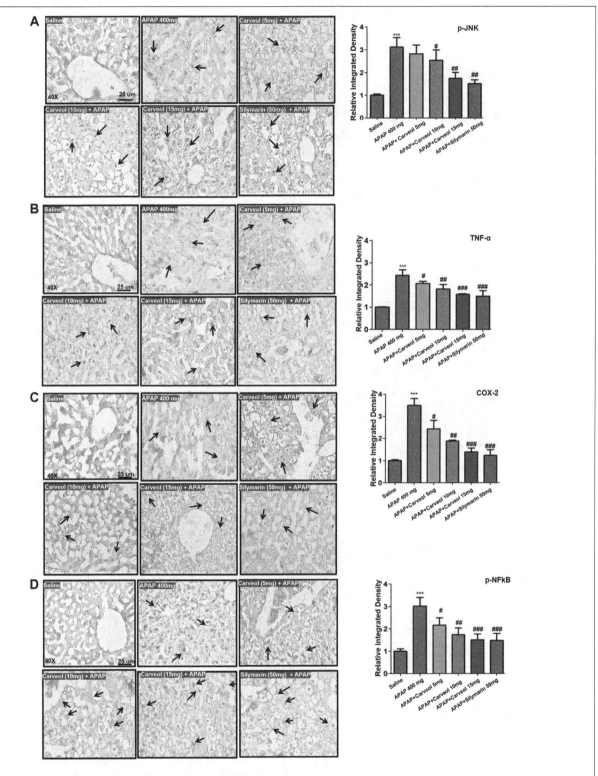

Figure 5 | Effect of carveol on inflammatory mediators. The presented images indicate immunoreactivity of **(A)** p-JNK **(B)** TNF-α **(C)** COX-2, and **(D)** p-NFκB. Scale bar = 25 μm, magnification ×40 with n = 7/group. The data presented are relative to saline and the number of experiments performed = 3. The data are presented as means ± SEM and were analyzed using one-way ANOVA followed by Tukey's multiple comparison test. The symbols ∗∗∗ and ### represent significant difference values of $p < 0.001$, while the symbol ## represent $p < 0.01$ values for significant differences and # represents $p < 0.05$. The slides were processed from cohort 1.

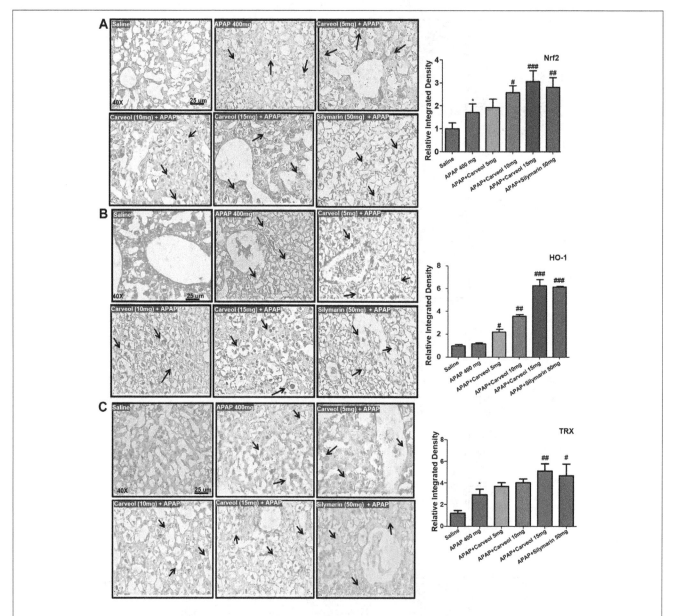

Figure 6 | Effect of carveol on immunohistochemistry expression **(A)** Nrf2 **(B)** HO-1, and **(C)** TRX with magnification ×40, and scale bar = 25 μm, n = 7/group. Representative histograms indicate a comparatively lower expression of **(A)** Nrf2 **(B)** HO-1, and **(C)** TRX in the APAP group than the carveol group. The data are presented as means ± SEM and were analyzed using one-way ANOVA followed by Tukey's multiple comparison test. The symbols ### represent significant difference values of $p < 0.001$, while the symbol ## represents $p < 0.01$ values of significant differences, and * or # represents $p < 0.05$. # is significantly different from APAP.

experimental groups. Representative images and densitometric analysis are shown in **Figure 6**.

Results of Experimental Design 2
Carveol Enhances the Antioxidant Capacity of the Liver via the Nrf2 Signaling Pathway

To further investigate whether the antioxidative effects of carveol against APAP-induced liver injury, *in vivo*, are Nrf2-dependent, we blocked the Nrf2 effect by using ATRA at a dose of 10 mg/kg. As shown in **Figure 7A**, Nrf2 gene expression was elevated by carveol at 15 mg dose, while ATRA downregulated this expression. To further validate the hepatoprotective effect, we

performed ELISA and we demonstrated similar results for Nrf2 (**Figure 7B**). The level of HO-1 was also decreased by ATRA ($p < 0.001$). Treatment with carveol at 15 mg/kg modulated the level of Nrf2 and HO-1, whereas ATRA treatment blocked the effects of carveol on Nrf2 ($p < 0.05$, **Figures 7B,C**). The expression of p-NFκB and TNF-α was also evaluated in these groups, and the results coincided with the Nrf2 findings, with hyperexpression in the ATRA + APAP group ($p < 0.001$). Moreover, carveol (15 mg/kg) attenuated the expression of p-NFκB and TNF-α in the carveol + ATRA + APAP group ($p < 0.05$, **Figure 7D**, $p < 0.001$, **Figure 7E**). The results were further validated using biochemical analysis (**Tables 4**) and H and E staining (**Figure 8**),

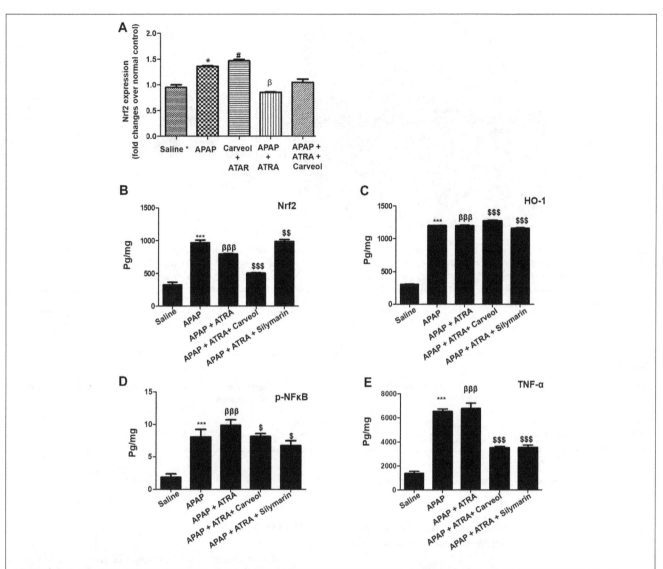

Figure 7 | Carveol produces Nrf2-dependent effects. **(A)** qPCR analysis, **(B)** Nrf2 **(C)** HO-1, **(D)** p-NFκB, and **(E)** TNF-α were quantified using ELISA. The data are expressed as mean ± SEM and were analyzed using one-way ANOVA followed by Tukey's multiple comparison test, and n = 5/group. The symbols ∗∗∗, βββ and represent significant difference values of $p < 0.001$, while the symbol $ represents significant difference values of $p < 0.05$. The symbol ∗ or β represents a significant difference relative to saline, while $ represents a significant difference relative to the APAP + ATRA group. The samples were collected 6 h later, for biochemical and morphological analyses. The samples were processed from cohort 2.

TABLE 4 | ATRA abrogated the effects of carveol.

Treatment	ALT (U/L)	AST (U/L)	TP (g/dl)	ALP (U/L)	LDH (mg/dl)
Saline	67 ± 5.4	89 ± 5.32	6.8 ± 1.56	110 ± 2.7	441.33 ± 14.46
APAP 400 mg/kg + ATRA 10 mg/kg	456 ± 13.25^{βββ}	634 ± 16.35^{βββ}	2.6 ± 1.7^{ββ}	545 ± 9.89^{βββ}	3653 ± 4.03^{βββ}
APAP + ATRA + Carveol 15 mg/kg	219 ± 12.56$^{\$\$\$}$	376 ± 3.45$^{\$\$\$}$	5.3 ± 1.21$^{\$\$}$	278 ± 7.89$^{\$\$\$}$	2162 ± 21.72$^{\$\$}$
APAP + ATRA + Silymarin 50 mg/kg	183 ± 14.23$^{\$\$\$}$	312 ± 8.64$^{\$\$\$}$	5.8 ± 2.1$^{\$\$}$	267 ± 5.78$^{\$\$\$}$	2017.66 ± 25.91$^{\$\$}$

ATRA augmented the serum level of LFTs and attenuated the TP, while carveol significantly reduced LFT levels compared to those in the ATRA + APAP group, and increased the total protein level. The symbols βββ and \$\$\$ represent significant difference values of $p < 0.001$, while the symbol \$\$ represents $p < 0.01$ values of significant differences, the symbol \$ represents a significant difference relative to APAP + ATRA, while β represents a significant difference relative to the saline group. The data are expressed as means ± SEM and were analyzed using one-way ANOVA followed by Tukey's multiple comparison test, n = 5. The samples were processed from cohort 2.

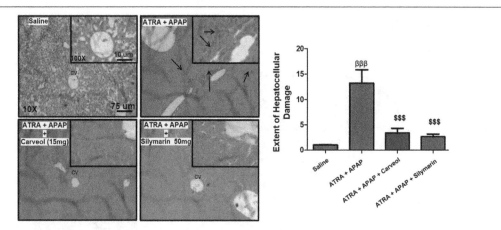

Figure 8 | Histological examination and morphological changes in liver tissues. Liver tissues stained with H and E (magnification ×10 and 40×) (n = 5/group). The necrotic cells are marked and shown by an arrow; abundant inflammatory cell infiltration can be seen in the APAP + ATRA group. The data are presented as means ± SEM and were analyzed using one-way ANOVA followed by Tukey's multiple comparison test. The symbols βββ and $$$ represent significant difference values of $p < 0.001$, the symbol β shows a significant difference relative to the saline, and the symbol $ shows a significant difference relative to the APAP + ATRA group. The slides were processed from cohort 2.

TABLE 5 | Binding energy values.

Groups	Hepatocytes necrosis	Inflammatory cells infiltration	Fatty degeneration/vacuolization
Saline	–	–	–
APAP 400 mg/kg + ATRA 10 mg/kg	+++	+++	++
APAP + ATRA + Carveol 15 mg/kg	–	–	–
APAP + ATRA + Silymarin 50 mg/kg	–	–	–

LEU, Leucine; ASP, Aspartate; ARG, Arginine; GLY, Glycine; GLU, Glutamic acid.

with amassing of inflammatory cell migration observed in the APAP + ATRA group ($p < 0.001$, **Supplementary Image S1**).

Docking Studies

Comprehensive docking studies were conducted to explore the possible targets of carveol. Cis-carveol was docked in the active catalytic pocket of COX-2, HO-1, IL-1, NFκB, inducible nitric oxide (iNOS), Nrf2, and TNF-α. **Table 5** shows the binding energies after docking analysis, and **Figure 9** shows the best pose of cis-carveol fitting to COX-2, HO-1, IL-1, NFκB, iNOS, Nrf2, and TNF-α after docking studies. The active sites of these proteins were retrieved from the literature. It was perceived that the hydroxyl group (OH-) of carveol participated in hydrogen bond formation with a protein molecule (**Figure 9**). The OH- groups of carveol, in these interactions, acted as hydrogen bond donors and the respective protein molecules were hydrogen bond acceptors. ASP-140 and ARG-136 of HO-1, LEU-80, and THR-79 of IL-1β, GLY 61 of NFκB, LEU-365 of Nrf2, and GLU-115 of TNF-α were involved in hydrogen bond interactions. In addition, non-covalent alkyl and Pi-alkyl interactions were observed, which are crucial for temporary interactions, specifically for the drug activity to be proficient in a system.

DISCUSSION

The clinical syndrome of a higher dose of APAP has long been established, and the potent natural antioxidant carveol attenuates APAP-induced detrimental outcomes in hepatic tissue; thus, this study further attested to our previously published data. We previously demonstrated that carveol treatment attenuated ischemic stroke-induced neurodegeneration, by positively affecting the Nrf2 pathway, thereby leading to a reduced infarction area (Malik et al., 2020). We demonstrated here that carveol reversed the oxidative and inflammatory cascades of APAP, possibly by triggering the Nrf2-dependent antioxidative mechanism, which is cross-linked to the pro-survival pathways (**Figure 10**). Moreover, the low energy values and relatively higher hydrogen bond formation further enhanced complex stability, as revealed through the molecular docking analysis. Additionally, previous studies have reported that targeting inflammation and oxidative stress-coupled targets could provide better therapeutic outcomes (Ali T et al., 2020; Ling et al., 2020), which opens several avenues for the use of natural drug substances.

Paracetamol is an established inducer of liver toxicity in laboratory animals, but the exact pathological mechanism for this toxicity is not well known, and several mechanisms have been

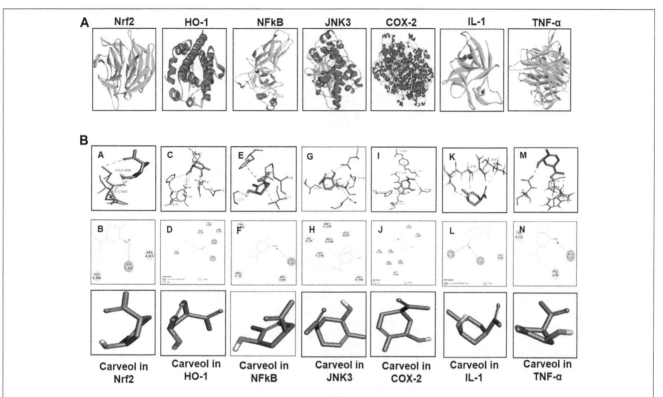

Figure 9 | Computational and docking analyses; **(A)** Tertiary structures of the proteins Nrf2, HO-1, NFκB, JNK3, COX-2, TNF-α, and IL-1β. **(B)** The docking results show the best pose of carveol that fitted to Nrf2, HO-1, NFκB, JNK3, COX-2, TNF-α, and IL-1β. The post-docking analysis was visualized using DSV in both 2D and 3D poses. The interaction between carveol and Nrf2 is shown in the panels **(A, B)**, HO-1 in the panels **(C, D)**, NFκB in the panels **(E, F)**, JNK in panels **(G, H)**, COX-2 in the panels **(I, J)**, IL-1 in the panels **(K, L)**, and TNF-α in the panels **(M, N)**. The 3D poses are shown in the panels **(A, C, E, G, I, K, M)** and the 2D in the panels **(B, D, F, H, J, L, N)**. Abbreviations: iNOS, inducible nitric oxide; TNF-α, tumor necrosis factor; IL-1β, interleukin; HO-1, heme oxygenase 1, COX-2, cyclooxygenase.

proposed. NAPQI, which is a highly reactive metabolite, is mostly attributed to this effect owing to its electrophilic nature, and it attacks several macromolecular targets (Shah et al., 2014; Sharma et al., 2016; Hellerbrand et al., 2017). The reactivity of NAPQI can be abolished by endogenous antioxidant enzymes, such as glutathione (James et al., 2003; Pastore et al., 2003; Lee et al., 2006). We observed a dose-dependent effect. Interestingly, carveol, at both doses, attenuated AST, ALT, and lactate dehydrogenase, along with favorable histological findings.

We have shown here that carveol treatment stimulates Nrf2, a key protein that combats various reactive oxygen species and other stress kinases, thereby halting necrotic and apoptotic cell death in the liver. The implications of inflammation, oxidative stress, and antioxidative mechanisms have been established previously. Our protein analysis using ELISA demonstrated that carveol alleviated the expression of different inflammatory mediators and cytokines, such as TNF-α and NFκB, which is further linked to increasing Nrf2 nuclear translocation and activation of the antioxidant machinery. Furthermore, such cascading events diminished the release of pro-inflammatory mediators and cytokines, by downregulating the NFκB signaling pathway, similar to previously reported data (Ali A et al., 2020). Nrf2 played a pivotal role in our model, as it reciprocally modulated the oxidative stress-induced inflammation. This notion was further demonstrated when ATRA treatment wore off the

hepatoprotective effects of carveol and elevated the expression of the inflammatory markers. These results are consistent with other experimental models, in which Nrf2 shields against inflammation (Mohsin Alvi et al., 2020). Thus, its activation, either pharmacological or signaling cascades, rescues the tissue from the hallmarks of inflammation and oxidative stress, while its pharmacological inactivation deteriorates the pathological conditions in several other related degenerative models. Furthermore, the downstream targets of Nrf2, such as HO-1 and TRX, later mediated the protective mechanism of Nrf2. It is worth mentioning here that natural drugs are frequently reported to activate the cleavage of Nrf2-Keap1 dimer and thus allow the translocation of Nrf2 to the nucleus, to stimulate antioxidant machinery, including HO-1 and NAPDH quinine dehydrogenase-1 (NQO1), and thus provide a notable antioxidative mechanism to reverse the oxidative stress-induced inflammation (Jaiswal, 2004).

GSH, SOD, and CAT are among the first-line defense antioxidants that are important and indispensable in the defense of oxidants, particularly in the liver. SOD catalyzes the conversion of superoxide free radicals to H_2O_2 and O_2, while CAT helps in protecting against the harmful effects of superoxide and lipid peroxidation in the liver. Our results demonstrated that carveol significantly attenuated hepatic MDA, a biomarker of lipid peroxidation, and leveled the GSH, SOD, and CAT contents,

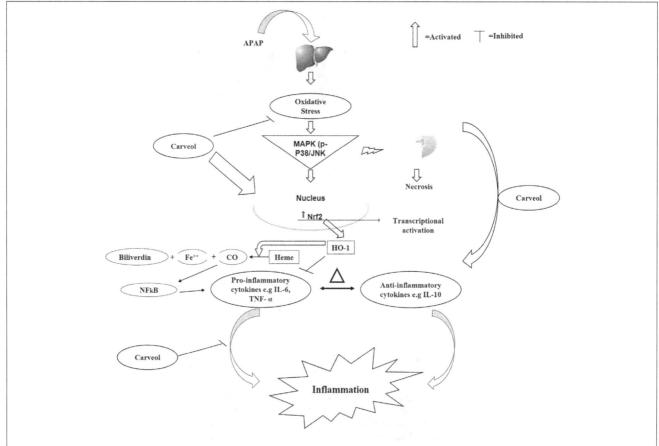

Figure 10 | The graphical representation indicates and elaborates the underlying antioxidant and anti-inflammatory mechanisms of carveol against the APAP-induced liver toxicity.

indicating a strong and complex effect of carveol in alleviating the APAP-induced oxidative stress. GSH activity is vital both for sustaining cellular homeostasis and for eliminating free radicals, such as superoxide. Furthermore, consistent studies have reported the detoxifying effect of GSH against electrophiles, such as NAPQI (Zai et al., 2018). Moreover, several protective agents act against liver insults, by normalizing GSH content. Thus, increased GSH, SOD, and CAT biosyntheses could account for the underlying mechanism of carveol against the NAPQI-induced oxidative stress and inflammation.

The Nrf2 pathway has a prominent protective role in the liver, while APAP exerts a detrimental effect on the Nrf2 pathway. A higher level of toxicity was observed in Nrf2-null mice than in wild-type mice when exposed to hepatotoxic agents (Aleksunes et al., 2008; Patterson et al., 2013; Guo and White, 2016). Previous studies on traditional Chinese drugs have shown their ability to activate Nrf2 and protect against the APAP-induced liver injury in mice. Consistent literature suggests that activation of the antioxidant machinery, such as Nrf2, could downregulate oxidative stress and the inflammatory cascade machinery, such as the NFκB pathway and cytokines (TNF-α and COX-2) (Ali A et al., 2020). The critical role of carveol in mediating the antioxidative effect of Nrf2 was further validated with the Nrf2 antagonist ATRA (Mohsin Alvi et al., 2020). ATRA

administration removed the hepatoprotective effect of carveol, abolished the increased levels of Nrf2 and HO-1, and further exaggerated p-NFκB and TNF-α levels.

Several studies have documented the cross-talk between oxidative stress and the inflammation process (Al Kury et al., 2019; Al Kury et al., 2020). Therefore, drug therapeutics should be designed to subside the inflammatory process and oxidative distress, by triggering the endogenous antioxidant defense system. We also studied the expression profile of a thiol-related protein, thioredoxin (TRX), an integral enzyme in hemostatic redox reactions (Patterson et al., 2013). Carveol treatment boosted the TRX level, which further validated the antioxidant nature of carveol in APAP-induced liver injury. However, the exact mechanism of how carveol abrogated liver injury needs to be explored in detail.

APAP provokes free radical formation and subsequent pro-inflammatory mediators. Moreover, role of the JNK pathway in inflammatory cascades and cellular death has been strongly established (Ali A et al., 2020), and ROS and inflammatory cytokines can trigger JNK activation (Ali A et al., 2020; Ali T et al., 2020; Ling et al., 2020). Furthermore, the p-JNK pathway has been implicated in various animal models and human diseases (Shah et al., 2018; Li and Liu, 2019; Ali A et al., 2020; Ling et al., 2020; Malik et al., 2020), and the downregulation or inhibition of this pathway has been found to contribute to the protective strategy (Shah et al., 2019). We observed similar activities in the APAP-intoxicated group, and carveol significantly reduced p-JNK expression. Furthermore, hepatic necrosis can be attenuated by downregulating p-NFκB expression, which may further act on the downstream COX-2 and iNOS and thus reduce ROS generation. Moreover, the expression of COX-2 and iNOS can be prevented by antagonizing p-NFκB expression (Ali A et al., 2020). Natural drug substances have significant anti-inflammatory potential, and we previously showed the inhibitory effect of carveol, polydatin, and Ginkgo biloba on NFkB, COX-2, and iNOS expression in different experimental models (Al Kury et al., 2019; Al Kury et al., 2020; Malik et al., 2020). We postulated here that carveol reduces hepatocellular necrosis by negatively modulating the expression of mitogen kinase and other inflammatory cytokines.

We performed docking analysis using the Autodock Vina program. The binding energy was evaluated for carveol and the respective proteins (**Figure 9**; **Table 5**). Different intermolecular interactive forces are vital for energetically stabilizing the drug-receptor complex. Carveol is flexibly complexed with protein targets, by establishing H-bonds and other hydrophobic interactions. Hydrogen bond formation is important for stabilization, recognition, and molecular movement (Baker and Hubbard, 1984; Desiraju and Steiner, 2001). Several studies have revealed the importance of this kind of bonding in ligand-protein complex stability, at a bond distance of 2.6Ao–3.2Ao (Glusker, 1995; Sarkhel and Desiraju, 2004; Panigrahi and Desiraju, 2007). We speculate that the formation of H-bonds between the ligand carveol and the respective protein supports the corresponding complex stability.

CONCLUSION

In summary, our *in vivo* results demonstrate that carveol could be a potent antioxidant and anti-inflammatory agent that mediates

protective properties in APAP-induced liver toxicity. Furthermore, our proposed mechanism suggests that carveol may activate the master endogenous antioxidant protein Nrf2 and may be associated with the negative modulation of p-JNK and other neuroinflammatory mediators; it may, thus, offer a new therapeutic option for preventing and managing oxidative stress and inflammation in degenerative disorders.

ETHICS STATEMENT

The animal study was reviewed and approved by Research and Ethical Committee of Riphah institute of Pharmaceutical Sciences, Riphah International University Islamabad Pakistan.

AUTHOR CONTRIBUTIONS

All authors made substantial contributions to conception and design, acquisition of data, or analysis and interpretation of data; took part in drafting the article or revising it critically for important intellectual content; agreed to submit to the current journal; gave final approval of the version to be published, and agree to be accountable for all aspects of the work.

ACKNOWLEDGMENTS

We are thankful to Alpha Genomics (PVT) LTD., PWD branch Islamabad for providing Paid excess to qPCR analysis.

REFERENCES

Abo-Haded, H. M., Elkablawy, M. A., Al-Johani, Z., Al-Ahmadi, O., and El-Agamy, D. S. (2017). Hepatoprotective effect of sitagliptin against methotrexate induced liver toxicity. *PLoS One.* 12, e0174295. doi:10.1371/journal.pone.0174295

Al Kury, L. T., Dayyan, F., Ali Shah, F., Malik, Z., Khalil, A. A. K., Alattar, A., et al. (2020). Ginkgo biloba extract protects against methotrexate-induced hepatotoxicity: a computational and pharmacological approach. *Molecules.* 25, 2540. doi:10.3390/molecules25112540

Al Kury, L. T., Zeb, A., Abidin, Z. U., Irshad, N., Malik, I., Alvi, A. M., et al. (2019). Neuroprotective effects of melatonin and celecoxib against ethanol-induced neurodegeneration: a computational and pharmacological approach. *Drug Des. Dev. Ther.* 13, 2715. doi:10.3390/molecules25112540

Al-Fartosi, K. G., Khuon, O. S., and Al-Tae, H. I. (2011). Protective role of camel's milk against paracetamol induced hepatotoxicity in male rats. *Int. J. Res. Pharm. Biomed. Sci.* 2, 1795–1799.

Aleksunes, L. M., Slitt, A. L., Maher, J. M., Augustine, L. M., Goedken, M. J., Chan, J. Y., et al. (2008). Induction of Mrp3 and Mrp4 transporters during acetaminophen hepatotoxicity is dependent on Nrf2. *Toxicol. Appl. Pharmacol.* 226, 74–83. doi:10.1016/j.taap.2007.08.022

Ali, A., Shah, F. A., Zeb, A., Malik, I., Alvi, A. M., Alkury, L. T., et al. (2020). NF-κB inhibitors attenuate MCAO induced neurodegeneration and oxidative stress—a reprofiling approach. *Front. Mol. Neurosci.* 13, 33. doi:10.3389/fnmol.2020.00033

Ali, J., Khan, A. U., Shah, F. A., Ali, H., Islam, S. U., Kim, Y. S., et al. (2019). Mucoprotective effects of Saikosaponin-A in 5-fluorouracil-induced intestinal mucositis in mice model. *Life Sci.* 239, 116888. doi:10.1016/j.lfs.2019.116888

Ali, T., Hao, Q., Ullah, N., Rahman, S. U., Shah, F. A., He, K., et al. (2020). Melatonin act as an antidepressant via attenuation of neuroinflammation by targeting Sirt1/Nrf2/HO-1 signaling. *Front. Mol. Neurosci.* 13, 96. doi:10.3389/fnmol.2020.00096

Ansari, S. F., Khan, A.-U., Qazi, N. G., Shah, F. A., and Naeem, K. (2019). *In vivo*, proteomic, and in silico investigation of sapodilla for therapeutic potential in gastrointestinal disorders. *BioMed Res. Int.* 2019, 4921086. doi:10.1155/2019/4921086

Baker, E., and Hubbard, R. (1984). Hydrogen bonding in globular proteins. *Prog. Biophys. Mol. Biol.* 44, 97–179. doi:10.1016/0079-6107(84)90007-5

Crowell, P. L., Kennan, W. S., Haag, J. D., Ahmad, S., Vedejs, E., and Gould, M. N. (1992). Chemoprevention of mammary carcinogenesis by hydroxylated derivatives of d-limonene. *Carcinogenesis.* 13, 1261–1264. doi:10.1093/carcin/13.7.1261

Dalaklioglu, S., Genc, G., Aksoy, N., Akcit, F., and Gumuslu, S. (2013). Resveratrol ameliorates methotrexate-induced hepatotoxicity in rats via inhibition of lipid peroxidation. *Hum. Exp. Toxicol.* 32, 662–671. doi:10.1177/0960327112468178

Desiraju, G. R., and Steiner, T. (2001). *The weak hydrogen bond: in structural chemistry and biology*, Oxford, United Kingdom: Oxford University Press.

Du, K., Ramachandran, A., and Jaeschke, H. (2016). Oxidative stress during acetaminophen hepatotoxicity: sources, pathophysiological role and therapeutic potential. *Redox Biol.* 10, 148–156. doi:10.1016/j.redox.2016.10.001

Ghaffar, U., and Tadvi, N. A. (2014). Paracetamol toxicity: a review. *J Contemp Med A Dent.* 2, 12–15. doi:10.18049/jcmad/232

Glusker, J. (1995). Intermolecular interactions around functional groups in crystals: data for modeling the binding of drugs to biological macromolecules. *Acta Crystallogr., Sect. D: Biol. Crystallogr.* 51, 418–427. doi:10.1107/S0907444995003313

Gopal, K. M., Mohan, J., Meganathan, M., Sasikala, P., Gowdhaman, N., Balamurugan, K., et al. (2011). Effect of dietary fish oil (omega-3-fatty acid) against oxidative stress in isoproterenol induced myocardial injury in albino wistar rats. *Global J. Pharmacol.* 5, 4–6.

Gorrell, M. D. (2005). Dipeptidyl peptidase IV and related enzymes in cell biology and liver disorders. *Clin. Sci.* 108, 277–292. doi:10.1042/CS20040302

Guo, J. Y., and White, E. (2016). Autophagy, metabolism, and cancer. *Cold Spring Harbor Symp. Quant. Biol.* 81, 73–78. doi:10.1101/sqb.2016.81.030981

Hellerbrand, C., Schattenberg, J. M., Peterburs, P., Lechner, A., and Brignoli, R. (2017). The potential of silymarin for the treatment of hepatic disorders. *Clin. Phytosci.* 2, 7. doi:10.1186/s40816-016-0019-2

Hennig, P., Garstkiewicz, M., Grossi, S., Di Filippo, M., French, L. E., and Beer, H.-D. (2018). The crosstalk between Nrf2 and inflammasomes. *Int. J. Mol. Sci.* 19, 562. doi:10.3390/ijms19020562

Imran, M., Al Kury, L. T., Nadeem, H., Shah, F. A., Abbas, M., Naz, S., et al. (2020). Benzimidazole containing acetamide derivatives attenuate neuroinflammation and oxidative stress in ethanol-induced neurodegeneration. *Biomolecules.* 10, 108. doi:10.3390/biom10010108

Iqbal, S., Shah, F. A., Naeem, K., Nadeem, H., Sarwar, S., Ashraf, Z., et al. (2020). Succinamide derivatives ameliorate neuroinflammation and oxidative stress in Scopolamine-induced neurodegeneration. *Biomolecules.* 10, 443. doi:10.3390/biom10030443

Jaiswal, A. K. (2004). Nrf2 signaling in coordinated activation of antioxidant gene expression. *Free Radic. Biol. Med.* 36, 1199–1207. doi:10.1016/j.freeradbiomed.2004.02.074

James, L. P., Mayeux, P. R., and Hinson, J. A. (2003). Acetaminophen-induced hepatotoxicity. *Drug Metab. Dispos.* 31, 1499–1506. doi:10.1124/dmd.31.12.1499

Lee, J. I., Kang, J., and Stipanuk, M. H. (2006). Differential regulation of glutamate-cysteine ligase subunit expression and increased holoenzyme formation in response to cysteine deprivation. *Biochem. J.* 393, 181–190. doi:10.1042/BJ20051111

Li, S., and Liu, F. (2019). Polydatin attenuates neuronal loss via reducing neuroinflammation and oxidative stress in rat MCAO models. *Front. Pharmacol.* 10, 663. doi:10.3389/fphar.2019.00663

Ling, L., Alattar, A., Tan, Z., Shah, F. A., Ali, T., Alshaman, R., et al. (2020). A potent antioxidant endogenous Neurohormone melatonin, rescued MCAO by attenuating oxidative stress-associated neuroinflammation. *Front. Pharmacol.* 11, 1220. doi:10.3389/fphar.2020.01220

Ma, Q., and He, X. (2012). Molecular basis of electrophilic and oxidative defense: promises and perils of Nrf2. *Pharmacol. Rev.* 64, 1055–1081. doi:10.1124/pr.110.004333

Malik, I., Shah, F. A., Ali, T., Tan, Z., Alattar, A., Ullah, N., et al. (2020). Potent natural antioxidant carveol attenuates MCAO-stress induced oxidative, neurodegeneration by regulating the Nrf-2 pathway. *Front. Neurosci.* 14, 659. doi:10.3389/fnins.2020.00659

Mohsin Alvi, A., Tariq Al Kury, L., Umar Ijaz, M., Ali Shah, F., Tariq Khan, M., Sadiq Sheikh, A., et al. (2020). Post-treatment of Synthetic polyphenolic 1, 3, 4 oxadiazole compound A3, attenuated ischemic stroke-induced neuroinflammation and neurodegeneration. *Biomolecules.* 10, 816. doi:10.3390/biom10060816

Ning, C., Gao, X., Wang, C., Kong, Y., Liu, Z., Sun, H., et al. (2018). Ginsenoside Rg1 protects against acetaminophen-induced liver injury via activating Nrf2 signaling pathway *in vivo* and *in vitro. Regul. Toxicol. Pharmacol.* 98, 58–68. doi:10.1016/j.yrtph.2018.07.012

Panigrahi, S. K., and Desiraju, G. R. (2007). Strong and weak hydrogen bonds in the protein-ligand interface. *Proteins.* 67, 128–141. doi:10.1002/prot.21253

Pastore, A., Federici, G., Bertini, E., and Piemonte, F. (2003). Analysis of glutathione: implication in redox and detoxification. *Clin. Chim. Acta.* 333, 19–39. doi:10.1016/s0009-9981(03)00200-6

Patterson, A. D., Carlson, B. A., Li, F., Bonzo, J. A., Yoo, M. H., Krausz, K. W., et al. (2013). Disruption of thioredoxin reductase 1 protects mice from acute acetaminophen-induced hepatotoxicity through enhanced NRF2 activity. *Chem. Res. Toxicol.* 26, 1088–1096. doi:10.1021/tx4001013

Rana, I., Khan, N., Ansari, M. M., Shah, F. A., Din, F., Sarwar, S., et al. (2020). Solid lipid nanoparticles-mediated enhanced antidepressant activity of duloxetine in lipopolysaccharide-induced depressive model. *Colloids Surf. B Biointerfaces.* 194, 111209. doi:10.1016/j.colsurfb.2020.111209

Sarkhel, S., and Desiraju, G. R. (2004). N. H. . . O, O. H. . . ON-H...O, O-H...O, and C-H...O hydrogen bonds in protein-ligand complexes: strong and weak interactions in molecular recognitionO hydrogen bonds in protein–ligand complexes: strong and weak interactions in molecular recognition. *Proteins.* 54, 247–259. doi:10.1002/prot.10567

Shah, F.-A., Gim, S.-A., Kim, M.-O., and Koh, P.-O. (2014). Proteomic identification of proteins differentially expressed in response to resveratrol treatment in middle cerebral artery occlusion stroke model. *J. Vet. Med. Sci.* 76, 1367–1374. doi:10.1292/jvms.14-0169

Shah, F. A., Zeb, A., Ali, T., Muhammad, T., Faheem, M., Alam, S. I., et al. (2018). Identification of proteins differentially expressed in the Striatum by melatonin in a middle cerebral artery occlusion rat model-a proteomic and. *Front. Neurosci.* 12, 888. doi:10.3389/fnins.2018.00888

Shah, F. A., and Rashid, S. (2020). Conformational ensembles of non-peptide ω-conotoxin mimetics and Ca$^+$ 2 ion binding to human voltage-gated N-type calcium channel Cav2. 2. *Comput. Struct. Biotechnol. J.* 18, 2357–2372. doi:10.1016/j.csbj.2020.08.027

Shah, F. A., Zeb, A., Li, S., and Al Kury, L. T. (2019). Pathological comparisons of the hippocampal changes in the transient and permeant middle cerebral artery occlusion rat models. *Front. Neurol.* 10, 1178. doi:10.3389/fneur.2019.01178

Sharma, S., Rana, S., Patial, V., Gupta, M., Bhushan, S., and Padwad, Y. (2016). Antioxidant and hepatoprotective effect of polyphenols from apple pomace extract via apoptosis inhibition and Nrf2 activation in mice. *Hum. Exp. Toxicol.* 35, 1264–1275. doi:10.1177/0960327115627689

Thompson Coon, J., and Ernst, E. (2002). Herbal medicinal products for non ulcer dyspepsia. *Aliment. Pharmacol. Ther.* 16, 1689–1699.

Ullah, U., Badshah, H., Malik, Z., Uddin, Z., Alam, M., Sarwar, S., et al. (2020). Hepatoprotective effects of melatonin and celecoxib against ethanol-induced hepatotoxicity in rats. *Immunopharmacol. Immunotoxicol.* 42, 255–263. doi:10.1080/08923973.2020.1746802

Wakabayashi, N., Skoko, J. J., Chartoumpekis, D. V., Kimura, S., Slocum, S. L., Noda, K., et al. (2014). Notch-Nrf2 axis: regulation of Nrf2 gene expression and cytoprotection by notch signaling. *Mol. Cell Biol.* 34, 653–663. doi:10.1128/MCB.01408-13

Zai, W., Chen, W., Luan, J., Fan, J., Zhang, X., Wu, Z., et al. (2018). Dihydroquercetin ameliorated acetaminophen-induced hepatic cytotoxicity via activating JAK2/STAT3 pathway and autophagy. *Appl. Microbiol. Biotechnol.* 102, 1443–1453. doi:10.1007/s00253-017-8686-6

18

Cellular Mechanisms of Liver Fibrosis

Pragyan Acharya[1]*, Komal Chouhan[1], Sabine Weiskirchen[2] and Ralf Weiskirchen[2]*

[1]Department of Biochemistry, All India Institute of Medical Sciences, New Delhi, India, [2]Institute of Molecular Pathobiochemistry, Experimental Gene Therapy and Clinical Chemistry, RWTH University Hospital Aachen, Aachen, Germany

*Correspondence:
Pragyan Acharya
pragyan.acharya@aiims.edu
Ralf Weiskirchen
rweiskirchen@ukaachen.de

The liver is a central organ in the human body, coordinating several key metabolic roles. The structure of the liver which consists of the distinctive arrangement of hepatocytes, hepatic sinusoids, the hepatic artery, portal vein and the central vein, is critical for its function. Due to its unique position in the human body, the liver interacts with components of circulation targeted for the rest of the body and in the process, it is exposed to a vast array of external agents such as dietary metabolites and compounds absorbed through the intestine, including alcohol and drugs, as well as pathogens. Some of these agents may result in injury to the cellular components of liver leading to the activation of the natural wound healing response of the body or fibrogenesis. Long-term injury to liver cells and consistent activation of the fibrogenic response can lead to liver fibrosis such as that seen in chronic alcoholics or clinically obese individuals. Unidentified fibrosis can evolve into more severe consequences over a period of time such as cirrhosis and hepatocellular carcinoma. It is well recognized now that in addition to external agents, genetic predisposition also plays a role in the development of liver fibrosis. An improved understanding of the cellular pathways of fibrosis can illuminate our understanding of this process, and uncover potential therapeutic targets. Here we summarized recent aspects in the understanding of relevant pathways, cellular and molecular drivers of hepatic fibrosis and discuss how this knowledge impact the therapy of respective disease.

Keywords: liver fibrosis, cytokines, chemokines, NASH, therapy, alcohol, cholestasis, drugs

INTRODUCTION

The liver is the largest solid organ in the human body, weighing about 1,200–1,500 g, and comprising about 1/50th of the total body weight in an adult (Dooley et al., 2018). Understanding the complex architecture of the liver is key to understanding liver fibrosis and its consequences.

The liver has two major sources of blood supply, namely (i) the portal vein and (ii) the hepatic artery. The portal vein brings venous blood from the intestines and spleen to the liver. The hepatic artery brings arterial blood to the liver from the celiac axis. The liver is encapsulated by the Glisson's capsule which is mainly composed of connective tissue (Junqueira and Carneiro, 2002). Within the Glisson's capsule, the liver is divided into polygonal sections called lobules which are also separated by connective tissue. Each lobule has a characteristic arrangement which is disturbed during liver fibrosis and is completely damaged during cirrhosis (**Figure 1A**) (Sasse et al., 1992). Since liver function is so intricately linked to this arrangement, hepatic function is completely disrupted during cirrhosis leading to complications. The liver lobule, which is roughly hexagonal, harbors the hepatic central vein at its center (Sasse et al., 1992; Junquiera and Carneiro 2002). Hepatocytes are the most abundant cell type in the liver, constituting about 60% of the total cell number and 80% of liver cell volume. Hepatocytes perform the major roles of the liver such as detoxification of xenobiotics, urea cycle and the synthesis of plasma proteins (Zhou et al., 2016). Hepatocytes are arranged in straight

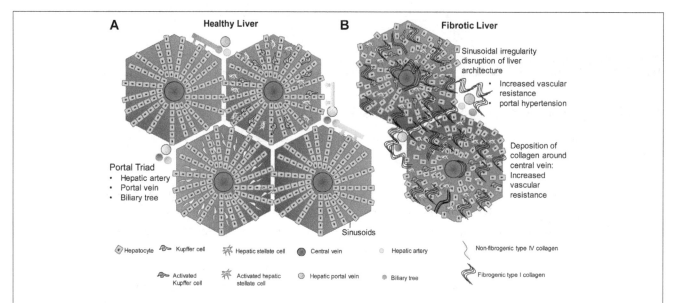

FIGURE 1 | Liver architecture in healthy liver and fibrosis. **(A)** In normal liver, hepatocytes are arranged in rows radiating outwards from the central vein, toward the edge of the lobule. The gaps between the hepatocyte rows are known as sinusoids which are lined with endothelial cells, and contain Kupffer cells, hepatic stellate cells, and contain extracellular material such as the non fibrogenic type IV collagen. Hepatic portal vein, hepatic artery and biliary tree are the three major vessels feeding into the sinusoids and the exchange of blood gases, nutrients and other signaling molecules occurs in the sinusoids. **(B)** Injury to hepatocytes due to any of several causes such as alcohol, drug, genetic predisposition, etc., activates the wound healing fibrogenic response. Chronic injury to the hepatocytes and chronic activation of the fibrogenic pathway in the liver leads to synthesis of fibrogenic type I collagen by the Hepatic stellate cells and its deposition within the sinusoids. Deposition around the central vein and around the portal vein leads to increase in vascular resistance and portal hypertension. Compensatory mechanisms such as esophageal varices and ascites follow.

lines radiating out from the central vein toward the edge of the lobule. The space between the radially arranged files of hepatocytes is commonly termed the sinusoids. Bile duct, lymphatics, neurons, as well as the branches of hepatic artery and portal vein line the periphery of the lobules and feed into the liver sinusoids. The portal vein and hepatic artery branch into the liver sinusoids, toward the central vein. Sinusoids are lined with fenestrated endothelial cells, and harbor immune cells such as Kupffer cells, hepatic stellate cells (HSCs) and hepatic natural killer cells (NK cells). These are known as the non-parenchymal cells of the liver. The space between the periphery of the hepatocyte lining and the endothelial cells is known as the space of Disse. The space of Disse is where the exchange of nutrients and other molecules occurs between the hepatocytes and blood flowing through the blood capillaries from the portal vein and the hepatic artery (Sasse et al., 1992). Interactions between the parenchymal and non-parenchymal cells in this carefully preserved architecture are central to efficient functioning of the liver.

Fibrogenesis is a normal wound healing response to tissue injury. All hepatocellular injuries activate the fibrogenic pathways. Once these pathways are activated, fibrogenic components of the extracellular matrix (ECM) are secreted into the space of Disse in order to encapsulate and isolate the damaged portion of the tissue for repair (Bataller and Brenner, 2005). During the encapsulation, there is an infiltration of immune cells that clear cellular debris and initiate tissue repair. The transition from a normal liver to fibrotic liver involves activation and modulation of complex signaling pathways, cell-cell communication between the hepatocytes and non-parenchymal cells, immune system, tissue repair pathways and the extracellular space. In the normal liver, the ECM present in the space of Disse is made up of glycoproteins like fibronectin and laminin, type IV collagen (non-fibrogenic) and proteoglycans such as heparan sulfate (**Figure 1A**). These components form a lattice-like matrix, which are essential for providing both mechanical support as well as molecular signals for the proper arrangement and functioning of liver cells. When there is hepatic injury, the composition and density of the ECM changes. There is almost a 6–8 fold increase in the production of ECM components. Non-fibrogenic type IV collagen is replaced by fibrogenic type I and II collagen (**Figure 1B**). There is additional secretion of fibronectin, hyaluronic acid and α-smooth muscle actin into the ECM. In addition, endothelial cell fenestrations as well as microvilli on the hepatocyte basal membrane are lost thereby compromising exchange of nutrients and metabolites as well as other signaling molecules between the circulation and hepatocytes. While the response to tissue injury is a rapid process and fibrogenesis is intended at promoting wound healing, repeated injury and activation of the fibrogenic pathways result in a chronic activation of fibrogenesis (Iredale et al., 2013). This leads to an increased synthesis and decreased degradation of type I collagen over a period of time. This results in deposition of type I collagen in the ECM

TABLE 1 | Genetic causes predisposing the liver to fibrosis.

Disease	Gene	Gene function	Cause of tissue injury	Clinical presentation with liver involvement
Wilson's Disease	ATP7B	Copper transport	Intra-hepatic Cu^{2+} accumulation	Variable presentation. Can be asymptomatic or accompanied by fibrosis, acute hepatitis, end stage liver disease
Progressive familial intrahepatic cholestasis type 3	ABCB4	Biliary phospholipid secretion	Accumulation of phospholipids and other xenobiotics; impairment of bile formation	Manifests in early childhood, jaundice, splenomegaly, portal hypertension and physical and mental retardation
Hereditary fructose intolerance	ALDOB	Converts fructose into trioses for entry into glycolysis and gluconeogenesis	Accumulation of fructose 1 phosphate and depletion of inorganic phosphate levels, inhibition of glycogenolysis, accumulation of high levels of fructose can be hepatotoxic	Hereditary fructose intolerance, hepatotoxicity, liver dysfunction progressing to cirrhosis
Glycogen storage disease type IV	GBE1	Glycogen branching enzyme	Accumulation of unbranched glycogen causing hepatotoxicity	Variable presentation. Hepatic classical presentation includes liver dysfunction progressing to cirrhosis, failure to thrive by 5 years of age. The non-progressive hepatic subtype present with hepatomegaly, liver dysfunction, myopathy, and hypotonia; but likely to survive without further progression to cirrhosis
Tyrosinemia type I	FAH	Last step in tyrosine catabolism	Accumulation of fumarylacetoacetate and tyrosine in the hepatocytes and oxidative damage to cells	Presentation as liver or renal failure; in early infancy; liver related symptoms are hypoalbunimea, lowering of synthetic functions of the liver, leading to steatosis, cirrhosis and HCC
Hemochromatosis	HFE	Interactions with the transferrin receptor and iron uptake	Intra-hepatic iron overload	Presentation as liver cirrhosis
Argininosuccinate lyase deficiency	ASL	Urea cycle enzyme that cleaves argininosuccinate into arginine and succinate	Accumulation of urea cycle intermediates, especially ammonia	Two forms:-Early onset in infancy associated with hyperammonimea and vomiting, failure to thrive, or late onset associated with hyperammonimea episodes, cirrhosis and neurological symptoms
Citrin deficiency	SLC25A13	Calcium binding mitochondrial carrier protein Aralar2 (exchange of cytoplasmic glutamate with mitochondrial aspartate across the inner mitochondrial membrane)	Citrullinemia and ammonia accumulation	Neonatal intrahepatic cholestasis: impaired bile flow, fibrosis, cirrhosis; late onset citrullinemia 2: neuropsychiatric symptoms
Cholesteryl ester storage disease	LIPA	Lysosomal acid lipase (LAL) catalyses the intracellular hydrolysis of triacylglycerols and cholesteryl ester	Intracellular accumulation of cholesteryl esters, triglycerides in the lysosomal compartment of hepatocytes	Early onset: hepatomegaly, splenomegaly and altered serum transaminases
α1 antitrypsin deficiency	SERPINA1	Inhibitor of various proteases including trypsin and therefore, protects cells from inflammatory proteases such as from neutrophils	Accumulation of mutant poly-AAT fibers leading to hepatotoxicity	Variable clinical severity ranging from chronic hepatitis and cirrhosis to fulminant liver failure
Cystic fibrosis	CFTR	Membrane chloride channel; expressed on the cholangiocytes	Pathogenesis unknown	Age of onset is late: elevation of serum liver enzymes, hepatic steatosis, focal biliary cirrhosis, multilobular biliary cirrhosis, neonatal cholestasis, cholelithiasis, cholecystitis and micro-gallbladder
Alström syndrome	ALMS1	Centrosome and basal body associated protein: microtubule organization	Pathogenesis unknown: likely to be involved in cellular Ca^{2+} signaling	Multiple organ dysfunction: liver involvement can range from steatohepatitis to portal hypertension and cirrhosis and can cause hepatic encephalopathy and life-threatening esophageal varices

(Continued on following page)

TABLE 1 | (*Continued*) Genetic causes predisposing the liver to fibrosis.

Disease	Gene	Gene function	Cause of tissue injury	Clinical presentation with liver involvement
Congenital hepatic fibrosis	Cryptogenic causes	NA	NA	Multiple organ fibrosis and dysfunction: Can present as the following in case of liver involvement: (i) portal hypertension (most common and more severe in the presence of portal vein abnormality), (ii) cholangitis with cholestasis and recurrent cholangitis, (iii) both portal hypertension and cholangitic symptoms; and (iv) latency that appears at a late age with hard hepatomegaly
Non-alcoholic fatty liver disease (NAFLD)	PNPLA3	Pleiotropic role with triglyceride lipase and retinyl esterase activity	Accumulation of triglycerides, impaired retinoic acid receptor signaling and activation of HSC fibrogenic pathway	Hepatic steatosis, fibrosis, cirrhosis, hepatocellular carcinoma

surrounding the lobules which is the hallmark of fibrosis. Large amounts of type I collagen deposition around the lobules and within the sinusoidal space disrupts the radial arrangement of the hepatocytes, interfering in the flow of nutrients and signaling molecules from the blood through the sinusoids to the hepatocytes, disrupting hepatocyte function. The deposition of collagen around the lobules causes major structural changes in the liver thereby disrupting liver function as well (Iwakiri, 2014). Accumulation of type I collagen fibers leads to mechanical rigidity in the ECM which puts pressure on the blood vessels flowing through the liver. This leads to intrahepatic vasoconstriction and vascular resistance (Pinzani and Vizzuti, 2005). Therefore, in a major vein like the hepatic portal vein, this leads to portal hypertension, which is a major clinical concern in liver fibrosis. The unchecked development of portal hypertension has two major consequences: (i) development of collateral blood vessels from the systemic and splanchnic circulation and, (ii) vasodilation of the hepatic artery (Bosch, 2007). This further increases blood flow into the hepatic portal vein leading to further portal hypertension. As a compensatory mechanism to relieve pressure, submucosal veins present at the lower portion of the esophagus dilate leading to esophageal varices that have the potential to rupture and can be fatal. Fluid begins accumulating within the peritoneal cavity, leading to ascites-the hallmark of advanced decompensated cirrhosis (Bolognesi, et al., 2014; Perri, 2013). These physiological processes are summarized in **Figure 1B**.

DRIVERS OF LIVER FIBROSIS

Genetic Disorders

Several genetic diseases predispose the liver to fibrosis (Scorza et al., 2014). In all of these diseases, the initiation of fibrosis begins with tissue injury due to a consequence of the genetic defect followed by a fibrogenic wound healing response, as discussed above. Genetic causes for liver fibrosis have come into light due to the advancements in molecular genetic and imaging techniques. Several genetic polymorphisms summarized in **Table 1**, have

been implicated in the occurrence of liver fibrosis, leading to cirrhosis (Pinzani and Vizzutti, 2005). Most of these mutations affect many different cell types but predispose the individual to liver fibrosis and in some cases, liver cirrhosis (Scorza et al., 2014). Many of the genes listed in **Table 1**, such as, *ABCB4*, *ALDOB*, *GBE1*, *FAH*, *ASL*, *SLC25A13*, and *SERPINA1* are highly expressed in the liver and therefore, mutations in these genes, the liver is the organ which is most affected. Most genetic disorders that lead to cirrhosis manifest in childhood and are a leading cause of pediatric liver cirrhosis, apart from childhood obesity (Pinto et al., 2015). In addition to the genetic mutations that predispose individuals to hepatic fibrosis that appear in childhood, mutations of the *PNPLA3* gene have been described as a major predisposing factor in non-alcoholic fatty liver disease (NAFLD) (Anstee et al., 2020). *PNPLA3* encodes for Patatin-like phospholipase domain-containing protein 3 or adiponutrin and is abundantly expressed in hepatocytes, adipocytes as well as HSCs (Dong, 2019). The *PNPLA3* I148M variant has been shown to have a positive association with hepatic fat content (steatosis), NAFLD, non-alcoholic steatohepatitis (NASH) as well as hepatocellular carcinoma (Dong, 2019). The global prevalence of NAFLD is about 25% and in obese individuals or in the presence of type 2 diabetes mellitus, it increases to about 60% (Younossi et al., 2016). Therefore, *PNPLA3* gene is a strong predisposing genetic factor for hepatic fibrosis. Although the PNPLA3 protein has been shown to have triacylglycerol lipase and acylglycerol transacylase enzymatic activities, its exact role in hepatocytes have been controversial (Jenkins et al., 2004; Dong, 2019). Other studies have demonstrated a retinyl esterase activity for PNPLA3 (Pirazzi et al., 2014). HSCs are reservoirs for retinoic acid, which activate the retinoic acid receptor (RAR) mediated transcription which keeps fibrogenesis under control (Hellemans, et al., 1999; Hellemans et al., 2004; Wang et al., 2002). Mutations in the *PNPLA3* gene that alter the retinyl esterase activity therefore, decrease the level of retinoic acid in the HSCs and therefore reduce the RAR mediated control of fibrogenesis in HSCs (Bruschi et al., 2017). However, it is now recognized that PNPLA3 has pleiotropic roles in the hepatocyte that are still

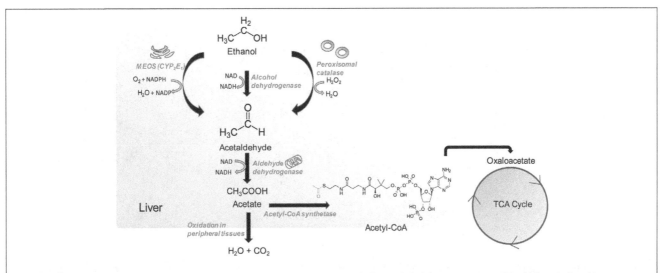

FIGURE 2 | Alcohol metabolism in the liver. Three pathways are involved in alcohol metabolism and all of them converge on the oxidation of ethanol to acetaldehyde. Acetaldehyde is further converted to acetate by aldehyde dehydrogenase in the mitochondria. Acetate can be rapidly oxidized into CO_2 and H_2O by peripheral tissues, or can be diverted to the tri-carboxylic acid (TCA) pathway. The oxidation of ethanol to acetaldehyde by microsomal ethanol oxidation system (MEOS) occurs in the smooth endoplasmic reticulum and changes the NADPH/NADP ratio which in turn influences the regeneration of glutathione thereby increasing cellular oxidative stress. The alcohol dehydrogenase pathway is the major pathway and occurs in the cytosol, generating large amounts of NADH. NADH in turn inhibits TCA cycle enzymes and leads to accumulation of acetyl CoA and increase in ketone body generation and acidosis. NADH also inhibits fatty acid oxidation leading to accumulation of fats and causing "fatty liver." A combination of the above factors leads to tissue injury and activation of the fibrogenic pathway.

under investigation such as in hepatocyte lipid droplet homeostasis, HSC quiescence and proliferation regulation (Dong, 2019). As several roles for PNPLA3 are suggested, PNPLA3 might be a good therapeutic target to control NAFLD related fibrosis and disease progression.

Alcohol

Excessive and continued alcohol intake over large periods of time, i.e., alcohol abuse, can lead to liver fibrosis followed by cirrhosis and liver cancer (Stickel et al., 2017). Alcoholic liver disease (ALD) comprises a spectrum of liver disorders ranging from fatty liver, steatosis, fibrosis with varying degrees of inflammation, cirrhosis. Alcohol abuse contributes to almost 50% of chronic liver disease related deaths globally (Rehm and Shield 2019). While the pathophysiology of alcohol induced cirrhosis is not completely understood, alcohol and its metabolic intermediates such as acetaldehyde are thought to play an important role in it. Alcohol is absorbed from the duodenum and upper jejunum by simple diffusion, reaching peak blood concentration by 20 min post ingestion after which it is quickly redistributed in vascular organs (Koob et al., 2014). Alcohol cannot be stored and needs to undergo obligatory oxidation which occurs predominantly in the liver (**Figure 2**) (Yang et al., 2019). The first step in alcohol oxidation converts alcohol into acetaldehyde. There are three enzymes in the liver that can carry out this reaction (i) alcohol dehydrogenase (ADH) which catalyzes the bulk of ethanol to acetaldehyde conversion, (ii) the alcohol inducible liver cytochrome P450 CYP2E1 (microsomal ethanol oxidizing system or MEOS) and, (iii) peroxisomal catalase. The ethanol to acetaldehyde conversion by ADH generates NADH (Berg et al., 2002). Oxidation of large amounts of alcohol therefore, leads to the

accumulation of NADH, which inhibits lactate to pyruvate conversion and promotes the reverse reaction. Lactate to pyruvate conversion is an important means of entry of lactate into gluconeogenesis. As a result, lactic acidosis and hypoglycemia may occur during excessive alcohol consumption. NADH/NAD$^+$ ratio also allosterically regulates fatty acid β-oxidation which breaks down long chain acyl CoA to acetyl CoA for entry into TCA cycle (Berg et al., 2002). Since NADH is a product of fatty acid oxidation, an increase in NADH/NAD$^+$ ratio provides an allosteric feedback to the fatty acid β-oxidation pathway thereby decreasing the catabolism of fatty acids and leading to their intracellular accumulation. This leads to "fatty liver." NADH also inhibits two enzymes of the TCA cycle-isocitrate dehydrogenase and α-ketoglutarate dehydrogenase thereby decreasing the consumption of acetyl CoA by the TCA cycle and leading to increase in intra-hepatic acetyl CoA levels. The accumulation of acetyl CoA, in turn, leads to the increased production and release of ketone bodies exacerbating the acidosis already present in the blood due to increased levels of lactate (McGuire et al., 2006). This is known as alcoholic ketoacidosis, which creates a medical emergency. At very high levels of ethanol consumption, the metabolism of acetate becomes compromised leading to the accumulation of acetaldehyde within the hepatocytes. Acetaldehyde can modify the functional groups of many proteins and enzymes irreversibly forming acetaldehyde adducts which leads to a global dysfunction of hepatocytes and eventually, to cell death (Setshedi et al., 2010). The second major pathway for ethanol metabolism is via the inducible cytochrome P450 CYP1E2, also known as the microsomal ethanol oxidizing system (MEOS) (Lieber, 2004). This is located in the smooth

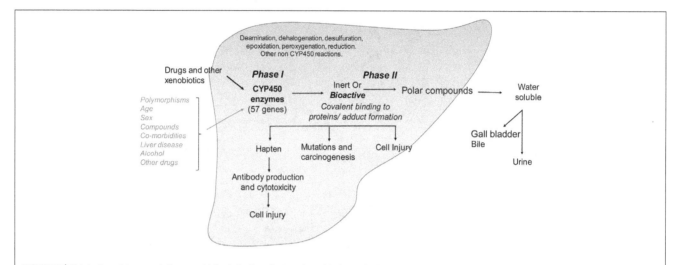

FIGURE 3 | Metabolism of drugs and other xenobiotics in the liver. Drug and xenobiotic metabolism occurs in two phases: (i) phase I is catalyzed by the cytochrome P450 family of monooxygenases which metabolize ingested small molecules to form inert or bioactive metabolic intermediates. (ii) These intermediates are further catalyzed in phase II reactions to form soluble polar compounds that can be further excreted through urine or bile. Accumulation of bioactive drug or xenobiotic intermediates can lead to the formation of protein or nucleic acid adducts causing autoimmune reaction, carcinogenesis or direct cellular injury.

endoplasmic reticulum of hepatocytes. In normal people with average to below average alcohol consumption, MEOS forms a minor pathway for intracellular alcohol metabolism (Lieber, 2004). However, it increases manifold upon chronic alcohol consumption. MEOS catalyzes a redox reaction converting molecular oxygen to water and NADPH to NADP (**Figure 2**). In the liver, glutathione plays an important role in maintaining the cellular redox status and participates in xenobiotic metabolism (Yuan and Kaplowitz, 2009). NADPH is essential in the regeneration of glutathione. The consumption of cellular NADPH leads to a decrease in regeneration of glutathione thereby leading to oxidative stress. This results in cell death and inflammation leading to alcoholic hepatitis which, in itself can be fatal (Morgan, 2007). Often, these processes occur hand in hand. Cellular depletion of glutathione has an additional consequence. Glutathione is required for the detoxification of several drugs including acetaminophen (van de Straat et al., 1987). In the hepatocytes, acetaminophen is modified to form a cytotoxic metabolite known as N-acetyl-p-benzoquinone imine (NAPQI) via CYP2E1 (van de Straat et al., 1987). Conjugation of NAPQI to glutathione results in an S-glutathione product that detoxifies the molecule and allows safe excretion in the urine. However, depletion of glutathione reserves allows unconjugated NAPQI to prevail in the cells which reacts with DNA and proteins to form adducts, thereby causing cytotoxicity and hepatocyte death (Macherey and Dansette, 2015). Long term alcohol use induces CYP2E1 and therefore facilitates rapid NAPQI formation when the liver encounters acetaminophen. At the same time, chronic alcohol abuse leads to low glutathione reserves. A combination of both these changes makes the liver highly susceptible to acetaminophen induced liver injury as well as injury due to other drugs or metabolites that go through the glutathione detoxification pathway. While drug overuse is, in itself a cause for liver injury, in a background

of alcoholic liver disease, it can lead to massive liver damage. Damage to hepatocytes, either due to chronic alcohol abuse, exacerbated by drug use, activates the fibrogenic pathway leading to hepatic fibrosis, cirrhosis and hepatocellular carcinoma.

Drugs

Drugs induce hepatic fibrosis by causing drug-induced liver injury (DILI) that causes the initiation of fibrogenic tissue repair mechanisms. While the prevalence of DILI is lower as compared to other causes of liver injury, such as alcohol, hepatisis or steatosis, it can lead to life-threatening complications. DILI can be of two types: (i) intrinsic (due to injury caused by a known on-target drug) or (ii) idosyncratic (due to injury caused by an unknown factor and cannot be explained by known pharmacological elements e.g., herbal preparations of unknown compositions) (DiPaola and Fontana, 2018). Among intrinsic causes, acetaminophen induced DILI is the most common. As described above, acetaminophen overload combined with alcohol abuse can exacerbate the liver injury that can occur due to either alcohol or acetaminophen alone. A major function of the liver is detoxification of xenobiotic compounds that enter our circulation either through diet or through intravenous drug usage. Detoxification mechanisms in the liver mainly involve the cytochrome P450 family (CYP gene families CYP1, CYP2, CYP3) (McDonnell and Dang, 2013) (**Figure 3**). Cytochrome P450s are a group of heme proteins that are involved in the initial detoxification reactions of small molecules such as dietary and physiological metabolites, as well as drugs (Zanger and Schwab, 2013; Todorovic Vukotic et al., 2021). The expression of the CYP genes is influenced by several factors such as age, sex, promoter polymorphisms, cytokines, xenobiotic compounds and hormones, to name a few (Zanger and Schwab, 2013). Cytochrome P450 mainly carry out a monooxygenation reaction and carry oxidation of drugs/xenobiotic compounds.

This can either convert the molecule into an inert or bioactive molecule.

Bioactive compounds can covalently modify intracellular proteins, leading to direct cellular injury, carcinogenesis or production of hapten-protein conjugates that can lead to antibody mediated cytotoxicity (**Figure 3**). Although the classical view of DILI is that drugs become hepatotoxic as a consequence of or defects in their metabolism, several factors may influence the final outcome of drug intake such as age, gender, comorbidities, intake of alcohol, other drugs or herbal preparations and polymorphisms of the *CYP* genes (Tarantino et al., 2009). The exact mechanism of DILI in specific cases depends on the nature of the molecule and its CYP-transformed metabolites. Drug metabolism can generate free radicals or electrophiles that can be chemically reactive. This can lead to the depletion of reduced glutathione, formation of protein, lipid or nucleic acid adducts and lipid peroxidation. Unless these metabolic intermediates are rapidly neutralized through phase II reactions, they can contribute to cellular stress and injury (**Figure 3**). They can also lead to modulation of signaling pathways, induce transcription factors, and alter gene expression profiles. In the liver, accumulation of large quantities of reactive drug metabolites can lead to hepatocellular injury, formation of protein adducts that can act as haptens and stimulate production of auto-antibodies or promote cellular transformation. Cellular injury then leads to induction of fibrogenic responses as described above.

Cholestasis

Cholestasis is emerging as a leading cause for liver injury and fibrosis. Cholestatic liver diseases can occur due to primary biliary cirrhosis and primary sclerosing cholangitis and involve injury to the intra- and extra-hepatic biliary tree (Penz-Österreicher et al., 2011). The pathogenesis of cholestasis is unclear but is believed to have an autoimmune component to it (Karlsen et al., 2017). I primary sclerosing cholangitis (PSC) several strictures appear around the bile ducts and cause bile duct injury. This activates the portal fibroblasts around the bile duct, which then differentiate into collagen secreting myofibroblasts (MFBs) similar to those derived from HSC activation. Recent studies have shown that fibrogenic MFBs have inherent heterogeneity and can be derived from both HSCs and portal fibroblasts (Karlsen et al., 2017). PSC has been shown to be associated with a varied manifestation of other diseases such as inflammatory bowel disease, cholangiocarcinoma, high IgG4 levels, autoimmune hepatitis and colonic neoplasia (Wee et al., 1985; Broomé et al., 1992; Perdigoto et al., 1992; Siqueira et al., 2002; Mendes et al., 2006; Berntsen et al., 2015). Due to its association with autoimmune responses, PSC is thought to involve a genetic predisposition which is activated by an as yet unidentified environmental trigger such as gut dysbiosis (Rossen et al., 2015). Although PSC is traditionally recognized as a rare disease, its incidence is on the rise due to an increase in unknown environmental triggers (Karlsen et al., 2017). Therefore, the pathogenesis of PSC is varied and injury to the bile ducts can occur through multiple pathways.

However, the resultant bile duct injury leads to activation of the portal fibroblasts and consequent fibrogenesis.

Metabolic Disorders: Non-alcoholic Fatty Liver Disease and Non-alcoholic Steatohepatitis

The metabolic syndrome is a group of associated diseases that increase cardiovascular risk factors and are linked with obesity and type 2 diabetes mellitus (Rosselli et al., 2014). Liver manifestations of the metabolic syndrome result in NAFLD (Rosselli et al., 2014). NAFLD is attaining epidemic proportions all over the world. The global prevalence of NAFLD is about 25% and in obese individuals or in the presence of type 2 diabetes mellitus, it increases to about 60% (Younossi et al., 2016). NAFLD is linked to increased risk of hepatic fibrosis, hepatocellular carcinoma and mortality due to cardiovascular disease. The more severe subtype of NAFLD is NASH, which has a global prevalence of about 2–6% and which is associated with severe hepatic inflammation, fibrosis leading to cirrhosis and HCC as well as end stage liver disease (Younossi et al., 2016; Younossi et al., 2019). Recently reported trends in the incidence of NAFLD over time suggest that NAFLD will become the leading cause of end stage liver disease in the decades to come. Emerging data from India, suggests that the national prevalence of NAFLD is about 9–32% in the general population and about 53% in obese individuals (Kalra et al., 2013; Duseja, 2010). Therefore, NAFLD is a global clinical concern. The molecular pathogenesis of NAFLD is complex. However, all pathways in NAFLD converge at the conversion of HSCs into profibrogenic MFBs, through the activation of the TGF-β pathway (Buzzetti et al., 2016) (**Figure 4**). TGF-β is a pleiotropic cytokine and is involved in various cellular processes like cell proliferation, survival, angiogenesis, differentiation, and the wound healing response (Mantel and Schmidt-Weber, 2011). TGF-β binds to the TGF-β receptor type II, which in turn phosphorylates TGF-β receptor type I thereby recruiting and phosphorylating the intracellular signal transducer proteins belonging to the SMAD superfamily. The SMAD superfamily is composed of intracellular signal transducers that specifically respond to the TGF-β receptor modulation. Phosphorylated SMADs subsequently translocate into the nucleus and control the expression of the TGF-β regulated target genes (Mantel and Schmidt-Weber, 2011) (**Figure 4**). The activation of HSCs via TGF-β plays a major role in the advanced NAFLD in both experimental animal models, as well as in human liver injury (Yang et al., 2014). In addition to HSC activation, TGF-β signaling followed by SMAD phosphorylation is known to cause hepatocyte death driving progression to NASH (Yang et al., 2017). Hepatocyte death via TGF-β signaling is accompanied by generation of reactive oxygen species as well as lipid accumulation in hepatocytes (Yang et al., 2017). Activation of the TGF-β pathway also leads to HSC differentiation into MFBs leading to formation of fibrillar collagen and exacerbating the combined effects of hepatocyte injury, fibrosis and inflammation, leading to NASH (Yang et al., 2014). While the TGF-β pathway is central to liver fibrogenesis, emerging proteome and transcriptome studies have suggested

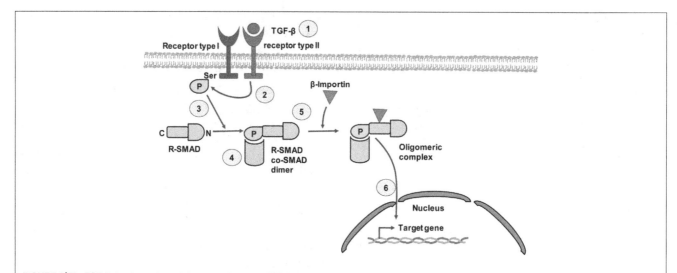

FIGURE 4 | The TGF-β signaling pathway in hepatic stellate cells. TGF-β binds to type II TGF-β receptor leading to receptor dimerization i.e. recruitment of the type I TGF-β receptor. The kinase domain of Type II TGF-β receptor then phosphorylates the Ser residue of type I TGF-β receptor. The phosphorylated receptor now recruits R-SMAD, which binds to receptor through its N-terminal region and gets phosphorylated by the Type II receptor. The C-terminal of R-SMAD has a DNA binding domain (DBD) that can act as a transcription factor. The co-SMAD now binds to R-SMAD and β-Importin binds to the dimer forming an oligomeric complex that guides the R-SMAD and Co-SMAD into the nucleus. The dimer enters the nucleus and the DBD of SMAD now acts as transcription factor that can transcribe target genes.

additional regulatory genes and pathways. These studies have been carried out in animal models of NAFLD or NASH and human liver biopsies obtained from patients. Comparative transcriptomic studies between mouse models of NAFLD and human liver biopsies obtained from NASH patients reveal major differences between human NASH liver transcriptome and mouse NAFLD transcriptomes even at severe stages (Teufel et al., 2016). This suggests major pathophysiological differences between human disease and animal models of the disease and the need to design studies in humanized models of disease or in liver organoid systems (Suppli et al., 2019). A meta-analysis of transcriptomic studies carried out with human liver biopsies suggests the upregulation of several genes within the lipogenesis pathway (**Table 2**). Interestingly, genes such as *ACACA* (Acetyl carboxylase 1) which catalyzes the synthesis of malonyl CoA from acetyl CoA, the rate limiting step in fatty acid biosynthesis and *ACACB* (Acetyl carboxylase 2) which regulates fatty acid oxidation, are associated with NAFLD liver tissue demonstrating the association of lipogenic functions within the tissue with active disease (**Table 2**) (Widmer et al., 1996; Locke et al., 2008). In several cases, NAFLD has been shown to be linked to progression toward hepatocellular carcinoma. Recent studies have led to the understanding that the evolution of NAFLD to NASH and HCC is multifactorial and involves the innate immune system to a great extent (Chen et al., 2019). Lipid accumulation and mitochondrial dysfunction have been identified as critical components of the pathways leading to NAFLD (Margini and Dufour, 2016). Many new genes and pathways have been implicated at every stage of NAFLD to NASH to HCC progression (**Figure 5**). Regulation in PPAR-γ, Insulin and p53-mediated signaling have been implicated in NAFLD development, whereas signatures of inflammatory signaling such as Toll-like receptor (TLR) and Nucleotide-binding, oligomerization domain (NOD) protein signaling

pathways, in addition to pathways reflecting mitochondrial dysfunction characterize NASH (**Figure 5**) (Ryaboshapkina and Hammar, 2017).

There are only a limited number of proteomics studies in human NAFLD. A comparative quantitative proteomics study between NAFLD and Metabolic Healthy Obese (MHO) individuals was carried out using liver tissue obtained during surgery (Yuan et al., 2020). This study demonstrated the relevance of PPAR signaling, ECM-receptor interaction and oxidative phosphorylation in resisting NAFLD. Proteins upregulated in NAFLD were involved in organization of the ECM, and proteins downregulated in NAFLD were involved in redox processes. A schematic of pathways relevant in NAFLD progression, as gleaned from various "omics" approaches is summarized in **Figure 5**.

Viral Hepatitis

In older children, autoimmune hepatitis and viral hepatitis are the leading causes of liver fibrosis followed by cirrhosis. Viral hepatitis can be caused by any one of the five viruses: Hepatitis A, B, C, D, and E of which A and E are usually acute, while B, C, and D are chronic (Zuckerman 1996). All hepatitis viruses are infectious, while alcohol, other toxins and autoimmune mediated hepatitis are usually non-infectious. HBV and HCV lead to hepatic inflammation (Gutierrez-Reyes et al., 2007). Several viral components are known to induce cellular damage in hepatocytes and liver constituents. For instance, the HCV core protein in chronic infections is known to interact with the TNF-α receptors (TNFRSF1A) which subsequently induces a pro-apoptotic signal in hepatocytes (Zhu et al., 1998). Polymorphisms in *TNFRSF1A* have been shown to be associated with HCV outcomes (Yue et al., 2021). The HCV core protein is also known to interact with ApoA1and ApoA2, thereby interfering with the assembly and secretion of

TABLE 2 | Summary of pathways from transcriptomics analyses implicated in NAFLD

Gene		Function/remarks	References
LEP	Leptin	Anti-steatotic, but also a proinflammatory and profibrogenic action	Polyzos et al. (2015)
PEMT	Phosphatidylethanolamine N-methyltransferase	Governs the secretion of hepatic triglycerides in the form of very low-density lipoprotein	Tan et al. (2016)
PPAR-γ2	Peroxisome proliferator activated receptor gamma	Ppary2 is expressed in the liver, specifically in hepatocytes, and its expression level positively correlates with fat accumulation induced by pathological conditions such as obesity and diabetes	Lee et al. (2018)
TNF-α	Tumor necrosis factor	Tumor necrosis factor (TNF)-α is associated with insulin resistance and systemic inflammatory responses	Seo et al. (2013)
PNPLA3	Patatin like phospholipase domain containing 3	Polymorphisms in PNPLA3 have been linked to obesity and insulin sensitivity	Chen et al. (2010)
CD14	CD14 molecule	Upregulation of CD14 in liver cells show increased sensitivity to LPS, changes in CD14 expression could represent a mechanism regulating liver sensitivity to LPS toxicity	Satoh et al. (2013)
ACACA	Acetyl-coa carboxylase α	Low level is correlated with long time survival	Liu et al, (2020)
ACACB	Acetyl-coa carboxylase β	Involved in insulin signaling pathway and adipokine metabolic pathway	Li et al. (2019)
ASPG	Asparaginase	The bacterial enzyme L-Asparaginase is a common cause of anti-neoplastic-induced liver injury with occurrence of jaundice and marked steatosis	Kamal et al. (2019)
CCS	Copper chaperone for superoxide dismutase	CCS expression is regulated by copper by modulating its degradation by the 26S proteosome	Bertinato and L'Abbé (2003)
CHEK1	Checkpoint kinase 1	This kinase is necessary to preserve genome integrity	Zhang and Hunter (2014)
HDAC9	Histone deacetylase 9	Downregulation of HDAC9 decrease TGF-β1-induced fibrogenic gene expression in hepatic stellate cells	Yang et al. (2017)
NADSYN1	NAD synthetase 1	Reduced NAD concentrations contribute to the dysmetabolic imbalance and consequently to the pathogenesis of NAFLD	Guarino and Dufour (2019)
NHP2L1	Small nuclear ribonucleoprotein 13	This genes encodes a protein of the spliceosome complex	Liu et al. (2020)
OAS3	2'-5'-oligoadenylate synthetase 3	OAS3 is an interferon-induced anivral enzyme	Zhang and Yu (2020)
PCNA	Proliferating cell nuclear antigen	PCNA encodes the protein which is found in the nucleus and is a cofactor of DNA polymerase delta and involved in the RAD6-dependent DNA repair pathway in response to DNA damage	Xing et al. (2018)
RPL10L	Ribosomal protein L10 like	The encoded protein shares sequence similarity with ribosomal protein L10	Liu et al. (2020)
RSL24D1	Ribosomal L24 domain containing 1	The encoded protein is involved in involved in the biogenesis of the early pre-60S ribonucleoparticle	Xie et al. (2020)
SRC	SRC proto-oncogene, non-receptor tyrosine kinase	SRC is a proto-oncogene encoding a non-receptor tyrosine kinase	Amanatidou and Dedoussis (2021)
TOP2A	DNA topoisomerase II alpha	Regulates the topologic states of DNA and controls tumor cell response	Wong et al. (2009)
TP53	Tumor protein p53	Induces apoptosis but the association between p53 and NAFLD remains controversial, P53 plays an essential role in the pathogenesis of NAFLD, whereas others have indicated that suppression of p53 activation aggravates liver steatosis	Yan et al. (2018)
TWISTNB	RNA polymerase I subunit F	This gene (i.e. TWIST Neighbor) is ubiquitous expressed in all tissues	Liu et al. (2020)
UMPS	Uridine monophosphate synthetase	Lack of this gene results in reduced cell membrane stability	Wortmann and Mayr (2019)
HORMAD2	HORMA domain containing 2	Decreases with advancing fibrosis	Liu et al. (2020)
LINC01554	Long intergenic non-protein coding RNA 1554	LINC01554, one kind of lncRNA, has been found specifically enriched in liver tissue and have strong association with pathogenesis and clinical evaluation of HCC	Ding et al. (2020)

very low density lipoprotein (VLDL), thus cause the accumulation of triglycerides in the liver through the interaction of both viral and metabolic factors and subsequent cell death (Gutierrez-Reyes et al., 2007). Furthermore, the viral core protein as well as the HCV non-structural protein 5A (NS5A) are known to cause mitochondrial ROS production and cellular stress leading to cell death (Bataller et al., 2004). Interestingly, HCV and NAFLD can co-exist and have been shown to have a more rapid disease progression than either disease alone (Patel and Harrison, 2012; Dyson et al., 2014). About 50% of HCV patients have steatosis with significant fibrosis and the HCV genotype 3 is mainly associated with the steatosis, however the exact mechanism leading to steatosis in HCV patients is not fully elucidated.

The association of hepatitis B virus (HBV) infection with NAFLD however, appears to be controversial. Some studies suggest that HBV infection is protective against steatosis, insulin resistance and metabolic syndrome (Morales et al., 2017; Xiong et al., 2017) while others suggest that chronic HBV infections can co-exist with NAFLD and can actively worsen the disease (Zhang et al., 2020). The presence of Hepatitis B protein X (HBx) in the cells has been shown to increase the production of reactive oxygen species (ROS) increasing the formation of lipids in the cells and therefore HBx could be a risk factor for the development of NAFLD (Wang et al., 2019). Therefore, an alternative mechanism by which viral hepatitis can induce fibrosis is through their ability to cause NAFLD.

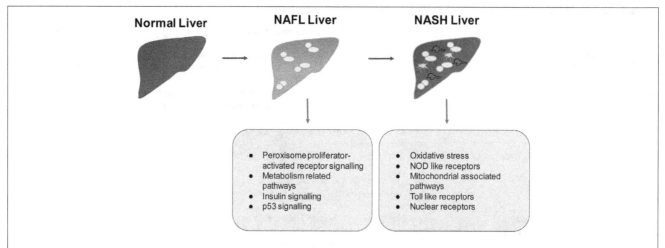

FIGURE 5 | Summary of pathways that may be important in the progression of NAFLD to NASH. The transition from healthy to NAFLD involves the activation of peroxisome proliferator activated receptor signaling, insulin signaling and p53 signaling whereas the switch to NASH involves activation of inflammatory pathways such as TLR and NOD like receptor mediated signaling, generation of intracellular oxidative stress and mitochondrial signaling.

Parasitic Infections

The liver is capable of hosting a wide range of parasites which vary in host cell requirement (extra or intracellular), sizes (unicellular to multicellular) and potential harm to the host cells or organs (Dunn, 2011). Parasites which have co-evolved with humans through centuries, such as the malaria parasites cause minimal injury to the host liver and move on to the blood with ease (Acharya et al., 2017). However, some parasites can cause injury to the cells of the liver and trigger the activation of the fibrogenic pathway. Some of these parasites are discussed below:

Leishmania is an intracellular protozoan parasite that infects the reticuloendothelial system (RES) in the body, i.e., circulating monocytes as well as tissue-resident macrophages (Magill et al., 1993). Leishmaniasis is transmitted by the bite of infected sandflies (Dunn, 2011). Visceral leishmaniasis (kala-azar) involves the RES infection of the visceral organs like the liver, spleen, bone marrow and other lymph nodes. Kupffer cells, the tissue resident macrophages of the liver, take up the amastigote stage of Leishmania from circulating infected reticuloendothelial cells. The parasite then replicates within the macrophages and activates the host inflammatory and Th1 and Th17 mediated adaptive immune responses in immunocompetent individuals (Pitta et al., 2009). Leishmaniasis is typically associated with increased liver fibrosis (Melo et al., 2009). Leishmania parasites have been shown to use host ECM components such as fibronectin and laminin to access Kupffer cells for infection (Wyler et al., 1985; Wyler, 1987; Vannier-Santos et al., 1992; Figueira et al., 2015). Visceral leishmaniasis has been frequently studied in dogs as a model system. These studies suggest that dogs infected with Leishmania have a significantly higher level of collagen and fibronectin deposition (Melo et al., 2009). Intralobular collagen deposition, appearance of MFBs and effacement of the space of Disse are characteristic of overt Leishmania infection in slightly or severely immunocompromised individuals (Dunn, 2011). Leishmania associated fibrosis is completely reversible once the parasitic infection has been treated. However, since overt disease and severe fibrosis usually occurs in immunocompromised individuals such as those infected with HIV, relapses typically occur once treatment ceases (Dunn, 2011).

Schistosomiasis is caused by Schistosoma species which are a group of blood flukes belonging to the trematode or flatworm family (Andrade, 2009). It is prevalent mainly in the tropical and sub-tropical regions of the world. Schistosoma use freshwater snails as intermediate hosts, which release eggs into water bodies which then come into contact with humans and infect them (WHO. World Health Organization, 2021). Schistosomiasis can be intestinal (wherein the liver is involved) or urogenital. Intestinal schistosomiasis can be caused by many different species such as Schistosoma mansoni (found in Africa, Middle East, Caribbean, Brazil, Venezuela and Suriname), S. japonicum (found in China, Indonesia and the Philippines), S. mekongi (Cambodia, and the Lao People's Democratic Republic), S. guineensis and S. intercalatum (found in the rain forests of central Africa). Urogenital infection is caused by S. hematobium (found in Africa, the Middle East and Corsica in France) (WHO. World Health Organization, 2021).

Schistosoma mansoni are associated with liver fibrosis (Andrade, 2009). Schistosome eggs are carried to the liver by the portal vein and stop in the pre-sinusoidal vessels (Andrade, 2004). The development of severe schistosomiasis is thought to have two components- (a) a major determinant is the high worm load and, (b) a secondary determinant is thought to be genetic predisposition. At low to moderate worm loads, many patients are asymptomatic and the lesions heal automatically due to the appropriate activation of T-cell mediated host immune responses (Andrade, 2004). A high worm load is also associated with damage to the portal vein and appearance of MFBs and collagen deposition around the portal stem leading to portal fibrosis called pipestem fibrosis (Andrade et al., 1999). Since all infected individuals do not develop severe liver disease, or liver fibrosis, schistosomiasis linked liver fibrosis development is also thought to have a genetic component. A metaanalysis of genetic polymorphisms associated with severe liver disease and fibrosis in schistosomiasis reveals several genetic polymorphisms (Dessein et al., 2020). Several polymorphisms in genes related to the TGF-β pathway were found to be associated with severe fibrosis in schistosomiasis e.g., *TGFBR1*, *TGFBR2*, *ACVRL1*, *SMAD3* and *SMAD9* (Dassein et al., 2020). Polymorphisms in the connective tissue growth factor (CTGF) as well as the IL-22 pathway were also observed. In addition, several associations have been reported between severe hepatic fibrosis during Schistosomiasis and genes encoding for IL-13, TNF-α, MAPKAP1, ST2, IL-10, M1CA, HLADRB1, IL-4, ECP, and IFN-γ, have been reported from various studies (Hirayama et al., 1998; Chevillard et al., 2003; Eriksson et al., 2007; Gong et al., 2012; Silva et al., 2014; Zhu et al., 2014; Long et al., 2015; Oliveira et al., 2015; Long et al., 2017; Silva et al., 2017). These observations suggest that while infectious agents such as schistosoma can drive hepatic fibrosis by mediating tissue damage, genetic predispositions to TGF-β pathway activation or a specific inflammatory response may make the hepatic environment conducive to fibrosis in the presence of an infectious agent.

Fasciola hepatica, also known as the liver fluke is also a trematode parasite that infects humans (Machicado et al., 2016). Fascioliasis is a neglected tropical disease. A recent meta-analysis has found an association of Fasciola infections with liver fibrosis, cirrhosis and hepatocellular carcinoma (Machicado et al., 2016). The mechanism of fibrosis development is thought to be due to the activation of HSCs by parasite encoded cathepsins (Marcos et al., 2011). As with schistosoma, worm-load seems to be an important determinant of fibrosis. However, there are a very limited number of studies available on the pathogenesis, molecular epidemiology and prevalence of fascioliasis with liver fibrosis and this area needs further investigation.

Cryptogenic Causes

Cryptogenic causes of liver fibrosis are cases with unknown causes but it is believed that a high proportion of the cryptogenic liver fibrosis cases could be linked to NAFLD or NASH (Caldwell, 2010; Patel et al., 2020). Other causes could include occult alcohol intake, viral hepatitis, autoimmune hepatitis, biliary disease, vascular disease, celiac disease, mitochondriopathies, systemic lupus erythematosus, Alstrom syndrome, Apolipoprotein B with LDL cholesterol, and genetic disorders such as short telomere syndrome, keratin 18 mutations and glutathione-S-transferase mutations (Caldwell, 2010; Patel et al., 2020).

SOLUBLE MEDIATORS IN LIVER FIBROSIS

The development of liver fibrosis occurs as a result of interaction between several different cell types including hepatocytes, HSCs, Kupffer cells, as well as infiltrating immune cells. These inter-cellular interactions involve several soluble and secreted mediators which regulate inflammatory pathways, chemotaxis

and HSC activation. Some of the known soluble mediators are briefly discussed below.

Cytokines and Chemokines

Cytokines are regulatory soluble small molecular weight proteins or glycoproteins released by several cells and mediate interaction, communication between different cell types. Cytokines play an important role in the progress of liver fibrosis (Xu et al., 2012). In liver they mediate the interactions of the various cell types and contribute to either the production of proinflammatory or hepatoprotective responses (Kong et al., 2012). Cells of the immune system such as Kupffer cells and neutrophils produce many cytokines and chemokines that can affect the gene expression, proliferation, contractility and activation of HSCs. The interaction between HSCs and immune cells are bidirectional, i.e., while immune cells produce cytokines to activate HSCs. HSCs also regulate immune cell chemotaxis and response by secreting soluble mediators themselves (Weiskirchen, 2016). For instance, the pro-inflammatory cytokines TGF-α increases HSC proliferation, TGF-β inhibits HSC apoptosis and promotes ECM remodeling leading to a pro-fibrogenic phenotype, TNF-α inhibits HSC apoptosis and induces chemokines and ICAM-1 in HSCs (Maher, 2001). IL-4 in concert with MMP-2 and ROS increase ECM synthesis and fibrosis. At the same time, anti-fibrogenic cytokines are also released from immune cells that can control the pro-fibrogenic HSC activation, such as IL-10, IFN-α, IFN-γ. A balance of these factors results in a net pro-or anti-fibrogenic effects on HSCs. The HSCs also secretes several molecules which are instrumental in recruiting immune cells at the site of activation such as M-CSF that causes macrophage proliferation and maintenance, PAF, MIP-2 and CINC/IL-8 which cause neutrophil chemotaxis and MCP-1 which recruits monocytes (Maher, 2001).

While activation of the TGF-β pathway is a central event in the induction of hepatic fibrosis, HSC activation is regulated by other pathways and molecular mechanisms as well, such as the Hippo pathway and autophagy (Tsuchida and Friedman, 2017). The Hippo signaling pathway is an evolutionarily conserved pathway that derives its name from its key player, the protein kinase "Hippo", which is involved in the regulation of cell and organ size (Saucedo and Edgar, 2007). However, Hippo pathway components such as the transcriptional co-activator Yes-associated protein 1 (YAP1) and the protein kinases macrophage stimulating 1 (MST1) and MST 2 have been shown to be important in initial HSC activation (Manmadhan and Ehmer, 2019). Inhibition or silencing of YAP1, and inactivation of MST1 and MST2 have been shown to have therapeutic effects in mouse models of fibrosis but the human clinical impact of such approaches is presently not known (Manmadhan and Ehmer, 2019).

Chemokines are a subgroup of cytokines that have chemotactic properties. They are synthesized by most liver cells as well as by infiltrating immune cells and their effects depend on their local concentrations at the site of injury (Sahin et al., 2010). Typically, chemokines bind G-protein coupled receptors (GPCRs) and induce signaling in target cells (Bonecchi et al., 2009). Stellate cells express several chemokines as well as chemokine receptors. HSCs have been shown to secrete CCL2, CCL3, CCL5, CXCL1, CXCL8, CXCL9 and CXCL10 (Holt et al., 2009; Wasmuth et al., 2009; Zaldivar et al., 2010; Marra and Tacke, 2014). Portal fibroblasts which are involved in cholestastis-associated fibrosis are also capable of secreting chemokines (Dranoff and Wells, 2010]. Targeting of chemokines and chemokine receptors in experimental models of fibrosis has been shown to control fibrosis and therefore warrants further investigation as a potential therapeutic anti-fibrosis strategy (Sahin et al., 2010).

In addition to these cytokines and chemokines, several miRNA have been recently identified to be involved in the HSC-immune cell cross-talk (Zhangdi et al., 2019).

Lipid Mediators

Lipid mediators in hepatic fibrosis are mainly studied in the context of NAFLD and NASH (Liangpunsakul and Chalasani, 2019). Several different types of lipid species have been shown to be associated with NAFLD such as saturated free fatty acids (FFA), diacylglycerols, ceramides, lysophosphatidylcholine, eicosanoids and free cholesterol (Feldstein et al., 2003; Caballero et al., 2009; Gorden et al., 2011; Luukkonen et al., 2016). Increased triglyceride accumulation is a hallmark of NAFLD and is associated mainly with hepatic steatosis (Yamaguchi et al., 2007). While triacylglycerol (TAG) accumulation has not been found sufficient for causing insulin resistance, excessive TAG accumulation can increase mechanical pressure on hepatic sinusoids leading to the impairment of hepatic blood flow, and generation of compensatory collateral flow (Wanless and Shiota, 2004). Excessive amounts of free fatty acids can act directly as TLR agonists in the liver or are taken up by the liver, converted into lipotoxic intermediates that activate the JNK, IKK pathway leading to cell injury, inflammation and apoptosis (Yu et al., 2002).

Extracellular Vesicles

Cellular injury to hepatocytes can lead to many outcomes. In addition to hepatocyte cell death, injured and stressed hepatocytes have been shown to release extracellular vesicles (EV) (Ibrahim et al., 2016; Schattenberg and Lee, 2016). EV are nanovesicles released by almost all cell types (Dooyle et al., 2018). They constitute two major size categories, namely plasma membrane derived microvesicles (50–1,000 nm) and endosome-derived exosomes (30–150 nm in diameter) as defined by the International Society for Extracellular Vesicles" (ISEV) and according to the Minimal Information for Studies of Extracellular Vesicles (MISEV) guidelines of 2014 (Lötvall et al., 2014). In fact, lipid overload has been shown to activate hepatocyte signaling through the death receptor 5 (DR5) followed by release of hepatocyte-derived pro-inflammatory EV containing TNF-α (Cazanave et al., 2011). These EV activated macrophage induced inflammation leading to further cellular injury and the development of NASH in experimental mouse models (Cazanave et al., 2011). Administration of EV isolated from high fat diet (HFD) mice into normal fed mice have been shown to result in exacerbation of hepatic steatosis and accumulation of activated myeloid cells in the liver through

the release of chemotactic EV (Ibrahim et al., 2016). In addition to hepatocyte-derived EV, extra-hepatic EV have also been implicated in the progression of NAFLD, NASH and associated fibrosis (Srinivas et al., 2021). Due to their ability to carry signal from one cell type to another, they can activate or modulate target cell responses and are therefore an emerging therapeutic targets in NAFLD and NASH.

Autophagy and Unfolded Protein Response

Autophagy in response to endoplasmic reticulum (ER) stress has also been recognized as an activator of HSCs. Under normal circumstances, autophagy is an important regulator of hepatic homeostasis (Mallat et al., 2014). While normally, autophagy is believed to have a protective effect on injured hepatocytes, recent studies demonstrate that ER stress signals activate autophagy and a profibrogenic phenotype in HSCs (Mallat et al., 2014). HSC activation is linked to increased flux in autophagy-related metabolic pathways and inhibition of this process can prevent HSC activation (Thoen et al., 2012). Similarly, there is evidence that the accumulation of misfolded or unfolded proteins in the ER triggering a process called unfolded protein response is a critical feature during early activation of profibrogenic cells such as HSCs (Mannaerts et al., 2019), suggesting that the development of interventions targeting the processes of autophagy or unfolded proteins response might be effective in therapy of hepatic fibrosis.

CELLULAR MEDIATORS OF HEPATIC FIBROSIS

The hallmark of hepatic fibrosis is the increased expression and deposition of ECM compounds. There are different resident and infiltrating cells that can either be activated or produced by progenitors that transform into a phenotype capable to synthesize ECM. Each of these cell types have specific pro-fibrogenic features and expression potential. Other cells invade the inflamed tissue and acquire a matrix-synthesizing phenotype by reprogramming their cell fate (**Figure 6**). In most cases, TGF-β regulated pathways contribute to the acquirement of fibrogenic features. However, this might be due to the fact that several cell types were only recently added to the list of profibrogenic progenitors and relevant signaling pathways still need to be defined. In the following we will discuss how the different cells contribute to hepatic fibrosis.

Hepatic Stellate Cells and Myofibroblasts

HSCs reside in the perisinusoidal space between hepatocytes and the sinusoids (i.e., the space of Disse). In the normal liver, these cells exhibit a quiescent phenotype with the main known function of storing vitamin A. During chronic hepatic disease, these cells progressively lose their vitamin A, become activated and transdifferentiate into fibrogenic MFBs that are supposed to be the central cellular drivers of hepatic fibrosis in experimental and human liver injury (Tsuchida and Friedman, 2017). In this process, the induction of α-SMA is the most reliable marker indicating cellular activation HSC. Fundamental fate tracing experiments in mice have demonstrated that HSCs are the

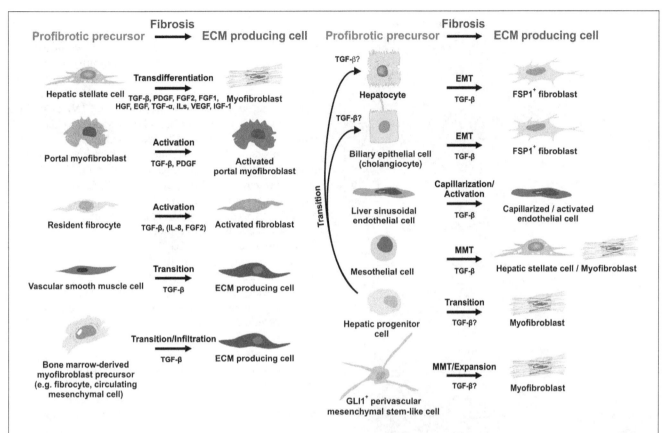

FIGURE 6 | Potential sources of extracellular matrix (ECM) producing cells in liver fibrosis. ECM producing cells during hepatic fibrosis can originate from many sources. Hepatic stellate cells (HSCs) that transdifferenatiate into myofibroblasts (MFBs), activated portal myofibroblasts and activated resident fibroblasts are rich sources of ECM. In addition, several other cell types that become activated, infiltrate the liver, or originate by diverse transition processes are suitable to express large quantities of ECM. Major pathways driving establishment of myofibrogenic features are indicated for each progenitor. Abbreviations used are: ECM, extracellular matrix; EGF, epithelial growth factor; EMT, epithelial-to-mesenchymal transition; FGF1/2, fibroblast growth factor 1/2; GLI1, glioma-associated oncogene homolog 1; HGF, hepatocyte growth factor; IGF-1, insulin growth factor-1; IL, interleukin; MMT, mesothelial-to-mesenchymal transition; PDGF, platelet-derived growth factor; TGF-α/β, transforming growth factor-α/β; VEGF, vascular endothelial growth factor. For details see text.

most important profibrogenic cell type in the liver giving rise to 82–96% of all MFBs in models of toxic, cholestatic and fatty liver disease (Mederacke et al., 2013). HSCs typically express desmin and vimentin, but other markers such as glial fibrillary acidic protein (GFAP), lecithin retinol acyltransferase (LRAT), synemin, platelet-derived growth factor receptor-β (PDGFRβ), p75 neurotrophin receptor peptide (p75NTR), heart- and neural crest derivatives-expressed 2 (HAND2), cytoglobin, and cysteine and glycine-rich protein 2 (CRP2) have been discussed as HSC specific markers within the liver (Weiskirchen et al., 2001; Suzuki et al., 2008; Iwaisako et al., 2014; Kisseleva 2017; Tsuchida and Friedman, 2017). However, the definition of general markers for HSCs is rather complex because reporter microarray analysis, gene mouse models and single cell RNA sequencing have demonstrated the existence of distinct and functionally relevant subsets of resting HSCs and activated MFBs, both *in vivo* and *in vitro* (Magness et al., 2004; D'Ambrosio et al., 2011; 9,; Krenkel et al., 2019). Nevertheless, the expression of α-SMA and collagen type I is significantly increased during progression of hepatic fibrosis confirming the view that MFBs are still most likely the most relevant cell population contributing to hepatic

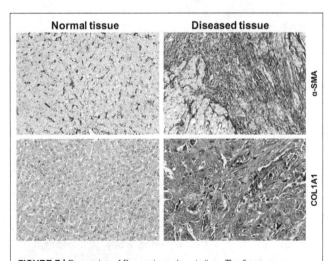

FIGURE 7 | Expression of fibrogenic markers in liver. The figure was compiled using immunohistochemical data from the Human Protein Atlas (www.proteinatlas.org/) (Uhlén et al., 2015). α-smooth muscle actin (α-SMA) and collagen type 1α1 (COL1A1) proteins were stained in normal and diseased livers.

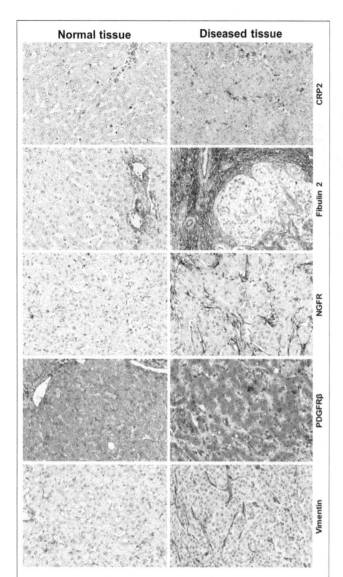

FIGURE 8 | Additional markers of hepatic stellate cells and portal myofibroblasts. The figure was compiled from data deposited from Human Protein Atlas (www.proteinatlas.org/) (Uhlén et al., 2015). Immunohistochemistry of the cysteine and glycine rich protein 2 (CRP2), Fibulin 2, nerve growth factor receptor (NGFR), platelet-derived growth factor-β (PDGFRβ) and Vimentin in normal and diseased liver tissue. Liver damage is associated with increased expression of these profibrogenic markers. Image credit: Human Protein Atlas.

Similarly, a very recent human liver scRNA-seq study has revealed HSC heterogeneity along the porto-central axis of the healthy liver lobule (Valery et al., 2021). Two major HSC sub-populations were obtained from the healthy human liver lobules. One sub-population (HSC1) expressed high levels of the cell surface proteoglycan glypican 3 (*GPC3*) and the neurotrophic tyrosine kinase receptor type 2 (*NTRK2*) along with other commonly expressed HSC markers, whereas the second sub-population (HSC2) expressed high levels of the genes encoding for dopamine-norepinephrine converting enzyme (*DBH*), hedgehog-interacting protein (*HHIP*), and the G-protein coupled receptors (GPCRs) vasoactive intestinal peptide receptor 1 (*VIPR1*), parathyroid hormone 1 receptor (*PTH1R*), receptor activity-modifying protein 1 (*RAMP1*), endothelin receptor type B (*EDNRB*), and angiotensin receptor 1A (*AGTR1A*) (Valery et al., 2021). In addition, beside the identification of novel quiescent markers such as Quiescin Q6 sulfhydryl oxidase 1 (*QSOX1*) and six-transmembrane epithelial antigen of prostate 4 (*STEAP4*), these scRNA-seq studies have also confirmed well-established HSC marker including the regulator of G protein signaling (*RGS5*), pleiotrophin (*PTN*), nerve growth factor receptor (*NGFR*), lecithin retinol acyltransferase (*LRAT*), fibulin 5 (*FBLN5*), dihydrolipoamide branched-chain transacylase (*DPT*), decorin (*DCN*), cytoglobin (*CYGB*), collectin 11 (*COLEC11*), olfactomedin-like 3 (*OLFML3*), and tropomyosin 2 (*TPM2*), respectively (Valery et al., 2021). All these findings established by scRNA-seq suggests this methodology as an emerging area and promising experimental tool to reveal deeper insights into HSC biology.

Portal Fibroblasts

In the normal liver, they encompass a quiescent phenotype with a spindle-shaped fibroblastic phenotype that surrounds the portal vein to maintain integrity of portal tract. In cholestatic liver injury, portal MFBs are supposed to be a more important source of activated MFBs than HSCs around proliferating bile ducts (Tsuchida and Friedman, 2017). However, in contrast to the well-characterized HSCs/MFBs the biology of these cells is only partially known. Studies on rat portal MFB cell lines and fibrotic mouse livers have shown that typical markers of this profibrogenic cells are elastin, type XV collagen α1, ectonucleoside triphosphate diphosphohydrolase-2 (ENTPD2/CD39L1) and cofilin 1, while these cells are negative for the HSC markers desmin, cytoglobin, and LRAT (Iwaisako et al., 2014; Fausther et al., 2015). However, likewise HSCs, these cells are positive for typical myofibroblastic markers including α-SMA, type I collagen α1, and tissue inhibitor of metalloproteinase-1 (Fausther et al., 2015). Other markers for portal MFBs were identified by immunohistochemistry of fibrotic liver and FACS sorting of liver cell preparations. These include Gremlin 1, Thy1/CD90, Fibulin 2, mesothelin, asporin, and Mucin-16 (Iwaisako et al., 2014; Kisseleva, 2017). Some of them are drastically induced during progression of hepatic fibrosis, while their expression signature might dependent on the hepatic insult analyzed (Iwaisako et al., 2014).

fibrosis (**Figure 7**). In addition, the expression of CRP2, Fibulin 2, NGFR, PDGFRβ, Vimentin and many other genes is often used as markers that become increased expressed during hepatic fibrosis (**Figure 8**).

Recent studies have shown that there exists complex cellular heterogeneity even within activated HSCs that convert into collagen-secreting MFBs. Recent single-cell RNA sequencing (scRNA-seq) studies in a CCl$_4$-induced hepatic fibrosis model in mice, clearly showed the presence of four sub-populations of MFBs in the fibrotic liver that all express collagen but differentially express chemokines (Krenkel et al., 2019).

Fibrocytes

Each organ has multiple populations of resident mesenchymal cells capable of producing ECM. In the liver, HSCs and portal fibroblasts are supposed to be the major cell types implicated in the pathogenesis of liver fibrosis. Nevertheless, dependent of the nature of hepatic insult, ECM producing cells may also originate from many other sources. Fibrocytes are defined monocyte-derived spindle-shaped cells having features of both macrophages and fibroblasts (Reilkoff et al., 2011). Animal experimentation using chimeric mice transplanted with donor bone marrow from collagen α1(I)-GFP$^+$ reporter mice has shown that collagen-producing fibrocytes are recruited from the bone marrow to the damage liver tissue when recipient mice were subjected to bile duct ligation (Kisseleva et al., 2006). Moreover, when treated in culture with TGF-β1, these cells differentiated into α-SMA and desmin positive collagen-producing MFBs.

Vascular Smooth Muscle Cells

Vascular smooth muscle cells (VSMCs) are integral components of the blood vessel wall contributing to structural stability and regulating vessel diameter. As such these contractile cells are highly responsive toward vasoactive stimuli and contain a large repertoire of specific contractile proteins facilitating their dynamic phenotype (Metz et al., 2012). In response to injury, VSMCs can shift from a contractile to a synthetic phenotype characterized by increased expression of ECM compounds such as collagen I and III and elevated expression of various non-muscle myosin heavy chain isoforms (Metz et al., 2012). In normal human liver, these cells are positive for α-SMA and smoothelin representing a 59-kD cytoskeletal protein that is found exclusively in contractile smooth muscle cells (Lepreux et al., 2013). During the pathogenesis of advanced human liver fibrosis, the cellular fraction of MFBs positive for both α-SMA and smoothelin expanses to 5–10% suggesting a progressive involvement of these resident cells in MFB recruitment (Lepreux et al., 2013). Comparative transcriptome profiling of endothelial cells and VSMCs from canine vessels revealed an enrichment of expression in genes associated with cytoskeleton composition and actin filament organization including transforming growth factor-β1 (*TGFB1*), collagen type I α1 (*COL1A1*), nephroblastoma overexpressed gene (*NOV*), Tenascin c (*TNC*), tissue factor pathway inhibitor 2 (*TFPI2*), Tubulin α-4A (*TUBA4A*), Retinol–binding protein (*RBP4*), insulin-like growth factor-binding protein 5 (*IGFBP5*), and Cingulin-like 1 (*CGNL1*) (Oosterhoff et al., 2019). Single cell transcriptomic further showed that VSMC in mouse and human livers can be differentiated from other pro-fibrogenic cells of mesenchymal origin (fibroblasts, HSCs) by their expression of Calponin 1 (*CNN1*) or Myosin heavy chain 11 (*MYH11*) (Dobie et al., 2019).

Bone Marrow-Derived Fibrocytes

The first hints for a unique population of collagen-producing fibrocytes derived from the bone marrow that could participate in the pathogenesis of hepatic fibrosis were established in chimeric mice transplanted with donor bone marrow from collagen α1(I)-GFP$^+$ reporter mice (Kisseleva et al., 2006). In livers of respective mice, a significant increase in GFP$^+$/CD45$^+$ positive myofibroblastic cells was observed when animals were subjected to bile duct ligation, that however, were not positive for the typical HSC markers α-SMA or vimentin underpinning their lymphoid origin (Kisseleva et al., 2006). However, these cells differentiated into α-SMA and desmin positive cells when cultured in the presence of TGF-β1. A relevant functional contribution of fibrocytes to the pathogenesis of hepatic fibrosis was demonstrated in a mouse model in which fibrocytes were specifically depleted utilizing a herpes simplex thymidine kinase/ganciclovir suicide approach in the thioacetamide-induced liver fibrosis model (Hempel et al., 2019). Although the depletion of fibrocytes resulted in reduced deposition of fibrillar collagen, the antifibrotic effect was not accompanied by a reduction of MFBs. In the multidrug resistance gene 2 knockout (*Mdr2*$^{-/-}$) mice spontaneously developing cholestatic fibrosis, fibrocytes only minimally contributed to the deposition of ECM in the injured livers (Nishio et al., 2019). It will now be of fundamental interest, to better define the autocrine and paracrine functions of fibrocytes during initiation and progression of hepatic fibrosis in these and other models.

Hepatocytes

Hepatocytes are specialized epithelial cells making up 80% of the total mass of the liver. They perform numerous vital functions, including protein synthesis, metabolism of lipids and carbohydrates, biotransformation and detoxification of xenobiotics that enter the body. In addition, hepatocytes synthesize and secrete bile and must therefore establish a unique polarity in which apical (canalicular) and basolateral (sinusoidal) plasma membranes are equipped with highly specialized surface proteins, channels, and receptors (Schulze et al., 2019). During liver injury these cells can contribute to fibrogenesis by acquiring myofibroblastic phenotypes/features by undergoing a process termed epithelial-to-mesenchymal transition (EMT) (Zeisberg et al., 2007). During this process the cells downregulate epithelial features, lose their apical-basal polarity, cell-cell adhesion properties and obtain migratory/invasive properties, and acquire mesenchymal characteristics allowing synthesizing ECM compounds (Yang et al., 2020). Lineage-tracing experiments performed in transgenic mice in which liver fibrosis were induced by repeated injections of carbon tetrachloride demonstrated that up to 45% of fibroblast-specific protein 1 (FSP1) positive fibroblasts originated from hepatocytes via EMT (Zeisberg et al., 2007). In line with the concept of EMT, primary mouse hepatocytes transit in culture to FSP1 positive fibroblasts when cultured in the presence of TGF-β1 (Zeisberg et al., 2007). However, the concept that fibrogenic cells capable to express type I collagen can originate *in vivo* from hepatocytes was challenged by other studies (Taura et al., 2010; Xie and Diehl, 2013). It was argued that potential interpretational pitfalls may arise from the fact that FSP1 is not only expressed in subsets of fibroblasts but is also expressed by cells of the myeloid-monocytic lineage (Scholten and Weiskirchen, 2011). However, the evidence for and against EMT for the generation of myofibroblastic cells from intrahepatic cells is still controversially discussed (Taura et al., 2016; Munker et al., 2017; Chen et al., 2020).

Biliary Epithelial Cells

Similar to hepatocyte it was proposed that biliary epithelial cells (i.e., cholangiocytes) can change their fate and transit to invasive fibroblasts by EMT. In particular, in primary cirrhosis it was demonstrated that bile duct epithelial cells express FSP1 and vimentin as early markers of fibroblasts in the ductular reaction (Robertson et al., 2007). In line, the stimulation of cultured human cholangiocytes with TGF-β induced expression of FSP1 and vimentin suggesting that these cells can contribute significantly to portal tract fibrosis (Rygiel et al., 2008). The resulting cells formed in this localized EMT showed coexpression of both cytokeratin-7 (CK-7) and FSP1 indicating that these cells have the capacity to migrate out of the ductular structure (Rygiel et al., 2008). Several reports suggested that sonic hedgehog signaling promotes EMT by inducing myofibroblast specific genes and repressing epithelial genes during the pathogenesis of chronic biliary injury and NAFLD (Omenetti et al., 2008; Syn et al., 2009). However, bile duct ligation experiments performed in adult mice tagged with a YFP reporter directed under regulatory control of the cholangiocyte marker keratin 19 (K19) showed that cholangiocytes that were positive for YFP revealed no expression of EMT markers α-SMA, desmin, or FSP1 (Scholten et al., 2010).

Hepatic Progenitor Cells

The liver is the only visceral organ that can replace lost or damaged tissue from the remaining tissue in a well-orchestrated program, in which progenitor cells derived from the biliary epithelium transdifferentiate to restore the hepatocyte compartment (Michalopoulos 2013). Therefore, the occurrence of resident hepatic progenitor cells (HPCs) was proposed that should contain a defined cell fraction located in the canal of Hering. The proposed cells should be characterized by a high cellular plasticity and proliferation potential, the ability to differentiate into hepatocytes and cholangiocytes, and to mediate liver repopulation after injury (Li W et al., 2020). However, also the conversion of hepatocytes to progenitor-like cells has been documented in vitro (Li W et al., 2020). HPCs isolated from chronically injured liver were shown to have trilineage differentiation potential serving as progenitors for hepatocytes, cholangiocytes and MFBs Sekiya et al., 2016). Although the frequency of MFBs from HPCs was very low, it can be speculated that HPCs can contribute to the MFB pool during hepatic fibrogenesis (Sekiya et al., 2016).

Sinusoidal Endothelial Cells

Liver sinusoidal endothelial cells (LSEC) are a fenestrated cell type without an organized basement membrane that forms the predominant population in the hepatic sinusoid. In normal liver, these cells form a selective barrier between the hepatocytes and blood, possess a high endocytotic capacity allowing them to act as an initial line of defense against invading pathogens, and are critically involved in regulating vascular tone and permeability

(Hutchins et al., 2013). Under certain conditions these cells can acquire an active phenotype characterized by swelling and bulging of the cell body combined with enlargement of the Golgi complex, increase of rough endoplasmic reticulum, and formation of hemidesmosome-like structures that are hallmarks of fibroblastic reticulum cells (Bardadin and Desmet, 1985). During liver injury LSEC lose their fenestration, form a continuous basal membrane, and develop inflammatory and fibrotic features, a process referred to as capillarization (Baiocchini et al., 2019). Noteworthy, capillarized LSECs can be an active contributor to the production of a fibrotic environment during fibrogenesis by synthesis of collagen and fibronectin (Natarajan et al., 2017).

Mesothelial Cells

Mesothelial cells are specialized pavement-like cells forming a protective layer of epithelial cells (i.e., the mesothelium) around serous cavities and internal organs. These cells facilitate transport of fluid across these compartments and produce a lubricating fluid that is helpful in protecting the body against infections (Mutsaers 2004). Observations from different animal models and organ systems have shown that the adult mesothelium of mice and humans contains a sub-population of quiescent cells with stem-like properties (Koopmans and Rinkevich, 2018). Upon peritoneal damage and appropriate stimulus, these cells can be triggered to undergo a transition process, termed "mesothelial-to-mesenchymal transition" (MMT). The molecular reprogramming is associated with morphological and functional changes and lead to cells producing ECM compounds and pro-fibrogenic mediators (Koopmans and Rinkevich, 2018). In line, TGF-β1 in vitro induced morphologic and functional reformation of differentiated human mesothelial cells to MFBs that become positive for α-SMA (Yang et al., 2003). In regard to liver fibrogenesis, conditional cell lineage tracing in mice confirmed that liver mesothelial cells can be driven by TGF-β to generate both HSCs and MFBs depending on injury signals in the liver (Li et al., 2013). While mesothelial cells preferentially transit into HSCs in biliary fibrosis induced by bile duct ligation, the cells majorly convert into MFBs in carbon tetrachloride-induced fibrosis (Li Y et al., 2016). On the basis of lineage tracing studies, it was supposed that mesothelial cells are triggered by TGF-β to undergo MMT and contribute to the MFB fraction in peritoneal fibrosis, in which up to 16.8% of all MFBs were derived from peritoneal mesothelial cells (Lua et al., 2015).

GLI1 Positive Perivascular Mesenchymal Stem-like Cells

The glioma-associated oncogene homolog 1 (GLI1) belongs to the family of three GLI C_2H_2-Kruppel type transcription factors that contain five zinc finger domains and either activate or repress gene expression by binding to specific consensus DNA sequences (**Figure 9**). Traditionally, GLI proteins are viewed as downstream effectors of the Hedgehog (HH) signaling pathways, but are now also known to be regulated transcriptionally and

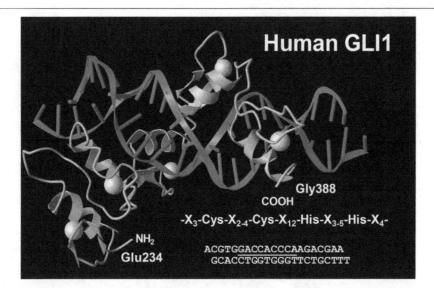

FIGURE 9 | Crystal structure of the five Zn fingers from human GLI1 in complex with a high-affinity DNA binding site. Shown is a complex of a peptide derived from the human GLI1 oncoprotein spanning region Glu 234 to Gly388 with a DNA fragment containing the specific binding site 5′-GACCACCCA-3′ (underlined). Each of the five zinc fingers has a conserved sequence motif that is characterized by the consensus sequence X_3-Cys-X_{2-4}-Cys-X_{12}-His-X_{3-5}-His-X_4 (where X is any acid residue). The structure has been determined at 2.6 Å resolution. Structure coordinates were taken from the PDB Protein Data Bank (access. no. 2GLI). For details see (Pavletich and Pabo 1993).

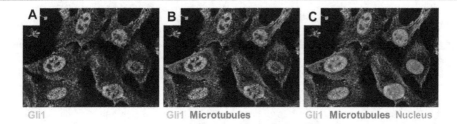

FIGURE 10 | Expression of GLI1 in human bone osteocarcoma cell line U-2 OS. The cell line U-2 OS originating from human mesenchymal tumors express large quantities of GLI1 (green), which is localized in the nucleus and the cytoplasm. Microtubuli (red) and nucleus (blue) are stained by a specific antibody or DAPI. The figure was compiled using immunocytochemical data taken from the Human Protein Atlas v.20 (www.proteinatlas.org/) (Uhlén et al., 2015). They can be found at: https://www.proteinatlas.org/ENSG00000111087-GLI1/cell#img.

post-transcriptionally through non-canonical mechanisms involving RAS-RAF-MEK-ERK and PI3K-AKT-mTOR (Dusek and Hadden, 2021). This zinc finger protein was originally identified as an oncogene that was amplified more than 50-fold and highly expressed in some cases of malignant glioma (Kinzler et al., 1987). GLI1 localize predominantly to the nucleus (**Figure 10**) and bind the 9-base-pair consensus DNA 5′-GACCACCCA-3′ with high affinity (Kinzler and Vogelstein, 1990). It has turned out that the individual GLI proteins play fundamental and distinct roles both in chronic inflammation and cancer. In some organs the lack of HH expression promotes chronic inflammation and tumor formation, while aberrantly activated HH/GLI signaling is also capable to foster tumor growth and simultaneously dampening inflammation and favoring immunosuppression (Grund-Gröschke et al., 2019). Genetic lineage tracing analysis in mice demonstrated that

tissue-resident, but not circulating, GLI1 positive mesenchymal-stem-cell-like cells can generate MFBs in kidney, lung, liver, or heart after injury (Kramann et al., 2015). Genetic ablation of GLI1 positive cells abolished bone marrow fibrosis and rescued bone marrow failure (Schneider et al., 2017). More recently it was demonstrated that the pro-fibrogenic activity of osteopontin in promoting HSC activation and ECM deposition during liver fibrogenesis is strongly dependent on GLI1 function (Rao et al., 2019). In the human HSC line LX-2, PAX6 binds to the promoter of the *GLI1* gene, thereby promoting fibrogenic activities and proliferation (Li C. et al., 2020). In the same cell line, GLI1 was further shown to be integrated in a complex network of Wnt/β-catenin, which regulates cellular contraction (Zhang F. et al., 2020). However, the significance of GLI1 positive perivascular mesenchymal stem-like cells for liver fibrogenesis is still unknown. Publicly available

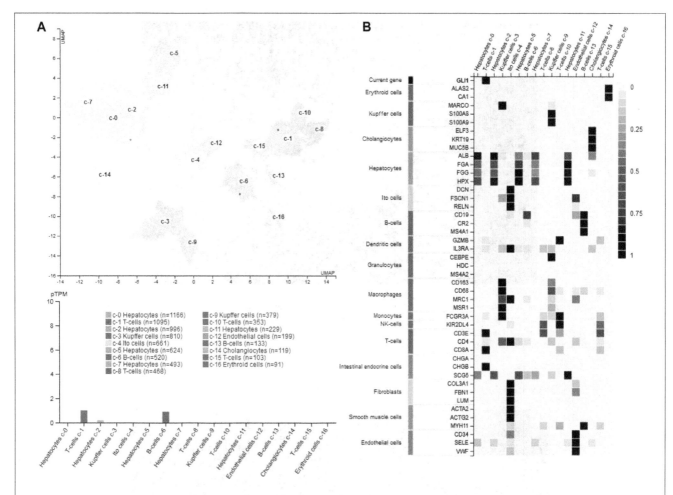

FIGURE 11 | GLI1 expression in liver **(A)** single cell PCR data shows that *GLI1* mRNA expression in normal human liver is rather low (<1 protein-coding transcript per million) and majorly restricted to a subpopulation of T-cells, B-cells and hepatocytes **(B)** Heatmap of marker gene expression in different hepatic cell types. The figure was compiled using expression data from the Human Protein Atlas (www.proteinatlas.org/) (Uhlén et al., 2015). Abbreviations used are: pTPM, protein-coding transcript per million; UMAP, uniform manifold approximation and projection.

data obtained by single cell PCR shows that *GLI1* mRNA expression in normal human liver is rather low (<1 protein-coding transcript per million) and restricted to some immune cells and hepatocytes (**Figure 11**), while not found in smooth muscle cells or endothelial cells. It will be now of particular interest to document the existence of respective cells and to clarify how these cells are triggered during hepatic fibrogenesis to generate the proposed large fraction of MFBs.

MECHANISMS OF FIBROSIS REGRESSION AND RESOLUTION

Liver fibrosis is potentially reversible (Ramachandran and Iredale, 2012). Patients undergoing treatment for HCV infection clearly demonstrate reversal of fibrosis upon complete HCV negativity (Brenner, 2013). However, liver fibrosis is reversible only in the early stages (Fibrosis grades 1 and 2). Once fibrosis crosses a threshold (Fibrosis grades 3 and 4), the fibrogenic type I collagen forms crosslinks and is

typically associated with cell damage and inflammation, making it harder to recover (Brenner, 2013). Two events are critical in directing the liver pro-fibrogenic phenotype to recovery - (i) Apoptosis of MFBs in the liver and, (ii) switching of macrophages from a pro-inflammatory to a tissue resolution phenotype (Pellicoro et al., 2014). During liver fibrogenesis, the ECM is extensively remodeled leading to accumulation of proteases such as matrix metalloproteinases (MMP) as well as collagenases (Iredale, 2008). However, at the same time, fibrotic liver also accumulates myofibroblast-derived tissue inhibitor of metalloproteinase 1 (TIMP1) which prevents the action of MMPs and ECM turnover (Iredale et al., 1996). As a result, there is an accumulation of collagen and pro-fibrotic ECM. Over a period of time, accumulation of a large number of crosslinked collagen and elastin fibers lead to sequestering of crosslinked fibers within the tissue beds, making them inaccessible for proteolytic digestion (Issa et al., 2004). As the cross links increase, the exposed fibers also become less susceptible to digestion themselves (Issa et al., 2004). The hallmark of a recovering

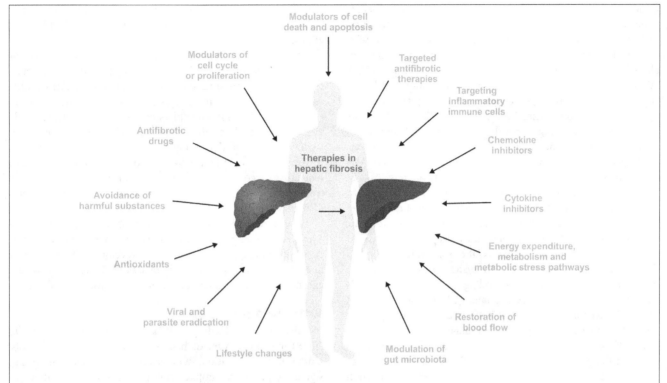

FIGURE 12 | Potential therapeutic options for liver fibrosis. Based on the fact that hepatic fibrosis is driven by different mediators and pathways, there is a plenitude of possibilities to interfere with this process. For more details see text or refer to (Schon et al., 2016; Weiskirchen 2016; Tacke and Weiskirchen, 2018; Weiskirchen et al., 2018; Levada et al., 2019).

fibrotic liver is the termination of cellular injury followed by the absence or disappearance of hepatic MFBs (Kisseleva et al., 2012). Studies show that at least 50% of the activated MFBs revert to less fibrogenic or quiescent HSCs (Kisseleva et al., 2012; Troeger et al., 2012). The role of macrophages and the trigger of switching from pro-inflammatory to pro-resolution macrophages during fibrosis is incompletely understood. However, macrophages in the resolving fibrotic liver have been shown to secrete increased levels of MMPs thereby contributing to ECM reorganization (Li H et al., 2016). Therefore, polarization of macrophages provides a therapeutic opportunity for the resolution of liver fibrosis.

THERAPY OF HEPATIC FIBROSIS

Although numerous drugs have beneficial anti-fibrotic effects *in vitro* and in animal models, none of these drugs has been ultimately shown to be efficacious in the clinic. Moreover, general anti-fibrotic therapies are not available. Instead, clinicians and professional associations have developed some clinical practice guidelines and recommendations for etiology-specific interventions. Most noticed are the guidelines published by the American Association for the Study of Liver Diseases (AASLD) and the European Association for the Study of Liver Diseases (EASL) that both develop evidence-based clinical practice guidelines on a regularly basis. These 'state-of-the-art' recommendations are intended to assist physicians and other

healthcare providers in the diagnosis and management of a specific etiology of liver injury. As such they typically contain information about disease definition, epidemiology, etiology, risk factors, incidence, recommended tests and examinations for disease detection, screening tools, preferred staging and grading systems, therapy strategies, surveillance tests/intervals, therapy outcome measures, prevention strategies, ongoing trials, and much other supporting information. From the view of basic scientists some generally applicable concepts should be effective in the therapy of hepatic fibrosis. These include the withdrawal of injurious stimuli, inhibition of ongoing hepatic damage, deactivation and elimination of ECM-producing cells, removal of superfluous scar tissue, counteracting biological mediators driving hepatic inflammation and fibrogenesis, and restoring the normal liver architecture (**Figure 12**). scRNA-seq and genetic cell tracing experiments have shown that the termination of hepatic fibrosis is associated with a reversal of HSC activation and expression of different inactivation markers (Troeger et al., 2012). However, reverted HSCs remain in a primed state maintaining a higher responsiveness toward fibrogenic stimuli.

Arrest of Chronic Liver Damage by Avoiding or Eradication of Harmful Substances and Replacement Therapies

As outlined, there are many genetic and environmental factors that can cause hepatic fibrosis. Most frequent inherited disorders associated with acute and chronic liver disease include hemochromatosis, Wilson disease, α1-antitrypsin deficiency, and cystic fibrosis. In the case of hemochromatosis, excessive iron can be removed from the body by regularly phlebotomy, or alternatively iron chelating therapy (Murphree et al., 2020). Wilson disease occurring as a consequence of impaired biliary copper excretion can be effectively treated with the chelators D-Penicillamine and trientine or by application of zinc preparations interfering with the gastrointestinal uptake of copper (Stremmel and Weiskirchen, 2021). Shortage of α1-antitrypsin in the lung can be partially overcome by intravenous replacement therapy, while this therapy is not appropriate to people with liver disease. In respective patients, there is emphasis on efforts to prevent progression of related liver injury by reducing of modifiable risk factors (overweight, tobacco, alcohol, non-steroidal anti-inflammatory drugs) or finally liver transplantation that still remains the sole curative option (Narayanan and Mistry, 2020). In cystic fibrosis resulting of mutations in the gene encoding the cystic fibrosis transmembrane conductance regulator (CFTR) the application of Ursodeoxycholic acid (UDCA) is the mainstay of therapy. This secondary bile acid is supposed to stimulate bile acid secretion, but its efficacy is therapy of cystic fibrosis-related liver disease is controversially discussed (Staufer, 2020). In addition, a large number of compounds restoring CFTR protein function (i.e., CFTR modulators) are actually under close investigation (Staufer, 2020).

In regard to alcoholic liver disease, the abstinence from drinking alcoholic beverages is quite the cornerstone of therapy. However, several studies have shown that glucocorticoids given alone or in combinations with antioxidants are beneficial to lower hepatic inflammation (Mitchell et al., 2020). In addition, drugs able to prevent the development of steatosis, modulate innate immune responses, targeting the microbiome, or stimulating liver regeneration are investigated in many clinical studies (Mitchell et al., 2020).

Antiviral treatment strategies are suitable to reduce the burden of chronic hepatitis B (HBV), hepatitis C virus (HCV), or hepatitis D (HDV) infections. In particular, the introduction of direct antiviral drugs offers nowadays a very competent way to obtain viral clearance with sustained virologic response rates greater than 95% (Do and Reau, 2020). Rigorous infant prophylaxis, early childhood and adult immunization programs as well as vaccination of high-risk individuals significantly contribute to prevalence of HBV transmission worldwide (Polaris Observatory Collaborators, 2018). Established interferon-based therapies are established and new encouraging drugs are currently under clinical evaluation for the treatment of HDV (Koh et al., 2019).

Autoimmune diseases of the liver typically affect either the liver parenchyma, which is termed autoimmune hepatitis, or alternatively the bile ducts provoking primary biliary cholangitis (PBC) or primary sclerosing cholangitis (PSC) (Weiskirchen, 2016). Immunosuppressive treatment consisting of either corticosteroids alone or in combination

with the purine analog azathioprine is the recommended first-line medical treatment in autoimmune hepatitis (Tanaka, 2020).

There are some pharmacological approaches available for the management of NAFLD and NASH, but an ultimate therapy is still missing and actual guidelines presently only recommend significant changes in lifestyle and nutrition, in particular weight loss and physical exercise (Drescher et al., 2019). Nevertheless, there are several drugs currently at various stages of development for the therapy of NASH, possessing anti-inflammatory activity, improve insulin resistance, reduce de novo lipogenesis, modulate lipid transport or oxidation, or evolve anti-apoptotic effects (Tacke and Weiskirchen, 2018).

Liver fibrosis resulting from Schistosomiasis (S. mansoni and S. japonicum) are presently treated with the pyrazinoisoquinoline derivative praziquantel, while several vaccines that are urgently needed are currently at differing phases of clinical development and not yet been accepted for public use (McManus et al., 2020).

Antioxidants

As discussed, elevated quantities of reactive oxygen species (ROS) are key drivers of hepatic inflammation and fibrosis. Under normal condition, ROS are required for many important signaling processes, impact cell proliferation, contribute to apoptotic pathways, and help phagocytic active cells to destroy and eliminate pathogens (Luangmonkong et al., 2018). They induce apoptosis and necrosis of parenchymal cells (i.e., hepatocytes) resulting in the release of harmful mediators (e.g., TGF-β, TNF-α), stimulate Kupffer cells to produce profibrogenic mediators, prompt recruitment of circulating inflammatory cells into the liver, and contribute to the activation of HSCs (Weiskirchen, 2016). Therefore, an imbalance between ROS production and degradation play an important role in the pathogenesis of liver fibrosis. Consequently, therapeutic interventions targeting elevated cellular oxidative stress should be beneficial for the treatment of liver fibrosis (Luangmonkong et al., 2018). In regard to therapy of liver fibrosis, many ROS inhibitors have been tested successfully in pre-clinical animal models (Weiskirchen, 2016). Most of these antioxidants are scavengers that unspecific alleviate ROS accumulation, while others are more selective by targeting defined molecular pathways involved in ROS generation. In particular, inhibitors of mitochondrial dysfunction (Coenzyme !0, Mitoquinone mesylate, NIM811), endoplasmic stress (Glycerol phylbutyrate), NADPH oxidases (GKT137831, Docosahexaenoic acid, losartan), and Toll-like receptors (Curcumin, Quercetin, various probiotics, Bicyclol) have attracted widespread attention in recent years (Luangmonkong et al., 2018). Most promising are drugs that interfere with the activity of different NADPH oxidase (NOX) subtypes. In experimental models, both the deficiency of NOX1 or NOX4 as well as the application of the dual NOX1/4 inhibitor GKT137831 was effective in attenuation of carbon tetrachloride-induced liver fibrosis (Lan et al., 2015). Likewise, the NOX inhibitor apocynin was therapeutically effective in preventing lipopolysaccharide/D-galactosamine-induced acute liver injury (Peng et al., 2020).

Inhibitors of Cytokine Signaling

Several cytokines play a crucial role in the pathogenesis of hepatic fibrosis. Commonly, they bind to specific cell-surface exposed receptors, thereby initiating intracellular signaling cascades ending in modified gene expression. Research performed during the last decades has identified a number of different cytokines relevant during the pathogenesis of hepatic fibrosis. Representative cytokines most prominent involved in disease initiation or progression are members belonging to the family of TGF-β, platelet-derived growth factors (PDGF), vascular endothelial growth factors (VEGF), interleukins (IL), fibroblast growth factors (FGF), interferons (IFN), insulin-like growth factors (IGF), TNF-α, epidermal growth factor (EGF), nerve growth factor (NGF), and hepatocyte growth factor (HGF) (Weiskirchen 2016). Their specific activities were comprehensively explored in many *in vitro* and *in vivo* models of hepatic fibrosis. However, proposed therapies by interfering with cytokine activities using small interfering RNAs, antisense oligonucleotides, aptamers, soluble receptors, scavenger molecules, therapeutic antibodies, or other biological agents have not been translated to the clinics yet (Borkham-Kamphorst and Weiskirchen, 2016; Weiskirchen, 2016; Schuppan et al., 2018).

Inhibitions of Chemokine Signaling

Chemokines are critical immunomodulatory mediators acting in humans through 20 different G-protein-coupled transmembrane receptors. They typically consists of 75–125 amino acids, share a similar tertiary structure, and based on the number and position of cysteine residues can be systematically categorized into four distinct subfamilies, namely CC, CXC, CX_3C, and XC followed by the letter L (standing for 'ligand') and a consecutive number indicating their temporal isolation (Hughes and Nibbs, 2018). The individual ligands and their cognate receptors (i.e., CCR, CXCR, CX_3CR, XCR) form an enormously complex network playing pivotal roles. By far the most studied functions are the control of cell recruitment, inflammation, wound healing, lymphoid trafficking, angiogenesis, and metastasis. For the formation of liver disease, there is now ample evidence that chemokines and their receptors have fundamental importance in both progression and regression of hepatic fibrosis (Marra and Tacke, 2014). Therefore, strategies for inhibiting common or individual chemokine activities are presently intensively investigated. Prototypically, the dual specific CC motif chemokine receptor 2/5 (CCR2/CCR5) antagonist cenicriviroc has been experimentally and clinically shown to block fat accumulation, Kupffer cell activation, monocyte recruitment, HSC activation, and fibrosis (Friedman et al., 2018; Krenkel et al., 2018; Ambade et al., 2019).

Other Anti-fibrotic Therapy Strategies

Besides the elimination of pathogenic causes, usage of replacement therapies, usage of antioxidants, or therapies targeting cytokine or chemokine activities, there are numerous other possibilities to interfere with hepatic fibrosis. In the past, many other drugs or herbal supplements or vitamins were experimentally tested in pre-clinical models of hepatic fibrosis (Weiskirchen, 2016). They act by inducing apoptosis, autophagy or senescence in ECM-producing cells, interfere with pro-fibrogenic target molecules, modulate cell cycle or proliferation synthesis, act hepatoprotective, or generally interfere with gene expression, replication, mitosis or meiosis. However, their efficacy was only successfully proven yet in experimental disease models. Clinical application is hindered in most cases because effective strategies that allow targeting these drugs to fibrogenic effector cells are not available (Schuppan et al., 2018). Other experimental approaches have identified the lysyl oxidase-like 2 (LOXL2) encoding an extracellular copper-dependent amine oxidase catalyzing the covalent cross-linking of collagen and elastin as a promising drug target (Khurana et al., 2021). In two experimental models of hepatic fibrogenesis, the selective LOXL2/3 inhibitor PXS-5153A was shown to dose-dependently diminish collagen content, thereby reducing disease severity and improve liver function (Schilter et al., 2019). In line, the preventive treatment with and anti-LOXL2 antibody was able to prevent ongoing experimental hepatic fibrosis (Ikenaga et al., 2017). Similarly, targeting Galectin-3 representing a 30 kDa protein with important functions in cell-cell adhesion, cell-matrix interaction, angiogenesis, macrophage activation, inflammation, and collagen synthesis has been identified as a suitable drug candidate.

Presently, there is much hope that engineered nanoparticles, magnetic-assisted drug delivery techniques, or therapeutic effective transgenes expressed under fibrosis-related promoters can be optimized in the near future to better target individual fibrogenic cell subpopulations (Herrmann et al., 2004; Schon et al., 2016; Levada et al., 2019).

CONCLUSION

Genetic disorders, alcohol abuse, drugs, cholestasis, metabolic disorders, chronic viral hepatitis, parasitic infections and several cryptogenic causes are major causes that provoke liver fibrosis. During this progressive process accumulation of ECM, disruption of the lobular structure, and progressive deterioration of hepatocellular function lead to fatal complications. In particular, the exuberant collagen deposition is one hallmark of fibrogenesis. Work from the last decades have identified a number of different resident and infiltrating cells that can either be activated or transform into a phenotype capable to synthesize ECM. In addition, cell- and animal-based experiments, clinical studies and complex integrated bioinformatics analysis have unraveled soluble mediators, molecular pathways, and pro-fibrogenic genes that are key drivers in the pathogenesis of hepatic disease. However, despite the important progress, there are currently no approved anti-fibrotic drugs that have been ultimately shown to be efficacious in the clinic. Presently, clinical practice guidelines are only etiology-specific. They intend to optimize patient care by withdrawal of injurious stimuli, consumption of antioxidant acting compounds, and lifestyle interventions including healthy food, exercised and controlled weight loss. Nevertheless, many experimental studies and clinical trials are currently being conducted to test drugs targeting more specifically inflammation, the cellular activation process, or the activity of inflammatory or fibrotic-acting cytokines or chemokines. There is hope that these compounds will be of fundamental importance in future treatments aiming at impeding or reversing the fibrogenic process.

AUTHOR CONTRIBUTIONS

All authors listed have made a substantial, direct, and intellectual contribution to the work and approved it for publication.

REFERENCES

Acharya, P., Garg, M., Kumar, P., Munjal, A., and Raja, K. D. (2017). Host-Parasite Interactions in Human Malaria: Clinical Implications of Basic Research. *Front. Microbiol.* 8, 889. doi:10.3389/fmicb.2017.00889

Amanatidou, A. I., and Dedoussis, G. V. (2021). Bioinformatics Analysis of the NAFLD Interactome: Revealing Candidate Biomarkers of Non-alcoholic Fatty Liver Disease. *Comput. Biol. Med.* 131. 104243. doi:10.1101/2020.12.01.406215

Ambade, A., Lowe, P., Kodys, K., Catalano, D., Gyongyosi, B., Cho, Y., et al. (2019). Pharmacological Inhibition of CCR2/5 Signaling Prevents and Reverses Alcohol-Induced Liver Damage, Steatosis, and Inflammation in Mice. *Hepatology* 69 (3), 1105–1121. doi:10.1002/hep.30249

Andrade, Z. A., Guerret, S., and Fernandes, A. L. (1999). Myofibroblasts in Schistosomal Portal Fibrosis of Man. *Mem. Inst. Oswaldo Cruz* 94 (1), 87–93. doi:10.1590/s0074-02761999000100018

Andrade, Z. A. (2004). Schistosomal Hepatopathy. *Mem. Inst. Oswaldo Cruz* 99 (5 Suppl. 1), 51–57. doi:10.1590/s0074-02762004000900009

Andrade, Z. A. (2009). Schistosomiasis and Liver Fibrosis. *Parasite Immunol.* 31 (11), 656–663. doi:10.1111/j.1365-3024.2009.01157.x

Anstee, Q. M., Darlay, R., Cockell, S., Meroni, M., Govaere, O., Tiniakos, D., et al. (2020). Genome-wide Association Study of Non-alcoholic Fatty Liver and Steatohepatitis in a Histologically Characterised Cohort☆. *J. Hepatol.* 73 (3), 505–515. doi:10.1016/j.jhep.2020.04.003

Baiocchini, A., Del Nonno, F., Taibi, C., Visco-Comandini, U., D'Offizi, G., Piacentini, M., et al. Liver Sinusoidal Endothelial Cells (LSECs) Modifications in Patients with Chronic Hepatitis C. *Sci. Rep.* 2019;9(1):8760. doi:10.1038/s41598-019-45114-1

Bardadin, K. A., and Desmet, V. J. (1985). Ultrastructural Observations on Sinusoidal Endothelial Cells in Chronic Active Hepatitis. *Histopathology* 9 (2), 171–181. doi:10.1111/j.1365-2559.1985.tb02433.x

Bataller, R., and Brenner, D. A. (2005). Liver Fibrosis. *J. Clin. Invest.* 115 (2), 209–218. doi:10.1172/JCI24282

Bataller, R., Paik, Y.-h., Lindquist, J. N., Lemasters, J. J., and Brenner, D. A. (2004). Hepatitis C Virus Core and Nonstructural Proteins Induce Fibrogenic Effects in Hepatic Stellate Cells. *Gastroenterology* 126 (2), 529–540. doi:10.1053/j.gastro.2003.11.018

Berg, J. M., Tymoczko, J. L., and Stryer, L. (2002). Section 30.5, Ethanol Alters Energy Metabolism in the Liver. *Biochemistry.* 5th edition. New York: W. H. Freeman. Available at: https://www.ncbi.nlm.nih.gov/books/NBK22524/ (Accessed February 23, 2021).

Berntsen, N. L., Klingenberg, O., Juran, B. D., Benito de Valle, M., Lindkvist, B., Lazaridis, K. N., et al. (2015). Association between HLA Haplotypes and Increased Serum Levels of IgG4 in Patients with Primary Sclerosing Cholangitis. *Gastroenterology* 148 (5), 924–927. doi:10.1053/j.gastro.2015.01.041

Bertinato, J., and L'Abbé, M. R. (2003). Copper Modulates the Degradation of Copper Chaperone for Cu,Zn Superoxide Dismutase by the 26 S Proteosome. *J. Biol. Chem.* 278 (37), 35071–35078. doi:10.1074/jbc.m302242200

Bolognesi, M., Di Pascoli, M., Verardo, A., and Gatta, A. (2014). Splanchnic Vasodilation and Hyperdynamic Circulatory Syndrome in Cirrhosis. *Wjg* 20 (10), 2555–2563. doi:10.3748/wjg.v20.i10.2555

Bonecchi, R., Galliera, E., Borroni, E. M., Corsi, M. M., Locati, M., and Mantovani, A. (2009). Chemokines and Chemokine Receptors: an Overview. *Front. Biosci.* 14, 540–551. doi:10.2741/3261

Borkham-Kamphorst, E., and Weiskirchen, R. (2016). The PDGF System and its Antagonists in Liver Fibrosis. *Cytokine Growth Factor. Rev.* 28, 53–61. doi:10.1016/j.cytogfr.2015.10.002

Bosch, J. (2007). Vascular Deterioration in Cirrhosis. *J. Clin. Gastroenterol.* 41 (Suppl. 3), S247–S253. doi:10.1097/MCG.0b013e3181572357

Brenner, D. A. (2013). Reversibility of Liver Fibrosis. *Gastroenterol. Hepatol. (N Y)* 9 (11), 737–739. doi:10.1007/0-387-26476-0_12

Broomé, U., Lindberg, G., and Löfberg, R. (1992). Primary Sclerosing Cholangitis in Ulcerative Colitis-A Risk Factor for the Development of Dysplasia and DNA Aneuploidy?. *Gastroenterology* 102 (6), 1877–1880. doi:10.1016/0016-5085(92)90308-1

Bruschi, F. V., Claudel, T., Tardelli, M., Caligiuri, A., Stulnig, T. M., Marra, F., et al. (2017). The PNPLA3 I148M Variant Modulates the Fibrogenic Phenotype of Human Hepatic Stellate Cells. *Hepatology* 65 (6), 1875–1890. doi:10.1002/hep.29041

Buzzetti, E., Pinzani, M., and Tsochatzis, E. A. (2016). The Multiple-Hit Pathogenesis of Non-alcoholic Fatty Liver Disease (NAFLD). *Metabolism* 65 (8), 1038–1048. doi:10.1016/j.metabol.2015.12.012

Caballero, F., Fernández, A., De Lacy, A. M., Fernández-Checa, J. C., Caballería, J., and García-Ruiz, C. (2009). Enhanced Free Cholesterol, SREBP-2 and StAR Expression in Human NASH. *J. Hepatol.* 50 (4), 789–796. doi:10.1016/j.jhep.2008.12.016

Caldwell, S. (2010). Cryptogenic Cirrhosis: what Are We Missing?. *Curr. Gastroenterol. Rep.* 12 (1), 40–48. doi:10.1007/s11894-009-0082-7

Cazanave, S. C., Mott, J. L., Bronk, S. F., Werneburg, N. W., Fingas, C. D., Meng, X. W., et al. (2011). Death Receptor 5 Signaling Promotes Hepatocyte Lipoapoptosis. *J. Biol. Chem.* 286 (45), 39336–39348. doi:10.1074/jbc.M111.280420

Chen, K., Ma, J., Jia, X., Ai, W., Ma, Z., and Pan, Q. (2019). Advancing the Understanding of NAFLD to Hepatocellular Carcinoma Development: From Experimental Models to Humans. *Biochim. Biophys. Acta (Bba) - Rev. Cancer* 1871 (1), 117–125. doi:10.1016/j.bbcan.2018.11.005C

Chen, W., Chang, B., Li, L., and Chan, L. (2010). Patatin-like Phospholipase Domain-Containing 3/adiponutrin Deficiency in Mice Is Not Associated with Fatty Liver Disease. *Hepatology* 52 (3), 1134–1142. doi:10.1002/hep.23812

Chen, Y., Fan, Y., Guo, D.-y., Xu, B., Shi, X.-y., Li, J.-t., et al. (2020). Study on the Relationship between Hepatic Fibrosis and Epithelial-Mesenchymal Transition in Intrahepatic Cells. *Biomed. Pharmacother.* 129, 110413. doi:10.1016/j.biopha.2020.110413

Chevillard, C., Moukoko, C. E., Elwali, N.-E. M. A., Bream, J. H., Kouriba, B., Argiro, L., et al. (2003). IFN-γ Polymorphisms (IFN-γ +2109 and IFN-γ +3810) Are Associated with Severe Hepatic Fibrosis in Human Hepatic Schistosomiasis (*Schistosoma Mansoni*). *J. Immunol.* 171 (10), 5596–5601. doi:10.4049/jimmunol.171.10.5596

D'Ambrosio, D. N., Walewski, J. L., Clugston, R. D., Berk, P. D., Rippe, R. A., and Blaner, W. S. (2011). Distinct Populations of Hepatic Stellate Cells in the Mouse Liver Have Different Capacities for Retinoid and Lipid Storage. *PLoS One* 6 (9), e24993. doi:10.1371/journal.pone.0024993

Dessein, H., Duflot, N., Romano, A., Opio, C., Pereira, V., Mola, C., et al. (2020). Genetic Algorithms Identify Individuals with High Risk of Severe Liver Disease Caused by Schistosomes. *Hum. Genet.* 139 (6-7), 821–831. doi:10.1007/s00439-020-02160-4

Ding, Y., Sun, Z., Zhang, S., Chen, Y., Zhou, B., Li, G., et al. (2020). Down-regulation of Long Non-coding RNA LINC01554 in Hepatocellular Cancer and its Clinical Significance. *J. Cancer* 11 (11), 3369–3374. doi:10.7150/jca.40512

DiPaola, F. W., and Fontana, R. J. (2018). "Drug-induced Liver Injury," in *Sherlock's Diseases of the Liver and Biliary System*. Editors J. S. Dooley, A. S. F. Lok, G. Garcia-Tsao, et al. (Hoboken, NJ: John Wiley & Sons), 468–493. doi:10.1002/9781119237662.ch24

Do, A., and Reau, N. S. (2020). Chronic Viral Hepatitis: Current Management and Future Directions. *Hepatol. Commun.* 4 (3), 329–341. doi:10.1002/hep4.1480

Dobie, R., Wilson-Kanamori, J. R., Henderson, B. E. P., Smith, J. R., Matchett, K. P., Portman, J. R., et al. (2019). Single-cell Transcriptomics Uncovers Zonation of Function in the Mesenchyme during Liver Fibrosis. *Cel Rep.* 29 (7), 1832–1847. doi:10.1016/j.celrep.2019.10.024

Dong, X. C. (2019). PNPLA3-A Potential Therapeutic Target for Personalized Treatment of Chronic Liver Disease. *Front. Med.* 6, 304. doi:10.3389/fmed.2019.00304

Dooley, J. S., Lok, A. S. F., and Garcia-Tsaqo, B. (2018). in *Sherlock's Diseases of the Liver and Biliary System*. Editors J. S. Dooley, A. S. F. Lok, B. Garcia-Tsaqo, and M. Pinzani. Thirteenth edition (Berlin: Springer).

Dranoff, J. A., and Wells, R. G. (2010). Portal Fibroblasts: Underappreciated Mediators of Biliary Fibrosis. *Hepatology* 51 (4), 1438–1444. doi:10.1002/hep.23405

Drescher, H., Weiskirchen, S., and Weiskirchen, R. (2019). Current Status in Testing for Nonalcoholic Fatty Liver Disease (NAFLD) and Nonalcoholic Steatohepatitis (NASH). *Cells* 8 (8), 845. doi:10.3390/cells8080845

Dunn, M. A. Parasitic Diseases. In: *Schiff's Diseases of the Liver* 11th Edition (2011). Chapter 39. pp. 1017–1033. ISBN: 9780470654682. doi:10.1002/9781119950509.ch39

Duseja, A. (2010). Nonalcoholic Fatty Liver Disease in India - a Lot Done, yet More Required!. *Indian J. Gastroenterol.* 29 (6), 217–225. doi:10.1007/s12664-010-0069-1

Dusek, C. O., and Hadden, M. K. (2021). Targeting the GLI Family of Transcription Factors for the Development of Anti-cancer Drugs. *Expert Opin. Drug Discov.* 16 (3), 289–302. doi:10.1080/17460441.2021.1832078

Dyson, J. K., Anstee, Q. M., and McPherson, S. (2014). Non-alcoholic Fatty Liver Disease: a Practical Approach to Diagnosis and Staging. *Frontline Gastroenterol.* 5 (3), 211–218. doi:10.1136/flgastro-2013-100403

Eriksson, J., Reimert, C. M., Kabatereine, N. B., Kazibwe, F., Ireri, E., Kadzo, H., et al. (2007). The 434(G>C) Polymorphism within the Coding Sequence of Eosinophil Cationic Protein (ECP) Correlates with the Natural Course of *Schistosoma Mansoni* Infection. *Int. J. Parasitol.* 37 (12), 1359–1366. doi:10.1016/j.ijpara.2007.04.001

Fausther, M., Goree, J. R., Lavoie, É. G., Graham, A. L., Sévigny, J., and Dranoff, J. A. (2015). Establishment and Characterization of Rat Portal Myofibroblast Cell Lines. *PLoS One* 10 (3), e0121161. doi:10.1371/journal.pone.0121161

Feldstein, A. E., Canbay, A., Guicciardi, M. E., Higuchi, H., Bronk, S. F., and Gores, G. J. (2003). Diet Associated Hepatic Steatosis Sensitizes to Fas Mediated Liver Injury in Mice. *J. Hepatol.* 39 (6), 978–983. doi:10.1016/s0168-8278(03)00460-4

Figueira, C. P., Carvalhal, D. G. F., Almeida, R. A., Hermida, M. d. E.-R., Touchard, D., Robert, P., et al. (2015). Leishmania Infection Modulates Beta-1 Integrin Activation and Alters the Kinetics of Monocyte Spreading over Fibronectin. *Sci. Rep.* 5, 12862. doi:10.1038/srep12862

Friedman, S. L., Ratziu, V., Harrison, S. A., Abdelmalek, M. F., Aithal, G. P., Caballeria, J., et al. (2018). A Randomized, Placebo-Controlled Trial of Cenicriviroc for Treatment of Nonalcoholic Steatohepatitis with Fibrosis. *Hepatology* 67 (5), 1754–1767. doi:10.1002/hep.29477

Gong, Z., Luo, Q.-Z., Lin, L., Su, Y.-P., Peng, H.-B., Du, K., et al. (2012). Association of MICA Gene Polymorphisms with Liver Fibrosis in Schistosomiasis Patients in the Dongting Lake Region. *Braz. J. Med. Biol. Res.* 45 (3), 222–229. doi:10.1590/s0100-879x2012007500024

Gorden, D. L., Ivanova, P. T., Myers, D. S., McIntyre, J. O., VanSaun, M. N., Wright, J. K., et al. (2011). Increased Diacylglycerols Characterize Hepatic Lipid Changes in Progression of Human Nonalcoholic Fatty Liver Disease;

Comparison to a Murine Model. *PLoS One* 6 (8), e22775. doi:10.1371/journal.pone.0022775

Grund-Gröschke, S., Stockmaier, G., and Aberger, F. (2019). Hedgehog/GLI Signaling in Tumor Immunity—New Therapeutic Opportunities and Clinical Implications. *Cell Commun. Signal* 17 (1), 172. doi:10.1186/s12964-019-0459-7

Guarino, M., and Dufour, J.-F. (2019). Nicotinamide and NAFLD: Is There Nothing New under the Sun?. *Metabolites* 9 (9), 180. doi:10.3390/metabo9090180

Gutierrez-Reyes, G., Gutierrez-Ruiz, M. C., and Kershenobich, D. (2007). Liver Fibrosis and Chronic Viral Hepatitis. *Arch. Med. Res.* 38 (6), 644–651. doi:10.1016/j.arcmed.2006.10.001

Hellemans, K., Grinko, I., Rombouts, K., Schuppan, D., and Geerts, A. (1999). All-trans and 9-cis Retinoic Acid Alter Rat Hepatic Stellate Cell Phenotype Differentially. *Gut* 45 (1), 134–142. doi:10.1136/gut.45.1.134

Hellemans, K., Verbuyst, P., Quartier, E., Schuit, F., Rombouts, K., Chandraratna, R. A. S., et al. (2004). Differential Modulation of Rat Hepatic Stellate Phenotype by Natural and Synthetic Retinoids. *Hepatology* 39 (1), 97–108. doi:10.1002/hep.20015

Hempel, F., Roderfeld, M., Savai, R., Sydykov, A., Irungbam, K., Schermuly, R., et al. (2019). Depletion of Bone Marrow-Derived Fibrocytes Attenuates TAA-Induced Liver Fibrosis in Mice. *Cells* 8 (10), 1210. doi:10.3390/cells8101210

Herrmann, J., Arias, M., Van De Leur, E., Gressner, A. M., and Weiskirchen, R. (2004). CSRP2, TIMP-1, and SM22alpha Promoter Fragments Direct Hepatic Stellate Cell-specific Transgene Expression In Vitro, but Not In Vivo. *Liver Int.* 24 (1), 69–79. doi:10.1111/j.1478-3231.2004.00891.x

Hirayama, K., Chen, H., Kikuchi, M., Yin, T., Itoh, M., Gu, X., et al. (1998). Glycine-Valine Dimorphism at the 86th Amino Acid ofHLA-DRB1Influenced the Prognosis of Postschistosomal Hepatic Fibrosis. *J. Infect. Dis.* 177 (6), 1682–1686. doi:10.1086/515299

Holt, A. P., Haughton, E. L., Lalor, P. F., Filer, A., Buckley, C. D., and Adams, D. H. (2009). Liver Myofibroblasts Regulate Infiltration and Positioning of Lymphocytes in Human Liver. *Gastroenterology* 136 (2), 705–714. doi:10.1053/j.gastro.2008.10.020

Hughes, C. E., and Nibbs, R. J. B. (2018). A Guide to Chemokines and Their Receptors. *FEBS J.* 285 (16), 2944–2971. doi:10.1111/febs.14466

Hutchins, N. A., Chung, C.-S., Borgerding, J. N., Ayala, C. A., and Ayala, A. (2013). Kupffer Cells Protect Liver Sinusoidal Endothelial Cells from Fas-dependent Apoptosis in Sepsis by Down-Regulating Gp130. *Am. J. Pathol.* 182 (3), 742–754. doi:10.1016/j.ajpath.2012.11.023

Ibrahim, S. H., Hirsova, P., Tomita, K., Bronk, S. F., Werneburg, N. W., Harrison, S. A., et al. (2016). Mixed Lineage Kinase 3 Mediates Release of C-X-C Motif Ligand 10-bearing Chemotactic Extracellular Vesicles from Lipotoxic Hepatocytes. *Hepatology* 63 (3), 731–744. doi:10.1002/hep.28252

Ikenaga, N., Peng, Z.-W., Vaid, K. A., Liu, S. B., Yoshida, S., Sverdlov, D. Y., et al. (2017). Selective Targeting of Lysyl Oxidase-like 2 (LOXL2) Suppresses Hepatic Fibrosis Progression and Accelerates its Reversal. *Gut* 66 (9), 1697–1708. doi:10.1136/gutjnl-2016-312473

Iredale, J. (2008). Defining Therapeutic Targets for Liver Fibrosis: Exploiting the Biology of Inflammation and Repair. *Pharmacol. Res.* 58 (2), 129–136. doi:10.1016/j.phrs.2008.06.011

Iredale, J. P., Benyon, R. C., Arthur, M. J., Ferris, W. F., Alcolado, R., Winwood, P. J., et al. (1996). Tissue Inhibitor of Metalloproteinase-1 Messenger RNA Expression Is Enhanced Relative to Interstitial Collagenase Messenger RNA in Experimental Liver Injury and Fibrosis. *Hepatology* 24 (1), 176–184. doi:10.1002/hep.510240129

Iredale, J. P., Thompson, A., and Henderson, N. C. (2013). Extracellular Matrix Degradation in Liver Fibrosis: Biochemistry and Regulation. *Biochim. Biophys. Acta (Bba) - Mol. Basis Dis.* 1832 (7), 876–883. doi:10.1016/j.bbadis.2012.11.002

Issa, R., Zhou, X., Constandinou, C. M., Fallowfield, J., Millward-Sadler, H., Gaca, M. D. A., et al. (2004). Spontaneous Recovery from Micronodular Cirrhosis: Evidence for Incomplete Resolution Associated with Matrix Cross-Linking☆. *Gastroenterology* 126 (7), 1795–1808. doi:10.1053/j.gastro.2004.03.009

Iwaisako, K., Jiang, C., Zhang, M., Cong, M., Moore-Morris, T. J., Park, T. J., et al. (2014). Origin of Myofibroblasts in the Fibrotic Liver in Mice. *Proc. Natl. Acad. Sci.* 111 (32), E3297–E3305. doi:10.1073/pnas.1400062111

Iwakiri, Y. (2014). Pathophysiology of Portal Hypertension. *Clin. Liver Dis.* 18 (2), 281–291. doi:10.1016/j.cld.2013.12.001

Jenkins, C. M., Mancuso, D. J., Yan, W., Sims, H. F., Gibson, B., and Gross, R. W. (2004). Identification, Cloning, Expression, and Purification of Three Novel Human Calcium-independent Phospholipase A2 Family Members Possessing Triacylglycerol Lipase and Acylglycerol Transacylase Activities. *J. Biol. Chem.* 279 (47), 48968–48975. doi:10.1074/jbc.M407841200

Junqueira, L. C., and Carneiro, J. (2002). *Basic Histology*. 10th edition Lange International Edition. London: McGraw-Hill/Appleton Lange, 332–343. 9780071378291.

Kalra, S., Vithalani, M., Gulati, G., Kulkarni, C. M., Kadam, Y., Pallivathukkal, J., et al. (2013). Study of Prevalence of Nonalcoholic Fatty Liver Disease (NAFLD) in Type 2 Diabetes Patients in India (SPRINT). *J. Assoc. Physicians India* 61 (7), 448–453. doi:10.21276/iabcr.2016.2.4.11

Kamal, N., Koh, C., Koh, C., Samala, N., Fontana, R. J., Stolz, A., et al. (2019). Asparaginase-induced Hepatotoxicity: Rapid Development of Cholestasis and Hepatic Steatosis. *Hepatol. Int.* 13 (5), 641–648. doi:10.1007/s12072-019-09971-2

Karlsen, T. H., Folseraas, T., Thorburn, D., and Vesterhus, M. (2017). Primary Sclerosing Cholangitis-a Comprehensive Review. *J. Hepatol.* 67 (6), 1298–1323. doi:10.1016/j.jhep.2017.07.022

Khurana, A., Sayed, N., Allawadhi, P., and Weiskirchen, R. (2021). It's All about the Spaces between Cells: Role of Extracellular Matrix in Liver Fibrosis. *Ann. Transl Med.* 11, 39. doi:10.21037/atm-20-2948

Kinzler, K., Bigner, S., Bigner, D., Trent, J., Law, M., O'Brien, S., et al. (1987). Identification of an Amplified, Highly Expressed Gene in a Human Glioma. *Science* 236 (4797), 70–73. doi:10.1126/science.3563490

Kinzler, K. W., and Vogelstein, B. (1990). The GLI Gene Encodes a Nuclear Protein Which Binds Specific Sequences in the Human Genome. *Mol. Cel. Biol.* 10 (2), 634–642. doi:10.1128/mcb.10.2.634

Kisseleva, T., Cong, M., Paik, Y., Scholten, D., Jiang, C., Benner, C., et al. (2012). Myofibroblasts Revert to an Inactive Phenotype during Regression of Liver Fibrosis. *Proc. Natl. Acad. Sci.* 109 (24), 9448–9453. doi:10.1073/pnas.1201840109

Kisseleva, T. (2017). The Origin of Fibrogenic Myofibroblasts in Fibrotic Liver. *Hepatology* 65 (3), 1039–1043. doi:10.1002/hep.28948

Kisseleva, T., Uchinami, H., Feirt, N., Quintana-Bustamante, O., Segovia, J. C., Schwabe, R. F., et al. (2006). Bone Marrow-Derived Fibrocytes Participate in Pathogenesis of Liver Fibrosis. *J. Hepatol.* 45 (3), 429–438. doi:10.1016/j.jhep.2006.04.014

Koh, C., Heller, T., and Glenn, J. S. (2019). Pathogenesis of and New Therapies for Hepatitis D. *Gastroenterology* 156 (2), 461–476. doi:10.1053/j.gastro.2018.09.058

Kong, X., Horiguchi, N., Mori, M., and Gao, B. (2012). Cytokines and STATs in Liver Fibrosis. *Front. Physio.* 3, 69. doi:10.3389/fphys.2012.00069

Koob, G. F., Arends, M. A., and Le Moal, M. (2014), Chapter 6—Alcohol, Editors: G. F. Koob, M. A. Arends, and M. Le. Moal, *Drugs, Addiction, and the Brain*, London: Academic Press, pp. 173–219. ISBN 9780123869371. doi:10.1016/B978-0-12-386937-1.00006-4

Koopmans, T., and Rinkevich, Y. (2018). Mesothelial to Mesenchyme Transition as a Major Developmental and Pathological Player in Trunk Organs and Their Cavities. *Commun. Biol.* 1, 170. doi:10.1038/s42003-018-0180-x

Kramann, R., Schneider, R. K., DiRocco, D. P., Machado, F., Fleig, S., Bondzie, P. A., et al. (2015). Perivascular Gli1+ Progenitors Are Key Contributors to Injury-Induced Organ Fibrosis. *Cell Stem Cell* 16 (1), 51–66. doi:10.1016/j.stem.2014.11.004

Krenkel, O., Hundertmark, J., Ritz, T., Weiskirchen, R., and Tacke, F. (2019). Single Cell RNA Sequencing Identifies Subsets of Hepatic Stellate Cells and Myofibroblasts in Liver Fibrosis. *Cells* 8 (5), 503. doi:10.3390/cells8050503

Krenkel, O., Puengel, T., Govaere, O., Abdallah, A. T., Mossanen, J. C., Kohlhepp, M., et al. (2018). Therapeutic Inhibition of Inflammatory Monocyte Recruitment Reduces Steatohepatitis and Liver Fibrosis. *Hepatology* 67 (4), 1270–1283. doi:10.1002/hep.29544

Lan, T., Kisseleva, T., and Brenner, D. A. (2015). Deficiency of NOX1 or NOX4 Prevents Liver Inflammation and Fibrosis in Mice through Inhibition of Hepatic Stellate Cell Activation. *PLoS One* 10 (7), e0129743. doi:10.1371/journal.pone.0129743

Lee, Y. K., Park, J. E., Lee, M., and Hardwick, J. P. (2018). Hepatic Lipid Homeostasis by Peroxisome Proliferator-Activated Receptor Gamma 2. *Liver Res.* 2 (4), 209–215. doi:10.1016/j.livres.2018.12.001

Lepreux, S., Guyot, C., Billet, F., Combe, C., Balabaud, C., Bioulac-Sage, P., et al. (2013). Smoothelin, a New Marker to Determine the Origin of Liver Fibrogenic Cells. *Wjg* 19 (48), 9343–9350. doi:10.3748/wjg.v19.i48.9343

Levada, K., Omelyanchik, A., Rodionova, V., Weiskirchen, R., and Bartneck, M. (2019). Magnetic-assisted Treatment of Liver Fibrosis. *Cells* 8 (10), 1279. doi:10.3390/cells8101279

Li, C., Tan, Y. H., Sun, J., Deng, F. M., and Liu, Y. L. (2020). PAX6 Contributes to the Activation and Proliferation of Hepatic Stellate Cells via Activating Hedgehog/GLI1 Pathway. *Biochem. Biophysical Res. Commun.* 526 (2), 314–320. doi:10.1016/j.bbrc.2020.03.086

Li, H., You, H., Fan, X., and Jia, J. (2016). Hepatic Macrophages in Liver Fibrosis: Pathogenesis and Potential Therapeutic Targets. *BMJ Open Gastroenterol.* 3 (1), e000079. doi:10.1136/bmjgast-2016-000079

Li, T., Yan, H., Geng, Y., Shi, H., Li, H., Wang, S., et al. (2019). Target Genes Associated with Lipid and Glucose Metabolism in Non-alcoholic Fatty Liver Disease. *Lipids Health Dis.* 18 (1), 211. doi:10.1186/s12944-019-1154-9

Li, W., Li, L., and Hui, L. (2020). Cell Plasticity in Liver Regeneration. *Trends Cel Biol.* 30 (4), 329–338. doi:10.1016/j.tcb.2020.01.007

Li, Y., Lua, I., French, S. W., and Asahina, K. (2016). Role of TGF-β Signaling in Differentiation of Mesothelial Cells to Vitamin A-Poor Hepatic Stellate Cells in Liver Fibrosis. *Am. J. Physiol.-Gastrointestinal Liver Physiol.* 310 (4), G262–G272. doi:10.1152/ajpgi.00257.2015

Li, Y., Wang, J., and Asahina, K. (2013). Mesothelial Cells Give Rise to Hepatic Stellate Cells and Myofibroblasts via Mesothelial-Mesenchymal Transition in Liver Injury. *Proc. Natl. Acad. Sci.* 110 (6), 2324–2329. doi:10.1073/pnas.1214136110

Liangpunsakul, S., and Chalasani, N. (2019). Lipid Mediators of Liver Injury in Nonalcoholic Fatty Liver Disease. *Am. J. Physiol.-Gastrointestinal Liver Physiol.* 316 (1), G75–G81. doi:10.1152/ajpgi.00170.2018

Lieber, C. S. (2004). The Discovery of the Microsomal Ethanol Oxidizing System and its Physiologic and Pathologic Role. *Drug Metab. Rev.* 36 (3-4), 511–529. doi:10.1081/dmr-200033441

Liu, J., Lin, B., Chen, Z., Deng, M., Wang, Y., Wang, J., et al. (2020). Identification of Key Pathways and Genes in Nonalcoholic Fatty Liver Disease Using Bioinformatics Analysis. *Aoms* 16 (2), 374–385. doi:10.5114/aoms.2020.93343

Locke, G. A., Cheng, D., Witmer, M. R., Tamura, J. K., Haque, T., Carney, R. F., et al. (2008). Differential Activation of Recombinant Human Acetyl-CoA Carboxylases 1 and 2 by Citrate. *Arch. Biochem. Biophys.* 475 (1), 72–79. doi:10.1016/j.abb.2008.04.011

Long, X., Chen, Q., Zhao, J., Rafaels, N., Mathias, P., Liang, H., et al. (2015). An IL-13 Promoter Polymorphism Associated with Liver Fibrosis in Patients with Schistosoma Japonicum. *PLoS One* 10 (8), e0135360. doi:10.1371/journal.pone.0135360

Long, X., Daya, M., Zhao, J., Rafaels, N., Liang, H., Potee, J., et al. (2017). The Role of ST2 and ST2 Genetic Variants in Schistosomiasis. *J. Allergy Clin. Immunol.* 140 (5), 1416–1422. doi:10.1016/j.jaci.2016.12.969

Lötvall, J., Hill, A. F., Hochberg, F., Buzás, E. I., Di Vizio, D., Gardiner, C., et al. (2014). Minimal Experimental Requirements for Definition of Extracellular Vesicles and Their Functions: a Position Statement from the International Society for Extracellular Vesicles. *J. Extracellular Vesicles* 3, 26913. doi:10.3402/jev.v3.26913

Lua, I., Li, Y., Pappoe, L. S., and Asahina, K. (2015). Myofibroblastic Conversion and Regeneration of Mesothelial Cells in Peritoneal and Liver Fibrosis. *Am. J. Pathol.* 185 (12), 3258–3273. doi:10.1016/j.ajpath.2015.08.009

Luangmonkong, T., Suriguga, S., Mutsaers, H. A. M., Groothuis, G. M. M., Olinga, P., and Boersema, M. (2018). Targeting Oxidative Stress for the Treatment of Liver Fibrosis. *Rev. Physiol. Biochem. Pharmacol.* 175, 71–102. doi:10.1007/112_2018_10

Luukkonen, P. K., Zhou, Y., Sädevirta, S., Leivonen, M., Arola, J., Orešič, M., et al. (2016). Hepatic Ceramides Dissociate Steatosis and Insulin Resistance in Patients with Non-alcoholic Fatty Liver Disease. *J. Hepatol.* 64 (5), 1167–1175. doi:10.1016/j.jhep.2016.01.002

Macherey, A.-C., and Dansette, P. M. (2015). "Biotransformations Leading to Toxic Metabolites," in *Rognan D. The Practice of Medicinal Chemistry*. Editors C. G. Wermuth, D. Aldous, and P. Raboisson. Fourth Edition (London: Academic Press), 585–614. doi:10.1016/B978-0-12-417205-0.00025-0

Machicado, C., Machicado, J. D., Maco, V., Terashima, A., and Marcos, L. A. (2016). Association of *Fasciola Hepatica* Infection with Liver Fibrosis,

Cirrhosis, and *Cancer*: A Systematic Review. *Plos Negl. Trop. Dis.* 10 (9), e0004962. doi:10.1371/journal.pntd.0004962

Magill, A. J., Grögl, M., Gasser, R. A., Jr, Sun, W., and Oster, C. N. (1993). Visceral Infection Caused by Leishmania Tropica in Veterans of Operation Desert Storm. *N. Engl. J. Med.* 328 (19), 1383–1387. doi:10.1056/NEJM199305133281904

Magness, S. T., Bataller, R. n., Yang, L., and Brenner, D. A. (2004). A Dual Reporter Gene Transgenic Mouse Demonstrates Heterogeneity in Hepatic Fibrogenic Cell Populations. *Hepatology* 40 (5), 1151–1159. doi:10.1002/hep.20427

Maher, J. J. (2001). Interactions between Hepatic Stellate Cells and the Immune System. *Semin. Liver Dis.* 21 (3), 417–426. doi:10.1055/s-2001-17555

Mallat, A., Lodder, J., Teixeira-Clerc, F., Moreau, R., Codogno, P., and Lotersztajn, S. (2014). Autophagy: a Multifaceted Partner in Liver Fibrosis. *Biomed. Res. Int.* 2014, 1–7. doi:10.1155/2014/869390

Manmadhan, S., and Ehmer, U. (2019). Hippo Signaling in the Liver - A Long and Ever-Expanding Story. *Front. Cel Dev. Biol.* 7, 33. doi:10.3389/fcell.2019.00033

Mannaerts, I., Thoen, L. F. R., Eysackers, N., Cubero, F. J., Batista Leite, S., Coldham, I., et al. (2019). Unfolded Protein Response Is an Early, Non-critical Event during Hepatic Stellate Cell Activation. *Cell Death Dis* 10 (2), 98. doi:10.1038/s41419-019-1327-5

Mantel, P.-Y., and Schmidt-Weber, C. B. (2011). Transforming Growth Factor-Beta: Recent Advances on its Role in Immune Tolerance. *Methods Mol. Biol.* 677, 303–338. doi:10.1007/978-1-60761-869-0_21

Marcos, L. A., Terashima, A., Yi, P., Andrade, R., Cubero, F. J., Albanis, E., et al. (2011). Mechanisms of Liver Fibrosis Associated with Experimental *Fasciola Hepatica* Infection: Roles of Fas2 Proteinase and Hepatic Stellate Cell Activation. *J. Parasitol.* 97 (1), 82–87. doi:10.1645/GE-2420.1

Margini, C., and Dufour, J. F. (2016). The Story of HCC in NAFLD: from Epidemiology, across Pathogenesis, to Prevention and Treatment. *Liver Int.* 36 (3), 317–324. doi:10.1111/liv.13031

Marra, F., and Tacke, F. (2014). Roles for Chemokines in Liver Disease. *Gastroenterology* 147 (3), 577–594. doi:10.1053/j.gastro.2014.06.043

McDonnell, A. M., and Dang, C. H. (2013). Basic Review of the Cytochrome P450 System. *J. Adv. Pract. Oncol.* 4 (4), 263–268. doi:10.6004/jadpro.2013.4.4.7

McGuire, L. C., Cruickshank, A. M., and Munro, P. T. (2006). Alcoholic Ketoacidosis. *Emerg. Med. J.* 23 (6), 417–420. doi:10.1136/emj.2004.017590

McManus, D. P., Bergquist, R., Cai, P., Ranasinghe, S., Tebeje, B. M., and You, H. (2020). Schistosomiasis-from Immunopathology to Vaccines. *Semin. Immunopathol.* 42 (3), 355–371. doi:10.1007/s00281-020-00789-x

Mederacke, I., Hsu, C. C., Troeger, J. S., Huebener, P., Mu, X., Dapito, D. H., et al. (2013). Fate Tracing Reveals Hepatic Stellate Cells as Dominant Contributors to Liver Fibrosis Independent of its Aetiology. *Nat. Commun.* 4, 2823. doi:10.1038/ncomms3823

Melo, F. A., Moura, E. P., Ribeiro, R. R., Alves, C. F., Caliari, M. V., Tafuri, W. L., et al. (2009). Hepatic Extracellular Matrix Alterations in Dogs Naturally Infected withLeishmania (Leishmania) Chagasi. *Int. J. Exp. Pathol.* 90 (5), 538–548. doi:10.1111/j.1365-2613.2009.00681.x

Mendes, F. D., Jorgensen, R., Keach, J., Katzmann, J. A., Smyrk, T., Donlinger, J., et al. (2006). Elevated Serum IgG4 Concentration in Patients with Primary Sclerosing Cholangitis. *Am. J. Gastroenterol.* 101 (9), 2070–2075. doi:10.1111/j.1572-0241.2006.00772.x

Metz, R. P., Patterson, J. L., and Wilson, E. (2012). Vascular Smooth Muscle Cells: Isolation, Culture, and Characterization. *Methods Mol. Biol.* 843, 169–176. doi:10.1007/978-1-61779-523-7_16

Michalopoulos, G. K. (2013). Principles of Liver Regeneration and Growth Homeostasis. *Compr. Physiol.* 3 (1), 485–513. doi:10.1002/cphy.c120014

Mitchell, M. C., Kerr, T., and Herlong, H. F. (2020). Current Management and Future Treatment of Alcoholic Hepatitis. *Gastroenterol. Hepatol.* 16, 178–189. doi:10.14218/jcth.2016.00006

Morales, M. R., Sendra, C., and Romero-Gomez, M. (2017). Hepatitis B and NAFLD: Lives Crossed. *Ann. Hepatol.* 16 (2), 185–187. doi:10.5604/16652681.1231556

Morgan, T. R. (2007). Management of Alcoholic Hepatitis. *Gastroenterol. Hepatol. (N Y)* 3 (2), 97–99. doi:10.3109/9780203301388-10

Munker, S., Wu, Y.-L., Ding, H.-G., Liebe, R., and Weng, H.-L. (2017). Can a Fibrotic Liver Afford Epithelial-Mesenchymal Transition? *Wjg* 23 (26), 4661–4668. doi:10.3748/wjg.v23.i26.4661

Murphree, C. R., Nguyen, N. N., Raghunathan, V., Olson, S. R., DeLoughery, T., and Shatzel, J. J. (2020). Diagnosis and Management of Hereditary Haemochromatosis. *Vox Sang* 115 (4), 255–262. doi:10.1111/vox.12896

Mutsaers, S. E. (2004). The Mesothelial Cell. *Int. J. Biochem. Cel Biol.* 36 (1), 9–16. doi:10.1016/s1357-2725(03)00242-5

Narayanan, P., and Mistry, P. K. (2020). Update on Alpha-1 Antitrypsin Deficiency in Liver Disease. *Clin. Liver Dis.* 15 (6), 228–235. doi:10.1002/cld.896

Natarajan, V., Harris, E. N., and Kidambi, S. (2017). SECs (Sinusoidal Endothelial Cells), Liver Microenvironment, and Fibrosis. *Biomed. Res. Int.* 2017, 1–9. doi:10.1155/2017/4097205

Nishio, T., Hu, R., Koyama, Y., Liang, S., Rosenthal, S. B., Yamamoto, G., et al. (2019). Activated Hepatic Stellate Cells and Portal Fibroblasts Contribute to Cholestatic Liver Fibrosis in MDR2 Knockout Mice. *J. Hepatol.* 71 (3), 573–585. doi:10.1016/j.jhep.2019.04.012

Oliveira, J. B., Silva, P. C. V., Vasconcelos, L. M., Gomes, A. V., Coêlho, M. R. C. D., Cahu, G. G. O. M., et al. (2015). Influence of Polymorphism (-G308A) TNF-α on the Periportal Fibrosis Regression of Schistosomiasis after Specific Treatment. *Genet. Test. Mol. Biomarkers* 19 (11), 598–603. doi:10.1089/gtmb.2015.0091

Omenetti, A., Porrello, A., Jung, Y., Yang, L., Popov, Y., Choi, S. S., et al. (2008). Hedgehog Signaling Regulates Epithelial–Mesenchymal Transition during Biliary Fibrosis in Rodents and Humans. *J. Clin. Invest.* 118 (10), 3331–3342. doi:10.1172/JCI35875

Oosterhoff, L. A., Kruitwagen, H. S., van Wolferen, M. E., van Balkom, B. W. M., Mokry, M., Lansu, N., et al. (2019). Characterization of Endothelial and Smooth Muscle Cells from Different Canine Vessels. *Front. Physiol.* 10, 101. doi:10.3389/fphys.2019.00101

Patel, A., and Harrison, S. A. (2012). Hepatitis C Virus Infection and Nonalcoholic Steatohepatitis. *Gastroenterol. Hepatol. (N Y)* 8 (5), 305–312.

Patel, N., Sharma, B., and Samant, H. (2020). Cryptogenic Cirrhosis. Available from: https://www.ncbi.nlm.nih.gov/books/NBK534228/ (Accessed February 23, 2021).

Pavletich, N., and Pabo, C. (1993). Crystal Structure of a Five-Finger GLI-DNA Complex: New Perspectives on Zinc Fingers. *Science* 261 (5129), 1701–1707. doi:10.1126/science.8378770

Pellicoro, A., Ramachandran, P., Iredale, J. P., and Fallowfield, J. A. (2014). Liver Fibrosis and Repair: Immune Regulation of Wound Healing in a Solid Organ. *Nat. Rev. Immunol.* 14 (3), 181–194. doi:10.1038/nri3623

Peng, X., Yang, Y., Tang, L., Wan, J., Dai, J., Li, L., et al. (2020). Therapeutic Benefits of Apocynin in Mice with lipopolysaccharide/D-Galactosamine-Induced Acute Liver Injury via Suppression of the Late Stage Pro-apoptotic AMPK/JNK Pathway. *Biomed. Pharmacother.* 125, 110020. doi:10.1016/j.biopha.2020.110020

Penz-Österreicher, M., Österreicher, C. H., and Trauner, M. (2011). Fibrosis in Autoimmune and Cholestatic Liver Disease. *Best Pract. Res. Clin. Gastroenterol.* 25 (2), 245–258. doi:10.1016/j.bpg.2011.02.001

Perdigoto, R., Carpenter, H. A., and Czaja, A. J. (1992). Frequency and Significance of Chronic Ulcerative Colitis in Severe Corticosteroid-Treated Autoimmune Hepatitis. *J. Hepatol.* 14 (2–3), 325–331. doi:10.1016/0168-8278(92)90178-r

Perri, G. A. (2013). Ascites in Patients with Cirrhosis. *Can. Fam. Physician* 59 (12), 1297–1299.

Pinto, R. B., Schneider, A. C., and da Silveira, T. R. (2015). Cirrhosis in Children and Adolescents: An Overview. *Wjh* 7 (3), 392–405. doi:10.4254/wjh.v7.i3.392

Pinzani, M., and Vizzutti, F. (2005). "Anatomy and Vascular Biology of the Cells in the Portal Circulation," in *Portal Hypertension Clinical Gastroenterology*. Editors A. J. Sanyal and V. H. Shah (London: Humana Press). doi:10.1007/978-1-59259-885-4

Pirazzi, C., Valenti, L., Motta, B. M., Pingitore, P., Hedfalk, K., Mancina, R. M., et al. (2014). PNPLA3 Has Retinyl-Palmitate Lipase Activity in Human Hepatic Stellate Cells. *Hum. Mol. Genet.* 23 (15), 4077–4085. doi:10.1093/hmg/ddu121

Pitta, M. G. R., Romano, A., Cabantous, S., Henri, S., Hammad, A., Kouriba, B., et al. (2009). IL-17 and IL-22 Are Associated with Protection against Human Kala Azar Caused by Leishmania Donovani. *J. Clin. Invest.* 119 (8), 2379–2387. doi:10.1172/JCI38813

Polaris Observatory Collaborators (2018). Global Prevalence, Treatment, and Prevention of Hepatitis B Virus Infection in 2016: a Modelling Study. *Lancet Gastroenterol. Hepatol.* 3 (6), 383–403. doi:10.1016/S2468-1253(18)30056-6

Polyzos, S. A., Kountouras, J., and Mantzoros, C. S. (2015). Leptin in Nonalcoholic Fatty Liver Disease: a Narrative Review. *Metabolism* 64 (1), 60–78. doi:10.1016/j.metabol.2014.10.012

Ramachandran, P., and Iredale, J. P. (2012). Liver Fibrosis: a Bidirectional Model of Fibrogenesis and Resolution. *QJM* 105 (9), 813–817. doi:10.1093/qjmed/hcs069

Rao, S., Xiang, J., Huang, J., Zhang, S., Zhang, M., Sun, H., et al. (2019). PRC1 Promotes GLI1-dependent Osteopontin Expression in Association with the Wnt/β-Catenin Signaling Pathway and Aggravates Liver Fibrosis. *Cell Biosci* 9, 100. doi:10.1186/s13578-019-0363-2

Rehm, J., and Shield, K. D. (2019). Global Burden of Alcohol Use Disorders and Alcohol Liver Disease. *Biomedicines* 7 (4), 99. doi:10.3390/biomedicines7040099

Reilkoff, R. A., Bucala, R., and Herzog, E. L. (2011). Fibrocytes: Emerging Effector Cells in Chronic Inflammation. *Nat. Rev. Immunol.* 11 (6), 427–435. doi:10.1038/nri2990

Robertson, H., Kirby, J. A., Yip, W. W., Jones, D. E. J., and Burt, A. D. (2007). Biliary Epithelial-Mesenchymal Transition in Posttransplantation Recurrence of Primary Biliary Cirrhosis. *Hepatology* 45 (4), 977–981. doi:10.1002/hep.21624

Rosselli, M., Lotersztajn, S., Vizzutti, F., Arena, U., Pinzani, M., and Marra, F. (2014). The Metabolic Syndrome and Chronic Liver Disease. *Cpd* 20 (31), 5010–5024. doi:10.2174/1381612819666131206111352

Rossen, N. G., Fuentes, S., Boonstra, K., D'Haens, G. R., Heilig, H. G., Zoetendal, E. G., et al. (2015). The Mucosa-Associated Microbiota of PSC Patients Is Characterized by Low Diversity and Low Abundance of Uncultured Clostridiales II. *J. Crohns Colitis* 9 (4), 342–348. doi:10.1093/ecco-jcc/jju023

Ryaboshapkina, M., and Hammar, M. (2017). Human Hepatic Gene Expression Signature of Non-alcoholic Fatty Liver Disease Progression, a Meta-Analysis. *Sci. Rep.* 7 (1), 12361. doi:10.1038/s41598-017-10930-w

Rygiel, K. A., Robertson, H., Marshall, H. L., Pekalski, M., Zhao, L., Booth, T. A., et al. (2008). Epithelial-mesenchymal Transition Contributes to Portal Tract Fibrogenesis during Human Chronic Liver Disease. *Lab. Invest.* 88 (2), 112–123. doi:10.1038/labinvest.3700704

Sahin, H., Trautwein, C., and Wasmuth, H. E. (2010). Functional Role of Chemokines in Liver Disease Models. *Nat. Rev. Gastroenterol. Hepatol.* 7 (12), 682–690. doi:10.1038/nrgastro.2010.168

Sasse, D., Spornitz, U. M., and Piotr Maly, I. (1992). Liver Architecture. *Enzyme* 46 (1–3), 8–32. doi:10.1159/000468776

Satoh, D., Yagi, T., Nagasaka, T., Shinoura, S., Umeda, Y., Yoshida, R., et al. (2013). CD14 Upregulation as a Distinct Feature of Non-alcoholic Fatty Liver Disease after Pancreatoduodenectomy. *Wjh* 5 (4), 189–195. doi:10.4254/wjh.v5.i4.189

Saucedo, L. J., and Edgar, B. A. (2007). Filling Out the Hippo Pathway. *Nat. Rev. Mol. Cel Biol.* 8 (8), 613–621. doi:10.1038/nrm2221

Schattenberg, J. M., and Lee, M.-S. (2016). Extracellular Vesicles as Messengers between Hepatocytes and Macrophages in Nonalcoholic Steatohepatitis. *Gastroenterology* 150 (4), 815–818. doi:10.1053/j.gastro.2016.02.064

Schilter, H., Findlay, A. D., Perryman, L., Yow, T. T., Moses, J., Zahoor, A., et al. (2019). The Lysyl Oxidase like 2/3 Enzymatic Inhibitor, PXS-5153A, Reduces Crosslinks and Ameliorates Fibrosis. *J. Cel Mol. Med.* 23 (3), 1759–1770. doi:10.1111/jcmm.14074

Schneider, R. K., Mullally, A., Dugourd, A., Peisker, F., Hoogenboezem, R., Van Strien, P. M. H., et al. (2017). Gli1 + Mesenchymal Stromal Cells Are a Key Driver of Bone Marrow Fibrosis and an Important Cellular Therapeutic Target. *Cell Stem Cell* 20 (6), 785–800. doi:10.1016/j.stem.2017.03.008

Scholten, D., Österreicher, C. H., Scholten, A., Iwaisako, K., Gu, G., Brenner, D. A., et al. (2010). Genetic Labeling Does Not Detect Epithelial-To-Mesenchymal Transition of Cholangiocytes in Liver Fibrosis in Mice. *Gastroenterology* 139 (3), 987–998. doi:10.1053/j.gastro.2010.05.005

Scholten, D., and Weiskirchen, R. (2011). Questioning the Challenging Role of Epithelial-To-Mesenchymal Transition in Liver Injury. *Hepatology* 53 (3), 1049–1051. doi:10.1002/hep.24191

Schon, H.-T., Bartneck, M., Borkham-Kamphorst, E., Nattermann, J., Lammers, T., Tacke, F., et al. (2016). Pharmacological Intervention in Hepatic Stellate Cell Activation and Hepatic Fibrosis. *Front. Pharmacol.* 7, 33. doi:10.3389/fphar.2016.00033

Schulze, R. J., Schott, M. B., Casey, C. A., Tuma, P. L., and McNiven, M. A. (2019). The Cell Biology of the Hepatocyte: A Membrane Trafficking Machine. *J. Cel Biol.* 218 (7), 2096–2112. doi:10.1083/jcb.201903090

Schuppan, D., Ashfaq-Khan, M., Yang, A. T., and Kim, Y. O. (2018). Liver Fibrosis: Direct Antifibrotic Agents and Targeted Therapies. *Matrix Biol.* 68–69, 435–451. doi:10.1016/j.matbio.2018.04.006

Scorza, M., Elce, A., Zarrilli, F., Liguori, R., Amato, F., and Castaldo, G. (2014). Genetic Diseases that Predispose to Early Liver Cirrhosis. *Int. J. Hepatol.* 2014, 1–11. doi:10.1155/2014/713754

Sekiya, S., Miura, S., Matsuda-Ito, K., and Suzuki, A. (2016). Myofibroblasts Derived from Hepatic Progenitor Cells Create the Tumor Microenvironment. *Stem Cel Rep.* 7 (6), 1130–1139. doi:10.1016/j.stemcr.2016.11.002

Seo, Y. Y., Cho, Y. K., Bae, J.-C., Seo, M. H., Park, S. E., Rhee, E.-J., et al. (2013). Tumor Necrosis Factor-α as a Predictor for the Development of Nonalcoholic Fatty Liver Disease: A 4-Year Follow-Up Study. *Endocrinol. Metab.* 28 (1), 41–45. doi:10.3803/enm.2013.28.1.41

Setshedi, M., Wands, J. R., and de la Monte, S. M. (2010). Acetaldehyde Adducts in Alcoholic Liver Disease. *Oxidative Med. Cell Longevity* 3 (3), 178–185. doi:10.4161/oxim.3.3.12288

Silva, P. C. V., Gomes, A. V., de Britto, L. R. P. B., de Lima, E. L. S., da Silva, J. L., Montenegro, S. M. L., et al. (2017). Influence of a TNF-α Polymorphism on the Severity of Schistosomiasis Periportal Fibrosis in the Northeast of Brazil. *Genet. Test. Mol. Biomarkers* 21 (11), 658–662. doi:10.1089/gtmb.2017.0133

Silva, P. C. V., Gomes, A. V., de Souza, T. K. G., Coêlho, M. R. C. D., Cahu, G. G. d. O. M., Muniz, M. T. C., et al. (2014). Association of SNP (-G1082A)IL-10with Increase in Severity of Periportal Fibrosis in Schistosomiasis, in the Northeast of Brazil. *Genet. Test. Mol. Biomarkers* 18 (9), 646–652. doi:10.1089/gtmb.2014.0098

Siqueira, E., Schoen, R. E., Silverman, W., Martini, J., Rabinovitz, M., Weissfeld, J. L., et al. (2002). Detecting Cholangiocarcinoma in Patients with Primary Sclerosing Cholangitis. *Gastrointest. Endosc.* 56 (1), 40–47. doi:10.1067/mge.2002.125105

Srinivas, A. N., Suresh, D., Santhekadur, P. K., Suvarna, D., and Kumar, D. P. (2021). Extracellular Vesicles as Inflammatory Drivers in NAFLD. *Front. Immunol.* 11, 627424. doi:10.3389/fimmu.2020.627424

Staufer, K. (2020). Current Treatment Options for Cystic Fibrosis-Related Liver Disease. *Ijms* 21 (22), 8586. doi:10.3390/ijms21228586

Stickel, F., Datz, C., Hampe, J., and Bataller, R. (2017). Pathophysiology and Management of Alcoholic Liver Disease: Update 2016. *Gut Liver* 11 (2), 173–188. doi:10.5009/gnl16477

Stremmel, W., and Weiskirchen, R. (2021). Therapeutic Strategies in Wilson Disease: Pathophysiology and Mode of Action. *Ann. Transl Med.* 13, 271. doi:10.21037/atm-20-3090

Suppli, M. P., Rigbolt, K. T. G., Veidal, S. S., Heebøll, S., Eriksen, P. L., Demant, M., et al. (2019). Hepatic Transcriptome Signatures in Patients with Varying Degrees of Nonalcoholic Fatty Liver Disease Compared with Healthy Normal-Weight Individuals. *Am. J. Physiology-Gastrointestinal Liver Physiol.* 316 (4), G462–G472. doi:10.1152/ajpgi.00358.2018

Suzuki, K., Tanaka, M., Watanabe, N., Saito, S., Nonaka, H., and Miyajima, A. (2008). p75 Neurotrophin Receptor Is a Marker for Precursors of Stellate Cells and Portal Fibroblasts in Mouse Fetal Liver. *Gastroenterology* 135 (1), 270–281. doi:10.1053/j.gastro.2008.03.075

Syn, W. K., Jung, Y., Omenetti, A., Abdelmalek, M., Guy, C. D., Yang, L., et al. (2009). Hedgehog-mediated Epithelial-To-Mesenchymal Transition and Fibrogenic Repair in Nonalcoholic Fatty Liver Disease. *Gastroenterology* 137 (4), 1478–1488. doi:10.1053/j.gastro.2009.06.051

Tacke, F., and Weiskirchen, R. (2018). An Update on the Recent Advances in Antifibrotic Therapy. *Expert Rev. Gastroenterol. Hepatol.* 12 (11), 1143–1152. doi:10.1080/17474124.2018.1530110

Tan, H.-L., Mohamed, R., Mohamed, Z., and Zain, S. M. (2016). Phosphatidylethanolamine N-Methyltransferase Gene Rs7946 Polymorphism Plays a Role in Risk of Nonalcoholic Fatty Liver Disease. *Pharmacogenet Genomics* 26 (2), 88–95. doi:10.1097/FPC.0000000000000193

Tanaka, A. (2020). Autoimmune Hepatitis: 2019 Update. *Gut and Liver* 14 (4), 430–438. doi:10.5009/gnl19261

Tarantino, G., Minno, M. N. D. D., and Capone, D. (2009). Drug-induced Liver Injury: Is it Somehow Foreseeable?. *Wjg* 15 (23), 2817–2833. doi:10.3748/wjg.15.2817

Taura, K., Iwaisako, K., Hatano, E., and Uemoto, S. (2016). Controversies over the Epithelial-To-Mesenchymal Transition in Liver Fibrosis. *Jcm* 5 (1), 9. doi:10.3390/jcm5010009

Taura, K., Miura, K., Iwaisako, K., Österreicher, C. H., Kodama, Y., Penz-Österreicher, M., et al. (2010). Hepatocytes Do Not Undergo Epithelial-Mesenchymal Transition in Liver Fibrosis in Mice. *Hepatology* 51 (3), 1027–1036. doi:10.1002/hep.23368

Teufel, A., Itzel, T., Erhart, W., Brosch, M., Wang, X. Y., Kim, Y. O., et al. (2016). Comparison of Gene Expression Patterns between Mouse Models of Nonalcoholic Fatty Liver Disease and Liver Tissues from Patients. *Gastroenterology* 151 (3), 513–525. doi:10.1053/j.gastro.2016.05.051

Thoen, L. F. R., Guimarães, E. L., and van Grunsven, L. A. (2012). Autophagy: a New Player in Hepatic Stellate Cell Activation. *Autophagy* 8 (1), 126–128. doi:10.4161/auto.8.1.18105

Todorović Vukotić, N., Đorđević, J., Pejić, S., Đorđević, N., and Pajović, S. B. (2021). Antidepressants- and Antipsychotics-Induced Hepatotoxicity. *Arch. Toxicol.* 95, 1–23. doi:10.1007/s00204-020-02963-4

Troeger, J. S., Mederacke, I., Gwak, G. Y., Dapito, D. H., Mu, X., Hsu, C. C., et al. (2012). Deactivation of Hepatic Stellate Cells during Liver Fibrosis Resolution in Mice. *Gastroenterology* 143 (4), 1073–1083. doi:10.1053/j.gastro.2012.06.036

Tsuchida, T., and Friedman, S. L. (2017). Mechanisms of Hepatic Stellate Cell Activation. *Nat. Rev. Gastroenterol. Hepatol.* 14 (7), 397–411. doi:10.1038/nrgastro.2017.38

Uhlén, M., Fagerberg, L., Hallström, B. M., Lindskog, C., Oksvold, P., Mardinoglu, A., et al. (2015). Tissue-based Map of the Human Proteome. *Science* 347 (6220), 1260419. doi:10.1126/science.1260419

Valéry, L. P., Arnaud, L., Niki, A. S., Megan, C., Latifa, K., Manon, D., et al. (2021). Single-cell RNA Sequencing of Human Liver Reveals Hepatic Stellate Cell Heterogeneity. *JHEP Rep.* 7, 184. doi:10.1016/j.jhepr.2021.100278

van de Straat, R., de Vries, J., Debets, A. J. J., and Vermeulen, N. P. E. (1987). The Mechanism of Prevention of Paracetamol-Induced Hepatotoxicity by 3,5-dialkyl Substitution. *Biochem. Pharmacol.* 36 (13), 2065–2070. doi:10.1016/0006-2952(87)90132-8

Vannier-Santos, M. A., Saraiva, E. M., Martiny, A., Neves, A., and de Souza, W. (1992). Fibronectin Shedding by Leishmania May Influence the Parasite-Macrophage Interaction. *Eur. J. Cel Biol* 59 (2), 389–397.

Wang, B., Li, W., Fang, H., and Zhou, H. (2019). Hepatitis B Virus Infection Is Not Associated with Fatty Liver Disease: Evidence from a Cohort Study and Functional Analysis. *Mol. Med. Rep.* 19 (1), 320–326. doi:10.3892/mmr.2018.9619

Wang, L., Rennie Tankersley, L., Tang, M., Potter, J. J., and Mezey, E. (2002). Regulation of the Murine α2(I) Collagen Promoter by Retinoic Acid and Retinoid X Receptors. *Arch. Biochem. Biophys.* 401 (2), 262–270. doi:10.1016/S0003-9861(02)00058-9

Wanless, I. R., and Shiota, K. (2004). The Pathogenesis of Nonalcoholic Steatohepatitis and Other Fatty Liver Diseases: a Four-step Model Including the Role of Lipid Release and Hepatic Venular Obstruction in the Progression to Cirrhosis. *Semin. Liver Dis.* 24 (1), 99–106. doi:10.1055/s-2004-823104

Wasmuth, H. E., Lammert, F., Zaldivar, M. M., Weiskirchen, R., Hellerbrand, C., Scholten, D., et al. (2009). Antifibrotic Effects of CXCL9 and its Receptor CXCR3 in Livers of Mice and Humans. *Gastroenterology* 137 (1), 309–319. doi:10.1053/j.gastro.2009.03.053

Wee, A., Ludwig, J., Coffey, R. J., Jr, LaRusso, N. F., and Wiesner, R. H. (1985). Hepatobiliary Carcinoma Associated with Primary Sclerosing Cholangitis and Chronic Ulcerative Colitis. *Hum. Pathol.* 16 (7), 719–726. doi:10.1016/s0046-8177(85)80158-1

Weiskirchen, R. (2016). Hepatoprotective and Anti-fibrotic Agents: It's Time to Take the Next Step. *Front. Pharmacol.* 6, 303. doi:10.3389/fphar.2015.00303

Weiskirchen, R., Moser, M., Weiskirchen, S., Erdel, M., Dahmen, S., Buettner, R., et al. (2001). LIM-domain Protein Cysteine- and Glycine-Rich Protein 2 (CRP2) Is a Novel Marker of Hepatic Stellate Cells and Binding Partner of the Protein Inhibitor of Activated STAT1. *Biochem. J.* 359 (Pt 3), 485–496. doi:10.1042/0264-6021:3590485

Weiskirchen, R., Weiskirchen, S., and Tacke, F. (2018). Recent Advances in Understanding Liver Fibrosis: Bridging Basic Science and Individualized Treatment Concepts. *F1000Res* 7, F1000. doi:10.12688/f1000research.14841.1

WHO. World Health Organization (2020). Schistosomiasis Fact Sheet. Available at: https://www.who.int/news-room/fact-sheets/detail/schistosomiasis (Accessed February 23, 2021).

Widmer, J., Fassihi, K. S., Schlichter, S. C., Wheeler, K. S., Crute, B. E., King, N., et al. (1996). Identification of a Second Human Acetyl-CoA Carboxylase Gene. *Biochem. J.* 316 (Pt 3), 915–922. doi:10.1042/bj3160915

Wong, N., Yeo, W., Wong, W.-L., Wong, N. L.-Y., Chan, K. Y.-Y., Mo, F. K.-F., et al. (2009). TOP2A Overexpression in Hepatocellular Carcinoma Correlates with Early Age Onset, Shorter Patients Survival and Chemoresistance. *Int. J. Cancer* 124 (3), 644–652. doi:10.1002/ijc.23968

Wortmann, S. B., and Mayr, J. A. (2019). Choline-related-inherited Metabolic Diseases-A Mini Review. *J. Inherit. Metab. Dis.* 42 (2), 237–242. doi:10.1002/jimd.12011

Wyler, D. J. (1987). Fibronectin in Parasitic Diseases. *Rev. Infect. Dis.* 9 (Suppl. 4), S391–S399. doi:10.1093/clinids/9.supplement_4.s391

Wyler, D. J., Sypek, J. P., and McDonald, J. A. (1985). *In vitro* parasite-monocyte Interactions in Human Leishmaniasis: Possible Role of Fibronectin in Parasite Attachment. *Infect. Immun.* 49 (2), 305–311. doi:10.1128/IAI.49.2.305-311.1985

Xie, G., and Diehl, A. M. (2013). Evidence for and against Epithelial-To-Mesenchymal Transition in the Liver. *Am. J. Physiology-Gastrointestinal Liver Physiol.* 305 (12), G881–G890. doi:10.1152/ajpgi.00289.2013

Xie, J.-Q., Lu, Y.-P., Sun, H.-L., Gao, L.-N., Song, P.-P., Feng, Z.-J., et al. (2020). Sex Difference of Ribosome in Stroke-Induced Peripheral Immunosuppression by Integrated Bioinformatics Analysis. *Biomed. Res. Int.* 2020, 1–15. doi:10.1155/2020/3650935

Xing, T., Yan, T., and Zhou, Q. (2018). Identification of Key Candidate Genes and Pathways in Hepatocellular Carcinoma by Integrated Bioinformatical Analysis. *Exp. Ther. Med.* 15 (6), 4932–4942. doi:10.3892/etm.2018.6075

Xiong, J., Zhang, H., Wang, Y., Wang, A., Bian, J., Huang, H., et al. (2017). Hepatitis B Virus Infection and the Risk of Nonalcoholic Fatty Liver Disease: a Meta-Analysis. *Oncotarget* 8 (63), 107295–107302. doi:10.18632/oncotarget.22364

Xu, R., Zhang, Z., and Wang, F.-S. (2012). Liver Fibrosis: Mechanisms of Immune-Mediated Liver Injury. *Cell Mol Immunol* 9 (4), 296–301. doi:10.1038/cmi.2011.53

Yamaguchi, K., Yang, L., McCall, S., Huang, J., Yu, X. X., au, S. K., et al. (2007). Inhibiting Triglyceride Synthesis Improves Hepatic Steatosis but Exacerbates Liver Damage and Fibrosis in Obese Mice with Nonalcoholic Steatohepatitis. *Hepatology* 45 (6), 1366–1374. doi:10.1002/hep.21655

Yan, Z., Miao, X., Zhang, B., and Xie, J. (2018). p53 as a Double-Edged Sword in the Progression of Non-alcoholic Fatty Liver Disease. *Life Sci.* 215, 64–72. doi:10.1016/j.lfs.2018.10.051

Yang, A. H., Chen, J. Y., and Lin, J. K. (2003). Myofibroblastic Conversion of Mesothelial Cells. *Kidney Int.* 63 (4), 1530–1539. doi:10.1046/j.1523-1755.2003.00861.x

Yang, J., Antin, P., Antin, P., Berx, G., Blanpain, C., Brabletz, T., et al. (2020). Guidelines and Definitions for Research on Epithelial-Mesenchymal Transition. *Nat. Rev. Mol. Cel Biol.* 21 (6), 341–352. doi:10.1038/s41580-020-0237-9

Yang, L., Roh, Y. S., Song, J., Zhang, B., Liu, C., Loomba, R., et al. (2014). Transforming Growth Factor Beta Signaling in Hepatocytes Participates in Steatohepatitis through Regulation of Cell Death and Lipid Metabolism in Mice. *Hepatology* 59 (2), 483–495. doi:10.1002/hep.26698

Yang, L., Yang, C., Thomes, P. G., Kharbanda, K. K., Casey, C. A., McNiven, M. A., et al. (2019). Lipophagy and Alcohol-Induced Fatty Liver. *Front. Pharmacol.* 10, 495. doi:10.3389/fphar.2019.00495

Yang, Y., Bae, M., Park, Y.-K., Lee, Y., Pham, T. X., Rudraiah, S., et al. (2017). Histone Deacetylase 9 Plays a Role in the Antifibrogenic Effect of Astaxanthin in Hepatic Stellate Cells. *J. Nutr. Biochem.* 40, 172–177. doi:10.1016/j.jnutbio.2016.11.003

Younossi, Z. M., Golabi, P., de Avila, L., Paik, J. M., Srishord, M., Fukui, N., et al. (2019). The Global Epidemiology of NAFLD and NASH in Patients with Type 2 Diabetes: A Systematic Review and Meta-Analysis. *J. Hepatol.* 71 (4), 793–801. doi:10.1016/j.jhep.2019.06.021

Younossi, Z. M., Koenig, A. B., Abdelatif, D., Fazel, Y., Henry, L., and Wymer, M. (2016). Global Epidemiology of Nonalcoholic Fatty Liver Disease-Meta-Analytic Assessment of Prevalence, Incidence, and Outcomes. *Hepatology* 64 (1), 73–84. doi:10.1002/hep.28431

Yu, C., Chen, Y., Cline, G. W., Zhang, D., Zong, H., Wang, Y., et al. (2002). Mechanism by Which Fatty Acids Inhibit Insulin Activation of Insulin Receptor Substrate-1 (IRS-1)-Associated Phosphatidylinositol 3-kinase Activity in Muscle. *J. Biol. Chem.* 277 (52), 50230–50236. doi:10.1074/jbc.M200958200

Yuan, L., and Kaplowitz, N. (2009). Glutathione in Liver Diseases and Hepatotoxicity. *Mol. Aspects Med.* 30 (1-2), 29–41. doi:10.1016/j.mam.2008.08.003

Yuan, X., Sun, Y., Cheng, Q., Hu, K., Ye, J., Zhao, Y., et al. (2020). Proteomic Analysis to Identify Differentially Expressed Proteins between Subjects with Metabolic Healthy Obesity and Non-alcoholic Fatty Liver Disease. *J. Proteomics* 221, 103683. doi:10.1016/j.jprot.2020.103683

Yue, M., Huang, P., Wang, C., Fan, H., Tian, T., Wu, J., et al. (2021). Genetic Variation on TNF/LTA and TNFRSF1A Genes Is Associated with Outcomes of Hepatitis C Virus Infection. *Immunological Invest.* 50 (1), 1–11. doi:10.1080/08820139.2019.1708384

Zaldivar, M. M., Pauels, K., von Hundelshausen, P., Berres, M.-L., Schmitz, P., Bornemann, J., et al. (2010). CXC Chemokine Ligand 4 (Cxcl4) Is a Platelet-Derived Mediator of Experimental Liver Fibrosis. *Hepatology* 51 (4), 1345–1353. doi:10.1002/hep.23435

Zanger, U. M., and Schwab, M. (2013). Cytochrome P450 Enzymes in Drug Metabolism: Regulation of Gene Expression, Enzyme Activities, and Impact of Genetic Variation. *Pharmacol. Ther.* 138 (1), 103–141. doi:10.1016/j.pharmthera.2012.12.007

Zeisberg, M., Yang, C., Martino, M., Duncan, M. B., Rieder, F., Tanjore, H., et al. (2007). Fibroblasts Derive from Hepatocytes in Liver Fibrosis via Epithelial to Mesenchymal Transition. *J. Biol. Chem.* 282 (32), 23337–23347. doi:10.1074/jbc.M700194200

Zhang, F., Wang, F., He, J., Lian, N., Wang, Z., Shao, J., et al. (2020). Regulation of Hepatic Stellate Cell Contraction and Cirrhotic Portal Hypertension by Wnt/β-catenin Signalling via Interaction with Gli1. *Br. J. Pharmacol.* 16, 59. doi:10.1111/bph.15289

Zhang, J., Lin, S., Jiang, D., Li, M., Chen, Y., Li, J., et al. (2020). Chronic Hepatitis B and Non-alcoholic Fatty Liver Disease: Conspirators or Competitors? *Liver Int.* 40 (3), 496–508. doi:10.1111/liv.14369

Zhang, Y., and Hunter, T. (2014). Roles of Chk1 in Cell Biology and Cancer Therapy. *Int. J. Cancer* 134 (5), 1013–1023. doi:10.1002/ijc.28226

Zhang, Y., and Yu, C. (2020). Prognostic Characterization of OAS1/OAS2/OAS3/OASL in Breast Cancer. *BMC Cancer* 20 (1), 575. doi:10.1186/s12885-020-07034-6

Zhangdi, H.-J., Su, S.-B., Wang, F., Liang, Z.-Y., Yan, Y.-D., Qin, S.-Y., et al. (2019). Crosstalk Network Among Multiple Inflammatory Mediators in Liver Fibrosis. *Wjg* 25 (33), 4835–4849. doi:10.3748/wjg.v25.i33.4835

Zhou, Z., Xu, M.-J., and Gao, B. (2016). Hepatocytes: a Key Cell Type for Innate Immunity. *Cel Mol Immunol* 13 (3), 301–315. doi:10.1038/cmi.2015.97

Zhu, N., Khoshnan, A., Schneider, R., Matsumoto, M., Dennert, G., Ware, C., et al. (1998). Hepatitis C Virus Core Protein Binds to the Cytoplasmic Domain of Tumor Necrosis Factor (TNF) Receptor 1 and Enhances TNF-Induced Apoptosis. *J. Virol.* 72 (5), 3691–3697. doi:10.1128/JVI.72.5.3691-3697.1998

Zhu, X., Zhang, J., Fan, W., Gong, Y., Yan, J., Yuan, Z., et al. (2014). MAPKAP1 Rs10118570 Polymorphism Is Associated with Anti-infection and Anti-hepatic Fibrogenesis in Schistosomiasis Japonica. *PLoS One* 9 (8), e105995. doi:10.1371/journal.pone.0105995

Zuckerman, A. J. Hepatitis Viruses. In: S. Baron, editor. *Medical Microbiology.* 4th edition. Galveston, TXUniversity of Texas Medical Branch at Galveston; 1996. Chapter 70. Available at: https://www.ncbi.nlm.nih.gov/books/NBK7864/ (Accessed February 23, 2021).

Permissions

The contributors of this book come from diverse backgrounds, making this book a truly international effort. This book will bring forth new frontiers with its revolutionizing research information and detailed analysis of the nascent developments around the world.

We would like to thank all the contributing authors for lending their expertise to make the book truly unique. They have played a crucial role in the development of this book. Without their invaluable contributions this book wouldn't have been possible. They have made vital efforts to compile up to date information on the varied aspects of this subject to make this book a valuable addition to the collection of many professionals and students.

This book was conceptualized with the vision of imparting up-to-date information and advanced data in this field. To ensure the same, a matchless editorial board was set up. Every individual on the board went through rigorous rounds of assessment to prove their worth. After which they invested a large part of their time researching and compiling the most relevant data for our readers.

The editorial board has been involved in producing this book since its inception. They have spent rigorous hours researching and exploring the diverse topics which have resulted in the successful publishing of this book. They have passed on their knowledge of decades through this book. To expedite this challenging task, the publisher supported the team at every step. A small team of assistant editors was also appointed to further simplify the editing procedure and attain best results for the readers.

Apart from the editorial board, the designing team has also invested a significant amount of their time in understanding the subject and creating the most relevant covers. They scrutinized every image to scout for the most suitable representation of the subject and create an appropriate cover for the book.

The publishing team has been an ardent support to the editorial, designing and production team. Their endless efforts to recruit the best for this project, has resulted in the accomplishment of this book. They are a veteran in the field of academics and their pool of knowledge is as vast as their experience in printing. Their expertise and guidance has proved useful at every step. Their uncompromising quality standards have made this book an exceptional effort. Their encouragement from time to time has been an inspiration for everyone.

The publisher and the editorial board hope that this book will prove to be a valuable piece of knowledge for researchers, students, practitioners and scholars across the globe.

List of Contributors

Paula Constanza Arriola Benitez, Ayelén Ivana Pesce Viglietti, Guillermo Hernán Giambartolomei and María Victoria Delpino
Instituto de Inmunología, Genética y Metabolismo (INIGEM), Universidad de Buenos Aires, CONICET, Buenos Aires, Argentina

Jorge Fabián Quarleri
Instituto de Investigaciones Biomédicas en Retrovirus y Sida (INBIRS), Universidad de Buenos Aires, CONICET, Buenos Aires, Argentina

Liuran Li, Qinghua Li, Yibing Han, Huiting Tan, Min An, Qianru Xiang and Yanzhen Cheng
Department of Endocrinology, Zhujiang Hospital, Southern Medical University, Guangzhou, China

Wenbin Huang
Department of Hepatobiliary Surgery II, Zhujiang Hospital, Southern Medical University, Guangzhou, China

Rui Zhou
Department of Pathology, School of Basic Medical Sciences, Southern Medical University, Guangzhou, China

Li Yang
Department of Endocrinology, Zhujiang Hospital, Southern Medical University, Guangzhou, China
Department of Nutrition, Zhujiang Hospital, Southern Medical University, Guangzhou, China

Jianqiang Zhang and Hui Chen
Department of Immunology, School of Medicine, Yangtze University, Jingzhou, China

Bing Zheng, Hao Nie and Quan Gong
Department of Immunology, School of Medicine, Yangtze University, Jingzhou, China
Clinical Molecular Immunology Center, School of Medicine, Yangtze University, Jingzhou, China

Heather Miller
Department of Intracellular Pathogens, National Institute of Allergy and Infectious Diseases, Bethesda, MD, United States

Chaohong Liu
Department of Pathogen Biology, School of Basic Medicine, Tongji Medical College, Huazhong University of Science & Technology, Wuhan, China

Sichen Ren, Ying Wei, Shizhang Wei, Jianxia Wen, Xing Chen and Shihua Wu
School of Pharmacy, Chengdu University of Traditional Chinese Medicine, Chengdu, China
Department of Pharmacy, The Fifth Medical Center of Chinese PLA General Hospital, Beijing, China

Manyi Jing, Haotian Li, Min Wang and Yanling Zhao
Department of Pharmacy, The Fifth Medical Center of Chinese PLA General Hospital, Beijing, China

Ruilin Wang
Integrative Medical Center, The Fifth Medical Center of Chinese PLA General Hospital, Beijing, China

Tao Yang
School of Clinical Medicine, Chengdu University of Traditional Chinese Medicine, Chengdu, China

Hannah K. Drescher and Lea M. Bartsch
Division of Gastroenterology, Massachusetts General Hospital and Harvard Medical School, Boston, MA, United States

Sabine Weiskirchen and Ralf Weiskirchen
Institute of Molecular Pathobio chemistry, Experimental Gene Therapy and Clinical Chemistry (IFMPEGKC), University Hospital, RWTH Aachen, Aachen, Germany
Institute of Molecular Pathobiochemistry, Experimental Gene Therapy and Clinical Chemistry, RWTH University Hospital Aachen, Aachen, Germany

Jing Xu and Yanyun Zhang
The First Affiliated Hospital of Soochow University, Institutes for Translational Medicine, State Key Laboratory of Radiation Medicine and Protection, Key Laboratory of Stem Cells and Medical Biomaterials of Jiangsu Province, Medical College of Soochow University, Soochow University, Suzhou, China
CAS Key Laboratory of Tissue Microenvironment and Tumor, Shanghai Institute of Nutrition and Health, Shanghai Institutes for Biological Sciences, University of Chinese Academy of Sciences, Chinese Academy of Sciences, Shanghai, China

Siyu Pei, Yan Wang, Junli Liu, Youcun Qian and Yichuan Xiao
CAS Key Laboratory of Tissue Microenvironment and Tumor, Shanghai Institute of Nutrition and Health, Shanghai Institutes for Biological Sciences, University of Chinese Academy of Sciences, Chinese Academy of Sciences, Shanghai, China

Mingzhu Huang
Department of Medical Oncology, Fudan University Shanghai Cancer Center, Shanghai, China

Nuria López-Alcántara
Department of Immunology, Ophthalmology and ENT, Complutense University School of Medicine, Madrid, Spain

Arantza Lamas-Paz, Beatriz Martín-Adrados, Eduardo Martínez-Naves and Francisco Javier Cubero
Department of Immunology, Ophthalmology and ENT, Complutense University School of Medicine, Madrid, Spain
12 de Octubre Health Research Institute (imas12), Madrid, Spain

Laura Morán
Department of Immunology, Ophthalmology and ENT, Complutense University School of Medicine, Madrid, Spain
Servicio de Aparato Digestivo del Hospital General Universitario Gregorio Marañón, Instituto de Investigación Sanitaria Gregorio Marañón (IiSGM), Madrid, Spain

Jin Peng
Department of Hepatobiliary Surgery, Nanjing Drum Tower Hospital, The Affiliated Hospital of Nanjing University Medical School, Nanjing, China

Beatriz Salinas
Servicio de Aparato Digestivo del Hospital General Universitario Gregorio Marañón, Instituto de Investigación Sanitaria Gregorio Marañón (IiSGM), Madrid, Spain
Centro Nacional de Investigaciones Cardiovasculares Carlos III, Madrid, Spain
Bioengineering and Aerospace Engineering Department, Universidad Carlos III de Madrid, Madrid, Spain
Centro de Investigación Biomédico en Red de Salud Mental (CIBERSAM), Madrid, Spain

Svenja Sydor and Lars Bechmann
Department of Internal Medicine, University Hospital Knappschaftskrankenhaus, Ruhr-University Bochum, Bochum, Germany

Iris Asensio, Javier Vaquero and Rafael Bañares
Servicio de Aparato Digestivo del Hospital General Universitario Gregorio Marañón, Instituto de Investigación Sanitaria Gregorio Marañón (IiSGM), Madrid, Spain
Centre for Biomedical Research, Network on Liver and Digestive Diseases (CIBEREHD), Madrid, Spain

Ramiro Vilchez-Vargas
Department of Gastroenterology, Hepatology, and Infectious Diseases, Otto von Guericke University Hospital Magdeburg, Magdeburg, Germany

Fengjie Hao
Department of Immunology, Ophthalmology and ENT, Complutense University School of Medicine, Madrid, Spain
12 de Octubre Health Research Institute (imas12), Madrid, Spain
Department of General Surgery, Hepatobiliary Surgery, Ruijin Hospital, Shanghai Jiao Tong University School of Medicine, Shanghai, China

Kang Zheng
Department of Immunology, Ophthalmology and ENT, Complutense University School of Medicine, Madrid, Spain
12 de Octubre Health Research Institute (imas12), Madrid, Spain
Department of Anesthesiology, Zhongda Hospital, School of Medicine, Southeast University, Nanjing, China

Laura Moreno and Angel Cogolludo
Department of Internal Medicine, University Hospital Knappschaftskrankenhaus, Ruhr-University Bochum, Bochum, Germany
Department of Pharmacology and Toxicology, Complutense University School of Medicine and Centre for Biomedical Research, Network on Respiratory Diseases (CIBERES), Madrid, Spain

Manuel Gómez del Moral
12 de Octubre Health Research Institute (imas12), Madrid, Spain
Department of Cell Biology, Complutense University School of Medicine, Madrid, Spain

Yulia A. Nevzorova
Department of Immunology, Ophthalmology and ENT, Complutense University School of Medicine, Madrid, Spain
12 de Octubre Health Research Institute (imas12), Madrid, Spain
Department of Internal Medicine III, University Hospital RWTH Aachen, Aachen, Germany

Min Zhong, Bota Cui, Xia Wu, Quan Wen, Qianqian Li and Faming Zhang
Medical Center for Digestive Diseases, The Second Affiliated Hospital of Nanjing Medical University, Nanjing, China
Key Lab of Holistic Integrative Enterology, Nanjing Medical University, Nanjing, China

Jie Xiang
Department of Gastroenterology, The Central Hospital of Enshi Autonomous Prefecture, Enshi, China

Min Zou
Department of Pharmacy and State Key Laboratory of Biotherapy, West China Hospital, Sichuan University, Chengdu, China

Shiyun Pu, Lei Chen, Rui Li, Jinhang Zhang, Tong Wu, Qin Tang, Xuping Yang, Zijing Zhang, Ya Huang, Jiangying Kuang, Hong Li and Jinhan He
Department of Pharmacy and State Key Laboratory of Biotherapy, West China Hospital, Sichuan University, Chengdu, China
Laboratory of Clinical Pharmacy and Adverse Drug Reaction, West China Hospital, Sichuan University, Chengdu, China

Yanping Li and Qinhui Liu
Laboratory of Clinical Pharmacy and Adverse Drug Reaction, West China Hospital, Sichuan University, Chengdu, China

Xu Zhang
Tianjin Key Laboratory of Metabolic Diseases and Department of Physiology, Tianjin Medical University, Tianjin, China

Wei Jiang
Molecular Medicine Research Center, West China Hospital of Sichuan University, Chengdu, China

Qinghua Meng
Department of Critical Care Medicine of Liver Disease, Beijing You-An Hospital, Capital Medical University, Beijing, China

Ran Xue
Department of Critical Care Medicine of Liver Disease, Beijing You-An Hospital, Capital Medical University, Beijing, China
Key Laboratory of Carcinogenesis and Translational Research (Ministry of Education), Department of Gastrointestinal Oncology, Peking University Cancer Hospital & Institute, Beijing, China

Maha M. Shouman
Department of Pharmacology and Toxicology, Faculty of Pharmacy, Modern Sciences and Arts University (MSA), Giza, Egypt

Sanaa A. Kenawy
Department of Pharmacology and Toxicology, Faculty of Pharmacy, Cairo University, Cairo, Egypt

Rania M. Abdelsalam
Department of Pharmacology and Toxicology, Faculty of Pharmacy, Cairo University, Cairo, Egypt
Department of Biology, Faculty of Pharmacy, New Giza University, Giza, Egypt

Mahmoud M. Tawfick
Department of Microbiology and Immunology, Faculty of Pharmacy (Boys), Al-Azhar University, Cairo, Egypt

Mona M. El-Naa
Department of Pharmacology and Toxicology, Faculty of Pharmacy, University of Sadat City, Sadat City, Egypt

Yueying Chen, Hanyang Li and Jun Shen
Division of Gastroenterology and Hepatology, Key Laboratory of Gastroenterology and Hepatology, Ministry of Health, Inflammatory Bowel Disease Research Center, Renji Hospital, School of Medicine, Shanghai Jiao Tong University, Shanghai Institute of Digestive Disease, Shanghai, China

Qi Feng
Department of Radiology, Renji Hospital, School of Medicine, Shanghai Jiao Tong University, Shanghai, China

Rodrigo C. O. Sanches, Cláudia Souza, Fabio Vitarelli Marinho, Suellen B. Morais and Erika S. Guimarães
Departamento de Bioquímica e Imunologia, Instituto de Ciências Biológicas, Universidade Federal de Minas Gerais, Belo Horizonte, Brazil

Fábio Silva Mambelli
Departamento de Genética, Ecologia e Evolução, Instituto de Ciências Biológicas, Universidade Federal de Minas Gerais, Belo Horizonte, Brazil

Sergio Costa Oliveira and Marco Tulio R. Gomes
Departamento de Bioquímica e Imunologia, Instituto de Ciências Biológicas, Universidade Federal de Minas Gerais, Belo Horizonte, Brazil
Instituto Nacional de Ciência e Tecnologia em Doenças Tropicais (INCT-DT), CNPq MCT, Salvador, Brazil

Shenghu Zhu, Guoquan Li and Bao Zhang
Jiangsu Hengshun Vinegar Industry Co., Ltd., Zhenjiang, China

Linshu Guan, Xuemei Tan, Changjie Sun and Meng Gao
College of Pharmacy, Dalian Medical University, Dalian, China

Lina Xu
College of Pharmacy, Dalian Medical University, Dalian, China
Key Laboratory for Basic and Applied Research on Pharmacodynamic Substances of Traditional Chinese Medicine of Liaoning Province, Dalian Medical University, Dalian, China

Qian Wang, Dehai Li, Jing Zhu, Mingyue Zhang, Hua Zhang, Guangchao Cao, Leqing Zhu, Jianlei Hao, Qiong Wen, Zonghua Liu, Hengwen Yang and Zhinan Yin
Zhuhai Precision Medical Center, Zhuhai People's Hospital (Zhuhai Hospital Affiliated with Jinan University), Jinan University, Zhuhai, China
The Biomedical Translational Research Institute, Faculty of Medical Science, Jinan University, Guangzhou, China

Qiping Shi
The First Affiliated Hospital of Jinan University, Guangzhou, China

Lumin Zhang and Meena B. Bansal
Divison of Liver Diseases, Icahn School of Medicine at Mount Sinai, New York, NY, United States

Zhen Tan and Jing Bo Li
Shenzhen University Clinical Research Center for Neurological Diseases, Health Management Center, Shenzhen University General Hospital, Shenzhen University Clinical Medical Academy, Shenzhen University, Shenzhen, China

Zaif Ur Rahman
Shenzhen University Clinical Research Center for Neurological Diseases, Health Management Center, Shenzhen University General Hospital, Shenzhen University Clinical Medical Academy, Shenzhen University, Shenzhen, China
Department of Pharmacy, Abdul Wali Khan University, Khyber Pakhtunkhwa, Pakistan

Haroon Badshah and Naveed Muhammad
Department of Pharmacy, Abdul Wali Khan University, Khyber Pakhtunkhwa, Pakistan

Lina Tariq Al Kury
College of Natural and Health Sciences, Zayed University, Abu Dhabi, United Arab Emirates

Abdullah Alattar and Reem Alshaman
Department of Pharmacology and Toxicology, Faculty of Pharmacy, University of Tabuk, Tabuk, Saudi Arabia

Imran Malik and Fawad Ali Shah
Riphah Institute of Pharmaceutical Sciences, Riphah International University, Islamabad, Pakistan

Zia Uddin
Department of Pharmacy, COMSATS University Islamabad, Abbottabad Campus, Abbottabad, Pakistan

Atif Ali Khan Khalil
Department of Biological Sciences, National University of Medical Sciences, Rawalpindi, Pakistan

Saifullah Khan
Department of Microbiology and Biotechnology, Abasyn University Peshawar, Khyber Pakhtunkhwa, Pakistan

Amjad Ali
Department of Botany, University of Malakand, Khyber Pakhtunkhwa, Pakistan

Shupeng Li
State Key Laboratory of Oncogenomics, School of Chemical Biology and Biotechnology, Shenzhen Graduate School, Peking University, Shenzhen, China

Pragyan Acharya and Komal Chouhan
Department of Biochemistry, All India Institute of Medical Sciences, New Delhi, India

Index